High Altitude Medicine and Physiology

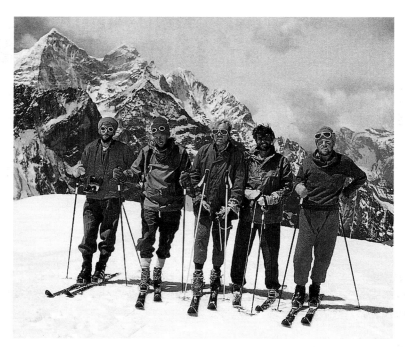

The authors, with two other colleagues, outside the Silver Hut at 5800 m in the Everest region during the Himalayan Scientific and Mountaineering Expedition, 1960–1961. Left to right: Dr. J.S. Milledge, Professor J.B. West, Dr. L.G.C.E. Pugh, Dr. M.P. Ward and Dr. M.B. Gill.

High Altitude Medicine and Physiology

3rd Edition

by

Michael P Ward CBE, MD, FRCS
Past Master, Society of Apothecaries of London, formerly Consultant Surgeon and Lecturer in Clinical Surgery, London Hospital Medical College, London, UK

James S Milledge MD, FRCP
Formerly Consultant Respiratory Physician and Medical Director, Northwick Park Hospital, Harrow, UK

John B West MD, PhD, DSc, FRCP, FRACP
Professor of Medicine and Physiology, the School of Medicine, University of California, San Diego, USA

A member of the Hodder Headline Group
LONDON
Co-published in the USA by
Oxford University Press Inc., New York

First published in Great Britain in 2000 by
Arnold, a member of the Hodder Headline Group,
338 Euston Road, London NW1 3BH

http://www.arnoldpublishers.com

Co-published in the USA by
Oxford University Press Inc.,
198 Madison Avenue, New York NY10016
Oxford is a registered trademark of Oxford University Press

Whilst the advice and information in this book are believed to be true and
accurate at the date of going to press, neither the author[s] nor the publisher
can accept any legal responsibility or liability for any errors or omissions
that may be made. In particular (but without limiting the generality of the
preceding disclaimer) every effort has been made to check drug dosages;
however, it is still possible that errors have been missed. Furthermore,
dosage schedules are constantly being revised and new side-effects
recognized. For these reasons the reader is strongly urged to consult the
drug companies' printed instructions before administering any of the drugs
recommended in this book.

British Library Cataloguing in Publication Data
A catalogue record for this book is available from the British Library

Library of Congress Cataloging-in-Publication Data
A catalog record for this book is available from the Library of Congress

ISBN 0 340 75980 1 (hb)

1 2 3 4 5 6 7 8 9 10

Commissioning Editor: Joanna Koster
Project Editor: Sarah de Souza
Production Editor: Wendy Rooke
Production Controller: Iain McWilliams
Cover design: Mouse Matt Design

Typeset in 10/12pt Minion and Ocean Sans by Phoenix Photosetting, Chatham, Kent
Printed and bound in Great Britain by Bath Press, Bath

Contents

Preface

New advances in the areas of high altitude medicine and physiology continue to occur at a rapid pace. As an example of the burgeoning number of publications, a Medline search using the term 'altitude' retrieves 1566 articles between 1995, when the last edition of this book was published, and May 2000. There is ample other evidence of continued growth in the field. For example, the International Hypoxia Symposia, which concentrate on high-altitude medicine and biology, have been held on alternate years for the past 20 years, with the next meeting scheduled for March 2001 in Jasper, Alberta, Canada. In addition, three World Congresses on Mountain Medicine have interdigitated with the International Hypoxia Symposia over the last 6 years, with a meeting in Arica, Chile, scheduled for October 2000. Previous World Congresses were held in La Paz, Bolivia, Cusco, Peru, and Matsumoto, Japan, emphasizing the breadth of international interest in high altitude studies. Furthermore there are now at least three journals exclusively devoted to high altitude life sciences: one in Japan, another in the People's Republic of China, and a third recently published in the United States with a large international editorial board. In addition, the International Society for Mountain Medicine publishes a quarterly newsletter.

A feature of high altitude life science studies over the last 5 years has been the increasing commercial use of high altitude sites. In the South American Andes, new mines are being developed at altitudes above 4500 m, and an interesting facet is that, increasingly, the miners live at sea level with their families but commute up to the mine for a period of perhaps a week, and then return to their families for the same time. This type of schedule raises many unanswered questions about the selection and health of the workers, and their degree of acclimatization.

Additionally, telescopes are being located at very high altitudes, up to 5000 m. There are now a number of telescopes at an altitude of about 4200 m in Mauna Kea, Hawaii, but more recently a 5000 m high plateau in north Chile at Chajnantor has been selected for additional telescopic sites. The advantages of the high altitude include the fact that the instruments are above much of the Earth's atmosphere, and also the Atacama region of north Chile is characterized by extreme dryness, which also improves telescope 'seeing.' During the present decade, the enormous multinational ALMA radio-telescope will be constructed at Chajnantor and, of course, the logistical problems of working at an altitude of 5000 m are daunting. A new chapter in this edition on commercial activities at high altitude reflects these advances.

All the material in this third edition has been updated, and there has also been some regrouping of material to reflect recent advances. New material has been added in every chapter. Our aim has been to produce a book that is useful to a wide range of readers from the ever-increasing number of climbers and trekkers who would like to know more about the hazards of high altitude, to expedition doctors faced with managing high altitude problems, to researchers who are studying cutting-edge aspects of high-altitude life sciences. We have tried to strike a balance between being too academic on the one hand, and competing with pocket guides on high altitude emergencies on the other. As far as we know, no other available text covers such a wide range of high-altitude life science topics, including cold injury, with the depth provided here.

As in the previous editions, we have tried to make each chapter readable in its own right even if this means a small amount of repetition of material, particularly historical points. Few people will read a book like this from cover to cover. We welcome constructive criticism, particularly the identification of factual errors, and will personally respond to every letter that we receive. We hope that this book will continue to improve the health and safety of all people who visit, or live at, high altitude.

Michael P. Ward
James S. Milledge
John B. West

Acknowledgments

We wish to acknowledge help from many friends and colleagues who have read and commented helpfully on parts of the text, especially, the late Michael J. Ball FRCS; F.E. Gallas; the late Eugene Grippenreiter; Surg. Rear-Adr. Frank Golden OBE, RN; Steven Hempleman PhD; Michael C. Holdan PhD; Professor W.R. Keatinge; Sukhamay Lahiri PhD; Robert Mahler FRCP; the late Betty A. Milledge MB; Odile Mathieu-Costello PhD; the late Hamish G. Nicol MB; David C. Poole PhD; Frank L. Powell PhD; Peter D. Wagner MD; E.J.M. Weaver FRCS; David C. Wellinford PhD; and Edward S. Williams FRCP.

We gratefully acknowledge the invaluable help of Amy Clay, Administrative Assistant to JBW, and Evelyn Denman MB, who read and corrected the chapters from JSM and MPW. Also we wish to thank the copy-editor, Kathleen Lyle, and the staff of Arnold Publishers, especially Joanna Koster and Wendy Rooke.

We would also like to thank all those who contributed to the original work on which much of this book is based. These include Sherpas, climbers, scientists and other supporters who made the projects possible.

We especially wish to thank John F. Nunn FFARCS and Stephen P.L. Travis FRCP who wrote sections in the previous edition that have been incorporated into this new edition.

Conversion tables

Table F.1 *Conversion of pressure units mm Hg (millimeters of mercury) to kPa (kilopascals)*

mm Hg	kPa
1	0.133
10	1.33
20	2.67
30	4.00
40	5.33
50	6.67
60	8.00
80	10.7
100	13.3
200	26.7
300	40.0
500	66.7
700	93.3
760	101.3

1 torr = 1 mm Hg

Table F.2 *Conversion of height units and barometric pressure according to the ICAO Standard Atmosphere. Note that in the great mountain ranges the actual pressure will usually be higher than given by the table (Chapter 2)*

Altitude		Pressure mm Hg
m	**ft**	
0	0	760
1000	3 281	674
2000	6 562	596
3000	9 843	526
4000	13 123	462
5000	16 404	405
6000	19 685	354
7000	22 966	308
8000	26 247	267
9000	29 258	231

Table F.3 *Conversion of temperature units, °C (degrees Celsius) to °F (degrees Fahrenheit)*

°C	°F
−40	−40
−30	−20
−25	−13
−20	−4
−15	5
−10	14
−5	23
0	32
5	41
10	50
15	59
20	68
25	77
30	86
35	95
40	104

Table F.4 *Conversion of energy units, kcal (kilocalories) to kJ (kilojoules)*

kcal	kJ
50	209.4
100	418.8
250	1 047
500	2 094
1000	4 188
2000	8 375
3000	12 563
4000	16 750
5000	20 938
6000	25 126

Abbreviations

17-OHCS	17-hydroxycorticosteroid	HAPE	high altitude pulmonary edema
2,3-DPG	2,3-diphosphoglycerate	HCVR	hypercapnic ventilatory response
A–a	alveolar–arterial	HVR	hypoxic ventilatory response
ACTH	adrenocorticotropic hormone	ICAO	International Civic Aviation Organization
ADH	antidiuretic hormone	iNOS	inducible nitric oxide synthase
AMREE	American Medical Research Expedition to Everest	LH	luteinizing hormone
		LVF	left ventricular failure
AMS	acute mountain sickness	MRI	magnetic resonance imaging
ANP	atrial natriuretic peptide	MVV	maximal voluntary ventilation
ARPE	Association pour la Recherche en Physiologie de l'Environnement	NST	nonshivering thermogenesis
		PA_{CO_2}	alveolar partial pressure of carbon dioxide
AVP	arginine vasopressin	Pa_{CO_2}	arterial partial pressure of carbon dioxide
BAL	bronchoalveolar lavage		
BCAA	branched-chain amino acid	PA_{O_2}	alveolar partial pressure of oxygen
BMR	basal metabolic rate	Pa_{O_2}	arterial partial pressure of oxygen
BTPS	body temperature, ambient pressure, saturated with water vapor	P_{CO_2}	partial pressure of carbon dioxide
		PCV	packed cell volume
CBF	cerebral blood flow	PD	potential difference
CCK	cholecystokinin	PDGF	platelet derived growth factor
CMS	chronic mountain sickness	PI_{O_2}	partial pressure of inspired oxygen
CNS	central nervous system	P_{N_2}	partial pressure of nitrogen
COLD	chronic obstructive lung disease	P_{O_2}	partial pressure of oxygen
CSF	cerebrospinal fluid	PRA	plasma renin activity
ECF	extracellular fluid	PRK	photorefractive keratectomy
ECG	electrocardiogram	PV	plasma volume
EEG	electroencephalogram	RCM	red cell mass
EMG	electromyelogram	NREM	non-REM (sleep)
EPO	erythropoietin	REM	rapid eye movement (sleep)
ERPF	effective renal plasma flow	RK	radial keratotomy
ET-1	endothelin-1	RQ	respiratory quotient
FEV_1	forced expiratory volume in 1 s	Sa_{O_2}	arterial oxygen saturation
FPA	fibrinopeptide A	SIDS	sudden infant death syndrome
FSH	follicle stimulating hormone	SiEp	serum immunoreactive EPO concentration
FVC	forced vital capacity		
GH	growth hormone	STPD	standard temperature and pressure, dry gas
HACE	high altitude cerebral edema		
HAGA	high altitude global amnesia		

SWS	slow wave sleep	TSH	thyroid stimulating hormone
T_4	thyroxine	UKIRT	United Kingdom Infrared Telescope
TBG	thyroxine binding globulin	VEGF	vascular endothelial growth factor
TGF	transforming growth factor	$\dot{V}_{O_2\,max}$	maximum oxygen consumption Kg^{-1}
TIA	transient ischemic attack		

History

SUMMARY

The effects of cold and high altitude are described by many early travelers in the highland regions of Central Asia, South America and elsewhere. Early balloonists and mountaineers accurately described acclimatization to altitude, mountain sickness, cold injury and their after effects.

The measurement of barometric pressure, the work of Paul Bert and the increasing interest in mountain regions gave high altitude medicine and physiology an increasingly scientific basis. Attempts on, and the first ascent of, Everest provided a catalyst and scientific expeditions and decompression chamber studies are increasingly common. More and more studies on high altitude populations are now being carried out.

The increased understanding of the oxygen transport system at altitude is important for the light it throws on many clinical conditions at sea level.

To the millions who trek, ski, climb and commute to altitude each year, together with those who live at altitude, the subject of high altitude medicine and physiology is one of increasing importance.

1.1 INTRODUCTION

The story of our attempts to climb higher and higher by our own unaided efforts is one of the most colorful and exciting in medicine and physiology, if only because scientists have been repeatedly astonished by mountaineers' ability to ascend higher than their confident predictions.

About 140 million people live at altitudes above 2500 m worldwide (WHO 1996), and each year some 40 million travel to similar altitudes. This means that over 180 million people are at risk, and this number is growing.

Over the centuries investigation into the effects of human hypoxia and the exploration of the world's highest mountain ranges have run a parallel and often overlapping course (Table 1.1).

Numerous clinical and physiological lessons have been learnt from altitude studies, which share a number of features found in the chronically hypoxic patient with cardiovascular and respiratory disorders (Chapter 31). The physiological problems of altitude are due in the main to hypoxia and cold: hypoxia because with gain in altitude there is reduction in

Table 1.1 *Chronology of some principal events in the development of high altitude medicine and physiology*

Year	Event
c. 30 BC	Reference to the Great Headache Mountain and Little Headache Mountain in the Tseen Han Shoo (classical Chinese history)
1590	Publication of the first edition (Spanish) of *Naturall and morall historie of the East and West Indies* by Joseph de Acosta with an account of mountain sickness
1644	First description of mercury barometer by Torricelli
1648	Demonstration of fall in barometric pressure at high altitude in an experiment devised by Pascal
1777	Clear description of oxygen and the other respiratory gases by Lavoisier
1783	Montgolfier brothers introduce balloon ascents
1786	First ascent of Mont Blanc by Balmat and Paccard
1878	Publication of *La Pression Barométrique* by Paul Bert
1890	Viault describes high altitude polycythemia
1890	Joseph Vallot builds high altitude laboratory at 4350 m on Mont Blanc
1891	Christian Bohr publishes *Uber die Lungenathmung*, giving evidence for both oxygen and carbon dioxide secretion by the lung
1893	Angelo Mosso completes the high altitude station, Capanna Regina Margherita, on a summit of Monte Rosa at 4559 m
1906	Publication of *Hohenklima und Bergwanderungen* by Zuntz et al.
1909	The Duke of Abruzzi reaches 7500 m in the Karakoram without supplementary oxygen
1910	Zuntz organizes an international high altitude expedition to Tenerife; members included C. G. Douglas and Joseph Barcroft
1910	August Krogh publishes *On the Mechanism of Gas-Exchange in the Lungs*, disproving the secretion theory of gas exchange
1911	Anglo-American Pikes Peak expedition (4300 m); participants C. G. Douglas, J. S. Haldane, Y. Henderson and E. C. Schneider
1913	T. H. Ravenhill publishes *Some Experiences of Mountain Sickness in the Andes*, describing puna of the normal, cardiac and nervous types
1920	Barcroft et al. publish the results of the experiment carried out in a glass chamber in which Barcroft lived in a hypoxic atmosphere for 6 days
1921	A. M. Kellas publishes *Sur les possibilites de faire l'ascension du Mt Everest* (Congrès de l'Alpinisme, Monaco 1920)
1921–2	International High Altitude Expedition to Cerro de Pasco Peru, led by Joseph Barcroft
1924	E. F. Norton ascends to 8500 m on Mount Everest without supplementary oxygen
1925	Barcroft publishes *Lessons from High Altitude*
1935	International High Altitude Expedition to Chile, scientific leader D. B. Dill
1946	Operation Everest I carried out by C. S. Houston and R. L. Riley
1948	Carlos Monge M. publishes *Acclimatization in the Andes*, describing the permanent residents of the Peruvian Andes
1949	H. Rahn and A. B. Otis publish *Man's Respiratory Response During and After Acclimatization to High Altitude*
1952	L. G. C. E. Pugh and colleagues carry out experiments on Cho Oyu near Mount Everest in preparation for the 1953 expedition
1953	First ascent of Mount Everest by Hillary and Tensing (with supplementary oxygen)
1960–1	Himalayan Scientific and Mountaineering Expedition in the Everest region, scientific leader L. G. C. E. Pugh. Laboratory at 5800 m, measurements up to 7440 m
1968–79	High altitude studies on Mount Logan (5334 m), scientific director C. S. Houston
1973	Italian Mount Everest Expedition with laboratory at 5350 m, scientific leader P. Cerretelli
1978	First ascent of Everest without supplementary oxygen by Reinhold Messner and Peter Habeler
1981	American Medical Research Expedition to Everest, scientific leader J. B. West
1985	Operation Everest II, scientific leaders C. S. Houston and J. R. Sutton
1983 to present	Research at Capanna Regina Margherita (4559 m) by O. Oelz, P. Bärtsch and co-workers from Zurich, Bern and Heidelberg
1984 to present	Studies at Observatoire Vallot (4350 m) on Mont Blanc by J.-P. Richalet and co-workers
1990 to present	Research at Pyramid Laboratory, Lohuje, Nepal by P. Cerretelli and co-workers
1994	British Mount Everest Medical Research Expedition, leaders S. Currin, A. Pollard, D. Collier
1997	Operation Everest III (COMEX), leader J.-P. Richalet
1998	Medical Research Expedition to Kangchenjunga, leaders S. Currin, D. Collier, J. Milledge

atmospheric and hence oxygen pressure (Chapter 2); cold because of the temperature lapse with altitude and wind chill (Chapter 23).

Frostbite is mentioned in a Tibetan medical text named the *Blue Beryl*, published in 1688. However, it seems possible that the text may have originated much earlier, and a date of 889 BCE has been suggested (Parfionovitch *et al.* 1992).

Early mountain travelers, like Xenophon, who crossed the mountains of Armenia following the battle of Cunaxa (401 BCE), were more concerned with cold than with altitude. Similarly Plutarch (46–120 CE) tells us that Alexander's army crossing the Hindu Kush to India in 326 BCE suffered severely from the 'state of the weather'. One of the earliest European accounts of the rarefied air of high altitude was given by the Greeks who, on their yearly ceremonial visit to the summit of Mount Olympus (2911 m), were not able to survive, we are told, unless they applied moist sponges to their noses (possibly soaked in vinegar) (Burnett 1983).

1.2 THE CHINESE HEADACHE MOUNTAIN STORY

The first documented description of mountain sickness comes from Chinese sources.

In the time of the Emperor Ching-Te (32–7 BCE) Ke-pin (possibly Afghanistan) again sent an envoy with offerings and an acknowledgement of guilt. The supreme board wished to send an envoy with a reply to escort the Ke-pin envoy home. Tookim (a Chinese official) addressed the Generalissimo Wang Fung to the following effect . . .

From Pe-shan southwards there are four to five kingdoms not attached to China. The Chinese Commission will in such circumstances be left to starve among the hills and valleys ... Again on passing the Great Headache Mountain, the Little Headache Mountain, the Red Land, and the Fever Slope, men's bodies become feverish, they lose colour and are attacked with headache and vomiting; the asses and cattle being all in like condition. (Wylie 1881; original Chinese text shown in West 1998 Figure 1.3)

Gilbert (1983a) considers that both the Kilik Pass and the Mintaka Pass across the Karakoram are possible candidates for the Great Headache Mountain,

but a pass is not a peak, and the Chinese are meticulous observers. Pe-shan, 37.6°N 78.2°S (*Mountains of Central Asia* 1987), mentioned as the starting place, is situated south-east of Shache (Yarkand) and west of Hotien (Khotan). From here to Afghanistan there are a great number of routes across the mountains, and the one followed has yet to be identified.

Gilbert also draws attention to a case of acute mountain sickness that was reported by Fa-Hsien (399–414 CE) who in 403 CE traveled in Kashmir and Afghanistan. He noted that his companion foamed at the mouth and later died as they were ascending a mountain pass. This was possibly a case of high altitude pulmonary edema (HAPE), as the clinical description is typical.

It has been suggested, too, that the occurrence of mountain sickness and its complications may have been taken by the Chinese as a sign for them not to transgress their natural boundaries (Needham 1954).

1.3 CENTRAL AND SOUTH AMERICA: DE ACOSTA

In each inhabited mountain region, whether it is in Asia, Europe or the Americas (Figure 1.1), there is a vast depository of legend and folklore. The peaks, passes and glaciers are deemed to have been created by a series of gods, Titans and tribal heroes, and individual peaks have been enshrined with virtues and defects, like any human. For instance, in South America there is the legend of the trauco found in southern Chile and Argentina, a mythical animal that feeds on the blood of animals and human beings. This is very similar to the yeti legend, found in the Himalayas and mountains of central Asia (Napier 1972, Reinhard 1983).

Well-built pre-Columbian structures have been found near the summit of Llullaillaco (6721 m) and are probably associated with mountain worship. Human sacrifice was carried out on these peaks, and an Inca body has been found at 6300 m on El Toro. The summits of a number of volcanoes, up to 6425 m and easily accessible from Arequipa, may have been used as the altars of sacrificial shrines. These peaks, with few glaciers and easy rounded slopes, present little technical difficulty other than altitude and South American highlanders were used to ascending to great heights for worship in the late fifteenth century. Altitudes in excess of 6000 m were probably not

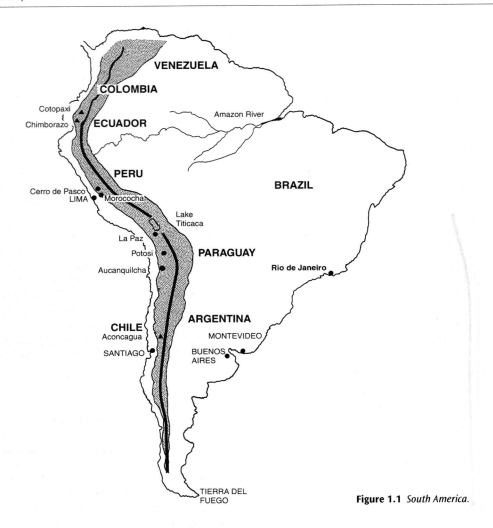

Figure 1.1 *South America.*

reached on foot in Asia until the later part of the nineteenth century (Echevarria 1968, 1979, 1983).

In Central America the Spanish Conquistadores were active in the sixteenth century and in 1519 Cortez sent Diego Ordaz to attempt the ascent of Mount Popocatepetl (5456 m). Ordaz and companions remarked, 'To increase their distress, respiration in these aerial regions became so difficult that every effort was attended with sharp pain in the head and limbs'. Two years later Francisco Montana and four Spaniards reached the summit and obtained sulfur from the crater for the manufacture of gunpowder (Prescott 1891).

Symptoms of mountain sickness were not described in any detail by these explorers and it was left to a Jesuit priest, Joseph de Acosta, to give the first account. The local names were *puna*, *soroche*, *mareo* and *veta*, and the cause thought to be emanations from the metal antimony. In other regions the vapors from rhubarb, primroses and roses were said to make men and animals ill. The government of the Incas clearly understood the effects of climate on health and it was known, for instance, that people who lived by the sea died in great numbers if transported to the mines at 3000–4000 m. The cause is unknown but it is likely to have been a combination of malnutrition, disease, altitude and cold.

The account of mountain sickness given by Joseph

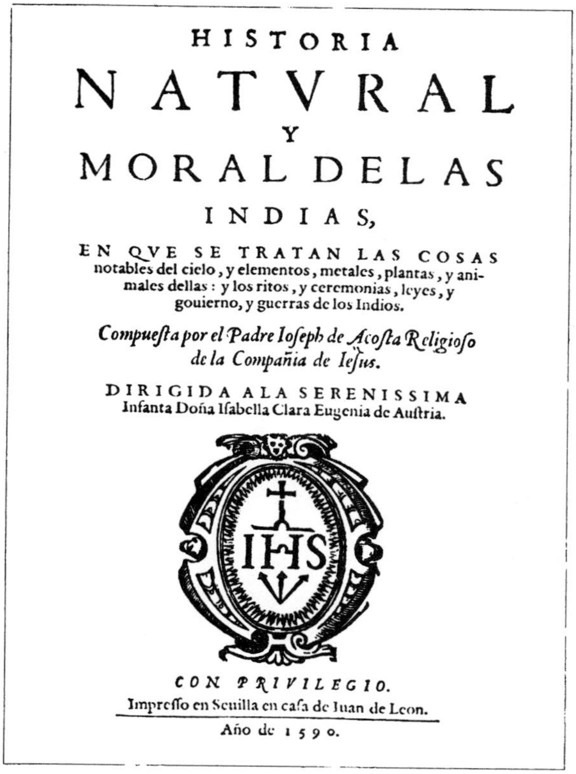

HISTORIA
NATVRAL
Y
MORAL DE LAS
INDIAS,

EN QVE SE TRATAN LAS COSAS
notables del cielo, y elementos, metales, plantas, y ani-
males dellas : y los ritos, y ceremonias, leyes, y
gouierno, y guerras de los Indios.

Compueſta por el Padre Ioſeph de Acoſta Religioſo
de la Compañia de Ieſus.

DIRIGIDA ALA SERENISSIMA
Infanta Doña Iſabella Clara Eugenia de Auſtria.

IHS

CON PRIVILEGIO.
Impreſſo en Seuilla en caſa de Iuan de Leon.

Año de 1 5 9 0.

Figure 1.2 *Title page of first edition of Joseph de Acosta's book published in Seville in 1590. (Reproduced with permission of the Bodleian Library.)*

de Acosta in *The Naturall and Morall Historie of the East and West Indies*, first published in 1590 in Seville (Figure 1.2), is worth quoting at length for his accuracy of description, feelings and cause of the symptoms:

> There is in Peru a high mountaine which they call Pariacaca . . . when I came to mount the degrees, as they call them, which is the top of this mountaine, I was suddenly surprized with so mortall and strange a pang, that I was ready to fall from the top to the ground and although we were many in company, yet everyone made haste (without any tarrying for his companion) to free himself speedily from this ill passage . . . I was surprised with such pangs of straining and casting as I thought to cast up my heart too: for having cast up meate, fleugme and choller both yellow and greene, in the end I cast up blood with the straining of my stomach. To conclude, if this had continued I should undoubtedly have died (de Acosta 1604 p. 146).

However, some reservations have been expressed as to whether de Acosta was describing acute mountain sickness (AMS). There is no mention of headache, and the vomiting in AMS is not usually so severe as to bring up bile and blood. The possibility that this was an attack of gastroenteritis should be considered although diarrhea is not mentioned.

De Acosta's route across the Andes has been investigated by Gilbert (1983b) and, of a number of alternatives, he considers that the pass of the Escaleras de Pariacaca (4800 m) is the most likely candidate. Bonavia *et al.* (1985) have made an on site inspection of the Pariacaca area and corrected a number of topographical misconceptions. Gilbert (1988) reported information from mountaineers who had climbed in the region that, whereas the peak Pariacaca is known by this name to inhabitants to the south-west (the direction from which de Acosta made his approach), it is also known as Tullujuto to those living to the north-east. The peak is named Tullujuto on the few maps on which it is marked. It is not unusual for a peak to have more than one name but this does give rise to confusion.

1.4 CENTRAL ASIA: MOGULS AND JESUITS

In 1531, the Moguls invaded Ladakh and western Tibet (Figure 1.3) and described mountain sickness which they called *yas*, and which the Tibetans called *damgiri* or *dam* (breath seizing), or *dugri* (poison of the mountain). The clinical features were vomiting, exhaustion, difficulty in sleeping, aphasia and swelling of the hands and feet. Death often occurred unless descent was rapid, and the Mogul sultan, Said Khan, died of *damgiri* on the Suget Pass on his way from Ladakh to Kashgar. This illness was made worse by cold, and horses also were severely affected. The Moguls recorded other central Asian names for mountain sickness: *tunk* (wakhi and badakhshi), *esh* (turki) and *bish-ka-hawa* (a term used by some Indian populations of the Himalayas) (Elias and Ross 1898).

In the middle of the seventeenth century there were rumours of Nestorian Christian colonies living in central Asia and a number of missionaries from Rome were sent out to contact them. These remarkable men established missions in Tibet and they were

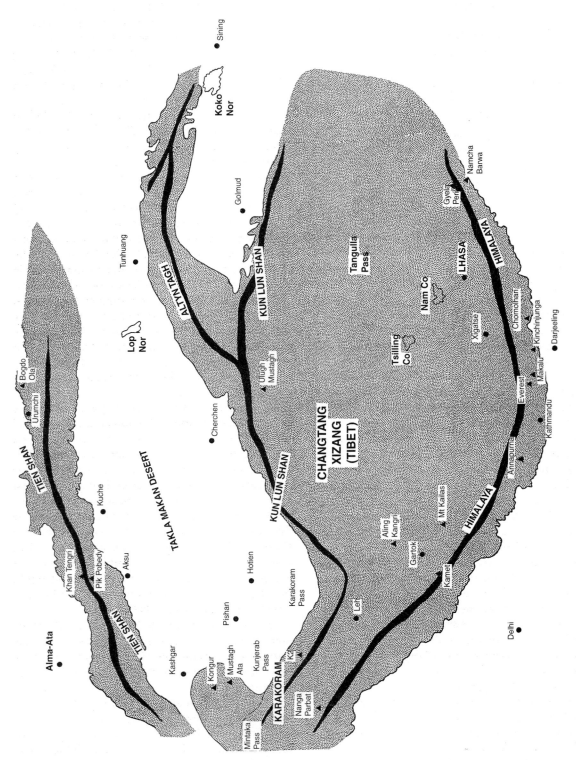

Figure 1.3 *Central Asia.*

among the first Europeans to bring back detailed information about this mysterious land from first hand knowledge. Inevitably they suffered from acute mountain sickness and had views on its cause.

The Jesuit, Father Andrade, was the first European to enter Tibet. He crossed the Himalayas by the Mana Pass (5450 m) in 1624 and was more concerned with hypothermia than with hypoxia:

> Many people die on account of the noxious vapours that arise, for it is a fact that people in good health are suddenly taken ill and die within a quarter of an hour, but I think it is rather owing to the intense cold and want of heat, which reduces the heat of the body (Wessels 1924).

In 1661, two Jesuit fathers, Grüber and D'Orville, left Peking, and crossed the Tibetan plateau to Lhasa. Staying a month in the capital they then crossed the Himalayas by the Thung La, arriving in Kathmandu several months after leaving Peking. Grüber called the Himalayas the Langur Mountains and comments that, 'man cannot breathe in the Langur mountains because the air is so subtle'. He adds that 'in summer certain poisonous weeds grow there which extrude such a bad smell and dangerous odour that one cannot stay up there without losing one's life'. It seems likely that he was applying Joseph de Acosta's experience to central Asia. Father Desiderei, another Jesuit who founded a mission in Lhasa in 1716, also comments on the 'reek of certain materials' but goes on to say that he believes that the unpleasant symptoms 'are due to sharp thin air'. He also suffered from excruciating headaches.

In 1739 Father Belligatti alludes to the 'singular influence which mountains exercise over both men and animals whether this arises from the rarefaction of the atmosphere or from deleterious exhalations' (Hedin 1913). This may have been a reference to *ladrak* as the 'poison of the pass' which was considered by the Tibetans to be the exhalation of mischievous gods who caused earthquakes and avalanches (Landon 1905). Rockhill (1891, p. 149) describes how mountain sickness was called *yen-chang* by the inhabitants of the Koko Nor and *chang-chi* in Szechuan. Both expressions mean a 'pestilential vapour' thought to be given off by the large quantities of rhubarb which grew in the mountains. Eating garlic and smoking tobacco were held to be antidotes.

In 1845–6 the Abbé Huc crossed the Burhan Buddha range into north Tibet (Pelliot 1928, Vol. 2, p. 138). He also complained of 'pestilential vapours and exhalations of carbonic acid' which made him feel ill and fire lighting difficult. The Russian traveler Prejavalski (1876) crossed the same pass 30 years later and correctly attributes his symptoms to 'the enormous elevation and rarefaction of the air'.

Tutek is another term used by central Asians for acute mountain sickness (Hedin 1903, Vol. 1, p. 25). Hedin also describes chronic mountain sickness occurring in gold miners in north Tibet which may be fatal (Hedin 1903, Vol. 2, p. 20). The Tibetan remedy for mountain sickness in ponies was to slit their noses (Bower 1893). In men an incision was made in the forehead at the hairline (Bonvalot 1891, p. 166).

Other clinical features ascribed to mountain sickness were described by Humboldt (1769–1859), who in 1802 climbed to 5500 m on Mount Chimborazo in the Andes of Ecuador (Maggilivary 1853). He and his companion suffered from bleeding of the lips and gums as well as malaise and nausea, thought to be due to low barometric pressure. De Saussure (Mathews 1898) on the third ascent of Mont Blanc in 1787 also suffered very considerably from fatigue, thought at the time to be the cause of mountain sickness.

The exploration of the Himalayas began in the early part of the nineteenth century and symptoms of mountain sickness were noted by many travelers including the Schlagintweit brothers, who, in 1855, climbed to 6785 m on Mount Ibi Gamin in the Garwhal Himal, a record that stood for 30 years (Von Schlagintweit and Von Schlagintweit 1862).

The pundits, secret native explorers employed by the Survey of India, who explored the Himalaya and Tibet in the nineteenth century (Ward 1998), describe the total exhaustion of altitude. In 1879 one pundit had to be carried to the foot of a 6400 m pass into Tibet, up which steps were cut with a kukri (a Nepali knife) (Freshfield 1903).

As in Central and South America there are many myths and much folklore associated with the Himalaya and mountains of central Asia. One of the most prevalent is that of the yeti. The yeti story was given a boost by the discovery in 1951 of the tracks of bare feet in the snow at about 5000 m in the Menlung glacier basin west of Everest. These have been attributed to the yeti, but despite much speculation and many expeditions the yeti has never been found. Ward (1997), who with Shipton discovered and photographed these footprints, suggests that they could have belonged to a native highlander with an untreated congenital or acquired abnormality of the foot, who was able, like many other high altitude people, to walk barefoot in the snow for many hours because of marked cold tolerance (see section 24.1.3). Schaller (1998) makes no mention of the yeti myth in his comprehensive work on wildlife of Tibet.

1.5 PAUL BERT

During the nineteenth century in Europe considerable interest in experimental physiology was being generated by Claude Bernard. Paul Bert, a pupil of his, was born in 1833 and the study of the medical aspects of low barometric pressure and resulting hypoxia was one of his many interests; he is recognized as the father of altitude physiology. He was the first to conduct experiments in a decompression chamber where he studied the effects of both reduced and increased barometric pressure in small animals and humans. He showed that breathing air under conditions of reduced barometric pressure as at altitude was dangerous because of oxygen lack, whereas breathing oxygen even under reduced pressure restored function.

Bert collected accounts from travelers and scientists from all over the world and, in addition to his work in steel decompression chambers, which were donated by his patron Dr Jourdanet, he became interested in the opportunities that balloon flights offered for the study of altitude physiology.

The first 350 or so pages of his classic work *La Pression Barométrique* are considered to be the most authoritative early account of the history of the physiological effects of decreased atmospheric pressure (Bert 1878) (Figure 1.4). His work did not go uncriticized, particularly by Mosso and Kronecker (Kellogg 1978). Kellogg also points out that Kronecker reviewed various case histories including one diagnosed as pulmonary edema at autopsy. Mosso (1898), who was Professor of Physiology at Turin, made good use of the Capanna Regina Margherita on the Punta Gnifetti (4560 m), one of the summits of Monte Rosa, constructed by the Club Alpino Italiano (Figure 1.5). He did not believe that mountain sickness was due to lack of oxygen but thought it was due to lack of carbon dioxide. He was a major figure in

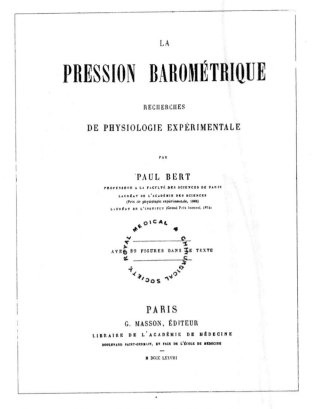

Figure 1.4 *Title page of Paul Bert's book* La Pression Barométrique, *published in Paris in 1878.*

altitude physiology, tracing the breathing pattern of periodic respiration; he also published the first clinical report of pulmonary edema.

1.6 ALPINE CLUB

In the middle of the nineteenth century mountain travel was becoming increasingly popular and the Alpine Club was founded in the UK in 1857. The *Alpine Journal*, 'a record of mountain adventure and scientific observation' contained a number of articles on mountain sickness in its early issues. Count Henry Russel (Russel 1871) comments that mountain sickness was 'known all over the world (though less in the tropics) … and in the Himalaya where the silly natives attribute it to the exhalations of a venomous plant'. Spinal anemia, the result of diminished atmospheric pressure, was suggested as a cause of the weakness of the lower limb 'which was so

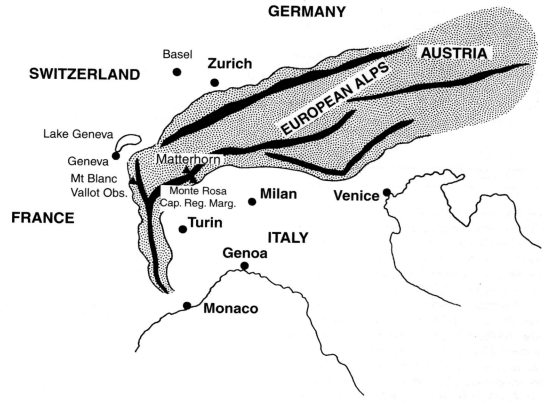

Figure 1.5 *European Alps.*

prominent a feature of mountain sickness' (Monro 1893).

A year later Thomas (1894) thought that the very dry air of Tibet and the Karakoram might be a factor, as the overall effect of altitude was felt there at a lower level than in damper Sikkim. A review of the eighteenth and nineteenth century theories on mountain sickness and its cause is given by Hepburn (1901, 1902). He suggests that following certain training, dietary and breathing routines, a man could climb to 30 000 ft (9144 m). He concludes: 'but even so we have yet to prove that dyspnoea and fatigue are dependent on lack of oxygen at any level either directly or indirectly, though the probabilities are in favour of such a theory'.

In a salutary article on alcohol and climbing, Marcet (1886–8b) writes that mountain sickness 'is certainly neither protected against nor relieved by the use of alcoholic beverages'. He ends by saying that, 'strong drinks do not give strength, and as a means of keeping the body warm they go in the opposite tack doing away with the natural powers that man possesses of resisting cold, thus acting as a delusion and snare'. Albutt (1876) in fact considered that the use of alcohol predisposed to frostbite. Earlier, Albutt (1870) had observed that the hard exercise of climbing accelerated the 'morning rise in temperature' (taken sublingually). However, rectal temperatures in two guides taken during the ascent of Monte Rosa showed a rise in one and a fall in the other (Payot 1881). Payot also considered that the increased respiration of climbing was associated with an increase in water loss from the lungs and poor urine output, a fact confirmed by Pugh in 1952.

Marcet (1886–8a) suggested that potassium chlorate be taken, as when it is heated it gives off oxygen and would combat the effects of altitude. He observed that it had been used by Sir Douglas Forsyth in the 'Cashmere mountains on the way to Kashgar' and by Whymper on the first ascent of Chimborazo. It is clear from Bellew (1875) that the salt was eaten! In 1879 Edward Whymper, the conqueror of the

Matterhorn, mounted an expedition to the Andes of South America specifically to study mountain sickness. He divided the clinical effects into permanent (which included poor appetite, fatigue and increased respiration) and transient (increase in blood pressure, temperature and heart rate) (Whymper 1892, pp. 366–84).

1.7   BALLOONISTS

Whilst observations on mountain sickness were being made by mountain travelers, more dramatic episodes were occurring to balloonists.

The Montgolfier brothers, Etienne and Joseph, the most famous pioneers of early ballooning, made the first ascent in a hot air balloon in November 1783, and, in the same month, De Rozier, a French apothecary, and the Marquis d'Arlandes, crossed Paris in a 'Montgolfier'. In the same year the physicist Charles, who had invented the hydrogen balloon, left the Tuileries and landed 2 h 45 min later in the plain of Nesles. Roberts, his companion, disembarked here and the lightened balloon rose to over 1500 fathoms (approximately 2740 m). Later Gay-Lussac ascended to over 7000 m, noticing that both his pulse and respiration were much increased.

Nearly a century later in September 1862, Coxwell and Glaisher, two English meteorologists were carried to 8800 m, escaping death only because Coxwell managed to pull the release valve with his teeth. Glaisher (Glaisher et al. 1871) made a number of further flights and considered that he had developed a tolerance to altitude. Though a decrease in barometric, and therefore oxygen, pressure had been demonstrated on these ascents, the early balloonists had still not fully grasped that the dangers at altitude were due to hypoxia.

In March 1874 Croce-Spinelli and Sivel came to Paul Bert's laboratory before an attempt on the balloon altitude record. Following decompression chamber experiments the balloonists were convinced of the effectiveness of oxygen but planned to carry too little for safety. Bert was alarmed and wrote indicating it was not enough but the letter arrived too late. On 15 April 1875, the balloon named Zenith rose to around 8000 m; Tissandier, the survivor, described in detail the features of hypoxia which killed his two companions and would have killed him

if he had not vented some hydrogen which caused Zenith to descend (Tissandier 1875) (Chapter 16).

1.8   LATE NINETEENTH AND EARLY TWENTIETH CENTURY EXPLORERS AND PHYSIOLOGISTS

In the late nineteenth and early twentieth centuries there was increasing medical and scientific interest in both the oxygen transport system and altitude adaptation, and many discoveries were made. Viault (1890) recorded the best known physiological response to altitude, namely an increase in the number of red cells. He found a rise from 5.0 million at sea level to 7.5–8.0 million at Morococha (4550 m) and observed that this change took place over a short period. By contrast, Bert had thought that it took place gradually over generations at altitude (Chapter 7). Later, Hingston (1914) considered that the symptoms of mountain sickness were due to failure to increase the number of red cells on ascent to high altitude.

Disorders of respiration that had the 'Stokes character' were also described at 4400 m (Egli-Sinclair 1891–2, 1894). A similar episode had been noted by Hirst in 1857 when he made an ascent of Mont Blanc with the well known physicist and mountaineer Professor J. Tyndall. Tyndall fell asleep on the summit and Hirst roused him saying 'I have listened for some minutes and have not heard you breathe once' (Tyndall 1860). Periodic respiration had, in fact, been described by the surgeon John Hunter in his case records in 1781 (Ward 1973) over 30 years before Cheyne's paper (Cheyne 1818) (Chapter 13).

Though a case of pulmonary edema due to altitude had been recorded by Kronecker at autopsy (Kellogg 1978), it is likely that the first full clinical description occurs in Mosso's book *Life of Man on the High Alps* (Mosso 1898, pp. 289–92). The victim, Dr Jacottet, died on Mont Blanc at 4300 m, and the autopsy report attributed the waterlogged lungs to pneumonia. Later, Ravenhill (1913), the medical officer of a mine in South America, differentiated between a cerebral and a cardiac form of mountain sickness, the latter being now regarded as pulmonary edema. Twenty years later Hurtado (1937) suggested that the pneumonia or pulmonary edema of altitude was not due to infection but altitude *per se* and Lundberg presented six cases of acute pulmonary edema to the Asociacion Medica de Yauli. Lizárraga (1955) published (in Spanish) the first series of cases of HAPE since Ravenhill, collected in Peru in 1951–2.

A case that was clearly HAPE, and in which the patient died, was reported in a letter to Pugh, commented on by him and published in the UK (Pugh 1955a). Pugh's comment indicated that the condition was unknown to him at the time.

In 1959 Hultgren visited Chulec General Hospital in Oroya, Peru, and found HAPE was a well known condition (Hultgren and Spickard 1960). Houston (1960) 'rediscovered' the condition, since when it has become widely recognized (Chapter 19).

Commercial groups were starting to build railways into the mountains to improve access and boost tourism, and plans were discussed for a railway to the top of the Jungfrau, in Switzerland. The scientific investigations were carried out on the Theodule Pass (3500 m) between Zermatt and Cervinia in 1894 (Kronecker 1903). Eventually this railway was built as far as the Jungfraujoch. The dangers to elderly travelers and those with angina pectoris of ascent by railway to even moderate altitude were discussed by Zangger (1899, 1903).

Though minor vascular disorders were often reported at altitude, the first major vascular accident to be reported occurred to a Russian traveler, Roborovsky (1896), while crossing the Mangur Pass (4270 m) in east Tibet. He suffered a transient stroke and it was 8 days before he could move (Chapter 22).

The tempo of Himalayan exploration accelerated in this period and Conway on Pioneer Peak (7000 m) in 1892 described the debilitating effects of long periods at high altitude. He also took sphygmograph pulse records at intervals up to and including the summit (Figure 1.6). His resting pulse remained between 90 and 100/min, but there is one reading at 6100 m when it was 48. Could this have been an incident of transient 2:1 heart block (Roy 1894)?

By contrast, the Duke of Abruzzi's expedition to the Karakoram in 1909 climbed to 7500 m with few of the symptoms due to altitude. Interestingly, however, Filippi (1912, p. 364) also reports 'the atmosphere of the expedition did work some evil effect revealing itself only gradually after several weeks of life above 17 500 ft', and he goes on to give a description of high altitude deterioration (section 4.2.2).

Anticipating the modern trend, some amazingly fast ascents were made, particularly by Longstaff, a

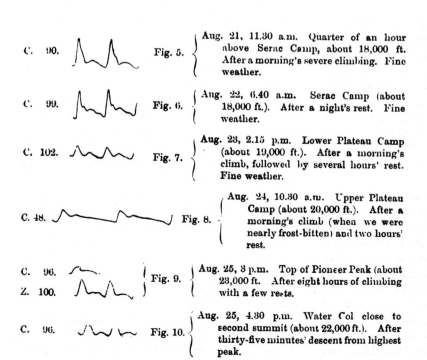

C. 90.   Fig. 5. { Aug. 21, 11.30 a.m. Quarter of an hour above Serac Camp, about 18,000 ft. After a morning's severe climbing. Fine weather.

C. 99.   Fig. 6. { Aug. 22, 6.40 a.m. Serac Camp (about 18,000 ft.). After a night's rest. Fine weather.

C. 102.   Fig. 7. { Aug. 23, 2.15 p.m. Lower Plateau Camp (about 19,000 ft.). After a morning's climb, followed by several hours' rest. Fine weather.

C. 48.   Fig. 8. { Aug. 24, 10.30 a.m. Upper Plateau Camp (about 20,000 ft.). After a morning's climb (when we were nearly frost-bitten) and two hours' rest.

C. 96.
Z. 100.   Fig. 9. { Aug. 25, 3 p.m. Top of Pioneer Peak (about 23,000 ft. After eight hours of climbing with a few rests.

C. 96.   Fig. 10. { Aug. 25, 4.30 p.m. Water Col close to second summit (about 22,000 ft.). After thirty-five minutes' descent from highest peak.

Figure 1.6 *Pulse sphygmograph records on Pioneer Peak (7000 m) taken by Conway in 1892 (from Roy 1894). Note resting pulse of 48 beats per minute in Figure 8, possibly due to 2:1 heart block. (Reproduced with permission of the Library of the Royal Geographical Society.)*

British physician, who ascended 2000 m to 7180 m in 10 h on Mount Trisul (section 1.11). He was also one of the first to recognize that sugar was of great importance in the diet at high altitude (Longstaff 1906, 1908).

Waddell, Medical Officer on the British Expedition to Lhasa 1903–4, supplies an amusing vignette:

> A peculiarity of the language of the Tibetans in common with the Russians and most arctic nations is the remarkably few vowels in their words and the extraordinarily large number of consonants. Indeed so full of consonants are Tibetan words that most of them could be articulated with an almost semi-closed mouth, evidently from the enforced necessity to keep the lips closed as far as possible against the cutting cold when speaking (Waddell 1905).

German contributions before and during World War I were considerable. Before the war Nathan Zuntz had worked on the relationship between barometric pressure and altitude in the European Alps (Zuntz et al. 1906) as well as on other aspects of altitude physiology with many well known physiologists of his time, including Durig, Douglas, Barcroft, Loewy and Pfluger. After the war, with the rise of National Socialism, aviation and high altitude medicine burgeoned, as did mountaineering. In 1931 a German expedition to Kangchenjunga had Hans Hartman as its physiologist and in the two German parties to Nanga Parbat in 1937 and 1938, Ulrich Luft took part. He later became an American citizen. Both Hartmann and Luft were interested in erythropoiesis at altitude. Luft also showed that altitude acclimatization could be preserved by daily exposure to 5000 m in a decompression chamber (Bauer 1938, Hartmann et al. 1942).

World War II played an important role in the history of high altitude medicine and physiology because it provided much increased activity in environmental and respiratory physiology. Individuals from different branches of medicine and physiology were brought together with a strong sense of common purpose and one remarkable combination was that of Wallace Fenn (plant physiologist), Herman Rhan (zoologist) and Arthur Otis (physiology of pressure breathing), who worked at the University of Rochester, New York. They carried out many studies for the US Air Force which culminated in the construction of the Rhan–Otis oxygen/carbon dioxide diagram which relates the composition of alveolar gas pressures in acclimatized and unacclimatized humans exposed to altitude (Rhan and Otis 1949). Also the foundation of the *Journal of Applied Physiology* can be traced to them.

1.9 COLD INJURY (HYPOTHERMIA, FROSTBITE AND NONFREEZING COLD INJURY)

For many centuries cold injury has been known to travelers in polar and highland regions and armies in the field, but it is relatively recently that specific disease patterns have been described. Local cold tolerance but not general acclimatization to cold is recognized amongst Inuit peoples, polar travelers, mountaineers and central Asian highlanders.

Hypothermia or general cold injury may affect climbers at extreme altitude even when fully clothed. It also occurs at sea level at temperatures above freezing when wetting and wind degrade the insulation of clothing. Nonfreezing cold injury (immersion injury) was common in the armed forces pinned down by trench warfare in World War I and in lifeboat survivors in World War II. Frostbite is described in early Tibetan medical texts dating back many centuries but its management by rapid rewarming is a relatively recent therapy (Mills and Whaley 1960, Marsigny 2000).

The term 'wind chill' was coined by Siple in 1945 to express the concept that on a windy day one feels much colder than on a calm day at the same temperature (Siple and Passell 1945, Paton 1999). The concept of wind chill was re-examined by Danielsson (1996), who considered that Siple and Passel had underestimated the effect of air speed.

1.10 THE OXYGEN SECRETION CONTROVERSY

The ascent to 7500 m by the Duke of Abruzzi's party amazed many physiologists, for it was thought that lung diffusion was inadequate for extreme exercise at low oxygen pressure. However, it was becoming apparent that in some organs 'chemicals' could move against the concentration gradient. If the lungs could secrete oxygen this might explain both the variability with which individuals reacted to altitude and also their ability to ascend so high.

The arguments deployed for and against this theory are reviewed in Chapter 6. Initially, in favor of secretion was the theoretical impossibility of the diffusion of 5–6 L of oxygen across the lung each minute during extreme exercise. However, at the turn of the century, Marie Krogh measured the diffusing capacity of the lung to carbon monoxide, from which the diffusing capacity of oxygen could be inferred. She showed that the lung was a very good diffuser of oxygen partly because of its enormous surface area and partly because of the affinity of hemoglobin for oxygen. However, her work was ignored, being rediscovered in the 1930s.

Haldane and Barcroft were both distinguished respiratory physiologists though they held opposing views. After a number of investigations, including the Cambridge 'glass box' experiment of Barcroft, and expeditions to high altitude by groups led by both workers, Barcroft finally showed conclusively that the arterial P_{O_2} was always lower than the alveolar P_{O_2}. The diffusion theory was correct and Barcroft's book, *Lessons from High Altitudes*, became a classic work on the subject (Barcroft 1925, Milledge 1985).

1.11   THE EVEREST STORY

In 1921, after years of prevarication, the government of Tibet gave permission for a British party to attempt Mount Everest from the northern Tibetan side.

The individual who knew most about the physical and physiological problems that would be encountered was Alexander Kellas, a lecturer in chemistry at the Middlesex Hospital Medical School. He had made a number of expeditions to the Sikkim Himal and the Tibetan border before World War I and had become increasingly interested in the problems of altitude (Kellas 1917).

Before he went on the first Everest reconnaissance expedition in 1921, Kellas wrote a paper entitled 'A consideration of the possibility of ascending Mount Everest'. Unfortunately he died on the approach march at Kampa Dzong on the Tibetan plateau, within sight of the mountain, and this paper was never published, though copies of the manuscript

were lodged in the archives of the Royal Geographical Society and the Alpine Club (West 1987). In it he considers both the difficulties of access and the physiological problems. The section of the 1921 manuscript entitled 'The process of acclimatisation to altitude' is of great interest because although there are many factual errors his insight in asking the correct questions was uncanny.

As Kellas saw it, the main issue was whether sufficient adaptation could occur to allow a climber to ascend from a camp at about 7700 m to the summit (8848 m) in one day without supplementary oxygen. His conclusion was that this was possible and, in fact, the first such ascent by Habler and Messner in 1978 started from a camp at 7950 m. He calculated too that the barometric pressure on the summit would be 251 mm Hg, a more accurate figure than estimates based on the 'standard atmosphere' (Chapter 2). The current value of 253 mm Hg was measured on the summit by the American Medical Research Expedition in 1981. Kellas estimated the maximum oxygen uptake on the summit to be 970 mL min^{-1} and the current value is thought to be about 1070 mL min^{-1}. As far as climbing rate near the summit, his estimate of 100–120 m h^{-1} closely parallels the rate of Habler and Messner: 'The last 100 m took us more than one hour to climb.' Finally, he thought that humans could live indefinitely at 6100 m.

Some of the few values for which Kellas's figures were too low were alveolar P_{O_2}, oxygen saturation and arterial pH; this was because he underestimated the degree of hyperventilation and assumed a normal arterial pH.

It is difficult to assess the probable effects of this paper had it been published, but at least it might have encouraged subsequent expeditions to consider more fully the scientific aspects of the ascent.

The series of expeditions between 1921 and 1953, the year of the first ascent, give a fascinating insight into the effects of altitude and cold and the attitude of mountaineers towards climbing the highest mountain in the world. It soon became obvious that the main obstacles to the ascent were altitude and weather, and not technical difficulty. The main controversy was whether supplementary oxygen should be used and this was compounded by personality clashes. The medical preparations for the first Everest expeditions in 1921, 1922, and 1924 were very thorough.

In 1920, Kellas and Morshead of the Survey of

India went to Kamet, a peak of over 7000 m in the western Himalayas, on behalf of the Everest Committee of the Alpine Club and Royal Geographical Society, to test primus stoves and oxygen equipment. At the suggestion of Professor Leonard Hill of Oxford, Oxylite bags containing sodium peroxide which when mixed with water gave off oxygen were also taken (Kellas 1921, Morshead 1921).

Because neither the primus stoves nor the oxygen cylinders worked satisfactorily, the stoves were tested in the decompression chamber at the laboratory of Professor Dryer at Oxford University in 1921. Dryer had strong views on the use of supplementary oxygen on Everest: 'I do not think that you will get up without, but if you do you might not get down again.' In March 1921, before the first reconnaissance of Everest left for India, Finch, a possible member of the party and later professor of physical chemistry at Imperial College London, and two members of the committee witnessed the stoves being tested in the decompression chamber. Dryer easily convinced Finch that supplementary oxygen should be used on Everest, and persuaded him to stay overnight. Next day he was decompressed to 6400 m and exercised both with and without supplementary oxygen. Not surprisingly, without the benefit of acclimatization, Finch was convinced of the benefit of supplementary oxygen at altitude.

As the 1921 expedition was for reconnaissance only, supplementary oxygen was not taken. In preparation for the 1922 attempt on the summit, Finch returned to Oxford in January 1922 with another party member, Somervell, a surgeon, and took part in further experiments, being decompressed to 7010 m. It was because of these experiments that supplementary oxygen was used in 1922. In 1922 four men ascended to 8250 m without supplementary oxygen and two men reached a similar height using it. Many clinical features of chronic hypoxia were recognized: poor appetite, loss of weight, dehydration, exhaustion and failure to recover from fatigue being the most obvious (Unna 1922).

Finch, confirming the observations of Paul Bert, noted the beneficial effects of using oxygen. However, in 1924 Odell spent 11 days above 7000 m, climbing on two occasions to 8300 m without supplementary oxygen (Bruce 1923, p. 237, Norton 1925, pp. 120–43). His performances were equal to those using supplementary oxygen; but when he used

supplementary oxygen at 1 L min^{-1} there was no improvement, and this observation clouded the clinical picture. Also, as Sherpa porters carrying loads without supplementary oxygen ascended as fast as those with it, an element of uncertainty was introduced which was not resolved until the work of Pugh in 1952 on the Menlung La (5800 m) in the Everest region (see below). Another feature of high altitude was emphasized by Mathews who considered that loss of heat could occur through increased respiration (Mathews 1932). However, it is now apparent that the upper respiratory tract acts as a very efficient heat exchanger.

Successive expeditions in 1933, 1935, 1936 and 1938 failed to ascend higher than 8500 m, mainly because supplementary oxygen at 2 L min^{-1} only was used and this failed to increase climbing rate. After World War II the Nepalese side of Everest was visited in 1950 by an Anglo-American party that included Houston and Tilman, and in 1951 a British party led by Shipton revealed a possible route. In 1951 too, investigations into the scientific problems posed by Everest were started in London by Pugh of the Medical Research Council under the general guidance of Professor Sir Bryan Mathews. The following year, 1952, a Sherpa, Tensing, and Lambert, on a Swiss attempt, reached 8500 m using oxygen intermittently, but not only was their flow rate of oxygen inadequate to compensate for the weight of the sets, they were also grossly dehydrated (Dittert *et al.* 1954).

In the same year a British mountaineering and scientific party visited a neighboring peak, Cho Oyu (8153 m), and Pugh carried out scientific work in a tented laboratory at 5800 m on the Menlung La which was vital to the subsequent ascent of Everest in 1953.

The most important outcome was the development of a reliable and not too heavy open-circuit oxygen apparatus which delivered oxygen at various flow rates between 2 and 6 L min^{-1}, much higher than the flow rates used on all previous expeditions. This compensated for the weight of the set and increased climbing rate sufficiently so that the mountaineer could ascend to the summit from a high camp and descend safely within the hours of daylight. The use of supplementary oxygen of 4 L min^{-1} above 7500 m was the single most important reason for the first ascent of Everest in 1953. It transformed climbers at extreme altitude from 'sick men walking in a dream' to individuals capable of overcoming reasonable difficulties, making good decisions and climbing through bad weather. Other causes for previous failures were the marked dehydration at extreme altitude (due partly to respiratory water loss through increased respiration and partly to inadequate fluid intake due to difficulty in melting enough snow); levels of food intake; and clothing insulation (Pugh 1952, 1954, Milledge 1992, Ward 1993a). The work of Pugh in 1951 and 1952 was one of the primary reasons for the success of the 1953 expedition.

The consecutive expeditions in 1951, 1952 and 1953 also enabled the basic clinical features of altitude exposure up to 8848 m to be established (Pugh and Ward 1956). On the first successful ascent of Everest, Hillary and Tensing removed their oxygen masks on the summit. Hillary (1954) remarks: 'I had now had my oxygen mask off for nearly eight minutes and was becoming rather clumsy fingered … We put on our oxygen masks and set off from the top down the way we had come.'

In 1978, Everest was climbed for the first time without using supplementary oxygen by Habeler and Messner (Messner 1979, pp. 174–80). They had little in reserve: 'After every few steps we huddled over our ice axes mouths agape struggling for sufficient breath', and the last 100 m took more than 1 h. Over 50 such ascents have now been made without supplementary oxygen both by sea level visitors and by high altitude residents, though the mortality rate amongst those attempting such an ascent is high.

In October 1981 the barometric pressure on the summit of Everest (8848 m) was measured for the first time by Pizzo. It was found to be 253 mm Hg and in May 1997 a further direct measurement on the summit was found to be within 1 mm Hg of this figure. Measurements on the South Col (7986m) in the summer of 1998 showed mean values in May of 284 mm Hg; June 285 mm Hg; July 286 mm Hg; and August 287 mm Hg. It appears therefore that on the days when Everest is usually climbed, that is between May and October, the barometric pressure on the summit is between 251 and 253 mm Hg (West 1999a).

A Sherpa, Ang Rita, has reached the summit on ten occasions and made the first winter ascent in December 1987, without supplementary oxygen (*Mountain* 1988).

By the end of 1992, 425 individuals had climbed Everest (Gillman 1993). By 1999 over 1000 people had made this ascent using supplementary oxygen,

including 54 women who had a mortality of 7.4%. The mortality rate in men was 3.2%. One hundred ascents have been made without supplementary oxygen, but with a mortality rate of 6%. By the end of 1999 the total number of deaths on Everest was 171 (Unsworth, 2000).

Following the example of Longstaff, some very rapid ascents and descents of Everest have been made. In 1986 two mountaineers climbed the North Face by the Hornbein Couloir without supplementary oxygen. They started from the West Rongbuk glacier (5800 m) at 22.00 h and in 12 h, overnight, reached a bivouac at 7800 m. Here they rested, then they ascended to the summit (8848 m), arriving at 14.30 h. After spending 1 h 30 min on the top they descended to their bivouac in 3 h. From there to the glacier (5800 m) took only 2 h (Everest 1987). The fastest Everest ascent took 22.5 h from Base Camp to summit (Gillman 1993).

In 1856 the height of Everest was estimated to be 29 002 ft, 8940 m (the average of six readings). Following the opening of Nepal in 1950, B.L. Gulatee of the Geodetic and Research branch of the Survey of India observed Everest from between 29 and 47 miles and computed a height of 29 028 (±0.8 ft), 8848 m. In 1999 a height of 29 035 ft (8850 m) was calculated using global positioning satellite equipment (Gulatee 1954, Ward 1995, *The Times* 1999a).

1.12 MEDICAL AND PHYSIOLOGICAL EXPEDITIONS

Although medical and physiological observations have been made on expeditions from the earliest times, probably the first series of investigations mounted primarily to study the physiology of high altitude was that of Angelo Mosso at the end of the nineteenth century. In the early years of the twentieth century Barcroft and Haldane, with their co-workers, were also involved in a series of research programs in Tenerife, the European Alps, Pikes Peak and Cerro de Pasco.

In 1935 the International High Altitude Expedition went to the Andes. They spent several months in Chile studying many aspects of acclimatization to altitude including lactacidosis on exercise, the acid–base status of the blood and arterial blood gases, both in members of the expedition and in local residents at various altitudes (Dill 1938).

In 1946 'Operation Everest' was carried out at Pensacola Naval Air Station in Florida. Four volunteers lived in a decompression chamber for 34 days, reaching 6600 m on day 27 after gradual decompression. On day 30 the chamber was decompressed to 235 mm Hg – equivalent to 8850 m on the standard atmosphere scale (Chapter 2).

Two men were able to tolerate this altitude for 30 min 'on the top of Everest'. The results strongly suggested a diffusion limitation of oxygen transfer during exercise (Houston and Riley 1947). A similar investigation, 'Operation Everest II', was completed in 1985 at the US Army Institute of Environmental Medicine at Natick, Massachusetts (Houston et al. 1987). The ascent profiles of Operation Everest and Operation Everest II were similar except that in the latter the ascent was more rapid and subjects spent longer at extreme altitude. Cardiac catheterization was possible at extreme altitude and important new information was obtained on pulmonary gas exchange. Muscle biopsies were also completed as well as psychometric tests and sleep studies.

Although Pugh made important physiological observations on Cho Oyu in 1952 and on Everest in 1953, the next expedition devoted to high altitude physiology was in 1960–1, which was led by Hillary

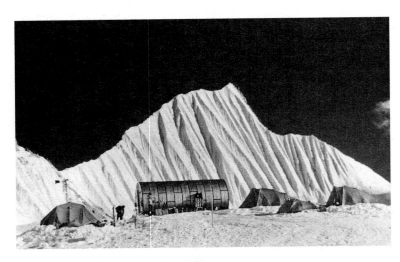

Figure 1.7 *The Silver Hut with Rakpa Peak in the background (taken at 5800 m during the Himalayan Scientific and Mountaineering Expedition in the Everest region, 1960–1).*

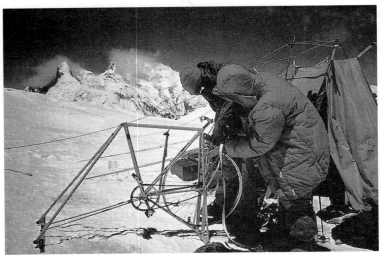

Figure 1.8 *Bicycle ergometer being assembled at 7400 m on the Makalu Col by Ward and West, 1961.*

with Pugh as scientific leader. A fully equipped physiological laboratory, the Silver Hut, was installed at 5800 m in the Everest region. The results from this expedition have formed the basis for much subsequent investigation into extreme altitude, and the expedition was an important landmark in high altitude studies. The Silver Hut was occupied for 6 months between November 1960 and May 1961 (Figure 1.7), and an attempt on Mount Makalu (8481 m) was also made when maximum work studies were completed at 7440 m by West and Ward (Figure 1.8). This still remains the highest altitude at which such studies have been made.

Projects included studies on exercise, lung diffusion, changes in the control of breathing, electrocardiograph (ECG) changes, basal metabolic rate, blood volume and hemoglobin changes, and psychomotor function. Two vascular accidents occurred – one cerebral, the other pulmonary; there was ample evidence to suggest that, despite good living conditions, all participants deteriorated during long-term residence at 5800 m (Pugh 1962a).

The next 20 years saw a number of field investigations into the physiology and medicine of high altitude and an increasing number of people – skiers, trekkers and tourists, as well as mountaineers – were going to high altitude all over the world.

In 1962 the Indian Defence Authorities arranged a 'symposium on the problems of high altitude' at Darjeeling (Symposium (Indian) 1962). This was during the period when China was threatening the northern Himalayan border of India. The Indians appreciated that the Chinese, who had acclimatized for long periods on the Tibetan plateau, would be at an advantage in any conflict in the Himalayas, as Indian soldiers, who lived at low altitude, would not have had time to acclimatize.

In 1964 China did invade India; the Indian soldiers suffered considerably from acute mountain sickness and HAPE. The work of Inder Singh and his colleagues dates from this period (Singh et al. 1969b). Since then the clash between India and Pakistan on the Siachen glacier of the Karakoram has provided an added stimulus to high altitude studies in both countries.

In 1967 a permanent laboratory was placed at 5300 m on Mount Logan in Alaska (Figure 1.9) and this was visited regularly by medical scientists until 1979. During these years, studies included retinal blood flow, the incidence of retinal hemorrhage and the value of acetazolamide in preventing acute mountain sickness. Evidence of subclinical pulmonary edema on ascending to the laboratory was found in many subjects (Houston 1980).

Studies on acute mountain sickness and the use of acetazolamide have also been carried out by groups from Birmingham, UK (Acute mountain sickness 1979, 1987).

On the successful Italian expedition to Everest in 1973, Cerretelli made an extensive series of measurements at 5350 m on climbers who had been to 8000 m. One of the many interesting observations was the failure of maximum oxygen uptake of subjects acclimatized to 5350 m to return to sea level values when pure oxygen was breathed. Noted also by Pugh and others, this finding has never been satisfactorily explained (Cerretelli 1976a).

In 1980–1 a Sino-British team explored the Kongur Massif in Southern Xinjiang, Chinese central Asia, climbing Kongur (7719 m), the highest peak in the Kun Lun range which runs along the northern edge of the Tibetan plateau (Ward 1983). Half the team were medical scientists and work was done on the cardiorespiratory response in elite mountaineers, on erythropoietin changes with ascent to altitude (Milledge and Cotes 1985), and on the renin–aldosterone system (Milledge 1984).

In 1981 West led the American Medical Research Expedition to Everest (AMREE). The barometric pressure, measured for the first time on the summit, was found to be 253 mm Hg. This was higher than predicted by some authorities (Chapter 2). Alveolar gas samples were taken on the summit of Everest for the first time by Pizzo and very low P_{CO_2} values were observed, indicating extremely high ventilation rates at rest. Pizzo and Hackett also obtained blood samples on the South Col from which it was deduced that there would have been extreme alkalosis on the summit (Chapter 12). In the Western Cwm a fully equipped laboratory was set up and important observations made on exercise, sleep, metabolism, nutrition, hormones and psychomotor function (West 1982a, 1985a). AMREE 1981, which developed from the Silver Hut Expedition (1960–1), and Operation Everest II (1985), which followed from Operation Everest I (1946), were both extremely successful and complemented each other.

Operation Everest II had the advantage that complex and invasive techniques could be carried out and any subjects who became ill could be removed from the chamber. Its disadvantage was the artificial

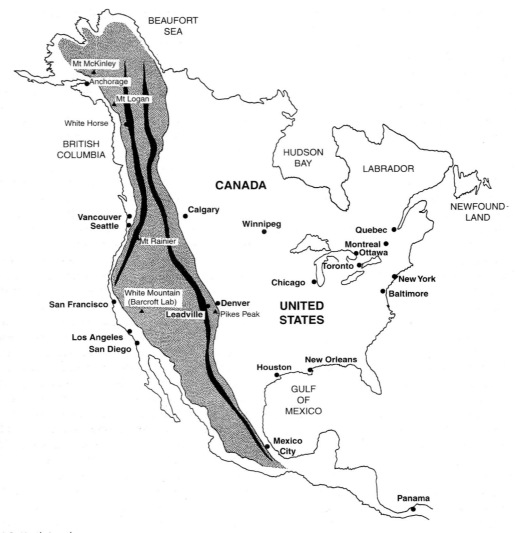

Figure 1.9 *North America.*

environment and shorter time available for acclimatization. AMREE 1981, of course, had to contend with the climatic factors of Everest. The cost of each investigation was similar, and taken together these four studies have made an enormous contribution to understanding the physiological and medical challenges of high altitude.

In the last 25 years too, numerous expeditions have been made on the Tibetan plateau by the Academia Sinica, including a traverse of the plateau by a Royal Society–Academica Sinica party in 1985 (Dong-Sheng 1981, Chang *et al.* 1986). In the course of these expeditions a number of peaks, including Everest, have been climbed and high altitude work carried out by members of the Shanghai Institute of Physiology led by Professor Hu Hsu-Tsu and other groups. During the Chinese ascent of Everest in 1975 telemetry of the heart was carried out and a number of other studies made (Shi *et al.* 1980, Hu 1983).

Russian contributions have been considerable. The most important early work on the effects of rarefied air on humans came from I.M. Sechenov after the deaths in the balloon Zenith in 1875. He studied the oxygen transport system, which formed the basis of later work on high altitude and in aviation.

At the end of the nineteenth century, P. Gorbachev, N. Tretiakov and O. Shlomm studied the effects of adaptation to altitude on soldiers in the Pamir and Tien Shan, probably in association with the 'great game' or rivalry with Britain for political influence in Central Asia.

The year 1923 saw the birth of Soviet mountaineering with the ascent of Mount Elbruz in the Caucasus. The first scientific expedition took place in 1926 and, between then and the outbreak of war with Germany in 1941, 25 expeditions from three main centers, Leningrad Military Medical Academy, Moscow and Kiev, took place in the Caucasus, Pamir, Altai and Tien Shan.

The father of Russian high altitude physiology is considered to be Nicolai Sirotinin (1897–1977), who built up the Institute of Physiology in Kiev, mainly to study the effects of hypoxia. His primary interest was in acid–base balance and he attributed the symptoms of mountain sickness to lack of carbon dioxide, as did Angelo Mosso. Between 1930 and 1940 he organized and took part in nine high altitude expeditions. Another very important physiologist was Z. I. Barbashova (1910–80) who studied the effects of hypoxia on the cells and peripheral tissues, and showed tissue adaptation to be present.

Postwar studies were stimulated by populations living at altitude for commercial reasons and the growth of space science. Good tolerance to hypoxic stress was considered an indication of the ability to combat the generalized stress of space flight.

In 1973 a permanent medical and biological station was opened in Terskol at the foot of Elbruz, at about 2000 m, and research expeditions have taken place in Tadzhikistan and Kirghizia, where M. M. Mubrakhimov has studied indigenous populations.

In 1983 rigorous exercise tests on potential Everest climbers revealed unsuspected cardiac abnormalities (Gippenreiter 1983, 1993 (personal communication); Gazenko 1987).

Many workers worldwide are now active in this field, including Japanese, French, German and Scandinavian workers as well as those from South America, India and Pakistan (Rivolier 1959, 1976, Brendel and Zink 1982, Richalet 1984, Richalet *et al.* 1992, Ueda *et al.* 1992).

1.13 PERMANENT HIGH ALTITUDE LABORATORIES

In 1890 Joseph Vallot built the Observatoire Vallot on Mont Blanc (4807 m) where studies on astronomy, glaciology and, later, physiology were carried out. Vallot used the hut until 1920. In 1983 it was updated by ARPE (Association pour la Recherche en Physiologie de l'Environment) but because it is close to the summit of Mont Blanc access on foot may be difficult and a helicopter is often used. The first high altitude laboratory dedicated to physiological studies was built by the Club Alpino Italiano on Monte Rossa (4559 m) in 1893, originally as a climbing hut with a room for use as a laboratory used by Anglo Mosso; a major rebuilding program was carried out in 1977 and field studies restarted in 1983. Almost every year since then it has been a center for studies by Oswald Oelz, Peter Bärtsch, Marco Maggiorini and others. Among other laboratories is one on Pikes Peak (4300 m), Colorado, USA. Earlier work was carried out in the railway station building (including Haldane's 1911 expedition). In recent times a modern laboratory has been built and is the responsibility of the US Army Research Institute of Environmental Medicine at Natick, Massachusetts. This provides excellent facilities for accommodation and physiological research. There are also facilities on Mount Evans (4350 m) and in the Barcroft Laboratory (3800 and summit hut at 4342 m) on White Mountain in North America. Facilities also exist at Morococha (4550 m) and Cerro de Pasco (4331 m) in Peru. In La Paz (3500 m) is the Instituto Boliviano de Biologia de Altura. A center for further study of cold and high altitude is situated at Anchorage, Alaska, and a Medical Research Center was opened at Xining on the northeast edge of the Tibet plateau in 1984. Studies are also being carried out in Lhasa (3658 m) and in Leh (3500 m) in Ladakh, India. In Shanghai a decompression chamber dedicated to long-term studies has been constructed. In the Sola-Khumbu, Nepal, the Ev-K2-CNR pyramid laboratory was built at just over 5000 m at Lobuche in 1990. In order to study large numbers of people at moderate altitude, the Colorado Altitude Research Institute was established in 1988 at 2500 m. Both India and Pakistan are concerned with high altitude studies as a result of their military confrontation at about 6000 m on the Siachen glacier in Kashmir.

Table 1.2 *Important high altitude research stations*

Location of station	Country	Altitude (m)
Cesar Tejos	Chile	6100
Laboratoro Fisica cosmica Chacaltaya (near La Paz)	Bolivia	5203
Ev-K2-CNR, Lobuche	Nepal	5050
Ticlio Pass	Peru	4700
Cab. Regina Margherita	Italy	4559
Inst. of Andean Biology, Morococha	Peru	4550
Inst. de Biological Mina, Aquilar de la Altura	Argentina	4503
Observatoire Vallot, Mont Blanc	France	4356
Mount Evans, Colorado	USA	4350
Summit Lab., White Mountain, California	USA	4342
Cerro de Pasco	Peru	4331
Pikes Peak, Colorado	USA	4300
Mauna Kea, Hawaii	USA	4209
La Oroya	Peru	3730
Inst. Boliviana de la Altura, La Paz	Bolivia	3500
Jungfraujoch	Switzerland	3476

French workers are active in South America and elsewhere. In 1991 an expedition supported by ARPE and led by J.-P. Richalet completed a project on the summit of an extinct volcano, Mount Sajama (6542 m) in Bolivia. Over 2 t of equipment was taken to the summit and solar cells and batteries provided electric power. More recently a long-term decompression chamber experiment, Operation Everest III (COMEX) has been completed by this group in Marseilles.

The locations of high altitude research stations are summarized in Table 1.2

1.14 STUDIES OF INDIGENOUS HIGH ALTITUDE DWELLERS

The extraordinary high work output of high altitude residents was emphasized by Barcroft (1925) when describing native miners at Cerro de Pasco (4328 m) in the Andes:

> Every few minutes like a bee out of some hive . . . someone would appear from the mouth of the mine. He would be much out of breath, he would take frequent pauses on the way up, but the weight on his back would be one hundred pounds.

Possibly with his tongue in his cheek, Barcroft commented that, 'All dwellers at altitude are persons of impaired physical and mental powers.' This drew an immediate and indignant response from Carlos Monge, a Peruvian physician:

> Andean man must be physically distinct from sea level man, requiring much further research before one may define let alone apply the terms inferior and superior.

Monge and his associates were stimulated to a study of Andean high altitude populations (Monge 1948, Hurtado 1964, Léon-Vellade and Arregui 1993). Studies have also been carried out in Ethiopia, the Himalayan valleys of Bhutan, and Nepal, as part of the International Biological Programme (Baker 1978), on the Tibetan plateau (Sun 1986) and in Lhasa. Work has also been done on Caucasian subjects in Leadville (3100 m), especially by a group from the University of Colorado, Denver (Winslow and Monge 1987 pp. 15–16).

Recently studies at sea level on elite Sherpas, born and bred at high altitude, who had had considerable experience of extreme altitude, showed that they had high aerobic capacities of 66 mL min^{-1} kg^{-1} and maximum heart rates of 199 beats min^{-1} (Garrod *et al.* 1997). Sun *et al.* (1970) reported a $V_{O_2 max}$ of 50–58 mL min^{-1} kg^{-1} in Tibetans born and bred at altitude and a high $V_{O_2 max}$ was found in Andean highlanders (Vogel *et al.* 1974).

The number of studies on the high altitude populations in Tibet has greatly increased in the last few years. These studies have compared Tibetans with

Han Chinese and more recently with highlanders of South America. Differences have been found in respect of hemoglobin concentration, arterial oxygen saturation, pulmonary hypoxic pressor response and susceptibility to various forms of mountain sickness. These are reviewed in Chapter 17.

A new category of people exposed to altitude hypoxia is those who commute to work at altitude. These include miners in the Andes, working, for instance, at the new Collahuasi mine (4400–4600 m)

in Chile, and scientists and technicians working on the telescopes on Mauna Kea (4200 m) in Hawaii (see Chapter 29).

The increasing number of national and international conferences held and societies established in the last two decades attests to increasing interest in the field of high altitude medicine and physiology. The first book devoted exclusively to the history of the subject was published in 1998 (West 1998).

2

The atmosphere

SUMMARY

An understanding of some of the physical principles of the atmosphere is important in high altitude medicine and physiology. This is because most of the problems that occur at high altitude are attributable to the hypoxia which is caused by the decrease in barometric pressure as altitude increases. The relationship between barometric pressure and altitude is discussed, particularly for regions of the world such as the Andes and Himalayas where large numbers of people reside at high altitude. Recent work has determined the pressure–altitude relationship with much better confidence than previously. Considerable confusion has occurred in the past by assuming that the relationship follows the standard atmosphere. In fact, the pressures are usually substantially higher at a given altitude because the relationship between barometric pressure and altitude is latitude dependent, and most of the high mountains of the world are relatively near the equator. At extreme altitudes, the variation of barometric pressure with season is sufficient to affect human performance. This is particularly true of the summit of Mount Everest where climbers are near the limit of tolerance to hypoxia. Other atmospheric factors such as temperature, humidity and solar radiation are also important.

2.1 INTRODUCTION

It has been known since the time of Paul Bert and the publication of *La Pression Barométrique* (Bert 1878) that most of the deleterious effects of high altitude on humans are caused by hypoxia. This in turn is a direct result of the reduction in atmospheric pressure. Yet in spite of the fact that we celebrated the centennial of Bert's book several years ago, there is still confusion in the minds of some physicians and physiologists about the relationship between barometric pressure and altitude, particularly at extreme heights. For example, some environmental physiologists are still surprised to learn that the barometric pressure at the summit of Mount Everest is considerably higher than that predicted by the standard pressure–altitude tables used by the aviation industry, and that humans can reach the summit without supplementary oxygen only because the tables are inapplicable.

Although most of the undesirable effects of high altitude are due to hypoxia, under some circumstances additional deterioration results from cold, dehydration, solar radiation, and even ionizing radiation. However, most of these hazards of the environment can be avoided by proper clothing or shelter. Only hypoxia is unavoidable unless, of course, supplementary oxygen is available. The low barometric pressure in itself has no physiological sequelae unless the decompression is rapid, for example in the case of the explosive decompression that occurs when a window fails in a pressurized aircraft. Rapid decompression causes so-called barotrauma as a result of the very rapid enlargement of airspaces within the body including the lungs and middle ear cavity. Such accidents can also occur in ascent from deep diving, but are not considered here.

That low pressure *per se* is innocuous was not always realized. Indeed, early theories of mountain sickness included a number of exotic explanations based on the reduced pressure itself (Bert 1878, pp. 342–7 in 1943 translation). One was weakening of the coxofemoral articulation; it was thought that barometric pressure was an important factor in pressing the head of the femur into its socket and that, at high altitudes, the necessary increase in action of the neighboring muscles resulted in fatigue. Another hypothesis was that superficial blood vessels would dilate and rupture if the barometric pressure which normally supported them was reduced. Indeed, modern day medical students occasionally raise issues of this kind when they are first introduced to high altitude physiology. A further theory was that distension of intestinal gas would interfere with the action of the diaphragm and also impede venous return to the heart. All these theories neglect the fact that, when humans ascend to high altitude, all the hydrostatic pressures in the body fall together. In other words, although the pressure outside the superficial blood vessels falls, the pressure inside the vessels falls to the same extent and therefore the pressure differences across the vessels are unchanged.

2.2 BAROMETRIC PRESSURE AND ALTITUDE

2.2.1 Historical

The notion that air has weight and therefore exerts a pressure at the surface of the Earth evaded the ancient Greeks and had to wait until the Renaissance. Galileo (1638) was well aware of the force associated with a vacuum and therefore the effort required to 'break' it, but he thought of this in the context of a force required to break a copper wire by stretching it, that is, the cohesive forces within the substance of the wire. In 1647, Otto von Guericke provided a graphic demonstration of the forces associated with a vacuum when he showed that teams of horses could not separate two carefully fitting hemispheres from which the air had been pumped. But it was left to Galileo's pupil Torricelli to realize that the force of a vacuum is due to the weight of the atmosphere. In his memorable letter addressed to Michelangelo Ricci in 1644 he wrote, 'We live submerged at the bottom of an ocean of the element air, which by unquestioned experiments is known to have weight' (Torricelli 1644). How simple and striking this is. Moreover, Torricelli wondered whether the air pressure became less on the tops of high mountains where the air 'begins to be distinctly rare . . .' as he put it. Torricelli is credited with making the first mercury barometer, though barometers filled with other liquids had apparently been constructed previously, for example by Gaspar Berti. These were unsatisfactory because of the effect of the vapor pressure of the liquid.

The Jesuit priest Joseph de Acosta, who accompanied the early Spanish explorers in Peru, gave his dramatic description of acute mountain sickness as early as 1590 (de Acosta 1590). This included the inspired guess that the deleterious effects of high altitude were caused by the thinness of the air. However, the landmark experiment took place in 1648 when the French philosopher and mathematician Blaise Pascal suggested that his brother-in-law, F. Périer, take a barometer to the top of the Puy de Dôme (1463 m) in central France to see whether the pressure fell (Pascal 1648). The results were communicated to Pascal in a delightful letter by Périer in which he described how the level of the mercury barometer fell some three pouces (about 75 mm) during the ascent of '500 fathoms' of altitude (probably about 900 m). The experiment had elaborate controls. For example, the Reverend Father Chastin, 'a man as pious as he is capable', stood guard over one barometer in the town of Clermont while Périer and a number of observers (including clerics, counselors, and a doctor of medicine) took another to the top of the mountain. On returning, it was found that the first barometer had not changed, and Périer even checked it again by filling it with the same mercury that he had taken up the mountain. Another observation was made the next day on the top of a high church tower in Clermont, and this also showed a fall in pressure, though of much smaller extent.

A few years later, Robert Boyle carried out experiments with the newly invented air pump and wrote his influential book *New Experiments Physico-Mechanicall Touching the Spring of the Air, and its Effects*. In the second edition of this book published in 1662 he formulated his famous law, which states that gas volume and pressure are inversely related (at constant temperature) (Boyle 1662).

An influential analysis of the relationships between altitude and barometric pressure was made by Zuntz *et al.* in 1906. They pointed out the important effect of temperature on the pressure–altitude relationship noting that, on a fine warm day, the upcurrents carry air to high altitudes and thus increase the sea level barometric pressure. Indeed, this is the basis for weather prediction based on barometric pressure.

Zuntz *et al.* (1906, pp. 37–9) gave the following logarithmic relationship for determining barometric pressure at any altitude:

$$\log b = \log B - \frac{h}{72\,(256.4 + t)}$$

where h is the altitude difference in meters, t is the mean temperature (°C) of the air column of height h, B is the barometric pressure (mm Hg) at the lower altitude, and b is the barometric pressure at the higher altitude. Note that this expression implies that the higher the mean temperature, the less rapidly does barometric pressure decrease with altitude. In addition, if temperature were constant, $\log b$ would be proportional to negative altitude, that is, the pressure would decrease exponentially as altitude increased. Zuntz *et al.* cite Hann's *Lehrbuch der Meteorologie* where the pressure–altitude relationship is given in a slightly different form (Hann 1901).

Zuntz *et al.*'s expression was used by FitzGerald (1913) in her study of alveolar P_{CO_2} and hemoglobin concentration in residents of various altitudes in the Colorado mountains during the Anglo-American Pikes Peak expedition of 1911. She showed that barometric pressures calculated from the Zuntz formula agreed closely with pressures observed in the mountains when a sea level pressure of 760 mm Hg and a mean temperature of the air column of +15 °C were assumed. Kellas (1917) used the same expression to predict barometric pressures in the Himalayan ranges, obtaining a value of 251 mm Hg for the summit of Mount Everest, assuming a mean temperature of 0 °C. This was almost the same as the pressure of

248 mm Hg given by Bert (Bert 1878, Appendix 1) in contrast to the erroneously low values used 70 years after Bert because of the inappropriate application of the standard atmosphere (section 2.2.3). However, a major difficulty with the use of the Zuntz formula is the sensitivity of the calculated pressure to temperature and the fact that the mean temperature of the air column is not accurately known. For example, the barometric pressure on the summit of Mount Everest was calculated by Kellas to be 267 mm Hg for a mean temperature of + 15 °C, but only 251 mm Hg for a mean temperature of 0 °C.

2.2.2 Physical principles

Barometric pressure decreases with altitude because the higher we go, the less atmosphere there is above us pressing down by virtue of its weight. If the atmosphere were incompressible, as is very nearly the case in a liquid, barometric pressure would decrease linearly with altitude, just as it does in a liquid. However, because the weight of the upper atmosphere compresses the lower gas, barometric pressure decreases more rapidly with height near the Earth's surface. If temperature were constant, the decrease in pressure would be exponential with respect to altitude, but because the temperature decreases as we go higher (at least, in the troposphere), the pressure falls more rapidly than the exponential law predicts.

The relationships between pressure, volume and temperature in a gas are governed by simple laws. These derive from the kinetic theory of gases which states that the molecules of a gas are in continuous random motion, and are only deflected from their course by collision with other molecules, or with the walls of a container. When they strike the walls and rebound, the resulting bombardment results in a pressure. The magnitude of the pressure depends on the number of molecules present, their mass and their speed.

- **Boyle's law** states that, at constant temperature, the pressure (P) of a given mass of gas is inversely proportional to its volume (V), or

  PV = constant   (temperature constant)

  This can be explained by the fact that as the molecules are brought closer together (smaller volume), the rate of bombardment on a unit surface increases (greater pressure).

- **Charles' law** states that at constant pressure, the volume of a gas is proportional to its absolute temperature (T), or

  V/T = constant (pressure constant)

  The explanation is that a rise in temperature increases the speed and therefore the momentum of the molecules, thus increasing their force of bombardment on the container.

  Another form of Charles' law states that at constant volume, the pressure is proportional to absolute temperature. (Note that absolute temperature is obtained by adding 273 to the Celsius temperature. Thus 37 °C = 310 K.)

- The **ideal gas law** combines the above laws thus:

  $PV = nRT$

  where n is the number of gram molecules of the gas and R is the 'gas constant'. When the units employed are mm Hg, liters and kelvin, then R = 62.4. Real gases deviate from ideal gas behavior to some extent under certain conditions because of intermolecular forces.

- **Dalton's law** states that each gas in a mixture exerts a pressure according to its own concentration, independently of the other gases present. That is, each component behaves as though it were present alone. The pressure of each gas is referred to as its partial pressure or tension (now obsolete). The total pressure is the sum of the partial pressures of all gases present. In symbols:

  $P_x = PF_x$

  where P_x is the partial pressure of gas x, P is the total pressure and F_x is the fractional concentration of gas x. For example, if half the gas is oxygen, F_{O_2} = 0.5. The fractional concentration always refers to dry gas.

- The **kinetic theory of gases** explains their diffusion in the gas phase. Because of their random motion, gas molecules tend to distribute themselves uniformly throughout any available space until the partial pressure is the same everywhere. Light gases diffuse faster than heavy gases because the mean velocity of the molecules is higher. The kinetic theory of gases states that the kinetic energy ($0.5\ mv^2$) of all gases is the same at a given temperature and pressure. From this it follows that the rate of diffusion of a gas is inversely proportional to the square root of its density (**Graham's law**).

On the basis of different diffusion rates, one might expect that very light gases such as helium would separate and be lost from the upper atmosphere. This does happen to some extent at extreme altitudes. However, at the altitudes of interest to us, say up to 10 km, convective mixing maintains the composition of the atmosphere constant.

Vertically, the atmosphere can be divided on the basis of temperature variations into the troposphere, the stratosphere and regions above that. The troposphere is the region where all the weather phenomena take place and is the only region of interest to high altitude medicine. Here, the temperature decreases approximately linearly with altitude until a low of about −60 °C is reached. The troposphere extends to an altitude of about 19 km at the equator but only to about 9 km at the poles. The average upper limit is about 10 km.

Above the troposphere is the stratosphere where the temperature remains nearly constant at about −60 °C for some 10–12 km of altitude. The interface between the troposphere and stratosphere is known as the tropopause.

Beyond the stratosphere, temperatures again vary with altitude. One of the important components of this region is the ionosphere where the degree of ionization of the molecules makes short-wave radio propagation possible.

2.2.3 Standard atmosphere

With the development of the aviation industry in the 1920s it became necessary to develop a barometric pressure–altitude relationship which could be universally accepted for calibrating altimeters, low pressure chambers and other devices. Although it had been recognized for many years that the relationship between pressure and altitude was temperature dependent and, as a result, latitude dependent, there were clear advantages in having a model atmosphere which applied approximately to mean conditions over the surface of the Earth. This is often referred to as the ICAO standard atmosphere (1964) or the US standard atmosphere (NOAA 1976). These two are identical up to altitudes of interest to us.

The assumptions of the standard atmosphere are a sea level pressure of 760 mm Hg, sea level temperature of +15 °C and a linear decrease in temperature with altitude (lapse rate) of 6.5 °C km^{-1} up to an altitude of 11 km (Table 2.1). Haldane and Priestley

(1935, p. 323) gave the following expression for the pressure–altitude relationship of the standard atmosphere in the second edition of their textbook *Respiration*:

$$\frac{P_0}{P} = \left(\frac{288}{288 - 1.98H}\right)^{5.256}$$

where P_0 and P are the pressures in mm Hg at sea level and high altitude respectively, and H is the height in thousands of feet. A more rigorous description is given in the *Manual of the ICAO Standard Atmosphere* (1964).

It should be emphasized that this model atmosphere was never meant to be used to predict the actual barometric pressure at a particular location. Rather it was developed as a model of more or less average conditions within the troposphere with full recognition that there would be local variations caused by latitude and other factors. Nevertheless, the standard atmosphere has assumed some importance in respiratory physiology because it is universally used as the standard for altimeter calibrations, and it has frequently been inappropriately used to predict the pressure at various specific points of the Earth's surface, particularly on high mountains.

Haldane and Priestley (1935) clearly understood that the standard atmosphere predicted barometric pressures considerably lower than those given by the expression of Zuntz *et al.* (1906), which had been shown by FitzGerald to predict accurately pressures in the Colorado mountains when a mean air column temperature of +15 °C was assumed.

Nevertheless, some physiologists have used the standard atmosphere for predicting the pressure at great altitudes, for example on Mount Everest (Houston and Riley 1947, Riley and Houston 1950–1, Rahn and Fenn 1955, Houston *et al.* 1987). The barometric pressure calculated in this way for the Everest summit (altitude 8848 m) is 236 mm Hg, which is far too low. In retrospect, one of the reasons for the indiscriminate use of the standard atmosphere was undoubtedly its very frequent employment in low pressure chambers during the very fertile period of research on respiratory physiology during World War II.

2.2.4   Variation of barometric pressure with latitude

The limited applicability of the standard atmosphere is further clarified when we look at the relationship between barometric pressure and altitude for different latitudes (Figure 2.1). This shows that the barometric pressure at the Earth's surface and at an altitude of 24 km is essentially independent of latitude. However, in the altitude range of about 6–16 km, there is a pronounced bulge in the

Table 2.1 *Barometric pressures (in mm Hg) from the standard atmosphere (ICAO 1964) and a model atmosphere (West 1996): the latter is a better fit for most sites where high altitude physiology and medicine are studied*

Altitude		Standard atmosphere		Model atmosphere	
km	ft	Barometric pressure	Inspired P_{O_2}[a]	Barometric pressure	Inspired P_{O_2}
0	0	760	149	760	149
1	3 281	674	131	679	132
2	6 562	596	115	604	117
3	9 843	526	100	537	103
4	13 123	462	87	475	90
5	16 404	405	75	420	78
6	19 685	354	64	369	67
7	22 966	308	54	324	58
8	26 247	267	46	284	50
9	29 528	231	38	247	42
10	32 810	199	31	215	35

[a] The P_{O_2} of moist inspired gas is 0.2094 $(P_B - 47)$.

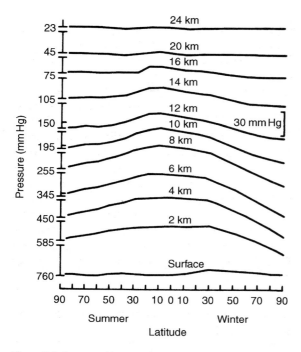

Figure 2.1 *Increase of barometric pressure near the equator at various altitudes in both summer and winter. Vertical axis shows the pressure increasing upwards according to the scale on the right. The numbers on the left show the barometric pressures at the poles for various altitudes; the altitude of Mount Everest is 8848 m. (From Brunt 1952.)*

2.2.5 Variation of barometric pressure with season

Not only does barometric pressure alter with latitude, but there are marked variations according to the month of the year. For example, Figure 2.2 shows the mean monthly pressures for an altitude of 8848 m as obtained from radiosonde balloons released from New Delhi, India, over a period of 15 years. Delhi has about the same latitude as Everest. Note that the mean pressures were lowest in the winter months of January and February (243.0 and 243.7 mm Hg, respectively) and highest in the summer months of July and August (254.5 mm Hg for both months). The monthly standard deviation showed a range of 0.65 mm Hg (July) to 1.66 mm Hg (December). The daily standard deviation was as low as 1.54 in the summer and as high as 2.92 in the winter. The standard deviation shown on Figure 2.2 is the mean of the monthly standard deviation for the 12 months of the year.

The single measurement of barometric pressure (253.0 mm Hg) made by Pizzo on the summit of Mount Everest on 24 October 1981 (West *et al.* 1983a) is also shown on Figure 2.2. This was 4.3 mm Hg higher than that predicted from the data shown in Figure 2.1, which is twice the daily standard deviation of barometric pressure for the month of

barometric pressure near the equator both in winter and summer. Since the latitude of Mount Everest is 28°N, the pressure at its summit (8848 m) is considerably higher than would be the case for a hypothetical mountain of the same altitude near one of the poles.

The cause of the bulge in barometric pressure near the equator is a very large mass of very cold air in the stratosphere above the equator (Brunt 1952, p. 379). In fact, paradoxically, the coldest air in the atmosphere is above the equator. This is brought about by a combination of complex radiation and convective phenomena. Another corollary of the same phenomenon is that the height of the tropopause is much greater near the equator than near the poles. These latitude-dependent variations of pressure are of great physiological significance for anyone attempting to climb Mount Everest without supplementary oxygen because they result in a barometric pressure on the Everest summit which is considerably higher than that predicted from the model atmosphere.

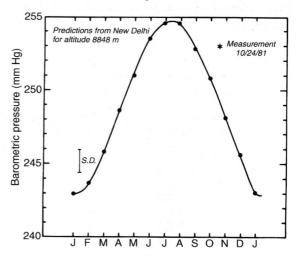

Figure 2.2 *Mean monthly pressures for 8848 m altitude as obtained from weather balloons released from New Delhi, India. Note the increase during the summer months. The mean monthly standard deviation (SD) is also shown. The barometric pressure measured on the Everest summit on 24 October 1981 (*) was unusually high for that month. (From West* et al. *1983a.)*

October. It should be added that Pizzo had an exceptionally fine day for his summit climb, the temperature on the summit being measured as −9 °C, much higher than expected for that altitude (section 2.3.1).

Figure 2.3 combines the effects of latitude and month of the year on the barometric pressure at an altitude of 8848 m. The data are for the northern hemisphere, and the pressures for the months of January (midwinter), July (midsummer) and October (preferred month for climbing in the post-monsoon period) are compared. The profile for the month of May, which is the usual month for reaching the summit in the pre-monsoon season, is almost the same as that for October. The data are the means from all longitudes (Oort and Rasmusson 1971). The data clearly show the marked effects of both latitude and season on barometric pressure. It is interesting that in midsummer the pressure reaches a maximum near the latitude of Mount Everest (28°35″N). Figure 2.3 shows that if Mount Everest was at the latitude of Mount McKinley (63°N), the pressure on the summit would be very much lower.

Radiosonde balloons are released from meteorological stations all over the world twice a day, and the resulting data on the relationship between barometric pressure and altitude are available from constant pressure charts. Details on how to obtain these are given in West (1993a). Using these data it can be shown that the barometric pressure on the Everest summit was 251 mm Hg when Messner and Habeler made their first ascent without supplementary oxygen in 1978. In August 1980, Messner made the first solo ascent without supplementary oxygen and he was fortunate that the barometric pressure was unusually high at 256 mm Hg; when Sherpa Ang Rita made the first winter ascent on 22 December 1987, the barometric pressure was only 247 mm Hg.

2.2.6 Barometric pressure–altitude relationship for locations of importance in high altitude medicine and physiology

We have seen that the standard atmosphere generally underestimates the pressures on high mountains, which are of interest to people concerned with high altitude medicine and physiology. Recently, it has been possible to define the barometric pressure–altitude relationship in the Himalayan and Andean ranges with some accuracy, and it transpires that the relationship holds for many other locations where high altitude medicine and physiology are studied.

As already stated, the first direct measurement of barometric pressure on the Everest summit was obtained by Pizzo in 1981 during the course of the American Medical Research Expedition to Everest (West *et al.* 1983a). The value was 253 mm Hg, as shown on Figure 2.2. During the same expedition, careful measurements of barometric pressure were made at two other locations on Mount Everest where the altitudes were accurately known. These were the Base Camp (altitude 5400 m) and at Camp 5, just above the South Col (altitude 8050 m). These points lay very close to a straight line on a log pressure–altitude plot and therefore allowed the barometric pressure–altitude relationship at very high altitudes on Mount Everest to be accurately described for the first time (Figure 2 in West *et al.* 1983a). This relationship is of great physiological interest because, as discussed in Chapter 12, the pressure near the summit is so low that the P_{O_2} is very near the limit for human survival.

More recently, additional measurements have been made at very high altitudes on Mount Everest (West 1999a). Another direct measurement was made on the summit in May 1997 and this agreed

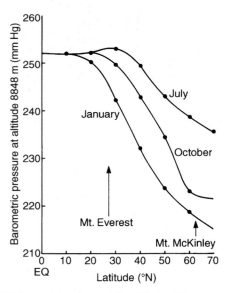

Figure 2.3 *Barometric pressure at the altitude of Mount Everest plotted against latitude in the northern hemisphere for midsummer, midwinter, and the preferred month for climbing in the post-monsoon period (October). Note the considerably lower pressures in the winter. The arrows show the latitudes of Mount Everest and Mount McKinley. (From West* et al. *1983a.)*

within 1 mm Hg of Pizzo's measurement of 253 mm Hg. In addition, a large number of measurements were reported from a barometer that telemetered information from the South Col (altitude 7986 m). When these points were added to those obtained during the 1981 expedition (Figure 2.4), they greatly increase our confidence in the barometric pressure–altitude relationship.

Two other pieces of data have recently come to light. Charles Corfield made a single measurement of the barometric pressure on the Everest summit at 10 a.m. on 5 May 1999. He used a Kollsman aneroid barometer and the value was 253 mm Hg (personal communication). The air temperature was −18 °C, and this had been shown not to affect the calibration of the barometer. The other data point comes from measurements made on the South Col by the Italian Ev-K2-CNR program. They reported 52 measurements of barometric pressure on 29 and 30 September and 1 October 1992 (personal communication). The mean value was 383.0 mbar (287 mm Hg). This is the same pressure as that found by the MIT group in August 1997 (West 1999a). These two additional pieces of data fit extremely well with the other measurements listed above.

2.2.7 Model atmosphere equation

It is now possible to provide a barometric pressure–altitude relationship that accurately predicts the pressure at most locations of interest to high altitude medicine and physiology (West 1996a). The data are shown in Figure 2.5. The prediction is particularly good if the locations lie within 30° of the equator, and especially if the pressure is measured in the summer months. Since many studies of high altitude medicine and physiology are carried out in locations and times that fulfill these criteria, the relationship is very useful in practice. The equation of the line is

$$P_\text{B} = \exp (6.63268 - 0.1112h - 0.00149h^2)$$

where P_B is the barometric presssure (in mm Hg) and h is the altitude in kilometers. This has been called the **model atmosphere equation,** and is useful for

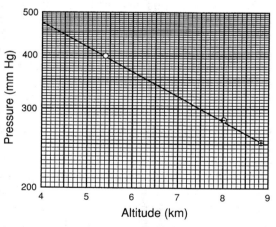

Figure 2.4 *Barometric pressure–altitude relationship for Mount Everest. The circles show data from the 1981 American Medical Research Expedition to Everest. The cross at the summit altitude (8848 m) is from the 1997 NOVA expedition. The cross at an altitude of 7986 m is from measurements made by the Massachusetts Institute of Technology in 1998. The standard deviations are too small to show on the graph. The line corresponds to the model atmosphere equation: $P_B = \exp (6.63268 - 0.1112h - 0.00149h^2)$ where h is in kilometers. (From West 1999a.)*

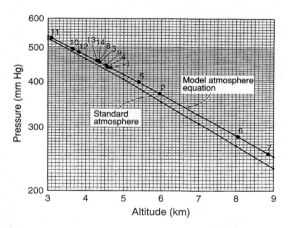

Figure 2.5 *Barometric pressure–altitude relationship corresponding to the model atmosphere equation. Note that it predicts the altitudes of many locations of interest in high altitude medicine and physiology very well. The lower line shows the standard atmosphere which predicts pressures that are too low. The locations and measured pressures are as follows: 1) Collahuasi mine, Chile, 438 mm Hg; 2) Aucanquilcha mine, Chile, 372 mm Hg; 3) Vallot observatory, France, 452 mm Hg; 4) Capanna Margherita, Italy, 440 mm Hg; 5) Mount Everest Base Camp, Nepal, 400 mm Hg; 6) Mount Everest South Col, 284 mm Hg; 7) Mount Everest summit, 253 mm Hg; 8) Cerro de Pasco, Peru, 458 mm Hg; 9) Morococha, Peru, 446 mm Hg; 10) Lhasa, Tibet, 493 mm Hg; 11) Crooked Creek, California, 530 mm Hg; 12) Barcroft laboratory, California, 483 mm Hg; 13) Pikes Peak, Colorado, 462 mm Hg; 14) White Mountain summit, California, 455 mm Hg. (From West 1996a.)*

theoretical calculations in high altitude physiology such as predicting the effects of oxygen enrichment at different altitudes.

2.2.8   Barometric pressure and inspired P_{O_2}

As we have seen, the composition of the atmosphere is constant up to altitudes well above those of medical interest so it is safe to assume that the concentration of oxygen in dry air is approximately 20.94 per cent. However, the effects of water vapor on the inspired P_{O_2} become increasingly important at higher altitudes.

When air is inhaled into the upper bronchial tree, it is warmed and moistened and becomes saturated with vapor at the prevailing temperature. The water vapor pressure at 37 °C is 47 mm Hg and this, of course, is independent of altitude. Thus the P_{O_2} of moist inspired gas is given by the expression

$$PI_{O_2} = 0.2094 \, (P_B - 47)$$

where P_B is barometric pressure.

This equation shows how much more important water vapor pressure becomes at very high altitudes. For example, at sea level, the water vapor pressure at 37 °C is only 6 per cent of the total barometric pressure. However, on the summit of Mount Everest, where the barometric pressure is about 250 mm Hg, the water vapor pressure is nearly 19 per cent of the total pressure, and the inspired P_{O_2} is correspondingly further reduced (see Table 2.1).

It has been pointed out from time to time that a relatively small reduction in body temperature at extreme altitude would confer a substantial increase in inspired P_{O_2}. For example, if the body temperature fell to 35 °C where the water vapor is 42 mm Hg, the P_{O_2} of moist inspired gas would be increased from 42.5 to 43.5 mm Hg. This increase of 1 mm Hg would be beneficial because the arterial P_{O_2} would increase by approximately the same extent, and since the oxygen dissociation curve is very steep at this point, there would be an appreciable gain in arterial oxygen concentration. However, there is no evidence that body temperature falls at extreme altitude. Nor is it reasonable to assume that the temperature in the alveoli where gas exchange takes place would be significantly less than the body core temperature.

2.2.9   Physiological significance of barometric pressure at high altitude

Since the barometric pressure directly determines the inspired P_{O_2}, it is clear that the variations of barometric pressure with latitude and season, as described in sections 2.2.4 and 2.2.5, will affect the degree of hypoxemia in the body. For example, a climber on Mount McKinley in Alaska, which is situated at a latitude of 63°N, will be exposed to a considerably lower barometric pressure on the summit than would be the case for a mountain of the same height located in the tropics (see Figure 2.3).

The variations of barometric pressure with latitude and season become particularly significant from a physiological point of view at extreme altitudes such as near the summit of Mount Everest. For example, it has been shown that if the pressure on the Everest summit conformed to the standard atmosphere, it would be impossible to climb the mountain without supplementary oxygen (West 1983). In addition, the variation of barometric pressure with month of the year shown in Figure 2.2 indicates that it would be considerably more difficult to reach the summit without supplementary oxygen in the winter as a result of the reduced inspired P_{O_2}, quite apart from the obvious difficulties of lower temperatures and high winds. Although there have now been many ascents of Everest without supplementary oxygen in the pre- and post-monsoon seasons, only one person has made a winter ascent without supplementary oxygen: Sherpa Ang Rita on 22 December 1987. This topic is considered in more detail in Chapter 11.

2.3   FACTORS OTHER THAN BAROMETRIC PRESSURE AT HIGH ALTITUDE

2.3.1   Temperature

Temperature falls with increasing altitude at the rate of about 1°C for every 150 m. This lapse rate is essentially independent of latitude. The consequence is that on a very high mountain, such as Mount Everest, the average temperature near the summit is predicted to be about −40 °C. Most climbers choose the warmer months of the year. In May, a temperature of −27 °C was measured at an altitude of 8500 m on Everest (Pugh 1957), although Pizzo obtained a temperature of −9 °C on the summit in October (West *et al.* 1983a). In the winter the temperatures are much lower. However, even then they do not approach the extremely low temperatures seen in northern Canada or Siberia during midwinter.

More important than temperature *per se* is the wind chill factor. Wind velocities on Himalayan peaks have often been estimated to be in excess of 150 km h^{-1}, though few measurements have been made. Such high winds result in extremely severe chill factors at low temperatures and can make climbing impossible. Cold injury is common in the mountains and is discussed in Chapters 25 and 26.

2.3.2   Humidity

Absolute humidity is the amount of water vapor per unit volume of gas at the prevailing temperature. This value is extremely low at high altitude because the water vapor pressure is so depressed at the reduced temperature. Thus even if the air is fully saturated with water vapor, the actual amount will be very small. For example, the water vapor pressure at +20 °C is 17 mm Hg but only 1 mm Hg at −20 °C.

Relative humidity is a measure of the amount of water vapor in the air as a percentage of the amount which could be contained at the prevailing temperature. This value may be low, normal or high at altitude. The disparity between absolute and relative humidities is explained by the fact that even saturated air is unable to contain much water vapor because of the very low temperature. If this air is warmed without allowing additional water vapor to form, its relative humidity falls.

The very low absolute humidity at high altitude frequently causes dehydration. First, the insensible water loss caused by ventilation is great because of the dryness of the inspired air. In addition, the levels of ventilation may be extremely high, especially on exercise (Chapter 11), and this increases water loss. For example, near the summit of Mount Everest, the total ventilation is increased some five-fold compared with sea level for the same level of activity. Pugh (1964b) found that during exercise at 5500 m altitude, the rate of fluid loss from the lungs alone was about 2.9 g water per 100 L of ventilation (body temperature and pressure, saturated with water vapor, or BTPS). This is equivalent to about 200 mL of water per hour for moderate exercise.

There is evidence that the dehydration resulting from these rapid fluid losses does not produce as strong a sensation of thirst as at sea level. As a result, climbers find it is necessary to drink large quantities of fluids at high altitude to remain hydrated even though they have little desire to do so. For men climbing 7 h a day at altitudes over 6000 m, 3–4 L of fluid are required in order to maintain a urine output of 1.5 L day^{-1} (Pugh 1964b). Even so, it appears that people living at very high altitude are in a state of chronic volume depletion. In a group of subjects living at an altitude of 6300 m during the American Medical Research Expedition to Everest, serum osmolality was significantly increased compared with sea level despite the fact that ample fluids were available and the lifestyle in terms of exercise and diet was not exceptional (Blume *et al.* 1984).

2.3.3   Solar radiation

The intensity of solar radiation increases markedly at high altitude for two reasons. First, the much thinner atmosphere absorbs less of the sun's rays, especially those of short wavelength in the near ultraviolet region of the spectrum. Second, reflection of the sun from snow greatly increases radiation exposure.

The reduced density of the air causes an increase in incident solar radiation of up to 100 per cent at an altitude of 4000 m compared with sea level (Elterman 1964). The fact that mountain air is so dry is another important factor because water vapor in the atmosphere absorbs substantial amounts of solar radiation.

The efficiency with which the ground reflects solar radiation is known as its albedo. This varies from less than 20 per cent at sea level to up to 90 per cent in the presence of snow at great altitudes (Buettner 1969). Mountaineers are familiar with the extreme intensity of solar radiation, especially on a glacier in a valley between two mountains. Here the sunlight is reflected from both sides as well as from the snow or ice on the glacier and the heat can be very oppressive despite the great altitude. A consequence of this is the extreme variation in temperature which has been noted in camps under these conditions.

2.3.4 Ionizing radiation

The intensity of cosmic radiation increases at high altitude because there is less of the Earth's atmosphere to absorb the rays as they enter from space. This is the reason why cosmic radiation laboratories are often located on high mountains. It has been shown that, at an altitude of 3000 m, the increased cosmic radiation results in an increased radiation dose to a human being of approximately 70 mrad (0.0007 Gy) per year. This should be considered in relation to the normal background radiation dose from all sources of 50–200 mrad (0.0005–0.002 Gy) per year. The increased ionizing radiation of high altitude has been cited as one of the factors causing acute mountain sickness (Bert 1878), but there is no scientific basis for this assertion.

3

Geography and the human response to altitude

SUMMARY

The highland areas of the world support considerable populations. The climate is harsh and methods of cultivation have to be adapted to the terrain. Terracing has been brought to a fine art in the mountain regions, although the South American altiplano and the Tibetan plateau allow normal methods of cultivation. Animal husbandry and mining are important, and tourism is becoming increasingly popular.

Mountains often form boundaries between cultures. Border peoples have developed a physique that enables them to survive under severe conditions of cold and hypoxia. Commerce in high valleys without roads depends on porters and without their remarkable capacity to carry loads the economy would remain static. Acclimatization to hypoxia is complex and far reaching and depends on the severity and rate at which oxygen lack is imposed. Local cold tolerance but not general cold acclimatization occurs, and protection is mainly by cultural methods.

3.1 INTRODUCTION

Although the expression 'high altitude' has no precise definition, the majority of individuals have certain clinical, physiological, anatomical and biochemical changes which occur at levels above 3000 m. Individual variation is, however, considerable and some people are affected at levels as low as 2000 m. For sea level visitors, an altitude of 4600–4900 m represents the highest acceptable level for permanent habitation; for high altitude residents 5800–6000 m is the highest so far recorded (West 1986a). At greater altitudes physical and mental deterioration occurs and permanent habitation is not possible (section 3.8.2, Chapter 17). In South America archaeological sites have been found at 6271 m on Llullaillaco, but there is no evidence that these were permanent dwellings.

The main areas of the world above 3000 m are:

- the Tibetan plateau
- the Himalayan range and its valleys
- the Tien Shan and Pamir
- the mountain ranges of east Turkey, Iran, Afghanistan and Pakistan
- the Rocky Mountains and Sierra Nevada of the USA and Canada
- the Sierra Madre of Mexico
- the Andes of South America
- the European Alps
- the Pyrenees between Spain and France
- the Atlas Mountains of North Africa
- the Ethiopian highlands

- the mountains of East and South Africa
- the plateau and mountains of Antarctica
- parts of New Guinea and other small regions such as Hawaii, Tenerife and New Zealand.

The European Alps do not support a large high altitude population, but the region is vitally important because of its position at the crossroads of Europe and because modern investigation into all aspects of mountain science originated there.

The three main regions that support large populations are the Tibetan plateau and Himalayan valleys, the Andes of South America and the Ethiopian Highlands. Although the plateau and peaks of Antarctica are a large area of high altitude there is no indigenous population.

3.1.1 European Alps

The early development of all branches of mountain science resulted from the increasing ability to travel in these inhospitable regions, due to developments in mountaineering and skiing.

The word 'alp' is based originally on a Celtic word meaning 'high mountain': the modern use of this word meaning 'high pasture' dates from the Middle Ages.

The history of the European Alps is the story of how this region, constrained by its geographical position and topography, became a vital and indispensable link in the communications of the whole of Europe.

The discovery of 'Similaun Man', some 5000 years old, at a height of 3210 m shows that considerable altitudes were reached by local people when crossing from one valley to another. The deposition of gold bracelets to propitiate the mountain gods was common from prehistory to the Middle Ages and many offerings have been found in the neighborhood of the Great St Bernard Pass. Here the Roman deity Poeninus presided over the crossing and he is commemorated in the present day name, Pennine Alps.

The century between 50 BCE and 50 CE was the first period in which the whole of the European Alps came into the orbit of one political system, the Roman Empire, with communications linking Rome via the Alpine passes with the periphery of that empire. Many of the names used for subregions, such as Alps Maritimae and Alps Cottiae, are still in use today.

The native population was neither static nor homogenous, but it was the Romans who established the main framework of communication in this region. However, their roads had little impact on the essential pasturalism of the Alpine economy and the mountains themselves were feared by the Romans as the abode of dragons and evil forces. The people, with their susceptibility to goitre, were not much admired either.

It was not until the nineteenth century that gradual easing of communications opened up the whole region to the outside world and ignorance turned to knowledge and understanding (Snodgrass 1993).

3.1.2 Himalayas and Tibetan plateau

The Himalayas form a topographically extremely complex region, extending 1500 miles from Nanga Parbat (8125 m) in the west to Namcha Barwa (7756 m) in the east. At their western extremity they are part of a confused mass of peaks, passes and glaciers where the western Kun Lun, Karakoram, Pir Panjal and Pamirs form an area the size of France. The Himalayas contain the world's highest mountain, Mount Everest (8848 m), and many other peaks over 7500 m. The main range forms the watershed between Central Asia and India, and there are middle ranges at intermediate altitudes. The outer Himalayas (up to 1500 m) form foothills rising from the plains of India.

The Tibetan plateau is an area occupied by Tibetans, who have a well defined culture. It extends in the south to the Himalayas and high Himalayan valleys. To the west the plateau is demarcated by the northward curve of the Himalayas which continues into Kashmir, Baltistan and then to Gilgit and the Karakoram. To the north the peaks (up to 7700 m) of the Kun Lun range, 1500 miles long, mark off the plateau of Tibet from Xinjiang (Chinese Turkestan); to the east it extends to the Koko Nor or Qinghai Lake and, further south, the valleys of Qinghai and Sikiang and the gorge country of south-east Tibet.

The area covers about 1.5 million square miles and is the largest and highest plateau in the world, much of it at an altitude of 4600–4900 m. It presents an enormous range of climate and topography. 'Every 10 li (3 miles) heaven is different.' The major climatic contrast is between the southern side of the

Himalayas and the high valleys exposed to the summer Indian monsoon with very high rainfall, particularly in the east, and the aridity and low rainfall of the Tibetan plateau. The change is so abrupt that in some passes in the eastern Himalayas, vegetation may change from tropical to subarctic within a few yards. .

The Tibetans believe that in the prehistoric era their land was a large sea, Tethys, which, according to the theory of plate tectonics, is correct. The Royal Society/Chinese Academy of Sciences Tibet Geotraverse in 1985–6 established that the thickness of the Tibetan plateau crust, which at 70 km is about twice as much as normal, is due mainly to folding and thrusting that has occurred as a result of India colliding with Asia, rather than India moving under Asia and elevating to a plateau (Chang *et al.* 1986). In mythology, Tibetans are descended from the union of a forest monkey and a female demon of the rocks, with the site of the first cultivated field being at Sothang in south-east Tibet, but other legends place their origin further east.

The Tibetans have always regarded themselves as living in the northern part of the world; the Indians, however, considered the Himalayas to be the abode of the gods and inhabited by a race of supermen gifted with special knowledge, particularly of magic, and this probably accounts for the popular European belief of Tibet as a place where the immortal sages dwell, guarding the ultimate secrets. Far from being isolated, however, Tibetans have been subject to influences from China, India, Central Asia and the Middle East for many centuries (Stein 1972).

With increasing numbers of Han Chinese immigrants there are more than 3.0 million people living over 3000 m, and it is estimated that the amount of this land available for agriculture is 5 per cent. In the valleys, fields are terraced; on the plateau, larger fields are found in sheltered areas on valley floors, but all are threatened by snow, hail, wind and erosion. Permanent buildings are found up to 3500 m with nomadic populations at higher levels. Neolithic human remains have been found near Lhasa (Ward 1990, 1991).

3.1.3   Andes of South America

The highland zone extends from Colombia in the north to central Chile in the south, and is flanked by an arid desert on its west, with a deeply eroded escarpment to the east, which adjoins the Amazon basin.

The central Andean region has three broadly defined areas running parallel with the Pacific Ocean: the cordillera occidentale, the altiplano, a broad undulating plain at 4000 m in the middle, and the cordillera orientale in the east.

The earliest archeological evidence for human occupation dates back 20 000 years (MacNeish 1971) and has been found at Ayacucho, Peru; at 2900 m; other early finds are recorded in central Chile, Venezuela and Argentina. The skeleton of a man who lived 9500 years ago has been found at Lauricocha (4200 m) in Peru (Hurtado 1971). The pre-Inca civilizations were situated mainly along the Pacific Coast and the population subsisted mainly on seafood. Little is known of the highland population during this period.

The Inca civilization only achieved a position of major importance in the 100 years preceding the Spanish invasion of 1532. Spanish settlement of highland areas was hindered by ecological restraints imposed by altitude and the nature of the terrain, and, after consolidation of Spanish rule, Peru remained under colonial domination for 300 years, achieving independence in 1824.

Both agriculture and stock raising dominate the subsistence economy, with the upper limit of agriculture at 4000 m and the upper limit of vegetation at 4600 m. Mining is carried out at even greater altitudes and tourism is increasingly popular.

3.1.4   Ethiopian highlands

No well circumscribed highland zone exists. The country is intersected by a number of rift valley systems, establishing a connection between the African rift valley in the south and the Red Sea. The valley systems divide the country into three reasonably well defined regions: the western highlands, the eastern highlands and the rift valley itself with the lowland area.

The northern part of the western highlands, the Amhara highlands, attains the greatest altitude (2400–3700 m). The highest peak of Ethiopia, Ras Dashau (4620 m), is a volcanic outcrop and Lake Tana, the origin of the Blue Nile, lies at the center of the region. Much of Ethiopian history centers on this area, which has been settled for many centuries. It is inhabited by the largest of Ethiopia's many population groups, the Amharas and Tigraeans, who are the descendants of people who came from southern Arabia prior to 1000 BCE (Sellassie 1972).

Gondar (3000 m), in the Amhara highlands, with a population of 100 000, became the second largest city in Africa, and it remained the capital of Ethiopia until the middle of the first century, when Addis Ababa was founded.

Much of the population of Ethiopia lives above 2000 m and in the highland area two types of cultivation, by plough and by hoe, predominate. Teff, a type of grass which produces a small seed, is grown up to 3000 m and is the mainstay of the agricultural economy.

3.2   TERRAIN

Although mountain country varies widely, there are two distinct types: the high, flat, plateaux (Tibet and the altiplano of South America) and deep valleys (Himalayas and Andes).

Plateaux can support large populations and large towns but they may be isolated by virtue of distance from lowland cities, which are usually the center of government, commerce and industry.

In mountain valleys, because flat ground is at a premium, populations tend to be smaller, with groups perched on slopes and ridges far from one another. The placing of houses in sunny positions is more difficult and isolation within the community is common. Communications are easily severed by land slips, avalanches and other natural disasters. The funneling effect of valleys on wind may increase its velocity with an ensuing stunting effect on vegetation and trees. This also restricts the placing of houses, as does the availability of water and the possibility of natural disasters (Figure 3.1).

3.3   CLIMATE

The climate near the ground at high altitude has several basic features. At any given latitude, seasonal variation of monthly temperature is less at high altitude than at sea level and, as the equator is reached, seasonal variation virtually disappears.

Diurnal variations are considerable, and can show a range of 30 °C. This is because of high levels of long-wave radiation that occur in cloudless skies during the day and escape to clear skies at night. In overcast conditions the diurnal variation decreases.

With increasing altitude the temperature falls. There is no uniform value for decline although the figure 1 °C for every 150 m is usually given.

Solar radiation is an important factor in maintaining thermal balance in humans at extreme altitude. High winds are also a feature of mountains. A gust of 231 miles/h has been recorded on Mount Washington (1917 m) in the eastern USA.

3.3.1   Rainfall

In Asia, the monsoon flows from east to west across India, cooling as it is forced to ascend by the Himalayas. Water vapor condenses and falls as rain, and as it passes to the west the monsoon becomes depleted of water; the eastern Himalayas are thus very wet, the western dry. In Darjeeling the annual rainfall is 2000–3000 mm a year; in the central Himalayas at Simla it is 1500 mm, but in the west at Ladakh it is only 75 mm. The Karakoram is arid whereas the eastern Himalayan region is tropical.

There is also considerable north–south variation with Palearctic species on the Tibetan plateau and tropical species often only a few hundred yards away to the south. This is particularly marked on some passes in the eastern Himalayas. On the plateau, although 'monsoon' clouds are seen on the Tangulla range, about 700 km north of Lhasa precipitation is small. In the deserts of the Tarim basin and Tsaidam to the north of the Tibetan plateau, annual rainfall may be less than 100 mm.

In the Andes the Pacific coastal strip is desert – 'It never rains in Lima.' Along the whole length of the coast the cold Humboldt current cools the air above the sea, reducing its capacity to retain moisture which normally falls as rain. Once air passes over the land, it is warmed again and increases its capacity to retain moisture, making rain unlikely.

The western slopes of the Andes are dry, cacti and eucalyptus trees flourish and only a few high mountains are snow covered. The eastern slopes which descend to the Amazon basin become progressively more humid and tree covered.

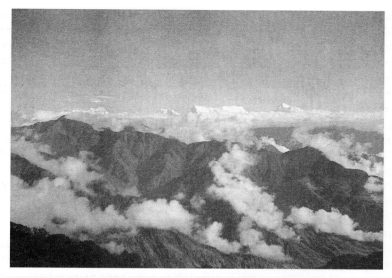

(a)

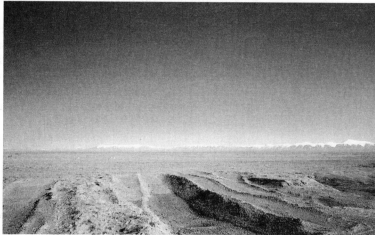

(b)

Figure 3.1 *Contrasting terrain and climate at altitude. (a) Rain clouds over the Himalayas during the monsoon period (September). (Reproduced with permission of the Library of the Royal Geographical Society.) (b) The north Tibetan plateau with the Kun Lun range in the background.*

The rainfall in the UK and Europe is influenced by the gulf stream. Records kept between 1884 and 1901 by the observatory on the summit of Ben Nevis, Scotland (1300 mm), the highest peak in the UK, show that the average daily sunshine was only 2 h and the annual rainfall was 3500 mm, as much or more as in Darjeeling (MacPhee 1936).

3.3.2 Temperature

The fall in temperature globally with altitude has been discussed in Chapter 2. However, the temperature of mountain regions is very variable and records of the observatory on the summit of

Ben Nevis (1300 m) between 1884 and 1901 show that the mean temperature over these 17 years was −0.1°C; the lowest temperature was −17°C and the highest +19°C. On the plateau of the Cairngorms in Scotland, which has an average height of around 1000 m, similar temperatures have been recorded with winds gusting to over 160 km h^{-1} (100 mph).

In North America, Alaska and the Yukon a number of peaks of 6000 m lie within the Arctic Circle. Because of their latitude the barometric pressure, and therefore alveolar P_{O_2}, is lower than on peaks of a corresponding altitude in the Himalayas, which are at a latitude of 28°N. They therefore appear to be 'higher', with all the corresponding dangers of mountain sickness and altitude deterioration (Chapter 2). Temperatures of −30 °C at 5500–6000 m have been recorded, with gale force winds, in the winter (Mills 1973b).

In the European Alps, the average temperature was −13 °C during a winter expedition up to 4000 m, carried out over several days, in the Bernese Oberland in Switzerland (Leuthold *et al.* 1975); gale force winds were not uncommon. Temperatures on the summit of Everest (8848 m) in winter are probably of the order of −60 °C; in summer the average temperature would be about −20 °C. Hillary recorded a temperature of −27 °C at 8500 m on Everest at 3 a.m. on 29 May 1953, the day the first ascent was made (Ward 1993b). On the Changthang (the northern part of the Tibetan plateau), which has an average height of 4900 m, there are few days when the temperature reaches as high as 10 °C and −25 °C has been recorded.

In Lhasa (3658 m) there are about 100 days a year when the temperature is around 10 °C; in summer it may rise as high as 27 °C but in the winter it falls to −15 °C.

In Antarctica, the lowest recorded temperature is −88.2 °C and the highest 15.2 °C. The dangers of cold injury, therefore, are likely to complicate accidents or illness in mountain regions.

3.3.3 Humidity

Ambient humidity influences heat loss from the body by evaporation and, in regions where the humidity is high, heat regulation is more difficult. In arid areas with a low humidity heat regulation is easier.

3.3.4 Solar radiation

Although temperature falls with altitude there is increased exposure to solar radiation (Chapter 2). The amount of radiation absorbed by the body depends on clothing and posture. The clear mountain air permits an increased degree of direct radiation which is enhanced by indirect radiation reflected from the snow. The altitude of the sun is also important (Chrenko and Pugh 1961). The solar heat absorbed depends on the type of clothing – dark clothing absorbs more radiation than light-colored clothing.

3.3.5 Ultraviolet radiation

There appears to be some increase in the level of ultraviolet radiation at high altitude.

Snow reflects up to 90 per cent of ultraviolet radiation, compared with 9–17 per cent reflected from ground covered by grass (Buettner 1969), so in snow-covered terrain the combination of direct (incident) and reflected ultraviolet radiation is considerable.

3.4 ECONOMICS

Most mountain communities depend on animal husbandry and agriculture; mining is important in some regions but more recently tourism has assumed a greater significance.

Animal husbandry predominates in regions above the limit of agriculture. On the Tibetan plateau, or Changtang, which covers two-thirds of Tibet, there are immense herds of yak, sheep and goats herded by nomads. In the bitter climate nomadic pastoralism is the only viable and economic way of life and this may have started between 9000 and 10 000 years ago. The survival of the animals depends exclusively on natural fodder, which creates problems as the sedges and grasses have only a short growing season between May and September. Because there are no areas on the plateau where grass will grow in the winter they cannot escape the climate and, as extensive migration would weaken the stock, only short distances, up to 40 miles, are traversed. Each family has a 'home base', which is sometimes a house, and migrates to set areas whose boundaries, though not fenced, are all well known. Here, tents made of yak and sheep's wool are used as dwellings. Further north camels are common (Goldstein and Beall 1989). In the upper Himalayan valleys the pattern is similar, with flocks spending the summer on pastures up to 5000 m, but below the snow line; in the winter they return to more permanent and protected locations at 4000 m.

The llama (*Lama glama*) and yak (*Bos grunniens*) are extremely important to the economy of the populations of the South American altiplano, and of Tibet and the Himalayan valleys. Both these species show genetic adaptation to high altitude (Chapter 17).

The limiting factor in agriculture is the number of months that the soil remains frozen; only a single period of the year may be available for cultivation. The type of crop may influence the size of population. Potatoes introduced into the high Himalayan valleys of Nepal between 1850 and 1860 increased the population of Sola Khumbu in the Everest region from 169 households in 1836 to 596 in 1957 (Fuhrer-Haimendorf 1964, p. 10). Immigrants came from Tibet over the Nangpa La, a glacier pass of 5800 m, and, because food was more abundant, were able to adopt the religious life and built many new monasteries. Increasing the productivity of the land, as well as the area under cultivation in Tibet, may change the pattern of life near the centers of population under the present Chinese-organized regime. Level land may have to be manufactured in the form of terraces, which range in size from a few square feet to a relatively large area, which is usually too small for pasture. Irrigation may involve ingenious construction of water conduits from surrounding streams. The task of building and maintaining terraces is considerable, especially as manure has to be carried up and placed manually. Despite this, terracing is a marked feature of populated mountain valleys and, as it involves ownership and maintenance by groups rather than individuals, the social implications are important. High grazing pasture (alps) is also communal pasture land and this too has social overtones.

Mining, which is often carried out above the pasture level or in rocky terrain, may involve the building of special towns and roads. Frisancho (1988) suggests that one reason for the relatively high hemoglobin concentration observed in Andean high altitude populations as opposed to those in the Himalayas is that miners (among whom respiratory disease is common) were included in some Andean samples. In Tibet gold mining has been carried on for centuries, often at 5000 m. However, shallow trenches were used and no deep mines were worked. Recently a gold mine has been established at 4500 m in northern Chile, and other mines are being opened at comparable altitudes.

Tourism, particularly skiing, may involve developing an area which has no natural amenities except good snow fields and glaciers. In 1992, 16 000 tourists visited the Everest region; as a result pollution, often in the form of nonbiodegradable rubbish, is a considerable problem.

Isolation, together with unexplained natural catastrophes, contributes to the undoubted tendency that mountain people have towards the religious life. Once this is established, the disinclination to accept change, so prevalent in religious-dominated communities, prevents the development of the communities, which then become easy prey to their more technically advanced neighbors.

3.5 LOAD CARRYING

Loads are carried by all who visit mountainous regions. In the valleys of the Himalayas professional porters carry much of the merchandise and the economy depends on them, together with yak and mule transport (Figure 3.2).

Observations by Pugh in 1952 and 1953 on the march in to Everest (Pugh 1955b) suggest that loads of 40–50 kg, with an addition of 10 kg personal baggage, are carried routinely by porters for 10–12 h over 10–12 miles each day. Often ascents and descents of 1000–1200 m are made, with loads of tea or paper weighing over 60 kg occasionally being carried.

As the body weight of porters is usually 45–60 kg, and the average height just over 150 cm, each porter carries his own weight in merchandise.

Where possible, loads are carried in a conical, light but strong, wicker basket, 22 cm × 30 cm at the base and 50 cm × 70 cm at the top, with a height of 60 cm. Larger sizes are available for carrying bulky loads such as leaf mould. Loads are supported by a strap passing over the forehead and under the lower end of the basket. When in position the upper end of the basket is level with the top of the porter's head. The center of gravity therefore is as close as possible to a vertical line passing through the center of the pelvis, thus reducing the angular momentum. The advantage of the head band is that it allows direct transmission of the load to the vertebral column, with muscles being used for balancing rather than support, as when shoulder straps are used. This method of carrying has to be learnt as a child, and the neck muscles in all such Himalayan porters are extremely well developed.

Marching technique depends on the weight of the load. With loads of 50 kg, stops are made every 2–3 min, with rests lasting 0.5–1.0 min after a distance of 70–250 m has been covered, depending on the gradient. With lighter loads, rests for 2–3 min

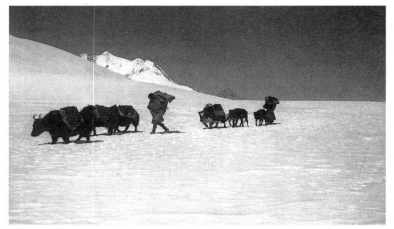

(a)

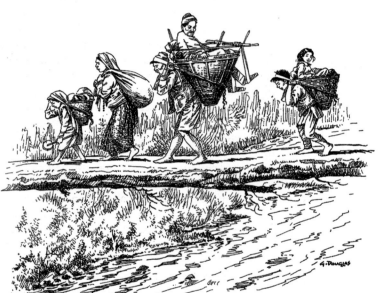

(b)

Figure 3.2 *Load carrying in the Himalayas. (a) Yaks carrying supplies over the Nanga La (5800 m). (Reproduced with permission of the Library of the Royal Geographical Society.) (b) Nepalese porters carrying people and supplies.*

every 10 min are normal. Longer pauses are made every hour.

During rests, the loads are supported on a T-stick about 1 m long, and the porter does not sit down. When longer rests are taken, loads are placed on the top of stone walls conveniently placed beside the track, usually in the shade of a large tree.

Heart rate in ascending porters varies between 140 and 160 beats min^{-1}: on the level between 100 and 124 beats min^{-1} and downhill between 80 and 104 beats min^{-1}.

At about 3700 m, porter loads are reduced to 25 kg (gross weight 35 kg) which are carried to 5700 m. Exhaustion, when it occurs, is due to overwork; that is, not enough rest days. Few porters have any

interest in climbing mountains and so tend to give up when the effects of hypoxia appear.

With high altitude Sherpas, load carrying ability is considerable. Without supplementary oxygen on Everest in 1933 eight porters carried loads weighing 10–15 kg to an altitude of 8300 m, as they did on the Swiss Everest Expedition in 1952.

Low altitude porters carry their own food, eating tsampa or ata, which is made into a paste or dough, three times a day. Four seers (4 kg) of tsampa is the standard ration for each man for 3.5 days, equivalent to 3500 kcal (14.6 kJ) man^{-1} day^{-1}.

Mountaineers also carry considerable loads to high altitude but use shoulder straps, climb more slowly and stop less frequently.

3.6 HOUSES AND SHELTER

Cultural mechanisms that provide a comfortable microclimate and reduce heat loss have been developed in all high altitude communities. The ideal house should be draught free with a low ratio of surface area to volume and well constructed of material which diminishes the daily extremes of temperature. The roof should be well insulated.

In the Andes the adobe (dried mud) building has the first meter or so of the walls made of stone, the roof is of tile, grass or tin and walls are plastered with mud to provide an airtight structure; the roof is tightly fitted and the floor may be wood or dirt. Because of the method of construction the diurnal change is reduced (Baker 1966). In the Himalayas the thermal protection of stone structures built for semi-nomadic occupation appears to be less. Sherpa houses often have only one floor, with stone walls and wooden roofs held on with stones. The ground floor is without windows and provides quarters for animals; the first floor is for human habitation. Windows usually have no glass, but have wooden shutters, and an open fire is placed in the center of one side, but this provides only a transient increase in temperature.

In north Bhutan houses are similarly constructed but animals are kept in a yard. Cracks between stones in both Bhutanese and Sherpa houses are filled with earth. Tibetan houses may be of more than one floor and are often in terraces. Glass is rare and the houses are heated by an open fire or stove. Nomads have tents with a loose wide weave which enables warm air to be entrapped but allows egress of smoke from open fires and is waterproof. However, some semi-nomadic families have a stove with a chimney.

3.7 CLOTHING

Because of the generally low temperature and loss of heat, particularly due to radiation and convection, clothing with good insulation is necessary to provide a warm microclimate. Trapped, still air is the best insulation and wool is the best naturally available insulating material; it resists compacting and loses only 40 per cent of its insulating value when wet. Garments that are loosely woven entrap more air than those that are tightly woven.

A multiple layered system for garments is preferable to one thick layer because insulation can be varied at will, thus minimizing perspiration. The outer layer should be as impermeable to wind as possible. A sheepskin coat is the best naturally available garment that has many of these characteristics, and is usually worn with cotton or wool undergarments.

In general, Andean clothing conforms to the above model and natural clothing is adequate for the conditions encountered. Measurements of insulation of normal clothing without hats, shawls and ponchos showed values for men slightly less than those for women (Little and Hanna 1978). The greatest increase in surface temperature occurred in the hands and feet. At night, Andean highlanders, who use a bedding of skins, can maintain their metabolic rate by light shivering that does not disturb sleep.

In the high Himalayan valleys and Tibet, clothing assemblies are similar. The main garment is a thick sheepskin 'chupa' with 15 cm (6 inch) sleeves which when extended keep the hands warm; gloves are never used. Normally the garment is gathered around the waist by a belt and hitched up to the knees so that there is a pocket for loose objects in front of the chest. When the belt is loosened the garment extends to the ground and thus can be used as a sleeping robe; often in warm conditions one or both shoulders are left bare. Under this is a woolen shirt and often long woolen, cotton or sheepskin trousers. Soft leather boots with decorative wool leggings extending to the knees are packed with grass, straw or leaves but a Tibetan often may walk in bare feet in the snow or through streams. Some wear a felt hat or balaclava and, to prevent snow blindness, yak hair is put in front of the eyes if goggles are not available (Desideri 1712–27, Moorcroft and Trebeck 1841, Vol. 1 p. 399) (Figure 3.3). Other methods used by Tibetans include blackening the eyelids and wearing masks with tiny eye holes, the rims of which are blackened (MacDonald 1929, p. 182). Cotton clothing is favored at high temperatures and low altitudes, but nomads wear wool or sheepskin. Many now wear wool sweaters and leather boots. Tibetan nomads sleep resting on their elbows and knees with all their clothes piled on their backs (Holditch 1907, Duff 1999). This 'fetal position' diminishes surface area and therefore heats loss: contact with the ground is also minimal.

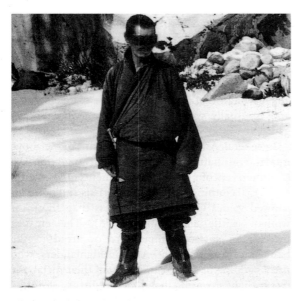

Figure 3.3 *Yak hair 'goggles'.*

Some Tibetan lamas have developed the ability to 'warm without fire'. The central core temperature is kept raised under cold conditions, both by increasing the metabolic rate, probably by continuous light shivering, and also by the practice of g-tum-mo yoga, which appears to involve peripheral vasodilatation (Pugh 1963, Benson *et al.* 1982).

Children have oil rubbed over their bodies and adults seldom wash, the natural skin oils forming a protective layer. Very few Tibetans living on the plateau are obese (Bell 1928).

3.8 POPULATION

Most of the high altitude areas of the world are in the economically least developed regions and for this reason population numbers in relation to altitude are difficult to obtain. Although the total population living in mountainous regions is estimated at 400 million, the majority live at low altitude in the valleys. De Jong (1968) 'guessed' that between 13 and 14 million people lived at altitudes above 3000 m. A more accurate figure is 38 million (Hultgren 1997). Worldwide, about 140 million people live over 2500 m (WHO 1996).

In South America large populations have lived at high altitude since prehistory and the Andean population at the time of the Spanish conquest was estimated as between 4.5 and 7.5 million. In 1980 it was considered that between 10 and 17 million were living at over 2500 m and in Peru 30–40 per cent of the population of 4 million lived at or above this height, with 1.5 per cent living at over 4000 m.

In Asia and Africa the estimates are less accurate. On the Tibetan plateau, which consists of the autonomous region of Tibet (Xizang) and Qinghai province, the population is estimated as between 4 and 5 million. Lhasa (3658 m), in 1986, had about 130 000 inhabitants, mainly Tibetan, but recent immigration of Han Chinese has increased this number. Relatively small groups, nomads (at up to 5450 m) and miners (at up to 6000 m), live at higher levels. Fairly large numbers live at altitudes exceeding 3000 m in the upper valleys of eastern Tibet, and in Nepal about 60 000 live above this level, with a number of villages in Dolpo being at 5000 m (Snellgrove 1961). In Ethiopia about 50 per cent of the total population of 26 million live above 2000 m. Small populations in Mexico, the USA and the former USSR live above 3000 m.

In the mainly subsistence economy of high mountain regions, survival means the capacity to perform physical work and high altitude natives living at altitude have a capacity similar to that of low altitude dwellers at low altitude. Many live to over 80 years of age; a Tibetan female hermit is said to have died at the age of 130 years (Taring 1970) (section 17.2.1), and the founder of traditional Tibetan medicine, Yu-Thog, is considered to have lived to the age of 125 years.

In tropical latitudes permanent settlements are usually placed where both pasture and timber can be used and the upper limit of habitation may fall between the two. Further from the equator the upper limit falls below the timber line and variation in temperature becomes seasonal; the upper pasture-lands are thus used for a semi-nomadic economy. Permanently inhabited villages are found at lower levels, with isolated groups of buildings or shelters on the pastures occupied for the grazing season and evacuated during the winter. Considerable migration may occur and part of the population may always be on the move. One mine, now closed, was worked at 5950 m in South America; although the miners lived at rather lower altitudes, the caretakers lived there permanently (West 1986a).

Those who spend periods at greater altitude are

mountaineers, who have evolved specialized techniques of movement above the snow line. In winter, movement across snow is essential for the feeding of livestock quartered in isolated shelters. Since prehistoric times boards have been placed on the feet to facilitate movement. The earliest references to primitive skis are found in the Nordic sagas of 3000 BCE and, in northern Norway, rock engravings of skiers are dated at around 2500 BCE. In the UK skis were used in Cumberland at the start of the eighteenth century. The modern sport dates from 1870. No historical evidence of the use of skis has been found in South American or Tibetan populations.

Highland populations, being strategically placed between prosperous lowland centers, play a vital role in trade. Because they are physiologically well adapted they are capable of crossing high mountain passes with heavy loads and use their animals to carry produce. Major mountain passes have for centuries been arteries for trade, the movement of people and ideas, and the dissemination of disease. The closing of passes such as the Nangpa La between the two different economies of Tibet and Nepal caused a fall in living standards until readjustments had been made.

3.9 HUMAN RESPONSE TO COLD AND ALTITUDE

The main environmental stresses of living in mountain regions are cold and the hypoxia of altitude.

3.9.1 Cold

Temperature is a more important factor than altitude in colonizing high mountainous regions; high altitude residents seem to withstand cold better than sea level visitors to altitude.

Most of the process of adaptation to cold consists of the adoption of clothing and housing which reduce cold stress by maintaining a microclimate as close as possible to the preferred temperature.

However, some studies have demonstrated different physiological responses in high altitude residents to experimental cold stress compared with low altitude controls. These have been summarized by Little and Hanna (1978) in drawing from work on Andean and Tibetan high altitude residents.

In response to abrupt exposure to cold, high altitude residents, when contrasted with sea level Caucasian control subjects, show the following responses:

- no dramatic fall of core temperature
- a slightly elevated basal metabolic rate
- consistently high surface temperatures in extremities
- a slightly greater loss of body heat.

These changes are probably the result of lifelong intermittent exposure to modest cold stress rather than cold plus altitude. Pugh (1963) found a number of these responses in a Nepalese pilgrim studied at 4500 m, who came from a village at only 1800 m. Benson et al. (1982) found similar changes in Tibetans practicing g-tum-mo yoga (an advanced form of Tibetan yoga). The elevation of basal metabolic rate may be the effect of hypoxia and cold acting together (Little and Hanna 1978). Further aspects of cold adaptation are considered in Chapter 24.

3.9.2 Hypoxia

In order to colonize the mountainous regions above about 3000 m, acclimatization to the chronic hypoxia of altitude is important. This response to hypoxia is discussed in detail in Chapter 4. People born and brought up at altitude have certain advantages over lowlanders and this is discussed in Chapters 4 and 17. However, long-term residence also carries the risk of chronic mountain sickness (Chapter 21). The question of whether altitude populations have undergone adaptation in the biological sense of genetic selection for that environment is hotly debated. There is some evidence that this has happened to a degree in the case of Tibetans (see Chapter 17, section 17.5).

4

Altitude acclimatization

SUMMARY

Altitude acclimatization is the physiological process which takes place on going to altitude. It comprises a number of responses by different systems in the body, which mitigate the effects of the fall in oxygen partial pressure so that the tissues of the body are defended against this fall to a remarkable degree. Probably the most important changes are the increase in breathing (total ventilation) due to stimulation of the peripheral chemoreceptors (carotid bodies) by hypoxia, and changes in the chemical control of breathing. Another is the well-known increase in hemoglobin concentration in the blood. The time courses of these responses vary but most of the changes take place over a period of days up to a few weeks. Individuals vary in the speed and extent to which they can acclimatize. Apart from past history of acclimatization there are no good predictors of future performance.

Deterioration is a condition that is evident after some time spent at extreme altitude. It comes on over weeks above about 5500 m, and over days above 8000 m. It is characterized by loss of appetite, weight loss, lethargy, fatigue, slowness of thought and poor judgment.

Adaptation is a term used to describe the changes that take place over generations by natural selection, enabling animals and humans to function better at altitude.

4.1 PHYSIOLOGICAL RESPONSE TO HYPOXIA

The response of the body to hypoxia depends crucially on the rate as well as the degree of hypoxia. For instance, the effect on a pilot of sudden loss of oxygen supply in an unpressurized aircraft at the height of the summit of Mount Everest is quite different from the effect of similar altitude on a climber who has spent some weeks at altitude. The pilot would probably lose consciousness in a few minutes (Figure 4.1) whereas the climber, though very breathless, will not only remain conscious but also be able to work out his route and climb slowly upward.

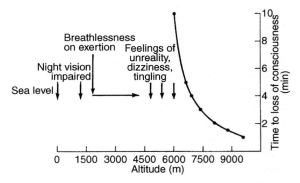

Figure 4.1 *The effect of sudden exposure to various altitudes. At extreme altitude consciousness will be lost after an average time indicated by the curve on the right. There is considerable variability in this time. (Data from Sharp 1978.)*

The symptoms of acute hypoxia are few and subtle (Figure 4.1). The effect of acute, often severe, hypoxia has been studied intensively since Paul Bert first pointed out the danger of ascent to high altitude to early balloonists (Chapter 1). Figure 4.1 shows the effect of sudden exposure to various increasing altitudes. At modest altitude breathlessness may be felt on exertion and some rise in heart rate noticed but the main effect is on the central nervous system. At levels as low as 1500 m night vision is impaired (Pretorius 1970). At 4000–5000 m some tingling of the fingers and mouth may be noticed but, although the subject would now definitely be hypoxic, there would be very little subjective sensation to indicate this fact. Above about 5000 m some subjects may become unconscious and above 7000 m most will do so (Sharp 1978). Figure 4.1 shows the average time to loss of consciousness after sudden exposure to given altitudes. It will be seen that, on acute exposure to the altitude equivalent to the summit of Everest, the unacclimatized subject remains conscious for only about 2 min.

By contrast, the effect of hypoxia on an acclimatized person is much less. The main symptom is shortness of breath on exertion. The preferred rate of climbing amongst mountaineers is at about 50 per cent $V_{O_2 max}$. This typically requires a ventilation of about 50 L min^{-1} at sea level, whereas at 6300 m the ventilation for this work rate will be about 160 L min^{-1}, close to the maximum voluntary ventilation at sea level. The difference between the pilot and the climber is due to a series of adaptive changes in the body known as acclimatization. The changes occur in various systems and with varying time courses. These are illustrated in Figure 4.2, which shows the futility of the frequently asked question, 'How long does it take to become acclimatized?'. However, the most important changes are in the cardiorespiratory system and the blood, with time courses of days or a few weeks.

In some cases the changes of acclimatization involve a biphasic response; for instance, the heart rate response to hypoxia shows a rise within a few minutes, followed by a fall over weeks at altitude (Chapter 7). The change measured can include two responses with different time courses. For instance, minute ventilation involves the rapid hypoxic ventilatory response within a few minutes, followed by slow changes in both central and peripheral chemoreceptor response over 1–20 days (Chapter 5).

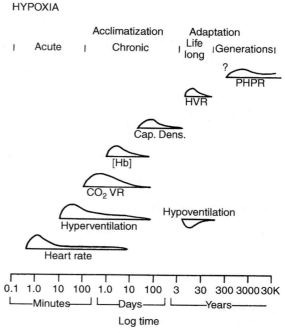

Figure 4.2 *Time courses of a number of acclimatization and adaptive changes plotted on a log time scale, the curve of each response denoting the rate of change, which is fast at first then tailing off. Included are: heart rate, hyperventilation and hypoventilation, the carbon dioxide ventilatory response (HCVR), hemoglobin concentration ([Hb]), changes in capillary density (Cap. Dens.), hypoxic ventilatory response (HVR) and the pulmonary hypoxic pressor response (PHPR).*

Similarly, the well-known increase in hemoglobin concentration is due to a rapid decrease in plasma volume, followed by a slow increase in red cell mass (Chapter 8).

4.2 ACCLIMATIZATION, DETERIORATION AND ADAPTATION

4.2.1 Acclimatization

The term 'altitude acclimatization' refers to the process whereby lowland humans and animals respond to the reduced partial pressure of oxygen (P_{O_2}) in the inspired air. It usually refers only to the changes in response to hypoxia seen as beneficial as opposed to changes which result in illness such as acute mountain sickness (AMS). Acclimatization is then a series of physiological processes. Other changes, resulting in illness, are pathological. The processes of acclimatization all tend to reduce the fall in P_{O_2} as oxygen is transported through the body from the outside air to the tissues.

4.2.2 Deterioration

The term 'high altitude deterioration' was first used by members of early Everest expeditions to denote deterioration in mental and physical condition as a result of prolonged stay at altitude. Filippi (1912, p. 364) noted the condition during an expedition to the Karakoram. He writes:

> The atmosphere of the expedition did work some evil effect revealing itself only gradually after several weeks of life above 17500 feet in a slow decrease of appetite and consequent lack of nourishment without, however, any disturbance of digestive function.

It is well known amongst climbers that staying at extreme altitudes for long is deleterious. Altitudes above 8000 m have been called 'the death zone' and summit bids on peaks over this height are wisely planned so as to spend as short a time as possible in this zone (Table 4.1). Deterioration can frequently be attributed to factors such as dehydration, starvation, physical exhaustion and cold. However, in the absence of such factors it seems that hypoxia *per se* can cause deterioration if sufficiently severe (Pugh 1962a). The altitude at which this becomes manifest is about 5000–6000 m, with considerable individual variation. Highlanders can probably tolerate prolonged periods at a higher altitude better than can most lowlanders (West 1986a).

High altitude deterioration (in the absence of dehydration, starvation, etc.) is characterized by weight loss, poor appetite, slow recovery from fatigue, lethargy, irritability and an increasing lack of willpower to start new tasks (Ward 1954).

The specific mechanisms underlying this deterioration are unknown. An attempt to investigate the mechanism underlying the recovery from fatigue of muscles under hypoxia was made by Milledge *et al.* (1977), who followed the resynthesis of muscle glycogen after depletion by exercise at sea level under normoxia and hypoxia. They showed that, although the rate of resynthesis was not significantly slowed by hypoxia in the muscle overall, there was an

Table 4.1 *Maximum period spent at varying altitudes without supplementary oxygen*

Height (m)	Period (days)
5791	90–100
6760–7315	11
7010	11
7467	8
7850	5
7925	4
8380	3
8450	1
8848	1

Source: Modified from Ward (1975, p. 238).

enhancement of the difference between the type I and type II fibers. This suggested that hypoxia depresses glycogen synthesis in type I though not type II fibers. This might contribute to the slowness of recovery from severe exercise at high altitude.

Over 5500 m malabsorption from the small gut (section 14.5) probably contributes to the weight loss as well as a negative energy balance so deterioration accelerates.

4.2.3 Adaptation

People born and bred at altitude have certain characteristics which distinguish them from even well acclimatized lowlanders. There is debate about whether these are due to environmental factors operating during early growth, or genetic causes. The term adaptation is used for characteristics thought to be due to natural selection working on the gene pool. Adaptation, in this sense, has certainly taken place in animals such as the yak and llama. In the case of the yak one example is the loss of the hypoxic pulmonary pressor response which seems to be due to a single dominant gene (Harris 1986). There is some evidence of a similar adaptation in Tibetans resident at high altitude for generations, but this is, at present, only suggestive (see section 17.5).

4.3 OXYGEN TRANSPORT SYSTEM

4.3.1 Introduction

Figure 4.3 shows the oxygen transport system at sea level and at high altitude. This diagram can be used as

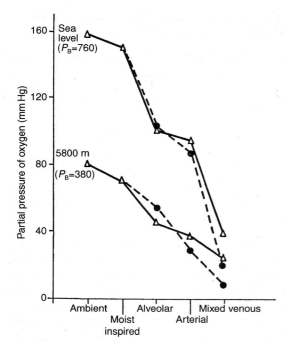

Figure 4.3 *The oxygen transport system from outside air through the body at sea level and at an altitude of 5800 m. P_B, barometric pressure; ●, rest; △, maximum work. (Reproduced with permission from Pugh 1964.)*

a 'table of contents' of changes due to acclimatization, which will be followed in succeeding chapters. P_{O_2} falls at each stage as oxygen is transported from outside air: ambient P_{O_2} to inspired, to alveolar, to arterial, to mixed venous. The latter approximates to the mean tissue P_{O_2}. This forms a staircase or cascade of P_{O_2}. The process of acclimatization can be thought of as reducing each step in this cascade as far as possible.

4.3.2 Ambient to inspired P_{O_2} (*PI_{O_2}*)

The ambient P_{O_2} of dry air at sea level is about 160 mm Hg (20.9 per cent of 760 mm Hg, the barometric pressure). At an altitude of 5800 m in the example shown in Figure 4.3 the barometric pressure is just half that at sea level (Chapter 2), so the ambient P_{O_2} is also half the sea level value, 80 mm Hg. The drop seen in the figure from ambient to inspired P_{O_2} of about 10 mm Hg is due to the addition of water vapor to the inspired air as it is wetted and warmed to body temperature in the nose, mouth, larynx and trachea. The water vapor pressure at body temperature is 47 mm Hg, and this displaces almost

10 mm Hg P_{O_2}. This physical cause of P_{O_2} reduction is beyond the control of the body and so applies equally at altitude, though its effect is proportionately more important there.

4.3.3 Inspired to alveolar P_{O_2} (*PA_{O_2}*)

At sea level there is a drop of about 50 mm Hg at this point in the oxygen transport system. This drop can be thought of as being due to the addition of carbon dioxide and the uptake of oxygen and so depends, in part, on the metabolic rate. However, it also depends on alveolar ventilation and for a given oxygen uptake and carbon dioxide output the size of this reduction is entirely due to ventilation. A doubling of ventilation results in a halving of this drop. If ventilation were infinite there would be no reduction and alveolar gas would be fresh air. After acclimatization at 5800 m resting alveolar ventilation is approximately doubled and this step in the system is halved, as shown in Figure 4.3.

This increase in ventilation is one of the most important aspects of acclimatization; the mechanisms underlying it, the changes in control of breathing, are dealt with in Chapter 5.

Figure 4.3 shows also the effect of exercise on the oxygen transport system (the dashed lines). At sea level the PA_{O_2} is little changed by exercise, but at altitude the increase of ventilation is far greater in response to exercise than at sea level so that with exercise the PA_{O_2} is increased and PA_{CO_2} decreased (Chapter 11).

4.3.4 Alveolar to arterial P_{O_2} (*Pa_{O_2}*)

Oxygen passes across the alveolar-capillary membrane by diffusion resulting in a small pressure drop but in the normal lung this accounts for less than 1 mm Hg. The total alveolar–arterial (A–a) P_{O_2} gradient at sea level is about 6–10 mm Hg. The major part of this gradient is due to ventilation/perfusion ratio (V/Q) inequalities. Even in the healthy lung the matching of ventilation to blood flow is not perfect. In lung disease such as emphysema or pulmonary embolism this mismatching results in much greater (A–a)PO_2 gradients and in significant hypoxemia. For a full discussion of this important topic see West (1986b).

At altitude, at rest there is little change in the (A–a)P_{O_2} gradient from its value at sea level. The V/Q ratio inequality is modestly reduced, because of the increase in pulmonary artery pressure due to hypoxia (Chapter 7), reducing the gravitational effect on the distribution of blood flow in the lung. However, this is not enough to cause any measurable increase in the diffusing capacity of the lung during acclimatization (West 1962a).

On exercise at altitude, however, the $(A–a)P_{O_2}$ gradient increases significantly and becomes important in limiting exercise performance. This is shown as the dashed line in Figure 4.3. This diffusion limitation, shown by West (1962), is explored more fully in Chapters 6, 11 and 12.

4.3.5 Arterial to mixed venous P_{O_2} (PvO_2)

The last drop in P_{O_2} shown in Figure 4.3 from arterial to mixed venous is due to the uptake of oxygen in the systemic capillaries. Its magnitude is influenced by the metabolic rate, the cardiac output and the oxygen-carrying capacity of the blood, i.e. the hemoglobin concentration. The increase in hemoglobin concentration is probably the best-known aspect of acclimatization. A modest increase is beneficial in that it increases the oxygen-carrying capacity of the blood, and at altitudes up to about 4000 m this is sufficient to balance the reduction in oxygen saturation due to reduced Pa_{O_2}. However, the increase in viscosity of the increased hemoglobin concentration is the price paid; if this is too great the cardiac output falls and so oxygen delivery is reduced. There is also the increased risk of vascular disorders. This aspect of acclimatization is the subject of Chapter 8.

Changes in cardiac output with acute and chronic hypoxia as well as other effects on the vascular system are discussed in Chapter 7. Changes in the oxygen dissociation curve at altitude, also important in this section of the oxygen transport system, are reviewed in Chapter 9.

Taking the body as a whole, the mixed venous P_{O_2} can be thought of as reflecting the mean tissue P_{O_2}. It can be seen (Figure 4.3) that the effect of these processes of acclimatization is to maintain this critical P_{O_2} as near as possible to the sea level value. Beyond this there is the possibility of adaptation at the tissue level involving the microcirculation and then intracellular mechanisms. These form the subject of Chapter 10.

4.4 PRACTICAL CONSIDERATIONS AND ADVICE

A very real problem in the study of acclimatization is that there is no single measure of the process. Respiratory acclimatization is very important and can be followed by measuring minute ventilation or the alveolar or end-tidal P_{CO_2}. The ventilation rises with acclimatization and the P_{CO_2} falls exponentially over the first few days at altitude. However, climbers find that their performance continues to improve over a longer period: presumably changes in other systems underlie this further acclimatization. This problem of how to measure the degree of acclimatization coupled with the very great individual variation in the rate and final degree of acclimatization means that we still do not have answers to apparently simple questions such as, 'Does exercise speed acclimatization?'. There is also the problem that the time of early and rapid acclimatization is also the risk time for AMS. It is hard, and perhaps futile, to try to separate the effect of any given strategy on preventing AMS and on speeding acclimatization since the two are inextricably commingled. Thus the advice given here is as much about preventing AMS as about acclimatization. In the absence of hard data, anecdotal evidence has to be relied on.

4.4.1 Rate of ascent

A rate of ascent which is slow enough to avoid AMS should be chosen. This will inevitably be dictated, in part, by the terrain, availability of camp sites, etc. A rule of thumb often given is that above 3000 m each night's camp should be about 300 m above the previous one and that every 2–3 days a rest day should be added when the party remains based at the same site for 2 nights. This is a rather slow ascent rate for many individuals but will prove too fast for some. Where a greater height gain has to be made, then a rest day should be taken. During the 'rest' day trips to higher altitude and back are considered beneficial by experienced climbers, probably because the greater altitude and exercise stimulate acclimatization. However, it should be noted that there is some evidence that exercise is a risk factor for AMS (Roach et al. 2000). See section 18.4.9 for a further discussion of exercise and AMS.

4.4.2 Individual variability and acclimatization

As already mentioned, there is great individual variation in the rate and degree of acclimatization. Some may acclimatize rapidly to moderate altitude but then find that they simply cannot tolerate an altitude above, say, 7000 m. Others may take time to acclimatize but then go well to extreme altitude. Usually, as with susceptibility to AMS, past experience is a good guide to future performance but apart from this there are no reliable predictors for good acclimatization.

4.4.3 Age, gender and experience

There are very few data to answer the frequently asked question about the effects of age or gender on acclimatization. If anything, older people are less susceptible to AMS than young people and seem to acclimatize just as well. There does not seem to be any important difference between men and women in this respect. There is a strong impression that experienced mountaineers acclimatize better than novices. (See Chapter 28 for further discussion of acclimatization in women, children and elderly people.)

4.4.4 Pre-acclimatization and carry-over acclimatization

There is increasing interest in methods by which people can achieve some degree of acclimatization before going to the mountains. Methods suggested include intermittent exposure to simulated altitude in chambers or by breathing low oxygen mixtures. There is no doubt that living in a chamber for a number of days at simulated altitude will achieve acclimatization. There is an impression that the degree of acclimatization is not as great as that achieved in the mountains, perhaps because of the lack of exercise. West (1998, pp. 358–63) argues the case for this being true for the long-term studies of Operation Everest I and II. However, incarceration in a chamber for days is not practicable or acceptable for most climbers. Intermittent exposure such as spending a few hours a day in a chamber, usually with exercise, i.e. training under hypoxia, or sleeping in a hypoxic environment has been suggested. At present there are no studies to show that these measures do produce beneficial effects. Savourey et al. (1998) studied the effect of 8 h daily for 5 days at 4500 m equivalent altitude on various hormones and biochemical measures but found very little effect with this dose of pre-acclimatization. Garcia et al. (1999) had their subjects breath 13 per cent oxygen (equivalent to 3800 m) for 2 h daily for 12 days. They found the hypoxic ventilatory response increased significantly, reaching a peak at 5 days but there was no change in ventilation, P_{CO_2} or arterial oxygen saturation (Sa_{O_2}). They found a reticulocytosis but no change in hemoglobin concentration or hematocrit. It seems that intermittent hypoxia has a qualitatively different effect than does chronic hypoxia. So one can only say that pre-acclimatization may well confer some benefit, but an extra few days at altitude would probably be as good and more pleasant.

If pre-acclimatization is attempted, how quickly should a climber get out to the mountains? In other words, how long does acclimatization last? There are very few hard data to guide us, though one study by Lyons et al. (1995) showed that a group of subjects who had been at 4300 m for 3 weeks retained some beneficial effect after 8 days at low altitude compared with a group who had had no altitude exposure. A later study by the same group (Beidleman et al. 1997) with a similar protocol helped to quantify this carry-over effect. After 8 days at sea level they calculated that on average the retained effect on Sa_{O_2} was 92 per cent, on plasma volume it was 74 per cent and on the lactate concentration at 75 per cent V_{O_2max} it was 58 per cent. These figures support anecdotal experience. The effect of acclimatization probably falls off exponentially with time over perhaps 2–3 weeks, though some feel there is some residual benefit even after months at sea level.

5

Ventilatory response to hypoxia and carbon dioxide

SUMMARY

Of all the changes that take place in the physiology of a person acclimatizing to altitude, those resulting in an increase in ventilation are probably the most important. There are changes in both the hypoxic ventilatory response (HVR) and the hypercapnic ventilatory responses (HCVR). The changes in HVR are more difficult to measure and there is still some debate about the details, but the consensus view is now that HVR increases with time at altitude over a period of days to a few weeks. The changes in HCVR were characterized 40 years ago and include a shift to the left and a steepening of the carbon dioxide response line. That is, a person when acclimatized responds to a lower P_{CO_2} and is more sensitive to carbon dioxide than when unacclimatized. The time course of these changes is exponential, with almost half taking place in the first 24 h and most of the change being complete in about 2 weeks. These changes in the chemical control of breathing underlie the well-known increase in ventilation and result in a lower P_{CO_2} and higher P_{O_2} characteristic of acclimatization. The mechanism underlying the increased carbon dioxide sensitivity is probably the documented reduction in bicarbonate concentration in cerebrospinal fluid (CSF) and presumably brain extracellular fluid (ECF).

High altitude residents have similar HCVR but generally have blunted HVR compared to acclimatized lowlanders. HVR does not predict susceptibility to acute mountain sickness (AMS), though subjects susceptible to high altitude pulmonary edema (HAPE) do have low HVR. Some studies have found a correlation between HVR and performance at extreme altitude but some elite climbers have HVR in the normal range, and high altitude residents (Sherpas and Andean peoples) who tend to have low HVR perform very well at extreme altitude.

5.1 INTRODUCTION

The increase in ventilation that takes place in the first few days at altitude is one of the most important aspects of the acclimatization process. It results in higher alveolar and arterial P_{O_2} and lower P_{CO_2} levels than would have obtained if the ventilation were unchanged. The cause of this increased ventilation is a change in the chemical control of breathing. Interest in the mechanisms underlying these changes goes back to the early years of the twentieth century. Haldane, who had shown that the level of carbon dioxide in the body was stable, soon realized that altitude resulted in depression of P_{CO_2} due to increased ventilation. He suggested that his colleague Mabel FitzGerald measure the alveolar P_{CO_2} in residents at mining camps at various altitudes in Colorado. She found that the P_{CO_2} fell linearly with altitude (FitzGerald 1913). Since then physiologists have continued to investigate these mechanisms and their work is reviewed in this chapter.

There are two sensing systems for the chemical control of breathing: the peripheral chemoreceptors (the carotid and aortic bodies), and central chemoreceptors situated in the medulla. There are three chemical drives to ventilation: hypoxia, pH and carbon dioxide. The peripheral chemoreceptors principally sense hypoxia, though they also respond to carbon dioxide and pH, whereas the central chemoreceptors sense changes in pH, which are frequently due to changes in P_{CO_2}.

5.2 HYPOXIC VENTILATORY RESPONSE (HVR)

The HVR is the increase in ventilation brought about by acute hypoxia. This is not a simple linear response and is complicated by the effect of ventilation on P_{CO_2}. As ventilation rises in response to hypoxia, P_{CO_2} falls. Thus the carbon dioxide drive to breathing is reduced and the hypoxic response is masked unless measures are taken to prevent this fall in P_{CO_2}.

If the inspired P_{O_2} is reduced acutely, i.e. over a period of a few minutes, either by breathing a low oxygen mixture or by decompression in a hypobaric chamber, the minute ventilation is increased. However, this increase in ventilation varies greatly

from individual to individual and does not usually begin until the inspired P_{O_2} is reduced to approximately 100 mm Hg (equivalent to about 3000 m altitude) (Rahn and Otis 1949). This corresponds to an alveolar P_{O_2} of about 50 mm Hg. Thereafter, as inspired P_{O_2} is further reduced ventilation increases more rapidly.

The relationship of ventilation to P_{O_2} is hyperbolic, as shown in Figure 5.1. However, if arterial saturation is measured by an oximeter the relationship between it and ventilation is found to be approximately linear (Figure 5.1). The Pa_{O_2} at which ventilation starts to increase corresponds to the P_{O_2} at which the oxygen dissociation curve begins to steepen.

The actual effect of acute hypoxia on ventilation will depend upon whether P_{CO_2} is allowed to fall or not. Unless the experimental arrangement allows control of PA_{CO_2}, a rise in ventilation will result in a fall of P_{CO_2}. As P_{CO_2} is reduced some drive to breathing will be lost so that the full hypoxic response is not seen.

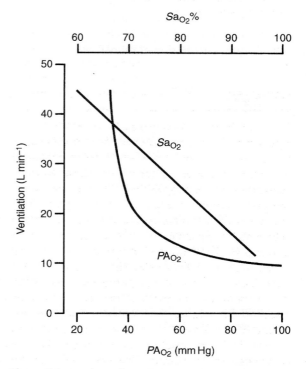

Figure 5.1 Hypoxic ventilatory response to PA_{O_2} and arterial oxygen saturation (Sa_{O_2}).

5.3   CAROTID BODY

Before considering HVR further, the transduction of the hypoxic response will be briefly considered. A transducer effects the conversion of one mode of signal to another, in this case from Pa_{O_2} to a neural signal by the carotid body.

5.3.1   Historical

The stimulating effect of oxygen lack on respiration had been known for many years before it became apparent at the turn of the century that, under normal sea level conditions, carbon dioxide was the main chemical stimulus to ventilation.

In the late 1920s, the father and son team of Heymans and Heymans in Belgium, using complex cross-circulation experiments in dogs, localized the main sensing organ for hypoxia to the carotid body (Heymans and Heymans 1927). Not long afterwards Comroe (1938) showed that the aortic bodies have a similar function. These bodies are known collectively as the peripheral chemoreceptors. However, in most animals, including humans, the main organ for transduction of the hypoxic signal is the carotid body and if this is removed or denervated, acute hypoxia actually causes depression of ventilation.

5.3.2   Anatomy and physiology of the carotid body

The human carotid body weighs about 10 mg and is situated just above the bifurcation of the common carotid artery. It has an extremely rich blood flow for its mass and oxygen consumption, and thus it is a very low extraction organ (i.e. it extracts only a very small percentage of the oxygen in the blood presented to it). This explains how it is able to respond to arterial P_{O_2} (or saturation) and not to oxygen content. Thus it responds to hypoxemia but not anemia or reduced flow. This is appropriate since an increase in ventilation would not help the organism overcome the tissue hypoxia caused by anemia or low cardiac output, but does help in a hypoxic environment.

Although an enormous amount of research work has been carried out on the carotid body, it is still not clear which cells or nerves actually sense the hypoxemia nor which transmitters are involved. It has been assumed that the glomus cells (type I), the characteristic cells of the carotid body, are the sites of chemoreception and that modulation of neurotransmitter release from the glomus cells by physiological and chemical stimuli affects the discharge rate of the carotid body afferent fibers. Undoubtedly the signal is modified, enhanced or suppressed by parts of the system not involved with the primary sensing process.

Two key observations need to be explained:

- Carotid body chemoreceptors are excited physiologically by hypoxia, hypercapnia and acidosis.
- Chemical agents which interfere with mitochondrial oxidative phosphorylation (and therefore reduce the ATP/ADP ratio) stimulate chemoreceptors.

There are two leading hypotheses:

- Hypoxia may slow down mitochondrial electron transport owing to the presence of a reduced affinity cytochrome in the oxygen transport chain. This could stimulate neurotransmitter release from glomus cells by progressive breakdown of the mitochondrial electrochemical gradient and release of mitochondrial calcium into the cytoplasm. The elevated intracellular calcium would then cause release of the neurotransmitter. Metabolic blockers which interfere with electron transport and oxidative phosphorylation would have a similar effect (Mulligan *et al.* 1981, Biscoe and Duchen 1990).
- Glomus cells may have potassium channels in their cell membranes that are modulated by the partial pressure of oxygen. The probability that the channel is open decreases with hypoxia and acidosis and the result is a reduction in overall potassium conductance which causes membrane depolarization. This could explain chemotransduction as follows: the membrane depolarizes, voltage sensitive calcium channels open, and these allow extracellular calcium to enter the cell. The elevated intracellular calcium then promotes neurotransmitter release.

The potassium channel has been demonstrated in submicron-sized membrane patches which continue to be modulated by oxygen when removed from the cell. It has been suggested that the channel itself contains a heme group which may interact with oxygen directly, thus modifying channel confirmation and the probability of its being open (Ganfornina and Lopez-Barneo 1991), but the heme group has not been identified (Lahiri and Delaney 1975).

The glossopharyngeal nerve carries sensory fibers from the carotid to the central nervous system (CNS) where the sensory input stimulates the respiratory center or centers in the pons. Another area of uncertainty is the existence or otherwise of efferent fibers in the glossopharyngeal nerve going to the carotid and modifying its response and the suggestion that sensory nerves and synapses can work both ways, i.e. as afferent or efferent.

Dopamine is the most abundant transmitter found in the carotid body, followed by norepinephrine (noradrenaline) and 5-hydroxytryptamine. There are also small quantities of acetylcholine and enkephalin-like peptides in some glomus cells. Hypoxia increases the rate of release of dopamine from glomus cells.

It should be noted that although the most important function of the peripheral chemoreceptors (carotid and aortic bodies) is to respond to hypoxia, they do also respond to any increase in Pa_{CO_2} and decrease in arterial pH. However, the greatest response to P_{CO_2} is via the central chemoreceptors in the brain stem (see section 5.13.1).

5.4   HVR AT SEA LEVEL

5.4.1   Methods for measuring HVR

A number of different methods have been used to measure HVR, each having its advantages and disadvantages. Probably the most popular method for studies involving large numbers of subjects is the rebreathing method using an oximeter to measure oxygen saturation continuously while the P_{CO_2} is held constant (Rebuck and Campbell 1974). More recently, Robbins and his group in Oxford have used a series of square wave pulses of hypoxia keeping the carbon dioxide constant and then fitting a single compartment model which yields a parameter G_p, the hypoxic sensitivity (Ren and Robbins 1999).

5.4.2   Variability of HVR

The range of HVR found in healthy sea level residents is wide. The coefficient of variation varies between 23 and 72 per cent in different studies (Cunningham *et al.* 1964, Weil *et al.* 1970, Rebuck and Campbell 1974).

Various groups of subjects at sea level have been shown to have lower HVRs than controls, for instance endurance athletes (Byrne-Quinn *et al.* 1971) and swimmers (Bjurstrom and Schoene 1986). With increasing age HVR becomes lower (Kronenberg and Drage 1973, Chapman and Cherniak 1986, Poulin *et al.* 1993) and respiratory depressant drugs and anesthetics inhibit HVR (Sahn *et al.* 1974, Davis *et al.* 1982).

5.5   HVR AT HIGH ALTITUDE

5.5.1   HVR and acclimatization

During the first few days at altitude, respiratory acclimatization takes place. This is shown by an increase in ventilation and a decrease in PA_{CO_2}. PA_{O_2} falls immediately on exposure to acute altitude and then rises (as PA_{CO_2} falls) over the next few days. The rise in ventilation on acute exposure to hypoxia is mediated by the HVR (by definition) but further increase in ventilation is due to changes in the ventilatory response to carbon dioxide (see section 5.12) and also in the sensitivity of the carotid body with more time at altitude.

The peripheral chemoreceptors are essential for normal respiratory acclimatization, and animals which have had their carotid bodies denervated fail to acclimatize normally (Forster *et al.* 1981, Lahiri *et al.* 1981, Smith *et al.* 1986). After denervation these animals have raised Pa_{CO_2}, which rises further with acute hypoxia. With chronic hypoxia, at least in some cases, there is a small fall in Pa_{CO_2} which has been taken by some workers as evidence of acclimatization (Sorensen and Mines 1970). This and other evidence suggests that chronic hypoxia produces some effect on ventilation via mechanisms other than the carotid body, possibly via cerebral metabolism. All agree, however, that denervated animals appeared ill at altitude and a number died.

It might be expected that exposure to hypoxia of some days or months would result in attenuation or sensitization of the HVR. Michel and Milledge (1963) found an increase in the hypoxic parameter A in three out of four subjects after 1–3 months at 5800 m. Parameter A is the 'shape' parameter of the hyperbola relating PA_{O_2} to ventilation (Figure 5.2). The larger the value the greater the response. There was no change in the other hypoxic parameter, C (the P_{O_2} at which theoretically ventilation becomes infinite, the P_{O_2} asymptote of the hyperbola). Cruz et al. (1980) also found an increase in parameter A after

74 h of altitude exposure; this was not seen in subjects whose PA_{CO_2} was not allowed to fall.

The question of a change in chemoreceptor responsiveness during acclimatization has been reviewed by Weil (1986), who points out that a number of studies have not found any change in HVR with acclimatization, although the presence of hypocapnic alkalosis, which has a depressant effect on HVR at sea level, may have obscured a real change. However, more recent studies have found an increase in responsiveness. Barnard et al. (1987) found neurophysiological evidence of increased sensitivity of the carotid body for hypoxia in cats after chronic hypoxia of 28 days but not after only 2–3 h. Vizek et al. (1987) also presented evidence from work in cats of an increase in HVR (parameter A) after 48 h hypoxia. Engwall and Bisgard (1990) found an increase in HVR after 4 h of hypoxia in awake goats. Yamaguchi et al. (1991), Sato et al. (1992, 1994) and Goldberg et al. (1992) found a significant increase in HVR in lowland subjects after acclimatization at 3730–4860 m compared with pre-exposure values. Masuda et al. (1992) measured HVR serially in seven lowland subjects after arrival at Lhasa (3658 m) as they acclimatized over 27 days. They found a biphasic response, i.e. a small decrease over the first 3–5 days then a considerable increase from day 5 to 27.

Robbins's group in Oxford have carried out a series of chamber studies in which the inspired gases can be controlled so as to keep the subject's end-tidal P_{CO_2} constant. Thus they are able to study the changes in HVR with hypoxia over first 8 h and later 48 h with or without the confounding effect of respiratory alkalosis mentioned above. They found that HVR did increase under isocapnia (Howard and Robbins 1995). They also showed that acclimatization had taken place even with isocapnia in that ventilation was raised under acute hyperoxia (Tansley et al. 1998). Using a 48 h chamber exposure, under either isocapnic or poikilocapnic hypoxia, the increase in hypoxic sensitivity started within 12 h and reached peak at about 36 h. That there was no difference between isocapnic and poikilocapnic results suggests that the respiratory alkalosis, normal in early acclimatization, is not an important part of the mechanism for this process, though it is for the changes in carbon dioxide sensitivity.

This increase in HVR over the period of a few days to a few weeks could explain the further increase in

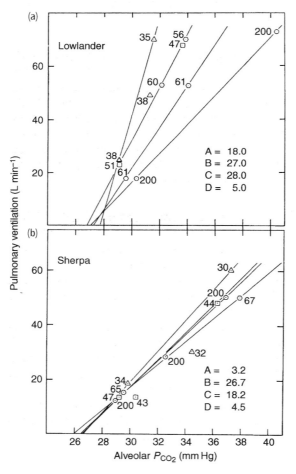

Figure 5.2 *Two steady-state inhalation experiments typical of a lowlander (upper panel) and a Sherpa highlander (lower panel). The numbers refer to the P_{O_2} of each point. There is no significant difference in HCVR but the 'closed fan' of the Sherpa indicates very little HVR. Letters A–D refer to the parameters relating HVR (A and C) and HCVR (B and D). (From Milledge and Lahiri 1967.)*

ventilation over this period of altitude exposure. The question of the role of HVR in effecting the change in carbon dioxide response and brain extracellular bicarbonate concentration is considered in section 5.13.

In humans, after decades at altitude, HVR becomes blunted (section 5.5.2). In cats this blunting is seen after 3–5 weeks if the hypoxia is sufficiently severe. Tatsumi *et al.* (1991) showed blunting of HVR after this time at a simulated altitude of 5500 m. They also found that HVR, measured by recording from the carotid sinus nerve, was blunted. They considered that both central and peripheral parts of the system contributed to the reduction in overall HVR.

5.5.2 HVR and altitude residents

Chiodi (1957) reported that altitude residents in the Andes had higher PA_{CO_2} than acclimatized lowlanders. Severinghaus *et al.* (1966a) showed that Andean Indians born and living at altitude had a blunted HVR and similar findings were reported in Sherpas, natives to high altitude in the Himalayas (Lahiri and Milledge 1967, Milledge and Lahiri 1967). Steady-state inhalation experiments typical of a lowlander and a Sherpa are shown in Figure 5.2. The 'opened-out fan' of the lowlander indicates a brisk HVR whereas the 'closed fan' of the Sherpa shows that changing PA_{O_2} between 200 and 30 mm Hg has very little effect on ventilation. These early reports have been confirmed and Lahiri (1977) has reviewed the data from these studies. There is considerable variability amongst these people, the HVR varying from almost zero response to values within the lowlander range. One study (Hackett *et al.* 1980) claimed that Sherpas did not show this blunted HVR. However, even this study showed that HVR was lower in Sherpas with the longest altitude exposure. More recently Zhuang *et al.* (1993) found HVR in Tibetan subjects at 3658 m to be lower than in acclimatized Han Chinese at the same altitude.

Recently there has been interest in comparing Tibetan with Andean high altitude residents. Beall *et al.* (1997a) studied 320 Tibetans and 552 Andean subjects. They found resting ventilation to be higher in Tibetans by a factor of about 1.5, and their HVR to be roughly double that of the Andean subjects. Comparison of these two populations is discussed further in Chapter 17.

Weil *et al.* (1971) showed blunting of HVR in white people born and living at Leadville, Colorado (3100 m), HVR being only 10 per cent of that found in the sea level controls.

5.5.3 Lowlanders resident at high altitude

Early studies of lowland subjects resident for a few years at high altitude suggested that HVR remained unchanged indefinitely (Sorensen and Severinghaus 1968, Lahiri *et al.* 1969). However, in a study of lowlanders resident at altitude for decades (Weil *et al.* 1971) it was shown that blunting did take place slowly.

5.5.4 Highlanders resident at sea level

The HVR was found not to change in high altitude natives who came down to live at low altitude (Lahiri *et al.* 1969), although Vargas *et al.* (1998), also from South America, found no difference in HVR between high and low altitude natives measured at low altitude, the high altitude natives having been at low altitude for only a few years.

5.5.5 The development of blunted HVR

Lahiri *et al.* (1976) found evidence in Andean Indians that HVR was normal in children and became blunted only as they grew into adulthood at altitude. They suggested the rate of blunting was more rapid the higher the place of residence. Weil *et al.* (1971) showed that in white subjects blunted HVR also developed only after decades of high altitude residence. In cats blunting can be induced in 3–4 weeks if the altitude is as high as 5500 m but not below 5000 m (Tatsumi *et al.* 1991).

These findings prove that the blunting of the HVR takes many years to develop in humans and is due to environmental and not genetic factors.

5.6 HVR AND ACUTE MOUNTAIN SICKNESS

AMS is a condition affecting otherwise fit people on ascending rapidly to altitude. For details of symptomatology, etiology and treatment, see Chapter 18. It would seem axiomatic that a brisk HVR by increasing ventilation reduces the degree of hypoxia and must be protective against AMS. There is some evidence that this may be the case, but it is by no means overwhelming.

Hu *et al.* (1982) showed that six good acclimatizers had brisk HVR whereas four poor acclimatizers had blunted responses. Richalet *et al.* (1988) found that in 128 climbers going to altitude on various expeditions a measure of HVR carried out before departure indicated that a low response was a risk factor for AMS. However, high altitude residents and peoples native to high altitude have blunted HVR (see section 5.5.2) and yet tend to be less subject to AMS than lowlanders. In lowland climbers of varying altitude experience, Milledge *et al.* (1988, 1991a) found no correlation between HVR measured before expeditions to Everest, Mount Kenya and Bolivia and the symptom score for AMS, in the first few days after arrival at altitude.

Masuda *et al.* (1992) found an initial decrease in HVR 1–5 days after arrival at Lhasa (3700 m) followed by an increase and suggested that this might explain why these first few days are the time of risk for AMS.

These studies all considered a correlation, or lack of it, between HVR and simple or benign AMS. Hackett *et al.* (1988b) studied seven male patients with HAPE and found HVR was low, especially in those with most severe hypoxemia. More recently Hohenhaus *et al.* (1995) measured HVR in 30 subjects proved to be HAPE susceptible compared with a control group. They concluded that a low HVR is associated with an increased risk of HAPE but not with simple AMS.

5.7 HVR AND ALTITUDE PERFORMANCE

Apart from AMS, some people 'go well' at altitude whereas others, just as athletically fit, seem much more adversely affected. In general, there is a good correlation between freedom from AMS and good altitude performance. Again, it would seem advantageous for a mountaineer to have a brisk HVR in order to maintain a better oxygen supply to the working muscles. However, the evidence for this is conflicting.

Climbers with a brisk HVR were found to suffer greater impairment of mental performance at altitude (Hornbein *et al.* 1989), presumably as a result of reduced brain blood flow due to lower Pa_{CO_2} (see Chapter 16 for details of this work).

Schoene (1982) showed that 14 high altitude climbers had significantly higher HVR than 10 controls. During the 1981 American Medical Research Expedition to Everest, Schoene *et al.* (1984) extended this work, showing again that the HVR measured before and on the expedition correlated well with performance high on the mountain (Figure 5.3). They also showed that, at altitude, the fall in oxygen saturation on exercise is greater in subjects with a low HVR and least in those with a brisk response. Thus, subjects with a blunt HVR are not only more hypoxic at rest but have even greater hypoxia on exercise than brisk responders. This is because there is a correlation between HVR and exercise ventilatory response (Martin *et al.* 1978).

Matsuyama *et al.* (1986) found that five climbers who reached an altitude of 8000 m on Kangchenjunga (8486 m) had a higher HVR than five climbers who did not.

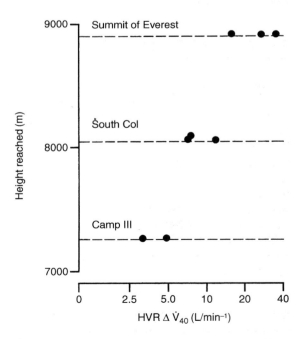

Figure 5.3 *HVR and height reached on Mount Everest by eight mountaineers on the American Medical Research Expedition to Everest 1981. (Redrawn from data of Schoene* et al. *1984.)*

However, the blunted HVR in peoples native to high altitude who perform at least as well as lowlanders argues against the necessity for a brisk HVR. They have probably adapted in other ways at a tissue level (Chapter 10). There is also evidence of not so brisk HVR in top level climbers. On the British Mount Kongur Expedition four elite climbers were found to have less HVR than four scientists on the same expedition (Milledge *et al.* 1983c). Schoene *et al.* (1987) studied one of the two climbers to first reach the summit of Mount Everest without supplementary oxygen and found him to have a low HVR. Oelz *et al.* (1986) also showed that six elite climbers who had all reached at least 8400 m without supplementary oxygen had HVRs no different from controls. In a prospective study of 128 climbers going on expeditions to the great ranges, Richalet *et al.* (1988) found that a measure of HVR did not correlate with the height reached, whereas maximal oxygen consumption ($\dot{V}_{O_2 max}$) measured at sea level did.

Serebrovskaya and Ivashkevich (1992) found that subjects with the highest HVR had higher physical capacity at moderate altitude but tolerated extreme hypoxia less well, in that the P_{O_2} at which they had a disturbance of consciousness was higher than subjects with less brisk HVR.

5.8   HVR AND SLEEP

A feature of sleep at high altitude is periodic breathing. This not only disturbs sleep, the subject often waking with a distressing sensation of suffocation, but also results in quite profound hypoxia for short but repeated periods following the apneic phase of the periodic breathing (see Chapter 13). It may be that these short but repeated periods of profound hypoxia are more detrimental than a steady moderate hypoxia, although the peak and average Sa_{O_2} tend to be higher during periodic breathing. Lahiri *et al.* (1984) have shown that to produce periodic breathing a brisk HVR is needed, so in this respect a brisk HVR may be a disadvantage.

5.9   HVR AT ALTITUDE: CONCLUSIONS

Animals that have had their carotid bodies denervated appear sick on being taken to altitude and have a high mortality, so an HVR sufficient to at least counter the central depressant effect of hypoxia is clearly beneficial. Whether a very brisk HVR is more advantageous than a more modest response is questionable on available evidence. Relative hypoventilation at altitude is probably a risk factor for AMS but the HVR measured at sea level is only one factor in determining the ventilation after a day or two at altitude. The speed of respiratory acclimatization may be more important than the HVR.

In subjects with a brisk HVR it seems likely that periodic breathing will begin at lower altitudes and be present for more of the night than in subjects with a more blunted HVR. Mental performance at altitude and even after return to sea level may be more impaired in subjects with a brisk HVR (see Chapter 16).

Lowlanders with little or no altitude experience may possibly acclimatize faster and be freer of AMS if they are endowed with a brisk HVR. Highlanders with decades of altitude living probably develop adaptations at the tissue level which allow them to dispense with this 'emergency' response to hypoxia and avoid the need for hyperventilation.

Highly experienced climbers may also have made some progress towards this adaptation and so may not require a brisk HVR to avoid mountain sickness and perform well at altitude.

5.10   ALVEOLAR GASES AND ACCLIMATIZATION

It has been pointed out that if PI_{O_2} is progressively reduced over a few minutes there is very little effect on ventilation until PI_{O_2} has fallen to about 100 mm Hg (equivalent to about 3000 m). However, in residents at altitudes lower than this, ventilation is increased. This effect of chronic hypoxia in increasing ventilation (over and above that due to acute hypoxia) is an important aspect of respiratory acclimatization.

Minute ventilation at rest is not easy to measure accurately because the placing of a mouthpiece or a mask on a subject itself tends to increase ventilation. Therefore it is usual to use PA_{CO_2} as an index of ventilation since during steady state there is a close (inverse) relationship between PA_{CO_2} and ventilation.

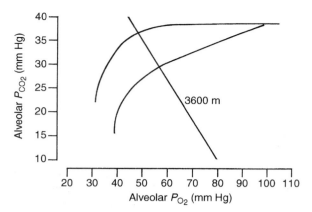

Figure 5.4 *Alveolar gas concentrations and altitude. The upper line represents the P_{O_2} and P_{CO_2} found in subjects actually exposed to increasing hypoxia in a chamber. The lower line is from residents at various altitudes and from acclimatized mountaineers. (After Rahn and Otis 1949.)*

The classical description of the effect of altitude on alveolar gases is by Rahn and Otis (1949) on the oxygen/carbon dioxide diagram (Figure 5.4). Alveolar gases in subjects acutely exposed to varying PI_{O_2} in a decompression chamber are compared with results from residents at various altitudes culled from the literature.

It will be seen that in chronic hypoxia P_{CO_2} falls in a linear fashion from sea level up to altitudes of about 5400 m, above which P_{CO_2} falls more rapidly so that the line dips down. These are altitudes above the highest permanent habitation and are from climbers who have been there for some days or weeks. At this altitude complete acclimatization is probably not possible; the physiology is further discussed in Chapter 12.

Figure 5.4 also shows that at about 5000 m the difference in alveolar gases between the two lines, i.e. acclimatized and unacclimatized subjects, is greatest. The PA_{CO_2} is 10–12 mm Hg lower in acclimatized subjects, indicating an increase in ventilation of over 40 per cent compared with unacclimatized subjects.

5.11 ACUTE NORMOXIA IN ACCLIMATIZED SUBJECTS

Respiratory acclimatization can be demonstrated by returning acclimatized subjects to normal (sea level) P_{O_2} either by rapid return to sea level or by breathing

a gas mixture appropriately enriched with oxygen. The ventilation is reduced and the PA_{CO_2} rises but does not return to sea level values. The remaining elevation of ventilation and depression of PA_{CO_2} indicate the degree of respiratory acclimatization. This is most accurately measured when ventilation is recorded during exercise.

Figure 5.5 shows results from two typical experiments (Milledge 1968). It will be seen that by breathing sea level PI_{O_2} the increase in ventilation at altitude compared with sea level is reduced by about 40 per cent at any given submaximal work rate.

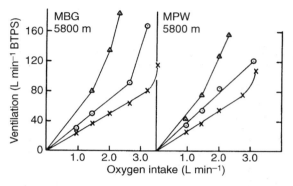

Figure 5.5 *Effect of breathing sea level PI_{O_2} on exercise minute ventilation in two acclimatized subjects (○) compared with their ventilation during air breathing at altitude (△) and at sea level (×). (Milledge 1968.)*

5.12 CARBON DIOXIDE VENTILATORY RESPONSE AND ACCLIMATIZATION

An important aspect of respiratory acclimatization is the change in carbon dioxide ventilatory response (HCVR) measured either by the steady state (Lloyd *et al.* 1958) or by a rebreathing method (Reed 1967).

The effect of time at altitude on the HCVR is shown in Figure 5.6, which is from the work of Kellogg (1963). The steady-state method was used in three subjects to measure the HCVR before ascent to White Mountain. The measurement was repeated a few hours after arrival by road at 4350 m and thereafter at intervals as indicated on the figure. It will be seen that the HCVR line shifts progressively leftwards and steepens. Voluntary hyperventilation of only 6 h duration breathing air has a significant effect in shifting the carbon dioxide response curve to the left (Ren and Robbins 1999).

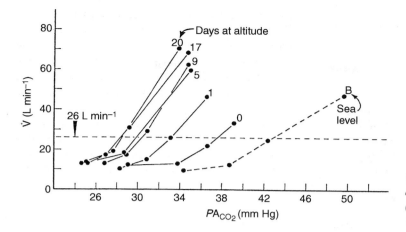

Figure 5.6 *Effect of acclimatization on HCVR at an altitude of 4340 m. V̇, ventilation. (Reproduced with permission from Kellogg 1963.)*

5.13   MECHANISM FOR RESETTING HCVR

5.13.1   Central chemoreceptors

Although the peripheral chemoreceptors are sensitive to changes in P_{CO_2} and hydrogen ion concentration, the main sensor for changes in P_{CO_2} is the central medullary chemoreceptor. This is a paired region of the CNS situated just beneath the surface of the fourth ventricle in the medulla. Work by Mitchell (1963) has shown that this area is sensitive to changes in hydrogen ion concentration in the brain ECF. Such changes are brought about primarily by changes in arterial P_{CO_2}.

The blood–brain barrier is readily permeable to dissolved carbon dioxide, less permeable to hydrogen ions and even less to bicarbonate. Thus, a rise in Pa_{CO_2} is rapidly reflected in CSF P_{CO_2} and causes a rapid increase in CSF hydrogen ion concentration. Increases in hydrogen ion concentration sensed by the chemoreceptors result in increased stimulation of the respiratory center and an increase in ventilation.

5.13.2   The importance of CSF bicarbonate

The chemoreceptors sense the hydrogen ion concentration in the brain ECF (or possibly some other extracellular or intracellular compartment) but since this cannot be sampled, the following discussion centers on the CSF acid–base changes which can be measured. See below (section 5.15.1) for further discussion of the differences between these two compartments.

The Henderson–Hasselbalch equation, which defines the relationship between P_{CO_2}, bicarbonate and pH (hydrogen ion concentration), is shown in Figure 5.7. This indicates that for hydrogen ion concentration to be held constant, a change of bicarbonate concentration must be followed by a change of P_{CO_2} in the same direction. Assuming the sensitivity of the central chemoreceptors to hydrogen ion concentration remains constant, a reduction in bicarbonate concentration will result in an increase in hydrogen ion concentration which will stimulate the central chemoreceptor and cause a rise in ventilation. This, in turn, will lower the P_{CO_2} and restore the hydrogen ion concentration to normal, but now with a lower P_{CO_2}. Thus a reduction in CSF bicarbonate concentration has the effect of resetting the chemoreceptor to start responding at a lower P_{CO_2} (a shift to the left of the HCVR line). A rise in CSF bicarbonate concentration has the opposite effect and is seen in patients with chronic bronchitis and hypercapnia. If the chemoreceptor responds to log hydrogen ion concentration (i.e. pH), then changes in P_{CO_2} at low values, e.g. 20–21 mm Hg, will have twice the effect as that at normal values, i.e. 40–41 mm Hg. This would then explain the steepening of the HCVR seen in acclimatized subjects.

These effects are shown in Figure 5.7. This is a theoretical representation of the effect on HCVR of a reduction in CSF bicarbonate concentration. A typical HCVR line at sea level is shown on the right. The CSF bicarbonate concentration is 24 mmol L^{-1}. If the CSF bicarbonate concentration is reduced to

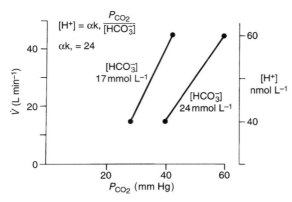

Figure 5.7 *Calculated effect of reducing CSF [HCO₃⁻] on the HCVR using the Henderson–Hasselbalch equation and assuming CSF pH is held constant by ventilatory induced changes in P_{CO_2}. $\dot{V}$, ventilation.*

17 mmol L⁻¹ the chemoreceptor now 'sees' an increased hydrogen ion concentration and ventilation is stimulated until hydrogen ion concentration is reduced to the previous value. The resulting P_{CO_2} values are plotted and joined by a line giving the new HCVR on the left. This looks very similar to the actual effect of acclimatization on HCVR.

It is suggested that the mechanism of the change in HCVR is a reduction in CSF bicarbonate concentration. Evidence for this is provided by the experiments of Pappenheimer *et al.* (1964) in which they perfused the cerebral ventricles of awake goats with artificial CSF, varying the pH and bicarbonate concentration. They showed that by simply reducing the bicarbonate concentration in the CSF, the HCVR was shifted to the left.

Bisgard *et al.* (1986) found evidence of the importance of CSF bicarbonate concentration in maintaining the residual ventilation of acclimatization on giving normoxia. These workers perfused the carotid body in awake goats with hypoxemic blood while the rest of the animal, including the brain, was normoxic. Carbon dioxide was added to the inspired gas to maintain normocapnia despite hyperventilation. There was a time-dependent increase in ventilation over the 4 h of the experiment, but since brain and body were normocapnic and normoxic there would have been no change in CSF bicarbonate concentration. Full respiratory acclimatization did not take place since, on switching the carotid perfusion to normoxia, ventilation promptly fell to normal.

5.13.3   Reduction in CSF bicarbonate concentration at altitude

In lowlanders going to an altitude of 3800 m the CSF bicarbonate concentration is reduced from a mean sea level value of 24.7 mmol L⁻¹ to 20.4 mmol L⁻¹ on the second day at altitude and 20.1 mmol L⁻¹ on day 8 (Severinghaus *et al.* 1963). Similar results (mean 20.1 mmol L⁻¹) were found at 4880 m (Lahiri and Milledge 1967). Residents at high altitude had similar values, 19.1–21.3 mmol L⁻¹ (Severinghaus and Carcelan 1964, Lahiri and Milledge 1967, Sorensen and Milledge 1971). Thus the reduction in CSF bicarbonate concentration of 4.5 mmol L⁻¹ measured at altitude sufficiently explains the shift of the HCVR line to the left, though respiratory acclimatization probably also involves contributions from other mechanisms such as changes in the hypoxic ventilatory response (see section 5.5.1).

5.14   MECHANISMS FOR REDUCTION IN CSF BICARBONATE CONCENTRATION

5.14.1   Possible mechanisms

Figure 5.8 shows three possible routes by which hypoxia could cause a reduction in CSF bicarbonate concentration. On the left is the 'classical' pathway. Hypoxia stimulates the peripheral chemoreceptors resulting in increased ventilation, decreased Pa_{CO_2} and hence respiratory alkalosis. The kidneys respond to the increased pH by excreting bicarbonate in the urine, and plasma bicarbonate concentration falls. A gradient develops for bicarbonate concentration across the blood–brain barrier and CSF bicarbonate concentration passes out slowly down the concentration gradient.

Severinghaus *et al.* (1963) reported that early in altitude acclimatization their subjects had less increase in CSF pH and a greater fall in CSF bicarbonate concentration than in the plasma. Thus bicarbonate appeared to pass out of the CSF against the concentration gradient, suggesting active transport of these ions out of, or hydrogen ion into, the CSF. This mechanism is shown in the center of the diagram (Figure 5.8).

On the right of Figure 5.8 is the third possible mechanism for CSF bicarbonate concentration

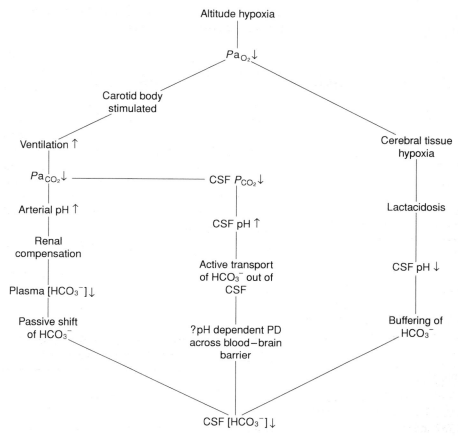

Figure 5.8 *Possible mechanisms by which altitude hypoxia could cause a reduction in CSF [HCO₃⁻]. PD, potential difference.*

reduction. With hypoxia there is a partial switch in cerebral metabolism of glucose from the aerobic to the anaerobic pathway. This results in formation of lactic and pyruvic acids. The hydrogen ion produced will directly buffer bicarbonate.

There is now abundant evidence supporting the conclusions of Severinghaus *et al.* (1963) that CSF acid–base changes are faster than renal compensation of plasma acid–base changes. Although the latter may contribute to the later changes of respiratory acclimatization, the major early changes are largely complete in 24 h and have little to do with renal compensation.

5.14.2 Active transport of CSF bicarbonate concentration

Severinghaus's postulate of an active transport of bicarbonate out of the CSF has stimulated a great deal of work aimed at disproving or proving this hypothesis. Fencl *et al.* (1966), using awake goats and ventricular perfusion, also presented data supporting the idea of active transport of bicarbonate out of the CSF.

However, we must consider not only ionic concentrations in blood and CSF but also the electrical potential difference (PD) across the blood–brain barrier. This PD between CSF and blood, normally about +6.4 mV in dogs and +3 mV in humans, becomes more positive as blood pH increases (Bledsoe and Hornbein 1981). The change is of the order of 32–53 mV per pH unit depending on the type of acid–base change. Changes in CSF pH do not affect PD. There is also a species difference in the magnitude and even direction of change so that extrapolation from experiments on animals to humans must be made with caution. To complicate the matter even further, PD is also affected by changes in plasma potassium concentration.

5.14.3 Passive transport of CSF bicarbonate concentration

Siesjo and Kjallquist (1969) proposed that the apparent disequilibrium of hydrogen ion concentration and bicarbonate concentration across the blood–brain barrier could be explained by these changes in PD. That is, that shifts of these ions across the barrier was by passive transport. Many papers have addressed this problem and are reviewed by Bledsoe and Hornbein (1981). Their conclusion is that neither the active nor the passive transport hypothesis is proven.

5.14.4 Cerebral tissue hypoxia and lactacidosis

It is well known that hypoxia increases lactate (and pyruvate) levels in the blood and CSF, and in their paper proposing active transport of bicarbonate Severinghaus *et al.* (1963) discussed the possibility that increased lactic acid in the CSF might account for the reduction in bicarbonate concentration. However, the increase in lactate was only about 1 mmol L^{-1} compared with 4–5 mmol L^{-1} reduction in bicarbonate concentration. Lactic acid dissociates to lactate and hydrogen ions in the cell. The two species then pass through the cell membrane to ECF, to CSF and across the blood–brain barrier, probably with different rates at each stage. There is no reason therefore to expect a simple one-to-one relationship between their concentrations in the CSF. In other words, production of hydrogen ion from lactic acid might well be greater than is indicated by the relatively small change in lactate concentration.

There is evidence that hypoxia produces respiratory acclimatization independent of increased ventilation or decreased Pa_{CO_2}.

- Eger *et al.* (1968) found that the effect of hyperventilation on the position of the carbon dioxide ventilatory response curve was greater when subjects breathed a hypoxic mixture than when they breathed air. This showed that hypoxia had an effect independent of any change in P_{CO_2}.
- Many high altitude residents having practically no ventilatory response to acute hypoxia nevertheless at altitude have Pa_{CO_2}, HCVR and CSF bicarbonate concentration very similar to lowlanders with a brisk HVR, indicating similar respiratory acclimatization.
- Sorensen and Mines (1970) showed that goats that had had their carotid bodies denervated, so that acute hypoxia actually depressed their respiration, nevertheless showed a reduction in PA_{CO_2} at altitude compared with sea level values. In a companion study (Sorensen 1970) it was shown that rabbits whose peripheral chemoreceptors were denervated had a reduction of CSF bicarbonate concentration similar to that of controls when taken to altitude. Steinbrook *et al.* (1983) also found evidence of good respiratory acclimatization in goats with ablated carotid bodies. However, in other studies in goats (Lahiri *et al.* 1981, Smith *et al.* 1986) respiratory acclimatization apparently did not take place in the denervated animals, in that Pa_{CO_2} did not fall significantly. Certainly animals with denervated or absent carotid bodies fare badly at altitude and most studies reported a number of deaths amongst their animals.
- Fencl *et al.* (1979), in the awake goat with perfused ventricles, showed that in the acclimatized animal lactate was higher and bicarbonate concentration lower in the brain ECF than in the CSF (at sea level there was no concentration difference).

These lines of evidence suggest that hypoxia *per se* has a role in respiratory acclimatization, presumably by its effect on cerebral metabolism.

5.15 BRAIN ACID–BASE BALANCE

5.15.1 Brain extracellular fluid

In the foregoing sections CSF pH has been discussed because that was what had been measured in the studies quoted. However, it must be remembered that the central chemoreceptor senses the hydrogen ion concentration in the fluid in its immediate vicinity, the local brain ECF. It has been calculated from studies in awake goats perfused with artificial CSF (Pappenheimer *et al.* 1964) that in the steady state this represents a point about three-quarters of the way along the concentration gradient for hydrogen ion and bicarbonate between CSF and plasma.

In a situation of changing acid–base balance, as for instance the developing respiratory alkalosis on going to altitude, the local brain ECF will change more rapidly than the bulk CSF. This is especially the case for respiratory as compared with metabolic changes. Within a few seconds of a fall in brain P_{CO_2}, brain bicarbonate concentration falls. The buffering capacity for brain ECF is greater by a third than the CSF so the compensation for pH change is faster and greater in this compartment than in the CSF (Dempsey and Forster 1982).

It must also be remembered that the brain ECF is affected by cerebral blood flow so that changes in Pa_{O_2} and Pa_{CO_2} will have secondary effects by changing cerebral blood flow. This makes interpretation of studies even more difficult.

5.15.2   The lack of stability of CSF pH

Since the sensitivity to P_{CO_2} is via the pH-sensitive central chemoreceptors and since Pa_{CO_2} is so closely regulated, it seemed reasonable to assume that CSF pH was extremely stable. At sea level a fall of pH of about 0.03 pH units results in a doubling of the resting ventilation. Even when this is converted to a change of hydrogen ion concentration concentration, it represents an increase of only 7 per cent. Thus we have a negative feedback loop of very high gain, suggesting very tight regulation of pH.

However, in fact during acclimatization the CSF pH rises by about 0.03–0.06 units while ventilation goes up. The reverse happens with acute normoxia (Dempsey and Forster 1982). The change in pH is, of course, much less than would have occurred without the change in bicarbonate concentration, as discussed in section 5.13.3. There are three possible explanations for this paradoxical change of CSF pH:

- The drive from peripheral chemoreceptors is sufficient to increase ventilation even when the central drive is reduced. In subjects with a brisk HVR this is the most important cause of CSF alkalosis.
- The brain ECF may well be different from the bulk CSF in respect of hydrogen ion concentration and bicarbonate concentration (see section 5.15.1), so that cerebral lactacidosis causes higher hydrogen ion concentration in

brain ECF than in CSF. This is suggested by the work on awake goats with perfused ventricles at altitude (Fencl et al. 1979).

- The effect of acute hypoxia on cerebral blood flow was studied by Crawford and Severinghaus (1978), who calculate that, at an altitude of 3810 m, hypoxia causes a 30 per cent rise in blood flow to the central chemoreceptor area, resulting in a rise in pH of 0.006 units. Acute normoxia causes a similar, though opposite, change.

These effects would seem to account for most of the 'negative correlation' of hydrogen ion concentration with ventilation pointed out by Dempsey et al. (1979). It is not necessary to invoke any change in sensitivity of the central chemoreceptor to hydrogen ion concentration, although this cannot be ruled out. Thus, it would seem that CSF pH is the result of the combined effects of peripheral and central drive and is not, in fact, very tightly controlled. Where peripheral drive is strong, as in lowlanders at altitude, the CSF pH is increased. Where peripheral drive is low, as at sea level, highlanders and even more in subjects with denervated carotid bodies, CSF pH is reduced.

5.15.3   Brain intracellular pH

Using magnetic resonance spectroscopy on unacclimatized lowland subjects in a hypobaric chamber, Goldberg et al. (1992) found that, after a week at 4267 m simulated altitude, there was no significant change in intracellular pH although on return to normobaria there was a significant intracellular acidosis.

5.16   DYNAMIC CARBON DIOXIDE RESPONSE

Carbon dioxide is eliminated only during expiration; during inspiration it is retained. Therefore the level of carbon dioxide in the blood leaving the lungs must oscillate in time with breathing. During exercise these oscillations will be increased. Yamamoto and Edwards (1960) suggested that these oscillations might be a signal to which the peripheral chemoreceptors could respond over and above the mean level of carbon dioxide in the arterial blood. The response to this putative signal of change in carbon dioxide with time is called the dynamic carbon dioxide ventilatory response. Datta and Nickol (1995) showed that this response could be demonstrated in exercising humans (it had been shown previously in anesthetized cats) by measuring the ventilation during the injection of a small bolus of carbon dioxide either early or late in inspiration. Ventilation was found to be greater with early pulses. Collier *et al.* (1995) showed that this response is absent in acute hypoxia and weak or absent on first arrival at altitude. It is enhanced with acclimatization and is greatest in subjects who have climbed to over 7000 m. This provides evidence that the ventilatory response of the peripheral chemoreceptor is increased for carbon dioxide as it is for hypoxia (section 5.5.1).

5.17 LONGER TERM ACCLIMATIZATION

5.17.1 Highlanders

People native to high altitude have lower ventilation and higher Pa_{CO_2} than acclimatized newcomers (Chiodi 1957). This is probably due to their blunted HVR (see section 5.5.2). The HCVR of Andean natives (Severinghaus *et al.* 1966a), Sherpas (Milledge and Lahiri 1967) and Tibetans (Shi *et al.* 1979) has the same slope as that of lowlanders at the same altitude. The position of the carbon dioxide ventilatory response line may be to the right (Severinghaus *et al.* 1966a) or not significantly different from lowlanders (Milledge and Lahiri 1967). That is, there is little difference between highlanders and lowlanders in their carbon dioxide ventilatory response.

5.17.2 Lowlanders

Although most of the respiratory acclimatization takes place within the first few hours and days at altitude, there may be further changes over the following weeks. In humans, there is a further increase in ventilation and Pa_{O_2} with a further decrease in Pa_{CO_2} (Forster *et al.* 1974), though in other animals, e.g. pony and goat, the Pa_{CO_2} reaches the lowest point at 8–12 h and then rises. The rat responds like humans with continued fall in Pa_{CO_2} up to 14 days (Dempsey and Forster 1982). There is no significant change in acid–base balance over this period to account for this further ventilatory adaptation. It is likely that there is an increase in sensitivity of the carotid body over this period (see section 5.5.1) and it is possible that changes in control from higher centers, such as have been demonstrated in cats by Tenney and Ou (1977), may be responsible.

Lung diffusion

SUMMARY

Diffusion of oxygen across the blood–gas barrier is a critical link in the oxygen cascade from the atmosphere to the mitochondria. In fact, exercise at high altitude is one of the few situations where oxygen transfer is diffusion limited in normal humans. On a historical note, up to the 1930s some physiologists believed that the lung secreted oxygen, but we now believe that all gases pass across the blood–gas barrier by passive diffusion. The distinction between a perfusion limited and diffusion limited gas such as carbon monoxide is emphasized. Diffusion across the blood–gas barrier is enhanced if the oxygen affinity of the hemoglobin is increased. This occurs in many animals that live in oxygen-deprived environments, and interestingly, the oxygen affinity of hemoglobin is greatly increased at extreme altitude because of the severe respiratory alkalosis. Lowlanders who go to high altitude have a small increase in the diffusing capacity of the lung for carbon monoxide but this can be explained by the polycythemia and the increased rate of reaction of carbon monoxide with hemoglobin as a result of the reduced P_{O_2}. Several studies show that high altitude natives have higher diffusing capacities than similar people at sea level. A possible explanation is the accelerated growth of the lung that occurs in a hypoxic environment. Diffusion limitation of oxygen transfer at extreme altitude, particularly on exercise, exaggerates the already severe hypoxemia. A relatively high diffusing capacity of the lung probably improves work capacity at very high altitudes.

6.1 INTRODUCTION

Diffusion refers to the process by which oxygen moves from the alveolar gas into the pulmonary capillary blood, and carbon dioxide moves in the reverse direction. That this step in the cascade of oxygen transfer from the air to the mitochondria might be a limiting factor at high altitude was suggested near the beginning of the twentieth century. However, it is only since about 1980 that the role of diffusion at high altitude has been clearly elucidated.

Diffusion as defined above refers to the movement of oxygen in solution through the tissues of the blood–gas barrier, and for convenience we also include the delay caused by the chemical combination of oxygen with hemoglobin in the pulmonary capillary blood (section 6.3.4). The term diffusion is also used in another context in the lung, that is the transport of gas in the small airways by the random movement of molecules in the gas phase. This process plays an important role in the movement of oxygen from the terminal bronchioles to the alveoli. It is unlikely that this process ever limits oxygen transfer in the normal lung at sea level, though the issue cannot be considered completely settled. At high altitude, diffusion in the gas phase becomes even less likely as a potential limiting factor because the mean free path of the molecules is increased as a result of the rarefaction of the gas. Consequently, diffusion in the gas phase will not be considered further.

6.2   HISTORICAL

The role of diffusion in the lungs was a topic of great controversy among respiratory physiologists in the last decade of the nineteenth century and the first two decades of the twentieth, and the arguments specifically involved the issue of diffusion at high altitude. Paradoxically much of the disagreement was generated by physiologists who contended that passive diffusion was not the primary mechanism of oxygen transfer through the blood–gas barrier, but that this process was achieved by active secretion. By this they meant that oxygen could be moved from a region of low partial pressure to one of high partial pressure as a result of some active process in the epithelial cells which required energy.

One of the strongest proponents of the secretion hypothesis was the Danish physiologist Christian Bohr. In a paper published in 1891 he compared the P_{O_2} and P_{CO_2} of alveolar gas with that of gas in a tonometer equilibrated with arterial blood taken at the same time. In some instances the alveolar P_{O_2} was reported to be as much as 30 mm Hg below, and the P_{CO_2} as much as 20 mm Hg above, the arterial blood values. Bohr's conclusion was:

> In general, my experiments have shown definitely that the lung tissue plays an active part in gas exchange; therefore, the function of the lung can be regarded as analogous to that of the glands (Bohr 1891).

Bohr referred to the secretion ability of the lung as its 'specific function'. In 1909 he published a long paper on this topic, claiming that the active secretion of oxygen and carbon dioxide could use large amounts of oxygen, up to 60 per cent of the total requirements of the body. If this were true, the Fick principle for deriving cardiac output from the oxygen consumption measured at the mouth would be invalid. Although the first part of his paper was devoted to active secretion, the second analyzed the basic principles of oxygen diffusion through the blood–gas barrier. Here Bohr introduced the mathematical process which is now known as the 'Bohr integration'. It forms the basis for modern calculations of the time course of oxygen transfer from the alveolar gas into the blood as it moves along the pulmonary capillary (Bohr 1909).

August Krogh was one of Bohr's students and assisted him in his experiments on gas secretion from 1899 to 1908. Krogh gradually became persuaded that passive diffusion rather than active secretion could account for the experimental data and in 1910 published a landmark paper on this topic. Since Bohr was his major professor and very jealous of the secretion theory, the introductory section of Krogh's paper required an unusually delicate touch. Part of it reads:

> I shall be obliged in the following pages to combat the views of my teacher Prof. Bohr on certain essential points and also to criticize a few of his experimental results. I wish here not only to acknowledge the debt of gratitude which I, personally, owe to him, but also to emphasize the fact, patent to everybody, who is familiar with the problems here discussed, that the real progress, made during the last twenty years in the knowledge of the processes in the lungs, is mainly due to his labours . . . (Krogh 1910).

The British physiologist J. S. Haldane visited Bohr in Copenhagen and also became convinced of the secretion theory, at least as far as oxygen was concerned. For example, in 1897 Haldane and Lorraine Smith wrote: 'The absorption of oxygen by the lungs thus cannot be explained by diffusion alone' (Haldane and Smith 1897). Haldane argued that oxygen secretion would be particularly beneficial at high altitudes, and in order to test the hypothesis the Anglo-American expedition to Pikes Peak was organized in 1911. Arterial P_{O_2} was calculated by an indirect method following the inhalation of carbon monoxide, and the results appeared strongly to support the secretion hypothesis.

However, the theory was also attacked by Marie Krogh (wife of August) when she developed a method for measuring the diffusing capacity of the lung using small concentrations of carbon monoxide

(Krogh and Krogh 1910). Her results indicated that the normal lung was capable of transferring very large amounts of oxygen by passive diffusion even when the inspired P_{O_2} was greatly reduced.

Various measurements in low pressure chambers and during climbs to great altitudes were used as evidence to support one or other of the two camps. For example, Zuntz and his co-workers made some measurements in the first high altitude research station, the Capanna Regina Margherita on the Monte Rosa in the Italian Alps, and Bohr used the results as evidence for active secretion of oxygen. In this experiment, the oxygen consumption of one subject was 1.52 L min^{-1} when the alveolar P_{O_2} was only 57 mm Hg (Zuntz et al. 1906, Appendix Tables XI and XVIII). Bohr had just described his mathematical integration procedure and he claimed that the experimental data were inconsistent with passive diffusion being the only mode of oxygen transfer (Bohr 1909).

In the same year that Bohr's paper appeared, the Duke of Abruzzi reached the extraordinary altitude of 7500 m in the Karakoram mountains without supplementary oxygen. This was an astonishing climb because only a few years before, experienced alpinists had reported that 21 500 ft (6500 m) was 'near the limit at which man ceases to be capable of the slightest further exertion' (Hinchliff 1876, p. 91). Indeed one of the reasons given for the Duke's expedition was 'to see how high man can go' (Filippi 1912).

Douglas, Haldane and their co-workers were duly impressed by the Duke's achievement and estimated from the reported barometric pressure of 312 mm Hg that the alveolar P_{O_2} was only 30 mm Hg. They therefore concluded that adequate oxygenation of the arterial blood would be impossible under these conditions without active secretion (Douglas et al. 1913). However, this conclusion was disputed by Marie Krogh (1915) who argued that Douglas and his colleagues had markedly underestimated the diffusing capacity of the lung. Incidentally we now know that Douglas et al.'s estimate of an alveolar P_{O_2} of 30 mm Hg for a barometric pressure of 312 mm Hg was much too low; the actual value is approximately 35 mm Hg (Gill et al. 1962) in a region of the oxygen dissociation curve where an increase of 5 mm Hg makes a world of difference.

Another physiologist who did not accept the secretion story was Joseph Barcroft. He conducted a heroic experiment on himself by living in a sealed glass chamber filled with hypoxic gas for 6 days (Barcroft et al. 1920). His left radial artery was exposed 'for an inch-and-a-half' and blood was taken for measurements of oxygen saturation. There was a 'somewhat dramatic moment' when the first blood sample was drawn because it 'looked dark', an observation which was believed to be inconsistent with oxygen secretion. The conclusion was that diffusion was the only mechanism necessary for oxygen transfer across the blood–gas barrier during hypoxia.

Barcroft and his colleagues subsequently tested the secretion hypothesis further on their expedition to Cerro de Pasco in the Peruvian Andes in 1921–2. The diffusing capacity of the lung for carbon monoxide was measured on five members of the expedition both at sea level and at Cerro de Pasco, and only a small increase was found. Barcroft therefore argued that the tendency for the arterial oxygen saturation to fall during exercise at high altitude could be explained by the failure of equilibration of P_{O_2} between alveolar gas and pulmonary capillary blood (Barcroft et al. 1923). This was one of the first direct demonstrations of diffusion limitation, a finding that has been confirmed many times since.

It is remarkable that J. S. Haldane remained a staunch supporter of oxygen secretion all his life. In the second edition of his book Respiration, written with J. G. Priestley and published in 1935, a year before Haldane's death, a whole chapter was devoted to evidence for oxygen secretion (Haldane and Priestley 1935). Haldane gradually shifted his position as evidence mounted against the secretion hypothesis. He initially thought that oxygen secretion occurred under all conditions, but later argued that it only became significant at high altitude, and later still that it required a period of acclimatization. His obsession with this theory long after seemingly overwhelming evidence had been provided against it was remarkable in this great physiologist.

6.3 PHYSIOLOGY OF DIFFUSION IN THE LUNG

6.3.1 Anatomical basis

The structure of the human lung is well suited to its role of allowing passive diffusion of oxygen from the alveolar gas to the interior of the red blood cell. The blood–gas barrier is extremely thin, being only

0.2–0.3 μm in many places, and the area of the blood–gas barrier available for diffusion is 50–100 m².

Figure 6.1 shows an electron micrograph of a pulmonary capillary and emphasizes the short distance over which oxygen diffuses in (or carbon dioxide diffuses out). The various tissues through which oxygen moves are: layer of surfactant (not shown in this preparation because of the method of fixation), type 1 alveolar epithelial cell (EP), interstitium (IN) (often much thinner on one side of the capillary than the other, as in the figure), capillary endothelial cell (EN), plasma and red cell. Note that the path length through the blood–gas barrier itself is only a small fraction of the total diffusion distance from the alveolar gas to the center of the red cell.

Recently, several morphometric studies have been

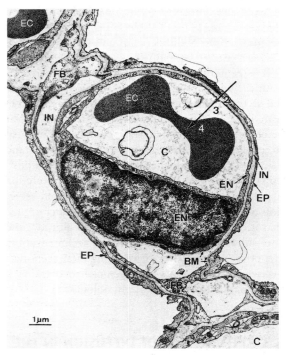

Figure 6.1 *Electron micrograph showing a pulmonary capillary (C) in the alveolar wall. Note that in many places, the thickness of the blood–gas barrier is less than 0.5 μm. The large arrow shows the diffusion path from the alveolar gas to the interior of the red blood cell (EC) and includes the alveolar epithelium (EP), interstitium (IN), and the capillary endothelium (EN), (these are grouped as (2) in the figure), plasma (3), and red blood cell (4). Other labeled structures include fibroblasts (FB) and the basement membrane (BM). (From Weibel 1970.)*

made of the pulmonary blood–gas barrier in humans and other animals. Since the diffusion rate of a gas through a tissue slice is inversely proportional to its thickness, the appropriate variable to be calculated for diffusion resistance is the harmonic mean of the width of the blood–gas barrier. An intriguing feature of these studies is that the calculated pulmonary diffusing capacity for the human lung is apparently higher than that found experimentally. For example, Gehr and his colleagues (1978) calculated a maximum diffusing capacity in the human lung of 263 mL min⁻¹ mm Hg⁻¹ by morphometry whereas the maximum values found experimentally are generally less than half of this (Riley *et al.* 1954, Shepard *et al.* 1958, Turino *et al.* 1963, Haab *et al.* 1965). The discrepancy may be related to artifacts of the morphometric techniques, for example assuming that all the pulmonary capillaries can take part in gas exchange at any instant of time, whereas in practice some of them may not be recruited even during maximum exercise. However, it should be noted that the measurement of the pulmonary diffusing capacity for oxygen is difficult and indeed some estimates have given values which are closer to the morphometric range (Wagner *et al.* 1987). Nevertheless, there still appears to be a disparity between the anatomical and functional estimates.

6.3.2 Fick's law of diffusion

Fick's law of diffusion states that the rate of transfer of a gas through a sheet of tissue is proportional to the area of the tissue and to the difference in gas partial pressure between the two sides, and inversely proportional to the tissue thickness. As indicated above, the area of the blood–gas barrier in the human lung is some 50–100 m², and the thickness is less than 0.3 μm in many places, so the dimensions of the barrier are well suited to diffusion.

In addition, the rate of gas transfer is proportional to a diffusion constant which depends on the properties of the tissue and the particular gas. The constant is proportional to the solubility of the gas and inversely proportional to the square root of its molecular weight. This means that carbon dioxide diffuses about 20 times more rapidly than oxygen through tissue sheets since its solubility is about 24 times greater at 37 °C and the molecular weights of carbon dioxide and oxygen are in the ratio of 1.375 to 1.

Fick's law can be written as

$$\dot{V}_{gas} = \frac{A}{T} D(P_1 - P_2)$$

where $\dot{V}$ is volume per unit time, A is area, T is thickness, D is the diffusion constant, and P_1 and P_2 denote the two partial pressures.

For a complex structure such as the blood–gas barrier of the human lung, it is not possible to measure the area and thickness during life. Instead, we combine A, T and D and rewrite the equation as

$$\dot{V}_{gas} = D_L(P_1 - P_2)$$

where D_L is the diffusing capacity of the lung.

The gas of choice for measuring the diffusing capacity of the lung is carbon monoxide (at very low concentrations) because the avidity of hemoglobin for this gas is so great that the partial pressure in the capillary blood is extremely small (except in smokers) and thus the uptake of the gas is solely limited by the diffusion properties of the blood–gas barrier. (The complication caused by finite reaction rates is considered below.) Thus if we rewrite the above equation as

$$D_L = \frac{\dot{V}_{CO}}{P_1 - P_2}$$

where P_1 and P_2 are the partial pressures of alveolar gas and capillary blood respectively, we can set P_2 to zero. This leads to the equation for measuring the diffusing capacity of the lung for carbon monoxide:

$$D_L = \frac{\dot{V}_{CO}}{P_{A_{CO}}}$$

In words, the diffusing capacity of the lung for carbon monoxide is the volume of carbon monoxide transferred in mL min^{-1} mm Hg^{-1} of alveolar partial pressure.

6.3.3 Measurement of diffusing capacity

Several techniques can be used for measuring the diffusing capacity of the lung for carbon monoxide. The popular single breath method is essentially a modification of that originally suggested by Marie Krogh (1915). The subject makes a vital capacity inspiration of a very dilute mixture of carbon monoxide, and the rate of its disappearance from alveolar gas during a 10 s breath-hold is calculated. This is often done by measuring the inspired and expired concentrations of carbon monoxide with an infrared analyzer. The alveolar concentration of carbon monoxide is not constant during the breath-holding period but allowance can be made for that; it is assumed that its disappearance is exponential with time. Helium is also added to the inspired gas so that by its dilution the lung volume in which the single breath has mixed can be calculated.

In the steady-state carbon monoxide method, the subject breathes a low concentration of the gas (about 0.1 per cent) for 30 s or so until a steady state of uptake has been reached. The constant rate of disappearance of carbon monoxide from alveolar gas is then measured for a further short period along with the alveolar concentration. The normal value of the diffusing capacity for carbon monoxide at rest is about 25 mL min^{-1} mm Hg^{-1}, and it increases to two or three times this value on exercise.

The measurement of the diffusing capacity for oxygen in humans is much more difficult. An early method was to measure the alveolar–arterial P_{O_2} difference during severe hypoxia (Riley et al. 1954, Shepard et al. 1958) but it is difficult to remove the contribution caused by ventilation/perfusion inequality. Another technique is to use an isotope of oxygen, for example oxygen-18 (Hyde et al. 1966). Other measurements have been made in experimental animals during severe hypoxia, assuming linearity of the oxygen dissociation curve, but this may introduce significant errors.

All methods of measuring pulmonary diffusing capacity are affected by the presence in the lung of ventilation/perfusion and diffusion/perfusion inequalities. No satisfactory way of allowing for these sources of error has yet been devised. However, studies using the multiple inert gas elimination technique can separate the hypoxemia caused by diffusion limitation from that due to ventilation/perfusion inequality (section 6.5).

6.3.4 Reaction rates with hemoglobin

Early workers assumed that all of the resistance to the transfer of oxygen from the alveolar gas into the capillary blood could be attributed to the diffusion process within the blood–gas barrier. However, when the rates of reaction of oxygen with hemoglobin were measured using a rapid reaction apparatus, it became clear that the rate of combination with hemoglobin might also be a limiting factor. If oxygen is added to deoxygenated blood, the formation of oxyhemoglobin is quite fast, being well on the way to completion in 0.2 s. However, oxygenation occurs so rapidly in the pulmonary capillary that even this rapid reaction significantly delays the loading of oxygen by the red cells. Thus the uptake of oxygen can be regarded as occurring in two stages:

- diffusion of oxygen through the blood–gas barrier (including the plasma and red cell interior)
- reaction of the oxygen with hemoglobin (Figure 6.2).

In fact it is possible to sum the two resulting resistances to produce an overall resistance (Roughton and Forster 1957).

We saw above that the diffusing capacity of the lung is defined as

$$D_L = \frac{\dot{V}_{gas}}{P_1 - P_2}$$

that is, as the flow of gas divided by the pressure difference. It follows that the inverse of D_L is pressure difference divided by flow and is therefore analogous to electrical resistance. Consequently the resistance of the blood–gas barrier in Figure 6.2 is shown as $1/D_M$ where M denotes membrane. The rate of reaction of oxygen with hemoglobin can be described by θ, which gives the rate in mL min^{-1} of oxygen which combine with 1 mL blood mm Hg^{-1} P_{O_2}. This is analogous to the 'diffusing capacity' of 1 mL of blood and, when multiplied by the volume of capillary blood (V_C), gives the effective 'diffusing capacity' of the rate of reaction of oxygen with hemoglobin. Again its inverse, $1/(\theta V_C)$, describes the resistance of this reaction.

It is possible to add the resistances offered by the membrane and the blood to obtain the total resistance. Thus the complete equation is

$$\frac{1}{D_L} = \frac{1}{D_M} + \frac{1}{\theta V_C}$$

In practice the resistances offered by the membrane and blood components are approximately equal in the normal lung.

6.3.5 Rate of oxygen uptake along the pulmonary capillary

By using Fick's law of diffusion, and data on reaction rates of oxygen with hemoglobin, it is possible to calculate the time course of P_{O_2} along the pulmonary capillary as the oxygen is loaded by the blood. The application of Fick's law to this situation is not trivial because of the chemical bond which forms between oxygen and hemoglobin. This means that the relationship between P_{O_2} and oxygen concentration in the blood is nonlinear, as shown by the oxygen dissociation curve. This problem was first solved by Bohr (1909) and the numerical integration procedure which he developed is known as the Bohr integration. A further complication occurs because, as oxygen is being taken up, carbon dioxide is given off, and this alters the position of the oxygen dissociation curve. A full treatment of this latter process should take into account not only the rate of diffusion of carbon dioxide through the blood–gas barrier, but also the rates of reaction of carbon dioxide in blood. Since not all the rate constants are known under all the required conditions, some assumptions and simplifications are necessary.

Figure 6.3 shows a typical time course calculated for the lung of a resting subject at sea level (Wagner and West 1972, West and Wagner 1980). The diffusing capacity of the blood–gas barrier itself (D_M) was assumed to be 40 mL min^{-1} mm Hg^{-1}, and the time spent by the blood in the pulmonary capillary was taken as 0.75 s (Roughton 1945). Other assumptions

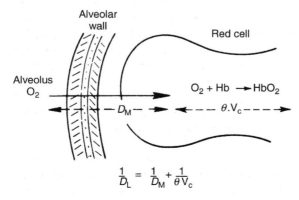

Figure 6.2 *How the measured diffusing capacity of the lung (D_L) is made up of two components, one due to the diffusion process itself (D_M), and one attributable to the time take for oxygen to react with hemoglobin (θV_c).*

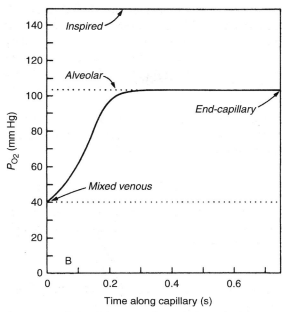

Figure 6.3 *Calculated time course for* P_{O_2} *in the resting human pulmonary capillary at sea level. Note that there is ample time for equilibration of the* P_{O_2} *between alveolar gas and end-capillary blood.* $\dot{V}_{O_2}$ *300 mL min^{-1}; DM$_{O_2}$ 40 mL min^{-1} mm Hg^{-1}. (From West and Wagner 1980.)*

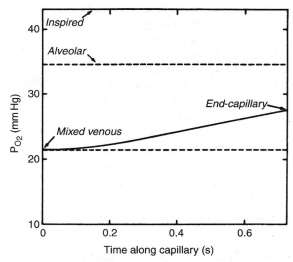

Figure 6.4 *Calculated time course of the* P_{O_2} *along the pulmonary capillary for a climber at rest on the summit of Mount Everest. Note that there is considerable diffusion limitation of oxygen uptake with a large alveolar end-capillary* P_{O_2} *difference.* P_B 253 mm Hg; $\dot{V}_{O_2}$ 350 mL min^{-1} (From West et al. 1983b.)

include a resting cardiac output of 6 L min^{-1} and oxygen uptake of 300 mL min^{-1}.

Note that the blood comes into the lung with a P_{O_2} of 40 mm Hg and the P_{O_2} rapidly rises to almost the alveolar P_{O_2} level by the time the blood has spent only about one-third of its available time in the capillary. The rate of rise of P_{O_2} in the latter two-thirds of the capillary is extremely slow, and there is a negligible P_{O_2} difference between alveolar gas and end-capillary blood.

This time course can be contrasted with that calculated for a resting climber breathing air on the summit of Mount Everest (Figure 6.4). Again, the membrane diffusing capacity of the blood–gas barrier was assumed to be 40 mL min^{-1} mm Hg^{-1} based on measurements made on acclimatized lowlanders at an altitude of 5800 m (West 1962a). The oxygen uptake was taken to be 350 mL min^{-1}, and other blood and alveolar gas variables were taken from measurements made on the American Medical Research Expedition to Everest (West *et al.* 1983b). The time spent by the blood in the pulmonary capillary was assumed to be unchanged at 0.75 s because this is determined by the ratio of capillary blood

volume to cardiac output (Roughton 1945). The capillary blood volume was shown to be unchanged at 5800 m (West 1962a), and the cardiac output is also the same as at sea level according to the measurements of Pugh (1964c) (Chapter 7).

It can be seen that the oxygen profile is very different at this extreme altitude. The blood comes into the lung with a P_{O_2} of only about 21 mm Hg, and the P_{O_2} rises very slowly along the pulmonary capillary, reaching a value of only 28 mm Hg at the end. Thus there is a large P_{O_2} difference of some 7 mm Hg between alveolar gas and capillary blood. This indicates marked diffusion limitation of oxygen transfer. It can be shown that this diffusion limitation becomes more striking as the oxygen consumption is increased by exercise.

The very different time courses for P_{O_2} shown in Figures 6.3 and 6.4 represent the extremes between sea level and the highest point on Earth for resting humans. At intermediate altitudes, the difference between alveolar and end-capillary P_{O_2} will be considerably reduced at rest and may be negligibly small. However, exercise will always tend to increase the alveolar end-capillary P_{O_2} difference.

Whether carbon dioxide elimination is ever limited by diffusion is still unknown. This is partly because some of the reaction rates of carbon dioxide in blood remain uncertain. Many physiologists believe that some diffusion limitation of carbon dioxide output may occur during heavy exercise.

6.3.6 Diffusion and perfusion limitation of oxygen transfer

It is clear from Figure 6.3 that a resting subject at sea level has no diffusion limitation of oxygen transfer because there is no P_{O_2} difference between alveolar gas and end-capillary blood. Under these conditions, the amount of oxygen which is taken up by the blood is determined by the pulmonary blood flow. This means that oxygen uptake is perfusion limited.

By contrast, Figure 6.4 shows a situation where oxygen uptake is, in part, diffusion limited. This is indicated by the large P_{O_2} difference between alveolar gas and end-capillary blood. However, under these conditions, oxygen uptake is also partly perfusion limited because increasing pulmonary blood flow will increase oxygen uptake.

The conditions under which diffusion and perfusion limitation occur have been clarified by Piiper and Scheid (1980). They used a simplified model with several assumptions including linearity of the oxygen dissociation curve in the working range. This is approached during conditions of severe hypoxia when the lung is operating very low on the oxygen dissociation curve, though even here it can be shown

that the rapid elimination of carbon dioxide in the early part of the capillary substantially increases the slope of the oxygen dissociation curve (West 1982b). This introduces appreciable errors; nevertheless, the model is valuable conceptually.

Using this simplified model, Piiper and Scheid showed that the total transfer rate $\dot{M}$ of a gas is given by the expression:

$$\dot{M} = (P_A - P_V)\, \dot{Q}\beta\, (1 - e^{-D/\dot{Q}\beta})$$

where P_A and P_V are the partial pressures of oxygen in the alveolar gas and venous blood respectively, $\dot{Q}$ is cardiac output, D is the diffusing capacity, and β is the slope of the oxygen dissociation curve (assumed to be linear). The total conductance G for gas exchange between alveolar gas and capillary blood may be defined as the transfer rate divided by the total effective partial pressure difference ($P_A - P_V$), or

$$G = \dot{Q}\beta\, (1 - e^{-D/\dot{Q}\beta})$$

This expression clarifies the factors responsible for diffusion and perfusion limitation. The equation shows that if D is very much larger than $\dot{Q}\beta$, the expression inside the large brackets tends to 1, and gas transfer is limited by perfusion only. In this case, the (perfusive) conductance is given by $G = \dot{Q}\beta$. The relative difference between the conductance without diffusion limitation and the actual conductance is an index of diffusion limitation, L_{diff} in Figure 6.5.

By contrast, diffusion limitation occurs if $\dot{Q}\beta$ is so

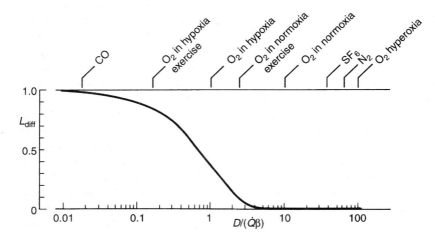

Figure 6.5 Conditions under which diffusion limitation of gas transfer in the lung occurs. L_{diff} is a measure of diffusion limitation; when its value is 1.0, gas transfer is entirely diffusion limited. It can be seen that L_{diff} is greatest for carbon monoxide, and least for oxygen under hyperoxic conditions. D, diffusing capacity; $\dot{Q}$, pulmonary blood flow; β, solubility of the gas in blood, or slope of its dissociation curve. See text for details. (Modified from Piiper and Scheid 1980.)

large that it greatly exceeds D, or to put it in another way, D becomes relatively very small. In this case the (diffusive) conductance is given by $G = D$. The relative difference between the conductance without perfusion limitation and the actual conductance is an index of perfusion limitation. Zero on the vertical axis of Figure 6.5 indicates complete perfusion limitation.

Figure 6.5 shows that oxygen uptake is entirely perfusion limited in hyperoxia (extreme right of diagram) and that this is also true for the uptake of the inert gases nitrogen and sulfur hexafluoride. However, oxygen transfer during hypoxia becomes diffusion limited to some extent (middle of diagram) and this is particularly the case during exercise when oxygen consumption is greatly increased. For carbon monoxide, gas transfer is essentially diffusion limited under all conditions (left of diagram).

The above analysis emphasizes that an important factor leading to diffusion limitation is an increase in β, that is the slope of the blood–gas dissociation curve. This is the reason why the uptake of carbon monoxide is entirely diffusion limited; the slope of its dissociation curve is extremely large. An increased slope of the oxygen dissociation curve tending to diffusion limitation occurs for three reasons at high altitude:

• First, the lung is working on a low part of the oxygen dissociation curve which is very steep.
• Secondly, the polycythemia of high altitude increases the change in blood oxygen concentration per unit change in P_{O_2}.
• Thirdly, the left shift of the curve caused by the respiratory alkalosis increases its slope. In fact, at extreme altitude, oxygen begins to resemble carbon monoxide to some extent.

For readers who prefer an intuitive explanation to the more formal analysis given above, the essential conclusion can be stated as follows. Diffusion limitation is likely when the 'effective solubility' of the gas in pulmonary capillary blood (that is, the slope of the dissociation curve) greatly exceeds the solubility of the gas in the tissues of the blood–gas barrier. This condition is met for carbon monoxide for which blood has an enormous avidity, and is approached for oxygen at high altitude because of the steepness of its dissociation curve at low P_{O_2} values, and the increased blood hemoglobin concentration.

6.3.7 Oxygen affinity of hemoglobin and diffusion limitation

It can be shown that increasing the affinity of hemoglobin for oxygen expedites the loading of oxygen in the pulmonary capillary under conditions of diffusion limitation at high altitude. The oxygen affinity of hemoglobin is conveniently expressed by the P_{50}, that is the P_{O_2} for 50 per cent saturation of the hemoglobin. The normal value is about 27 mm Hg.

Numerical analysis shows that increasing the affinity (leftward shift of the oxygen dissociation curve) results in more rapid equilibration between the P_{O_2} of alveolar gas and pulmonary capillary blood. A simplified way of looking at this is that the left-shifted curve keeps the blood P_{O_2} low in the initial stages of oxygen loading and thus maintains a large P_{O_2} difference between alveolar gas and capillary blood during much of the oxygenation time. This increased P_{O_2} difference therefore maintains the driving pressure and accelerates loading.

However, a left-shifted oxygen dissociation curve interferes with the unloading of oxygen in peripheral capillaries because, for a given P_{O_2} in venous blood (required to maintain the diffusion head of pressure to the tissues), the blood unloads less oxygen. It is therefore not intuitively obvious whether the advantages of a left-shifted curve in assisting the loading of oxygen in the pulmonary capillaries outweigh the disadvantages of unloading the oxygen in the peripheral capillaries.

Several pieces of evidence suggest that a high oxygen affinity of hemoglobin is beneficial under hypoxic conditions. For example, the llama and vicuna, animals native to the Peruvian highlands, have left-shifted oxygen dissociation curves (Figure 6.6), as do some burrowing animals whose environment becomes oxygen depleted (Hall *et al.* 1936). The human fetus, which is believed to have arterial P_{O_2} in the descending aorta of less than 25 mm Hg, has a greatly increased oxygen affinity by virtue of its fetal hemoglobin which has a P_{50} at pH 7.4 of about 17 mm Hg. Experimental studies have shown that rats with artificially left-shifted oxygen dissociation curves tolerate severe acute hypoxia better than rats with normal dissociation curves (Eaton *et al.* 1974). Again, Hebbel and his colleagues (1978) described a family in which two of the four children had an abnormal hemoglobin (Andrew-Minneapolis) with a P_{50} of 17 mm Hg. These two siblings had a higher

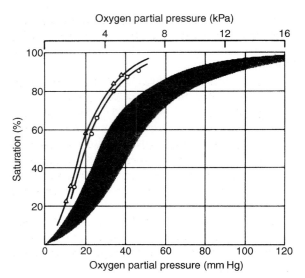

Figure 6.6 *Oxygen dissociation curves for blood of llama (○) and vicuna (△) compared with other mammals. The left-shifted curve for these high altitude native animals indicates an increased affinity of the hemoglobin for oxygen which assists in oxygen loading along the pulmonary capillaries. (From Hall et al. 1936.)*

$V_{O_2 max}$ at an altitude of 3100 m than the two with normal hemoglobin.

Numerical modeling gives some basis for these findings by showing that the increased oxygen affinity of the hemoglobin improves oxygenation in the pulmonary capillaries under conditions of diffusion limitation more than it interferes with the release of oxygen by peripheral capillaries (Bencowitz *et al.* 1982). Table 6.1 lists some of the strategies used by animals (including humans) to increase the oxygen affinity of their hemoglobin under hypoxic conditions.

Table 6.1 *Strategies for increasing oxygen affinity in chronic hypoxia*

Strategy	Subject
Different sequence in globin chain	Human fetus, bar-headed goose, toadfish
Decrease in red cell 2,3-DPG	Fetus of dog, horse, pig
Decrease in ATP	Trout, eel
Different hemoglobin, small Bohr effect	Tadpole
Mutant hemoglobin (Andrew-Minneapolis)	Family in Minnesota
Respiratory alkalosis	Climber at extreme altitude

Climbers at very high altitude tend to have an increased arterial blood pH, which causes a leftward shift of the oxygen dissociation curve. This is caused by a partially compensated respiratory alkalosis and was the case for members of the 1981 American Medical Research Expedition to Everest who spent several weeks at an altitude of 6300 m. The mean arterial pH of three subjects was 7.47 (Winslow *et al.* 1984), which is well above the normal range.

At extreme altitudes, there is evidence of extraordinary degrees of respiratory alkalosis. For example, when Pizzo took alveolar gas samples on the summit of Mount Everest, there is good evidence that his arterial pH exceeded 7.7. This value is based on a measured alveolar P_{CO_2} of 7.5 mm Hg, and a base excess measured in venous blood taken on the following morning of −5.9 mmol L^{-1}. This extreme respiratory alkalosis caused a marked leftward shift of the oxygen dissociation curve with a calculated *in vivo* P_{50} of about 19 mm Hg. Thus a climber on the summit of Mount Everest develops conditions rather similar to those in the human fetus where the arterial P_{O_2} is less than 30 mm Hg and the P_{50} is less than 20 mm Hg.

6.4 PULMONARY DIFFUSING CAPACITY AT HIGH ALTITUDE

6.4.1 Acclimatized lowlanders

Barcroft and his colleagues measured the diffusing capacity for carbon monoxide in five members of the expedition to Cerro de Pasco in the Peruvian Andes in 1921–2. They used the single breath method which had recently been described by Krogh (1915) and the measurements were made at rest. There was no consistent change from the sea level values though the investigators believed that there was a slight tendency for the diffusing capacity to rise. They pointed out, however, that this small change would not be an important element in acclimatization (Barcroft *et al.* 1923). Subsequent investigators have confirmed the absence of change or found only a very small (less than 10 per cent) increase in diffusing capacity for carbon monoxide in resting subjects after periods of up to several months at altitudes of up to 4560 m (Kreuzer and

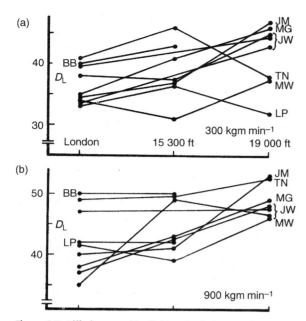

Figure 6.7 *Diffusing capacities (D_L) in mL min^{-1} mm Hg^{-1} measured at sea level (London), 15 300 ft (4700 m) and 19 000 ft (5800 m) in acclimatized lowlanders exercising at: (a) 300 kgm min^{-1} and (b) 900 kgm min^{-1}. Note the moderate increase in diffusing capacity of carbon monoxide with altitude. (From West 1962.)*

van Lookeren Campagne 1965, DeGraff *et al.* 1970, Guleria *et al.* 1971, Dempsey *et al.* 1978).

Measurements on exercising subjects at altitudes up to 5800 m showed that after 7–10 weeks of acclimatization, there was an increase in pulmonary diffusing capacity of 15–20 per cent (Figure 6.7). However, this small change could be wholly accounted for by the increased rate of reaction of carbon monoxide with hemoglobin due to hypoxia and by the increased blood hemoglobin concentration (West 1962a).

The mechanism of this increase can be explained by reference to Figure 6.2. The 'resistance' attributable to the rate of combination of oxygen with hemoglobin is given by $1/(\theta V_C)$. It has been found experimentally that the value of θ varies depending on the ambient P_{O_2}. At low P_{O_2} values, θ is increased and therefore the resistance to oxygen transfer is decreased. An additional factor is the increased blood hemoglobin concentration which, for a given value of V_C (capillary blood volume), increases the amount of hemoglobin present. Thus these factors completely accounted for the small observed increase in diffusing capacity for carbon monoxide at high

altitude and indicated that there was no change in the diffusion properties of the lung itself after 7–10 weeks of acclimatization at an altitude of 5800 m.

Acute mountain sickness (AMS) has been shown to reduce the diffusing capacity for carbon monoxide at high altitude (Ge *et al.* 1997). Presumably the mechanism is subacute pulmonary edema. Interestingly, the diffusing capacity was also reduced following a Himalayan expedition to altitudes of 4900 m and above compared with measurements made prior to the expedition. The fall in diffusing capacity was accompanied by small reductions in maximal cardiac index and $\dot{V}_{O_2 max}$. A possible explanation was the wasting of skeletal muscle which resulted in a reduced cardiac output and therefore diffusing capacity.

6.4.2 High altitude natives

Several studies have shown that people who live permanently at high altitude (high altitude natives or highlanders) have pulmonary diffusing capacities that are about 20–50 per cent higher than the predicted values, or than in lowlander controls (Figure 6.8). One of the first studies was by Velásquez (1956) who studied 12 native residents of Morococha (altitude 4550 m) and showed that the diffusing capacity for oxygen was consistently higher than in similar subjects at sea level. Remmers and Mithoefer (1969) showed that Andean Indians at an altitude of 3700 m had a diffusing capacity for carbon monoxide which was some 50 per cent higher than predicted. High diffusing capacities have also been reported in Caucasians living at an altitude of 3100 m (DeGraff *et al.* 1970, Dempsey *et al.* 1978). The increased diffusing capacities were demonstrated both during rest and exercise.

A potential problem in such studies is the appropriateness of the predicted values for diffusing capacity. For example, in the study by Remmers and Mithoefer (1969), predicted values were obtained from Caucasian North Americans and were applied to the South American high altitude Indian population. This may introduce errors because of ethnic differences in body build. However, in other studies such as that by Dempsey *et al.* (1971), diffusing capacities were compared between lowlanders and highlanders in similar ethnic groups (Figure 6.8).

The increased diffusing capacities can presum-

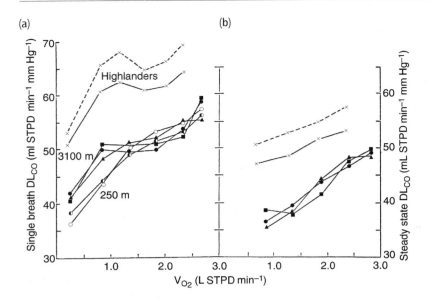

(a)   (b)

Figure 6.8 *Diffusing capacities for carbon monoxide as obtained by the single breath method (a) and steady-state method (b) in three groups of subjects; lowlanders at 250 m (○ and ◐), lowlanders sojourning at 3100 m (●, ▲ and ■ indicate different periods at this altitude), and native highlanders at 3100 m. The broken line indicates the measured data for highlanders; the continuous line shows the results after correction for 1/θ. All the measurements are on white people, the 3100 m data being from Leadville, Colorado. Note the higher diffusing capacities of the highlanders both at rest and on exercise. (From Dempsey* et al. *1971.)*

ably be explained by the larger lungs which result in an increased alveolar surface area and capillary blood volume. Barcroft *et al.* (1923) commented on the remarkable chest development of the Peruvian natives in Cerro de Pasco and these early investigators made chest radiographs to confirm this. The radiographs showed that the ratio of chest width to height was greater in the high altitude natives than in the Anglo-Saxon lowlanders (expedition members). Children who are raised at altitudes of 3000 m have been shown to have increased lung volumes and diffusing capacities (de Meer *et al.* 1995). It has been shown experimentally that animals exposed to low oxygen partial pressures during their active growth phase develop larger lungs and bigger diffusing capacities than animals reared in a normoxic environment (Figure 6.9) (Bartlett and Remmers 1971, Burri and Weibel 1971). This appears to be an adequate explanation for the observed high diffusing capacities, and would also account for the persistence of an increased diffusing capacity for carbon monoxide in highlanders after a prolonged period spent at sea level as observed by Guleria and his co-workers (1971). However, Lechner *et al.* (1982) presented evidence that the lungs only grow faster in a hypoxic environment and the end result is the same lung volume as in normoxic animals. The issue is unresolved.

6.5   DIFFUSION LIMITATION OF OXYGEN TRANSFER AT HIGH ALTITUDE

The significance of pulmonary diffusion at high altitude is that it may be a limiting factor in oxygen uptake. A considerable amount of evidence now supports this.

One of the first groups to suggest diffusion limitation of oxygen uptake at altitude was Barcroft and his colleagues (1923). They concluded from their measurements of pulmonary diffusing capacity for carbon monoxide at an altitude of 4300 m that P_{O_2} equilibration between alveolar gas and the blood at the end of the capillary would not be achieved, especially on exercise. Subsequently Houston and Riley (1947) measured alveolar–arterial P_{O_2} differences in four subjects who spent 32 days in a low pressure chamber in which the pressure was gradually reduced from 760 to 320 mm Hg (Operation Everest I). Measurements were made during rest and during relatively low levels of exercise (oxygen uptakes less than 1200 mL min^{-1} at simulated high altitude). During exercise, the alveolar–arterial P_{O_2} difference was increased to about 10 mm Hg, which they correctly ascribed to diffusion limitation.

During the Silver Hut Expedition of 1960–1, measurements of arterial oxygen saturation by ear oximetry were made on five subjects who lived for

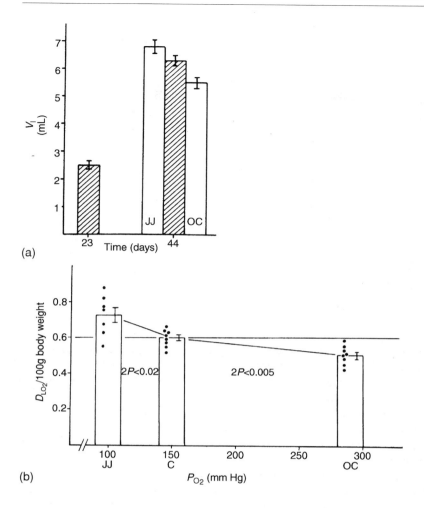

(a)

(b)

Figure 6.9 *(a) Increase in lung volume V_l from day 23 to day 44 of life in three groups of rats exposed to an altitude of 3450 m (JJ), sea level (cross-hatched), and 40 per cent oxygen at sea level (OC). Note that lung volume increased most in the hypoxic and least in the hyperoxic animals. (b) Pulmonary diffusing capacity estimated morphometrically in the same three groups of animals at the 44th day. Note that the diffusing capacities reflected the changes in lung volume. C shows a control group. (From Burri and Weibel 1971.)*

4 months at an altitude of 5800 m (P_B380 mm Hg) in a prefabricated hut. The average arterial oxygen saturation at rest was 67 per cent and this fell at work levels of 300 and 900 kgm min^{-1} to 63 per cent and 56 per cent respectively (West *et al.* 1962). The progressive fall in arterial oxygen saturation as the work level was raised occurred in the face of an increasing alveolar P_{O_2} and was strong evidence for diffusion limitation of oxygen transfer. Alveolar–arterial differences were calculated and nine measurements at the maximal exercise level gave a mean P_{O_2} difference of 26 mm Hg with a standard deviation of 4 mm Hg. Calculations based on the Bohr integration procedure showed that the results were consistent with a maximum pulmonary diffusing capacity for oxygen of about 60 mL min^{-1} mm Hg^{-1}.

Further evidence for diffusion limitation of oxygen transfer during exercise at very high altitudes was obtained on the 1981 American Medical Research Expedition to Everest. Fifteen subjects spent up to 4 weeks at an altitude of 6300 m (P_B 350 mm Hg) and arterial oxygen saturation was measured by oximeter at rest and during increasing levels of work (Figure 6.10). Again there was a progressive fall in arterial oxygen saturation as the work level was increased from rest to 1200 kg min^{-1}, equivalent to an oxygen consumption of about 2.3 L min^{-1}. The calculated alveolar–arterial P_{O_2} difference at this highest work level was 21 mm Hg (West *et al.* 1983c).

Figure 6.10 also shows that additional measurements were made with subjects breathing 16 per cent and 14 per cent oxygen at this very high altitude. The latter gave an inspired P_{O_2} of 42 mm Hg, equivalent to that encountered by a climber breathing air on the summit of Mount Everest. Note the very abrupt fall

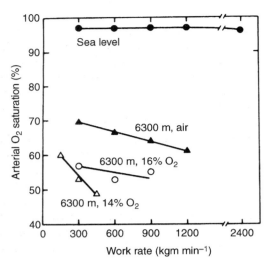

Figure 6.10 *Arterial oxygen saturation as measured by ear oximetry plotted against work rate at sea level and 6300m altitude. The two lower lines were obtained with subjects breathing 16 per cent and 14 per cent oxygen at 6300m. (From West* et al. *1983c.)*

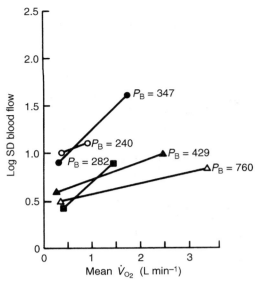

Figure 6.11 *Relationship between the degree of ventilation/perfusion inequality in the lung and oxygen uptake in subjects during a simulated ascent of Mount Everest in a low pressure chamber (Operation Everest II). The ordinate shows the log SD of blood flow which is a measure of ventilation/perfusion inequality. Note that both a reduction of barometric pressure (P_B, measured in mm Hg) and increase in work rate tended to increase the degree of ventilation/perfusion inequality. (From Wagner* et al. *1987.)*

in arterial oxygen saturation as work rate was increased at this highest altitude on Earth. Two subjects performed maximum exercise while breathing 14 per cent oxygen and in one of them the oximeter reading fell to less than 10 per cent oxygen saturation at one point during the experiment! Although the calibration of the oximeter at such values is unreliable, the actual saturation must have been extremely low.

A possible criticism of the measurements described so far is that no account was taken of ventilation/perfusion inequalities within the lung, and these may have contributed to the observed fall in arterial oxygen saturation and the increased alveolar–arterial P_{O_2} difference. Allowance for this possible factor can only be made if there is an independent measurement of ventilation/perfusion inequality. This was done by Wagner and his colleagues, both in an acute low pressure chamber study, and in a 40-day simulated ascent of Mount Everest (Operation Everest II). These studies are important because they show that some increase in ventilation/perfusion inequality occurred at rest and on exercise both during acute exposure to low pressure and in subjects acclimatized to high altitude for periods up to 40 days. The measurements of ventilation/perfusion inequality were made using the multi-

ple inert gas elimination technique (Wagner *et al.* 1974). Inert gas exchange is not diffusion limited, even during maximal exercise.

Figure 6.11 shows the increase in ventilation/perfusion inequality caused both by increasing altitude and increasing work level in the 40-day low pressure chamber experiment (Wagner *et al.* 1987). The vertical scale shows the mean log standard deviation of the blood flow distribution which is one measure of ventilation/perfusion inequality. It can be seen that this index was about 0.5 during rest at sea level but increased slightly when the oxygen consumption was raised to over 3 L min⁻¹ during exercise at sea level. At very high altitude, where the barometric pressure was 347 mm Hg, the resting standard deviation rose to approximately 0.9 and it increased further to over 1.5 with exercise. The explanation of these intriguing data is uncertain but may be subclinical pulmonary edema. There was evidence that rapid ascent was more likely to result in ventilation/perfusion inequality than slow ascent, suggesting that inadequate acclimatization may have been an important factor.

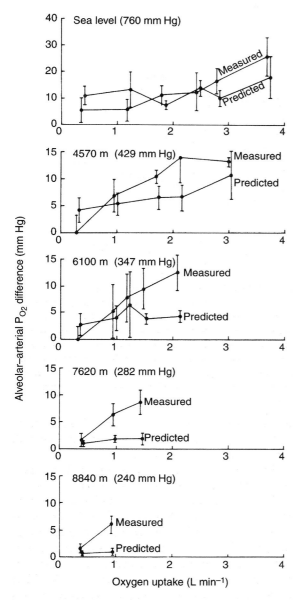

Figure 6.12 *Relationship between alveolar–arterial P$_{O_2}$ difference and the oxygen uptake in Operation Everest II (compare Figure 6.11). The predicted difference refers to that calculated from the measured amount of ventilation/perfusion inequality. Note that, at the highest altitudes, the measured differences considerably exceeded the predicted values, indicating diffusion limitation of oxygen uptake. For the measurements at 240 mm Hg, the subjects breathed an oxygen mixture to give an inspired P$_{O_2}$ of 43 mm Hg. (From Wagner et al. 1987.)*

Using these independent measurements of the amount of ventilation/perfusion inequality present, it was possible to separate the contribution of diffusion limitation and ventilation/perfusion inequality to the observed increase of the alveolar–arterial P$_{O_2}$ difference at high altitude. The results are shown in Figure 6.12. The arterial P$_{O_2}$ was directly measured on arterial samples. It can be seen that the measured alveolar-arterial P$_{O_2}$ difference increased to a mean of about 13 mm Hg during maximal exercise at a barometric pressure of 347 mm Hg where the oxygen consumption was a little over 2 L min^{-1}. At higher simulated altitudes, the maximum alveolar–arterial P$_{O_2}$ differences were smaller. This can be explained by the smaller maximum oxygen uptakes, and the fact that the subjects were operating on the lower, steeper region of the oxygen dissociation curve.

Also shown in Figure 6.12 are the predicted alveolar–arterial P$_{O_2}$ differences for the degree of ventilation/perfusion inequality measured at the same time by means of the multiple inert gas elimination technique. These predicted P$_{O_2}$ differences decreased as the altitude increased despite the broadening of the distributions of ventilation/perfusion ratios as shown in Figure 6.11. Again, the reason is that the P$_{O_2}$ values are lower on the curvilinear oxygen dissociation curve. The data allow the total alveolar–arterial P$_{O_2}$ difference to be divided into two components, one caused by ventilation/perfusion inequality, and the rest presumably attributable to diffusion limitation. The results show that, at sea level, essentially all of the alveolar–arterial P$_{O_2}$ difference was attributable to ventilation/perfusion inequality up to an oxygen consumption of nearly 3 L min^{-1}. Above that high exercise level, some diffusion limitation apparently occurred. By contrast, at a barometric pressure of 429 mm Hg, the measured alveolar–arterial P$_{O_2}$ difference exceeded that predicted from the amount of ventilation/perfusion inequality when the oxygen uptake was above about 1 L min^{-1}. This was also true at a barometric pressure of 347 mm Hg. At the higher simulated altitudes, with barometric pressures of 282 and 240 mm Hg, almost all of the observed alveolar–arterial P$_{O_2}$ difference during exercise could be ascribed to diffusion limitation. These elegant studies go a long way towards elucidating the role of diffusion in the hypoxemia of high altitude during exercise.

6.6   DIFFUSION IN THE PLACENTA AT HIGH ALTITUDE

The fetus derives its oxygen via the placenta rather than the lung. Gas exchange in the placenta is much less efficient than in the lung and, for example, the P_{O_2} in the descending aorta of the human fetus is less than 25 mm Hg. The fetus must be even more hypoxic at high altitude and it is known that birth weight is reduced at high altitude, and that smaller birth weights at high altitude are associated with increased infant morbidity and mortality (Lichty *et al.* 1957, Moore *et al.* 1998a).

An interesting question is whether the diffusion properties of the placenta are improved at high altitude, just as the diffusing capacity in high altitude natives is apparently raised. There is some evidence for this. Reshetnikova *et al.* (1994) examined 10 normal term placentas from women in Kirghizstan up to altitudes of 2800 m and found that there was an increase in capillary volume, and that the harmonic mean thickness of the maternal–fetal barrier fell from 6.9 μm in controls to 4.8 μm at high altitude. They calculated that the morphometric diffusing capacity of the villous membrane for oxygen was significantly increased, by about 80 per cent. However, Mayhew (1991) found somewhat different results in placentas from populations living at 3600 m compared with 400 m altitude in Bolivia. Although there was some improvement in diffusion properties on the maternal side of the placenta, these did not extend to the fetal side. Other research on this important topic is continuing.

7

Cardiovascular system

SUMMARY

Important changes in the cardiovascular system occur at high altitude. Cardiac output increases following acute exposure to high altitude, but in acclimatized lowlanders and high altitude natives, the cardiac output for a given work rate is the same as at sea level. Nevertheless, because of the polycythemia, hemoglobin flow is increased. Heart rate for a given work rate is higher than at sea level, with the result that stroke volume is reduced at high altitude. However, this is not caused by a reduced myocardial contractility; on the contrary, this is preserved up to very high altitudes in normal subjects. Abnormal heart rhythms, such as premature ventricular or atrial contractions, are unusual despite the severe hypoxemia. However, sinus arrhythmia accompanying periodic breathing is very common at high altitude. Changes in systemic blood pressure are small and variable; some studies report a reduction in hypertension when lowlanders move to high altitude. Pulmonary hypertension is striking at high altitude, in both newcomers and high altitude natives, particularly on exercise. There is some evidence that Tibetans have smaller degrees of pulmonary hypertension than other highlanders. The hypertension is relieved by oxygen breathing when the exposure to high altitude is acute, but after a few days the response to oxygen is less, apparently because of vascular remodeling. Right ventricular hypertrophy and corresponding electrocardiographic changes are seen.

7.1 INTRODUCTION

The cardiovascular system is an essential link in the process of transporting oxygen from the air to the mitochondria, and it therefore has an important role in acclimatization and adaptation to the oxygen-depleted environment of high altitude. However, aspects of the cardiovascular system at high altitude have not been as extensively studied as their importance may suggest. The chief reason for this is the difficulties of measurement, especially the invasive investigations necessary reliably to measure cardiac output and pulmonary artery pressure.

In this chapter we look at available data on many aspects of the cardiovascular system, though, as will be seen, there are still many areas of ignorance. This chapter is closely related to some others. The cerebral circulation is discussed in Chapter 16, and changes in the capillary circulation in high altitude acclimatization and adaptation are considered in Chapter 10. High altitude pulmonary edema and high altitude cerebral edema are discussed in Chapters 19 and 20 respectively.

7.2 HISTORICAL

Early travelers to high altitudes frequently complained of symptoms related to the cardiovascular system. Many of these accounts were collected by Paul Bert and set out in the first chapter of his classical book *La Pression Barométrique* (Bert 1878, p. 29 in the 1943 translation). For example, he quotes the great explorer Alexander von Humboldt at an altitude of 2773 'fathoms' (about 5070 m) on Chimborazo in the South American Andes complaining that 'blood issued from our lips and eyes'. Many other travelers gave accounts of bleeding from the mouth, eyes and nostrils, and they often attributed this to the low barometric pressure which, they argued, did not balance the pressures within the blood vessels. Of course this is fallacious reasoning because all vascular pressures fall along with the ambient atmospheric pressure (section 2.1). These early reports of bleeding are intriguing because this is not a typical feature of mountain sickness as we see it today.

Another common complaint of these early mountain travelers was cardiac palpitations, especially on exercise. Typical is the passage quoted by Bert (Bert 1878, p. 37 in 1943 translation) from the explorer D'Orbigny who stated when he was on the crest of the Cordilleras that 'at the least movement, I felt violent palpitations'. The most observant travelers measured their pulse rate and noted that mild exercise such as riding caused it to increase dramatically although it was normal at rest. Cloves of garlic were frequently eaten to relieve these symptoms, which often seem exaggerated to the modern reader.

An interesting historical vignette was the occurrence of edema in cattle while grazing at high altitude in Utah and Colorado early in the twentieth century (Hecht *et al.* 1962). The condition is known as brisket disease because the edema is most prominent in that part of the animal between the forelegs and neck (brisket). The condition is caused by right heart failure as a result of severe pulmonary hypertension caused, at least in part, by hypoxic pulmonary vasoconstriction.

Early climbers on Mount Everest who became fatigued were sometimes diagnosed as having 'dilatation' of the heart. This was thought to be one of the signs of failure to acclimatize. As late as 1934, Leonard Hill stated that 'degeneration of the heart and other organs due to low oxygen pressure in the tissues, is a chief danger which the Everest climbers have to face' (Hill 1934).

7.3 CARDIAC FUNCTION

7.3.1 Cardiac output

It is generally accepted that acute hypoxia causes an increase in cardiac output both at rest and for a given level of exercise compared with normoxia. These responses are seen at sea level following inhalation of low oxygen mixtures, and on acute exposure to high altitude (Asmussen and Consolazio 1941, Keys *et al.* 1943, Honig and Tenney 1957, Kontos *et al.* 1967, Vogel and Harris 1967). There is also good evidence that, in well acclimatized lowlanders at high altitude, the relationship between cardiac output and work rate returns to the sea level value (Pugh 1964c, Reeves *et al.* 1987). On the other hand, there is some uncertainty about the changes following short periods of acclimatization.

Perhaps the first systematic studies of cardiac output at high altitude were made by Douglas, Haldane and their colleagues (1913) on the Anglo-American Pikes Peak Expedition where they made measurements on themselves by means of ballisto-cardiography. No consistent changes in stroke volume of the heart were noted. They therefore concluded that cardiac output at rest was proportional to heart rate, which they showed increased over the first 11 days at 4300 m and subsequently decreased towards normal. Barcroft and his colleagues (1923) used an indirect Fick technique to measure cardiac output in their study of themselves at Cerro de Pasco in the Peruvian Andes at an altitude of 4330 m. They reported essentially no difference in acclimatized subjects compared with sea level.

Grollman (1930) made an impressive series of measurements on Pikes Peak in 1929 using the acetylene rebreathing method. He reported that the cardiac output increased soon after reaching high altitude, with a maximum value approximately 5 days later. However, by day 12 it had returned to its sea level value. Similar changes were found by Christensen and Forbes (1937) during the International High Altitude Expedition to Chile.

Most recent investigators have reported similar findings. Figure 7.1 shows the increase in cardiac output during the first 40 h of acute exposure to simulated high altitude (Vogel and Harris 1967). Klausen (1966) showed an increase in cardiac output following ascent to an altitude of 3800 m but after

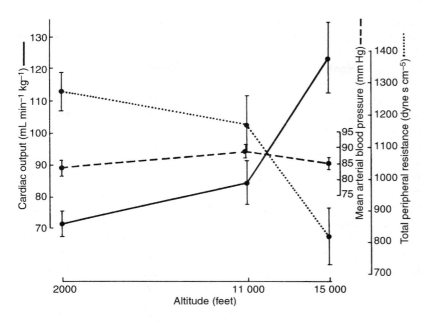

Figure 7.1 *Cardiac output (solid line), mean systemic arterial pressure (dashed line), and calculated peripheral resistance (dotted line) during acute exposure to simulated altitude of 2000 ft (610 m), 11 000 ft (3353 m) and 15 000 ft (4572 m). Measurements were made on 16 subjects after 10, 20, 30 and 40 h at each altitude. The results from the different altitude exposures were pooled. Mean ± SE indicated by vertical bars (1 dyne = 10^{-5} N). (From Vogel and Harris 1967.)*

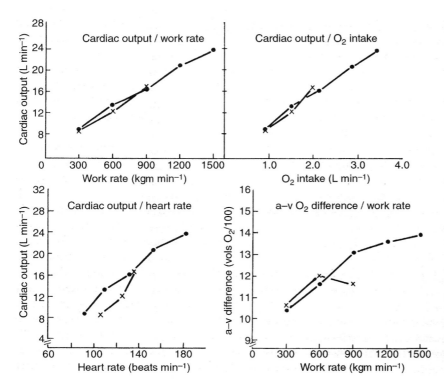

Figure 7.2 *Cardiac output in relation to work rate and related variables as obtained from four well acclimatized subjects during the Himalayan Scientific and Mountaineering Expedition. Note that the cardiac output/work rate relationship is the same at an altitude of 5800 m (×, barometric pressure 380 mm Hg) as at sea level (●). (From Pugh 1964a.)*

3–4 weeks it had returned to its sea level value. Similar findings were reported by Vogel and his colleagues (1967) on Pikes Peak at an altitude of 4300 m. However, Alexander et al. (1967) reported a decrease in cardiac output during exercise after 10 days at 3100 m compared with sea level. The decrease was caused by a fall in stroke volume.

In well acclimatized lowlanders at high altitude, and in high altitude natives, cardiac output in relation to work level is the same as at sea level. This was shown by Pugh (1964c) during the Silver Hut Expedition at an altitude of 5800 m where the measurements were made by acetylene rebreathing (Figure 7.2). Further measurements were made by Cerretelli (1976a) at the Everest Base Camp where the subjects had acclimatized for 2–3 months. Reeves et al. (1987) reported the same finding on subjects during Operation Everest II where a remarkable series of measurements was made down to an inspired P_{O_2} of 43 mm Hg, equivalent to that of the Everest summit (Figure 7.3).

High altitude natives also show the same relationship between cardiac output and oxygen consumption during exercise as at sea level. Vogel et al. (1974) studied eight natives of Cerro de Pasco, Peru, at an altitude of 4350 m and again after 8–13 days at Lima (sea level) and showed that the results were almost superimposable (Figure 7.4).

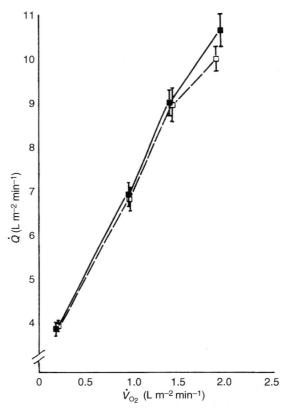

Figure 7.4 *Cardiac index ($\dot{Q}$) against oxygen uptake ($\dot{V}_{O_2}$) (both related to body surface area) in high altitude natives at 4350 m ($\square$) and again after 8–13 days at sea level ($\blacksquare$). (From Vogel et al. 1974.)*

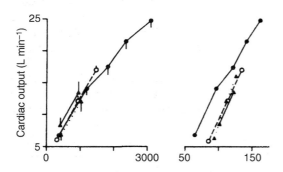

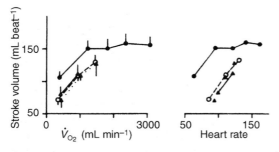

Figure 7.3 *Cardiac output (by thermodilution) and stroke volume plotted against oxygen uptake ($\dot{V}_{O_2}$) and heart rate at barometric pressures of 760 (●, n = 8), 347 (○, n = 6), 282 (△, n = 4) and 240 (▲, n = 2) mm Hg during Operation Everest II. For the measurements at 240 mm Hg, the subjects breathed an oxygen mixture to give an inspired P_{O_2} of 43 mm Hg. (From Reeves et al. 1987.)*

It is perhaps surprising that cardiac output in well acclimatized lowlanders and high altitude natives bears the same relationship to work rate (or power) as it does at sea level. After all, there is plenty of evidence of severe tissue hypoxia during exercise at high altitude, and at first sight it seems that one way of increasing the tissue P_{O_2} would be to raise cardiac output and thus peripheral oxygen delivery. However, in a theoretical study, Wagner (1996) has shown that although increasing cardiac output improves calculated maximal oxygen consumption at sea level, the improvement becomes progressively less as altitude increases. In fact, calculations done for a subject on the summit of Mount Everest show that $\dot{V}_{O_2 max}$ was essentially unchanged as cardiac output was increased from 50 per cent to 150 per cent of its expected value (Figure 7.5).

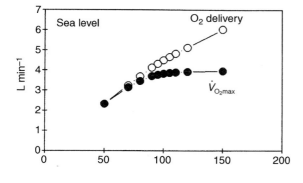

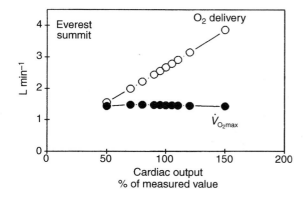

Figure 7.5 *Theoretical study of the effects of changing cardiac output on maximal oxygen consumption ($\dot{V}_{O_2 max}$) at sea level and at extreme altitude. Note that although $\dot{V}_{O_2 max}$ improves at sea level, there is essentially no change at extreme altitude. This is explained by diffusion limitation in the lung and tissues. (From Wagner 1996.)*

A very similar picture emerged when hemoglobin concentration was varied between 50 per cent and 150 per cent of its expected value. Note that in the case of both cardiac output and hemoglobin concentration, calculated oxygen delivery to the tissues was greatly increased. The reason for the lack of improvement in $\dot{V}_{O_2 max}$ with increases in cardiac output and hemoglobin concentration (and therefore oxygen delivery) is that diffusion impairment of oxygen, both in the lungs and in the muscles, reduces its

availability. At medium altitudes, the calculated improvement in $\dot{V}_{O_2 max}$ that accompanies an increase in cardiac output or hemoglobin concentration is intermediate between the values at sea level and extreme altitude.

Although cardiac output in relation to work level is unchanged in acclimatized subjects at high altitude, and in high altitude natives, hemoglobin flow is appreciably increased because of the polycythemia. As long ago as 1930, Grollman suggested that the return of cardiac output to its sea level value was related in some way to the increase in hemoglobin concentration of the blood.

7.3.2 Heart rate

Acute hypoxia causes an increase in heart rate both at rest and for a given level of exercise, just as is the case for cardiac output. The higher the altitude, the greater the increase in heart rate. At simulated altitudes of 4000–4600 m where acute exposure depresses the arterial P_{O_2} to 40–45 mm Hg, resting heart rates increase by 40–50 per cent above the sea level values (Kontos *et al.* 1967, Vogel and Harris 1967).

In acclimatized subjects at high altitude, resting heart rates return to approximately the sea level value up to an altitude of about 4500 m, though there is some individual variation (Rotta *et al.* 1956, Peñaloza *et al.* 1963). On exercise, heart rate for a given work rate or oxygen consumption exceeds the sea level value. Figure 7.6 shows comparisons of heart rate at sea level and at an altitude of 5800 m in four subjects from the Himalayan Scientific and Mountaineering Expedition who were well acclimatized to that altitude (Pugh 1964c). It can be seen that the sea level values were generally lower than the high altitude measurements. However, in three of the four subjects the data points crossed at the highest work level that was tolerated at the high altitude. Note that, in every instance, this crossover was associated with a reduction in measured oxygen consumption, suggesting that at the high work rate, an increasing amount of work was being accomplished anaerobically.

Maximal heart rate, that is the heart rate at maximal exercise, is reduced in acclimatized subjects at high altitude. This is clearly seen from Figure 7.6. In Operation Everest II, maximal heart rates

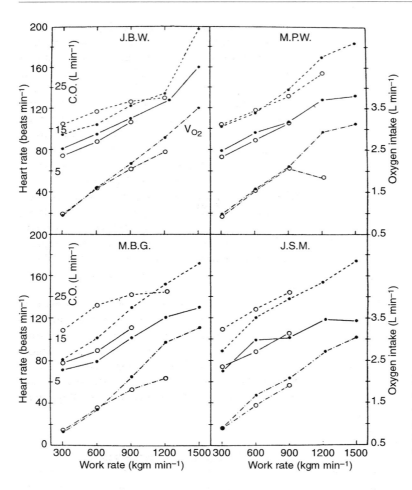

Figure 7.6 *Heart rate (HR, – – –), cardiac output (CO, —), and oxygen uptake ($\dot{V}_{O_2}$, – . – .) against work rate in four well acclimatized subjects at an altitude of 5800 m. Measurements taken at sea level (●) and 5800 m (○, P_B 380 mm Hg). (From Pugh 1964a.)*

decreased from 160 ± 7 at sea level to 137 ± 4 at a simulated altitude of 6100 m, 123 ± 6 at 7620 m and 118 ± 3 at 8848 m (Reeves *et al.* 1987). For a given work level, heart rates were greater at high altitude compared with sea level, though, interestingly, there seemed to be little difference between the measurements made at barometric pressures of 347, 282 and 240 mm Hg, as shown in Figure 7.7. This is possibly a reflection of the limited degree of acclimatization of the subjects at the higher altitudes (West 1988a).

Richalet (1990) has argued that the reduction of maximal heart rate in acclimatized subjects at high altitude represents a physiological adaptation which reduces cardiac work under conditions of limited oxygen availability. There is good evidence that hypoxia induces downregulation of β-adrenergic receptors in animal hearts (Voelkel *et al.* 1981, Kacimi *et al.* 1992). The role of the autonomic

nervous system in controlling heart rate and cardiac output is well established. Short periods of exposure to hypoxia increase the plasma concentration of epinephrine and norepinephrine (Richalet 1990) and the increase in heart rate caused by hypoxia is abolished by beta-blockers (Kontos and Lower 1963).

However, the reduction of maximal heart rate in acclimatized subjects at high altitude can be interpreted differently. Since heart rate is actually increased both at rest and at a given work level compared with sea level (except perhaps at the highest work level; Figure 7.6), it seems reasonable to regard the reduced maximal heart rate simply as a reflection of the reduced maximal work level. For example, it does not seem reasonable that a climber on the summit of Mount Everest where the $\dot{V}_{O_2 max}$ is only 1 L min^{-1} should have a maximal heart rate as

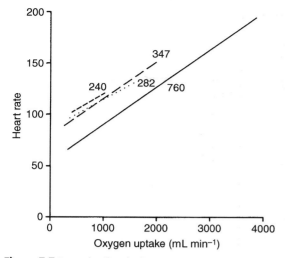

Figure 7.7 *Regression lines for heart rate on oxygen uptake at barometric pressures of 760, 347, 282, and 240 mm Hg during Operation Everest II. For the measurements at 240 mm Hg, the subjects breathed an oxygen mixture to give an inspired P_{O_2} of 43 mm Hg. (From Reeves* et al. *1987.)*

high as the same person at sea level when the $\dot{V}_{O_2 max}$ is 4–5 L min⁻¹.

Oxygen breathing in acclimatized subjects at high altitude reduces the heart rate for a given work level (Pugh *et al.* 1964). This is shown in Figure 11.4 where it can be seen that the heart rate for a given work level was actually lower than the corresponding measurements at sea level. Possible explanations include the fact that the arterial P_{O_2} at this altitude of 5800 m with 100 per cent oxygen breathing is higher than at sea level, and the fact that these subjects had much higher hemoglobin levels than at sea level because of the high altitude polycythemia. It is known that heart rate for a given work rate at sea level is inversely related to hemoglobin concentration (Richardson and Guyton 1959).

7.3.3   Stroke volume

Since stroke volume is determined by cardiac output divided by heart rate, its changes at high altitude can be deduced from those variables described in the last two sections.

Acute hypoxia causes approximately the same increase in cardiac output as in heart rate. The result is no consistent change in stroke volume. This is true for both rest and exercise (Vogel and Harris 1967).

After a few weeks' exposure to high altitude, the cardiac output response to work rate is the same as at sea level (Figures 7.2 and 7.3) but heart rate remains high (Figures 7.6 and 7.7). This means that stroke volume is reduced. The fall in stroke volume has been attributed to depression of myocardial function as a result of myocardial hypoxia (Alexander *et al.* 1967) but, as the next section shows, myocardial contractility is apparently well maintained up to extremely high altitudes. The reduction of stroke volume was also confirmed in Operation Everest II where it was shown that oxygen breathing did not increase stroke volume for a given pulmonary wedge or filling pressure. This suggested that the decline in stroke volume was not caused by severe hypoxic depression of contractility (Reeves *et al.* 1987). A possible contributing factor is a fall in plasma volume.

Studies of high altitude natives at an altitude of 4350 m gave results similar to those found in acclimatized lowlanders. Cardiac output against oxygen consumption at high altitude was almost identical to the sea level measurements (Figure 7.4), whereas heart rate was higher at high altitude and stroke volume was up to 13 per cent less (Vogel *et al.* 1974).

7.3.4   Myocardial contractility

As indicated above, stroke volume is reduced at high altitude both in acclimatized lowlanders and in high altitude natives compared with sea level. The reduced stroke volume could be caused by either reduced cardiac filling or impaired myocardial contractility. A fall in filling pressures could result from either an increased heart rate or a reduction of circulating blood volume, or both.

During Operation Everest II, it was possible to measure both right atrial mean pressure (filling pressure for the right ventricle) and pulmonary wedge pressure (as an index of the filling pressure of the left ventricle). Both these measurements tended to fall as simulated altitude increased (Reeves *et al.* 1987). It was interesting that the right atrial pressures tended to be low despite pulmonary hypertension (section 7.5). In general the relationship between stroke volume and right atrial pressure was maintained. This finding suggests maintenance of contractile function. In addition, as indicated above, oxygen breathing did not increase stroke volume for a given filling pressure, suggesting that the reduced stroke volume was not caused by hypoxic depression of contractility.

Additional evidence to support the finding of normal myocardial contractility came from a two-dimensional echocardiography study during Operation Everest II (Suarez *et al.* 1987). It was found that the ventricular ejection fraction, the ratio of peak systolic pressure to end-systolic volume, and mean normalized systolic volume at rest were all sustained at a barometric pressure of 282 mm Hg, corresponding to an altitude of about 8000 m. Indeed the surprising observation was made that during exercise at the level of 60 W, the ejection fraction was actually higher (79 per cent $\pm$ 2 compared with 69 per cent $\pm$ 8) at a barometric pressure of 282 mm Hg compared with sea level. The conclusion was that, despite the decreased cardiac volumes, the severe hypoxemia and the pulmonary hypertension, cardiac contractile function appeared to be well maintained.

7.3.5 Abnormal rhythm

Abnormal rhythms (apart from sinus arrhythmia during periodic breathing) are uncommon at high altitude and perhaps this is surprising in view of the very severe arterial hypoxemia. A resting climber on the summit of Mount Everest has an arterial P_{O_2} of less than 30 mm Hg (West *et al.* 1983b, Sutton *et al.* 1988). During exercise, the arterial P_{O_2} falls, principally because of diffusion limitation across the blood–gas barrier in the lung (West *et al.* 1983b). Thus the myocardium is exposed to extremely low oxygen levels and it is known that the hypoxic myocardium is prone to rhythm abnormalities (Josephson and Wellens 1984).

In an electrocardiographic study of 19 subjects during the 1981 American Medical Research Expedition to Everest, only one subject had premature ventricular contractions and these were recorded at an altitude of 5300 m. Another climber showed premature atrial contractions at 6300 m (Karliner *et al.* 1985). One subject on the 1960–1 Himalayan Scientific and Mountaineering Expedition showed premature ventricular contractions after exercise at an altitude of 5800 m (Figure 7.8). However, no other member of the

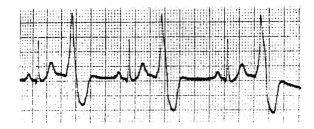

Figure 7.8 *Electrocardiogram showing premature ventricular contractions occurring after exercise at 5800 m. (From Milledge 1963.)*

expedition showed any dysrhythmia (Milledge 1963). Occasional premature ventricular contractions and premature atrial contractions have been observed by others (Cummings and Lysgaard 1981). Thus it appears that extreme hypoxia of the otherwise normal myocardium causes little abnormal rhythm, even at the most extreme altitudes. This conclusion is consistent with the maintenance of normal myocardial contractility even during the extreme hypoxia of very great altitudes (Reeves *et al.* 1987), as discussed in section 7.3.4.

Sinus arrhythmia accompanying the periodic breathing of sleep is extremely common at high altitude (Chapter 13). Indeed, the periodic slowing of the heart can be reliably used to identify the presence of periodic breathing at sea level (Guilleminault *et al.* 1984) and was used in this way with a Holter monitor to detect periodic breathing in climbers at an altitude of 8050 m during the American Medical Research Expedition to Everest (West *et al.* 1986). It is likely that the most extreme arterial hypoxemia for a given altitude occurs during the periodic breathing of sleep following the periods of apnea. It is not surprising that occasional premature ventricular and premature atrial contractions are then sometimes seen. For example, during the four sleep studies at 8050 m, one individual had occasional premature ventricular contractions, another had atrial bigeminy and a third had occasional premature atrial beats (Karliner *et al.* 1985).

7.3.6 Coronary circulation

The myocardium normally extracts a large proportion of the oxygen from the coronary arterial blood, with the result that the venous P_{O_2} has one of the lowest values of all organs in the body. It is perhaps surprising therefore that coronary blood flow has been shown to be reduced in permanent residents of high altitude compared with people at sea level. Moret (1971) measured coronary flow in two groups of people at La Paz (3700 m) and Cerro de Pasco (4375 m) and compared them with a group at sea level. The flow per 100 g of left ventricle was some 30 per cent less in the high altitude natives. A reduction of coronary blood flow in lowlanders following ascent to high altitude was found by Grover et al. (1970).

Despite this, there appears to be little evidence of myocardial ischemia in people living at high altitude (Arias-Stella and Topilsky 1971). These authors showed that casts of the coronary vessels had a greater density of peripheral ramifications than those of sea level controls. This might be part of the explanation for the apparent low incidence of angina and other features of myocardial ischemia.

7.4 SYSTEMIC BLOOD PRESSURE

Acute hypoxia causes essentially no change in the mean systemic arterial blood pressure in humans, at least up to altitudes of 4600 m (Kontos et al. 1967, Vogel and Harris 1967). This is in contrast to the dog, in which acute hypoxia results in a rise of mean arterial pressure (Kontos et al. 1967). Some measurements show that acclimatized lowlanders develop a rise in diastolic pressure with a corresponding decrease in pulse pressure (Brendel 1956). However, other studies suggest that the systemic blood pressure is lower in lowlanders living at high altitude than in sea level residents (Rotta et al. 1956, Marticorena et al. 1969, Peñaloza 1971). In one study, it was shown that a stay of 1 year at an altitude of 4500 m resulted in a decrease of systemic systolic and diastolic pressures (Rotta et al. 1956). In another study it was found that some patients with systemic hypertension who moved to an altitude of 3750 m had a reduction in their level of systemic blood pressure (Peñaloza 1971). A study of the prevalence of systemic hypertension at altitudes of 4100–4360 m in Peru, compared with two communities at sea level, showed a prevalence of hypertension in men at least 12 times greater at sea level than at high altitude

(Ruiz and Peñaloza 1977). The difference was even more marked in women.

In high altitude natives living at 4350 m, Vogel et al. (1974) found that the mean brachial arterial blood pressure was consistently higher during exercise than in the same subjects at sea level. The increase in mean systemic arterial pressure which occurs during the course of heavy exercise is apparently the same in acclimatized lowlanders as it is in sea level residents.

7.5 PULMONARY CIRCULATION

7.5.1 Pulmonary hypertension

One of the most striking cardiovascular changes at high altitude is the occurrence of pulmonary hypertension caused by an increase in pulmonary vascular resistance. This is seen in subjects exposed to acute hypoxia, in acclimatized lowlanders at high altitude and in most high altitude natives. The pulmonary hypertension of acute hypoxia is alleviated by oxygen breathing, but this is not the case in acclimatized lowlanders or high altitude natives. In normal subjects at sea level who are given low oxygen mixtures to breathe, mean pulmonary artery pressure almost always increases. In early studies, Motley et al. (1947) reported an increase of 13–23 mm Hg as a result of breathing 10 per cent oxygen in nitrogen for 10 min. This study followed the initial demonstration by von Euler and Liljestrand (1946) that the pulmonary arterial pressure in the cat increased when the animals breathed 10 per cent oxygen in nitrogen. The increase in pulmonary vascular resistance is caused by vasoconstriction, probably mainly as a result of contraction of smooth muscle in small pulmonary arteries.

Extensive studies of the effects of acute hypoxia on the pulmonary circulation have been made in humans and in a variety of animals. Figure 7.9 shows a typical study by Barer et al. (1970) in anesthetized cats in which the left lower lobe of the lung was made hypoxic and its blood flow was plotted against the alveolar P_{O_2}. Note the typical nonlinear stimulus–response curve. When the alveolar P_{O_2} was altered in the region above 100 mm Hg, little change in blood flow and therefore vascular resistance was seen. However, when the alveolar P_{O_2} was reduced to approximately 70 mm Hg, obvious vasoconstriction

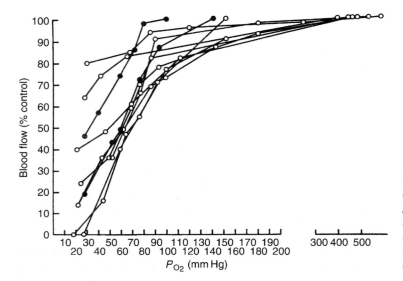

Figure 7.9 *Blood flow from left lower lobe of open-chest anesthetized cats against* P_{O_2} *of the pulmonary venous blood from the lobe. The lobe was ventilated with different inspired gas mixtures while the rest of the lung was breathing air (○) or 100 per cent oxygen (●). (From Barer et al. 1970.)*

occurred, and at very low P_{O_2} values approaching those of mixed venous blood, the local blood flow was almost abolished.

There are differences among species in the stimulus–response curves. In humans, the vasoconstrictor response to acute hypoxia shows considerable variation between individuals, leading Read and Fowler (1964) to refer to 'responders' and 'nonresponders'. Indeed, some people believe that the phenomenon of hypoxic pulmonary vasoconstriction is vestigial in the adult and that its most important function occurs in neonatal life. Here there is a release of pulmonary vasoconstriction when the newborn baby starts to breathe air, and the circulation transforms from the fetal placental mode to the adult lung mode. Presumably this is where the primary evolutionary pressure for the phenomenon comes from.

Acclimatized lowlanders show pulmonary hypertension with a mean pulmonary arterial pressure increasing from its sea level value of about 12 mm Hg to about 18 mm Hg after 1 year at 4540 m (Rotta *et al.* 1956, Sime *et al.* 1974). This resting pulmonary arterial pressure increases considerably during exercise. Figure 7.10 shows the relationship between mean pulmonary vascular pressure gradient across the lung (mean pulmonary arterial pressure minus pulmonary wedge pressure) and cardiac output in the subjects of Operation Everest II (Groves *et al.* 1987). Note that the resting values of the gradient (determined primarily by the mean pulmonary artery pressure) increased, but the most dramatic change was in the slope of the pressure gradient with respect to cardiac output. This indicates the very striking increase in pulmonary vascular resistance at these great simulated altitudes.

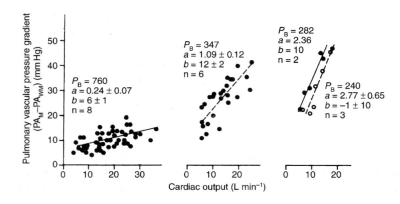

Figure 7.10 *Mean pulmonary artery pressure* (PA_M) *minus mean pulmonary wedge pressure* (PA_{WM}) *plotted against cardiac output (by thermodilution) at various barometric pressures* (P_B) *during Operation Everest II. For the measurements at 240 mm Hg, the subjects breathed an oxygen mixture to give an inspired* P_{O_2} *of 43 mm Hg;* ●, *282 mm Hg;* ○, *240 mm Hg. (From Groves et al. 1987.)*

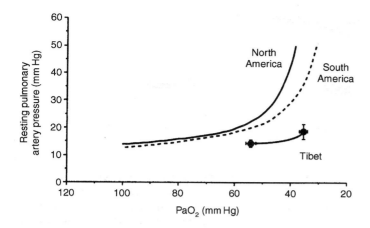

Figure 7.11 *Change in mean pulmonary artery pressure during alveolar hypoxia in five Tibetans compared with high altitude residents of North and South America. (From Groves et al. 1993.)*

High altitude natives also show a substantial increase in mean pulmonary artery pressure during exercise. In one study, mean pulmonary artery pressure increased from 26 to 60 mm Hg during exercise at an altitude of 4500 m (Sime *et al.* 1974). This was a greater increase than that found in acclimatized lowlanders.

In contrast to the dramatic effect of oxygen breathing in acute hypoxia, which causes pulmonary vascular resistance to return to its pre-hypoxic level, oxygen breathing has relatively little effect in acclimatized lowlanders and high altitude natives. For example, in Operation Everest II, 100 per cent oxygen breathing was shown to lower cardiac output and pulmonary artery pressure but there was no significant fall in pulmonary vascular resistance (Groves *et al.* 1987). In interpreting this result it should be recognized that a fall in cardiac output normally results in an *increase* in pulmonary vascular resistance because the reduction in capillary pressure causes derecruitment of capillaries and a reduction in caliber of those which remain open (Glazier *et al.* 1969). Thus the fact that pulmonary vascular resistance did not change when it was expected to rise indicated that oxygen breathing probably reduced vascular resistance to some extent. Nevertheless, it is remarkable that the subjects who were hypoxic for only 2–3 weeks when the measurements were made had a substantial degree of irreversibility of the increased pulmonary vascular resistance. This implies that there were structural changes in the pulmonary blood vessels, in addition to simple contraction of vascular smooth muscle, and is consistent with more recent studies on rapid remodeling of the pulmonary circulation (Tozzi *et al.* 1989).

High altitude natives also show little response of their increased pulmonary vascular resistance to 100 per cent breathing. In this case it is known that there are substantial structural changes in the lungs including a large increase in smooth muscle in the small pulmonary arteries (section 7.5.2).

A study of a small sample of Tibetans suggested that they may have an unusually small degree of hypoxic pulmonary vasoconstriction compared with other high altitude natives (Groves *et al.* 1993). Five normal male residents of Lhasa (3658 m) were studied at rest and during near-maximal ergometer exercise. The resting mean pulmonary arterial pressure and pulmonary vascular resistance were within normal values for sea level. Alveolar hypoxia resulted in a smaller rise of mean pulmonary artery pressure than in other high altitude residents of North and South America (Reeves and Grover 1975) (Figure 7.11). Exercise increased cardiac output more than threefold but did not elevate pulmonary vascular resistance; 100 per cent oxygen breathing during exercise did not reduce pulmonary arterial pressure or vascular resistance. The authors argued that elevated pulmonary arterial pressure in high altitude residents may be a maladaptive response to chronic hypoxia, and the findings indicated improved adaptation in a group that has been at high altitude for a very long period.

7.5.2 Mechanisms and structural changes

In acute hypoxia, the mechanism of hypoxic pulmonary vasoconstriction remains obscure despite a great deal of research. Since the phenomenon occurs in excised isolated lungs, it clearly does not depend on central nervous connections. Furthermore, excised segments of pulmonary artery can be shown to constrict if their environment is made hypoxic (Lloyd 1965), so the response appears to be due to local action of the hypoxia on the artery itself. It is also known that it is the P_{O_2} of the alveolar gas, not the pulmonary arterial blood, which chiefly determines the response (Duke 1954, Lloyd 1965). This can be proved by perfusing a lung with blood of a high P_{O_2} while keeping the alveolar P_{O_2} low. Under these conditions the response is well seen.

The site of the vasoconstriction is still not certain but several pieces of evidence suggest that it is predominantly in the small pulmonary arteries (Kato and Staub 1966, Glazier and Murray 1971). Some studies indicate that the alveolar vessels may be partly responsible for the increased resistance, and contractile cells have been described in the interstitium of the alveolar wall, which could conceivably distort capillaries and increase their resistance (Kapanci et al. 1974). However, the fact that the pulmonary arterial pressure can increase to levels of 50 mm Hg or more in subjects at high altitude without the occurrence of pulmonary edema suggests that the main site of constriction is upstream of the pulmonary capillaries from which the fluid leaks.

Having said this, it is also true that pulmonary edema does occur at high altitude from time to time (Chapter 19) and a likely mechanism is that the hypoxic pulmonary vasoconstriction is uneven (Hultgren 1978), with the result that those capillaries which are not protected from the increased pulmonary arterial pressure develop ultrastructural damage to their walls. This results in a high permeability type of edema. This topic is considered in more detail in section 19.7.5.

As indicated earlier, the mechanism of hypoxic pulmonary vasoconstriction is still unclear. Chemical mediators which have been studied in the past include catecholamines, histamine, angiotensin and prostaglandins (Fishman 1985). Recently, a great deal of interest has been generated by the observation that inhaled nitric oxide reverses hypoxic pulmonary vasoconstriction.

Nitric oxide has been shown to be an endothelium-derived relaxing factor for blood vessels (Ignarro et al. 1987). Nitric oxide is formed from L-arginine via catalysis by endothelial nitric oxide synthase (eNOS)

and is a final common pathway for a variety of biological processes (Moncada et al. 1991). Nitric oxide activates soluble guanylate cyclase, which leads to smooth muscle relaxation through the synthesis of cyclic GMP. Several studies suggest that potassium ion channels in smooth muscle cells may be involved, leading to increased intracellular concentration of calcium ions. Nitrovasodilators, such as nitroprusside and glycerol trinitrate, which have been used clinically for many years, are thought to act by these same mechanisms.

Inhibitors of nitric oxide synthesis have been shown to augment hypoxic pulmonary vasoconstriction in isolated pulmonary artery rings (Archer et al. 1989), and attenuate pulmonary vasodilatation in intact lambs (Fineman et al. 1991). Inhaled nitric oxide reduces hypoxic pulmonary vasoconstriction in humans (Frostell et al. 1993) and sheep (Pison et al. 1993), and lowers pulmonary vascular resistance in patients with high altitude pulmonary edema (HAPE) (Anand et al. 1998). The required inhaled concentration of nitric oxide is extremely low (about 20 µg g^{-1}), and the gas is highly toxic at high concentrations. The recognition of the role of nitric oxide has opened up a new era in our understanding of hypoxic pulmonary vasoconstriction.

Hypoxic pulmonary vasoconstriction has the effect of directing blood flow away from hypoxic regions of lung, caused, for example, by partial obstruction of an airway. Other things being equal, this will reduce the amount of ventilation/perfusion inequality in a lung and limit the depression of the arterial P_{O_2}. This is a useful response. However, the pulmonary hypertension that is seen at high altitude appears to have no value except to cause a more uniform topographical distribution of blood flow (Dawson 1972). In fact, the improvement in ventilation/perfusion relationships resulting from this more uniform distribution of blood flow is trivial in terms of overall gas exchange (West 1962b) and we must conclude that the pulmonary hypertension of high altitude has no useful function, but in fact is deleterious because it is responsible for the occurrence of HAPE. As stated earlier, the evolutionary pressure for the mechanism of hypoxic pulmonary vasoconstriction presumably comes from its value in the perinatal period.

The lungs of long-term residents at high altitude show changes related to pulmonary hypertension (Heath and Williams 1995). Bands of smooth muscle

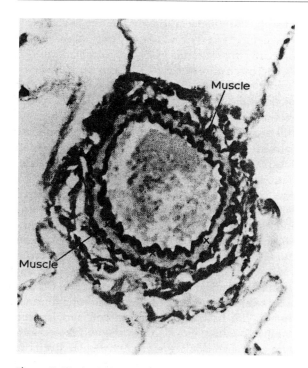

Figure 7.12 *Histological section of a pulmonary arteriole from a Quechua Indian living at high altitude in the Peruvian Andes. Muscle tissue is seen between internal and external elastic laminae. Normally there is a single elastic lamina and no muscle tissue in a vessel of this size at sea level. (Elastic van Gieson stain × 375.) (From Heath and Williams 1977.)*

develop in the small pulmonary arteries (arterioles) of approximately 500 μm diameter which normally have a wall consisting only of a single elastic lamina. The result is that these small vessels develop a media of circularly oriented smooth muscle bonded by internal and external elastic laminae (Figure 7.12). These changes are associated with narrowing of the lumen and an increase in pulmonary vascular resistance. Medial hypertrophy of the parent muscular pulmonary arteries is not a common feature (Arias-Stella and Saldaña 1963), though it occurs in some individuals (Wagenvoort and Wagenvoort 1973). Occlusive intimal fibrosis apparently does not occur. However, longitudinal muscle fibers developing in the intima of pulmonary arterioles in highlanders have been described (Wagenvoort and Wagenvoort 1973). Some authors have also described an increase in mast cell density in experimental animals exposed to long-term hypoxia (Kay *et al.* 1974). This is of

interest because at one stage it was thought that mediators from mast cells, for example histamine, might be involved in the vasoconstrictor response.

These structural changes are consistent with the fact that the pulmonary arterial pressure of high altitude natives falls only slightly (by 15–20 per cent) when oxygen is breathed (Peñaloza *et al.* 1962). These authors showed that inhabitants of Cerro de Pasco (4330 m) who moved to sea level had their mean pulmonary arterial pressure halved from 24 to 12 mm Hg after 2 years of residence at sea level. The fact that lowlanders who are exposed to high altitude for 2–3 weeks develop pulmonary hypertension which is not completely reversed by 100 per cent oxygen breathing (Groves *et al.* 1987) suggests that their pulmonary blood vessels may also have developed some increased smooth muscle.

The structural changes that occur in pulmonary arteries when the pulmonary arterial pressure is raised as a result of exposing an animal to hypoxia are referred to as vascular remodeling (Riley 1991). Meyrick and Reid (1978, 1980) exposed rats to half the normal barometric pressure for 1–52 days. The result was an increase in pulmonary artery pressure as a result of hypoxic pulmonary vasoconstriction. After 2 days they saw the appearance of new smooth muscle in small pulmonary arteries, and after 10 days there was doubling of the thickness of the media and adventitia of the main pulmonary artery due to increased smooth muscle, collagen and elastin, and also edema. There was some recovery after 3 days of normoxia, and after 14–28 days the thickness of the media was normal. However, some increase in collagen persisted up to 70 days.

The molecular biology of the responses of the pulmonary blood vessels has been studied by several groups. Mecham *et al.* (1987) looked at the response of the pulmonary arteries of newborn calves to alveolar hypoxia. There was a twofold to fourfold increase in elastin production in pulmonary arterial wall and medial smooth muscle cells. This was accompanied by a corresponding increase in elastin messenger RNA consistent with regulation at the transcriptional level. Poiani *et al.* (1990) exposed rats to 10 per cent oxygen for 1–14 days. Within 3 days of exposure there was increased synthesis of collagen and elastin, and an increase in mRNA for $\alpha_1(I)$ pro-collagen.

Tozzi *et al.* (1989) placed rat main pulmonary artery rings in Krebs–Ringer bicarbonate. They applied mechanical tension equivalent to a transmural pressure of 50 mm Hg for 4 h, and found increases in collagen synthesis (incorporation of $[^{14}C]$-proline), elastin synthesis (incorporation of $[^{14}C]$-valine), mRNA for $\alpha_1(I)$ procollagen, and mRNA for proto-oncogene v-*sis*. The last may implicate platelet-derived growth factor (PDGF) or transforming growth factor (TGF)-β as a mediator. They were able to show that these changes were endothelium dependent because they did not occur when the endothelium was removed from the arterial rings.

It is possible that this vascular remodeling is a general property of pulmonary vascular endothelium. It has been pointed out that the capillary wall has a dilemma in that it must be extremely thin for gas exchange but immensely strong to withstand the wall stresses when the capillary pressure rises during heavy exercise (West and Mathieu-Costello 1992b). There is good evidence that the extracellular matrix of the blood–gas barrier, at least on the thin side, is responsible for its strength, and it is known that in mitral stenosis, where the capillary pressure rises over long periods of time, there is an increase in thickness of the extracellular matrix (Kay and Edwards 1973). Thus it may be that the capillary is continually regulating the structure of the wall in response to the capillary pressure which is sensed by the endothelium. The capillaries appear to be the most vulnerable vessels in the pulmonary circulation when the pressure rises. Thus vascular remodeling, which has been largely studied in larger blood vessels,

may be a general property of the pulmonary vasculature, and its evolutionary advantage may be primarily to protect the walls of the capillaries.

The mechanism of capillary wall remodeling in response to increased wall stress has been the subject of three recent studies. Berg *et al.* (1997) exposed rabbit lungs to high levels of lung inflation because this is known to increase the wall stress of pulmonary capillaries (Fu *et al.* 1992). Increased gene expression for $\alpha_1(III)$ and $\alpha_2(IV)$ procollagens, fibronectin, basic fibroblast growth factor (bFGF), and TGF-$\beta 1$ was found in peripheral lung parenchyma compared with control animals in normal states of lung inflation. However, mRNA levels for $\alpha_1(I)$ procollagen and vascular endothelial growth factor (VEGF) were unchanged. Parker *et al.* (1997) raised capillary transmural pressure by increasing the venous pressure in isolated perfused rat lungs. There were significant increases in gene expression for $\alpha_1(I)$ and $\alpha_1(III)$ procollagens, fibronectin and laminin compared with controls in which the venous pressure was normal. Berg *et al.* (1998) placed rats in 10 per cent oxygen for periods from 6 h up to 10 days, and the hypothesis was that because the pulmonary vasoconstriction caused by alveolar hypoxia may be uneven, some capillaries may be exposed to a high transmural pressure, and therefore have increased wall stress. Levels of mRNA for $\alpha_2(IV)$ procollagen increased sixfold after 6 h of hypoxia, and sevenfold after 3 days of hypoxia. However, the levels decreased after 10 days of

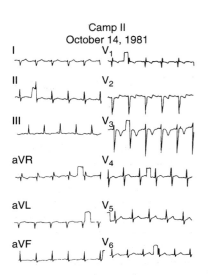

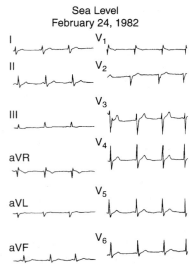

Figure 7.13 *Twelve-lead electrocardiogram obtained at Camp 2 (6300 m) and about 3 months after return of the subject to sea level. Sinus tachycardia and diffuse T-wave flattening present at altitude; the T waves in leads V_2 and V_3 exhibit terminal inversion. (From Karliner* et al. *1985.)*

exposure. mRNA levels for PDGF-B, $\alpha_1(I)$ and $\alpha_3(III)$ procollagens and fibronectin also increased. All the above results are consistent with capillary wall remodeling in response to increased wall stress, but the overall picture is still far from clear.

The environment of the human fetus is similar in some respects to that of the high altitude dweller in that the arterial P_{O_2} is less than 30 mm Hg, based on measurements on experimental animals (Itskovitz *et al.* 1987). The fetus also has pulmonary hypertension because the pulmonary artery is connected to the systemic arterial system through the patent ductus arteriosus. In keeping with this, the fetal lung shows a high degree of muscularization, of the pulmonary arteries. Babies born at a high altitude show persistence of this muscularization, whereas the pulmonary arteries of those born at sea level assume the adult appearance after only a few weeks.

7.5.3 Right ventricular hypertrophy

The pulmonary hypertension of high altitude causes right ventricular hypertrophy both in acclimatized lowlanders and in high altitude natives. In one study of children of 2–10 years of age it was shown that at sea level the ratio of left to right ventricular weights was about 1.8, whereas at high altitude it was less than 1.3 (3700–4260 m) (Arias-Stella and Recavarren 1962). Experimental studies on rats exposed to an altitude of 5500 m showed that they developed right ventricular hypertrophy within 5 weeks (Heath *et al.* 1973).

Data on acclimatized lowlanders are not generally available, though there is abundant indirect evidence of right ventricular hypertrophy from electrocardiographic changes (section 7.5.4). Occasionally, climbers returning from high altitude have shown evidence of right heart enlargement on the chest radiograph (Pugh 1962a).

7.5.4 Electrocardiographic changes

Electrocardiographic changes are considered here because most of the changes are attributable to pulmonary hypertension. An extensive study was carried out during the 1981 American Medical Research Expedition to Everest (Karliner *et al.* 1985) when recordings were made at sea level, 5400 m,

6300 m, and again at sea level. A total of 19 subjects were studied, though complete data were not obtained from all. Resting heart rate increased from a mean of 57 at sea level to 70 at 5400 m and 80 at

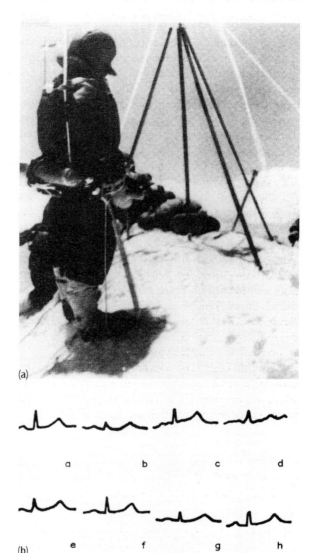

Figure 7.14 (a) Ms Phantog, deputy leader of the 1975 Chinese Expedition to Everest, lying under the tripod that was placed on the summit. Lead 1 of her electrocardiogram was telemetered to Base Camp (from Another Ascent of the World's Highest Peak, Qomolangma 1975). (b) Standard lead 1 of the ECG of Ms Phantog from 50 m altitude to 8848 m (Everest summit) and back to 50 m: a, 50 m; b, 500 m; c, 6500 m; d, 8848 m (summit); e, back at 500 m; f, 1 month after returning to 50 m; g, 2 months after returning to 50 m; h, 3 months after returning to 50 m. No obvious changes are seen. (From Zhongyuan et al. 1980.)

6300 m (compare section 7.3.2). The amplitude of the P wave in standard lead 2 of the electrocardiogram increased by over 40 per cent from sea level to 6300 m, consistent with right atrial enlargement. Right axis deviation of the QRS axis was seen. The mean frontal plane QRS axis increased from +64° to +78° at 5400 m and +85° at 6300 m. Three subjects showed abnormalities of right bundle branch conduction at the highest altitude and three others showed changes consistent with right ventricular hypertrophy (posterior displacement of the QRS vector in the horizontal plane). Seven subjects developed flattened T waves and four showed T-wave inversions (Figure 7.13). All the changes returned to normal in tracings obtained at sea level after the expedition.

Other investigators have reported similar findings in acclimatized lowlanders, though generally on smaller numbers or at lower altitudes. Milledge (1963) made measurements during the 1960–1 Himalayan Scientific and Mountaineering Expedition and reported data on subjects who spent several months at an altitude of 5800 m. In addition some recordings were made as high as 7440 m in climbers who never used supplemental oxygen. He found T-wave inversions on the right pre-cordial leads in six subjects; two had left pre-cordial T-wave inversion as well. Oxygen breathing had no effect on these changes. Das *et al.* (1983) reported on over 40 subjects who were rapidly transported to either 3200 or 3771 m. There was a tendency for a rightward axis shift which, interestingly, tended to resolve in most subjects after 10 days at high altitude.

A particularly remarkable measurement was made on Ms Phantog, deputy leader of the successful 1975 Chinese ascent of Mount Everest. She lay down on the summit under the newly erected tripod while her standard lead 1 was telemetered down to Base Camp (Figure 7.14). Note that there were no changes from sea level to 8848 m and back again (Zhongyuan *et al.* 1980). Other electrocardiographic studies at high altitude include those made by Peñaloza and Echevarria (1957), Jackson and Davies (1960), Aigner *et al.* (1980), Kapoor (1984), Halperin *et al.* (1998), Malconian *et al.* (1990) and Chandrashekhar *et al.* (1992).

8

Hematology

SUMMARY

The best known aspects of altitude acclimatization are the increase in red cell numbers per unit volume and the increase in hemoglobin concentration. These are achieved, initially, by a reduction in plasma volume and later by an increase in red cell mass (RCM). Hypoxia induces the release of erythropoietin (EPO), which stimulates the bone marrow to increase red cell output. The EPO gene is induced by hypoxia through a nuclear factor, the hypoxia-inducible factor-1 (HIF-1). Although EPO levels rise within a few hours, the increase in RCM takes weeks and only reaches a steady state after some 6 months. Plasma volume is restored to near sea level values after a few weeks. The rise in hemoglobin concentration is roughly linear with altitude and is similar in acclimatized lowlanders and residents of high altitude, though with wide individual variation. Evidence is accumulating that Tibetans have lower hemoglobin concentration than Andean residents at similar altitudes. Extreme polycythemia among residents or lowlanders staying at altitude for many years, is considered pathological and termed chronic mountain sickness (Chapter 21).

The effect of altitude on white cells has been little studied. Changes are variable, though increase in CD16 natural killer cells has been reported.

The effects of altitude on platelets and clotting are considered in Chapter 22.

8.1 INTRODUCTION

Probably the best-known adaptation to high altitude is the increase in the number of red cells per unit volume of blood. Paul Bert suggested in his book *La Pression Barométrique* (1878) that adaptation to high altitude might include an increase in the number of red cells and in the quantity of hemoglobin. Thus the blood would be able to carry more oxygen. A few years later he was sent samples of blood from a number of domestic animals from La Paz, Bolivia (3500 m). He showed that these samples combined with 16.2–21.6 volumes of oxygen per 100 volumes of blood compared with 10–12 volumes per cent in the blood of animals in France (West 1981).

Viault, in 1890, made the first blood counts of men at high altitude. His own blood count at sea level in Lima was 5 million mL^{-1} and after 3 weeks at Morococha, a mining township at 4372 m in the Andes, the value had increased to 7.1 million mL^{-1}. We now know that most of this increase, early in altitude exposure, would be due to reduced plasma volume rather than an increase in RCM. Viault found these elevated counts present in a companion doctor from Lima and also in a number of the local Indian residents at altitude. He also noted that in a male llama the value was 16 million mL^{-3}. He called the llama, 'l'animal par excellence des grandes altitudes', although, in fact, since the llama has very small red cells, the hemoglobin concentration of the blood is the same as in humans. In 1891 Viault published further observations which confirmed Bert's work on the oxygen-carrying capacity of high altitude animals. He showed in two sheep and one dog that their oxygen-carrying capacity was increased compared with similar animals in France.

Since then, almost all expeditions with any pretence at carrying out physiological research at high altitude have observed this increase in red cell count, packed cell volume, or hemoglobin concentration. ∆ The increase in red cell number and hemoglobin concentration increases the oxygen-carrying capacity in such a way that, up to about 5300 m, fully acclimatized humans have the same oxygen content in their blood as at sea level (Figure 8.1). ⋆ The increased carrying capacity compensates for the reduced oxygen saturation. This affords physiology teachers a classical example of beneficial adaptation. However, it is unlikely that the mechanism of this adaptation evolved primarily to serve humans at high altitude (section 8.2.1). The extent to which benefit can be gained by increasing hemoglobin concentration is fairly limited and indeed has been questioned as beneficial at all (Winslow and Monge 1987, p. 203; section 8.5.4).

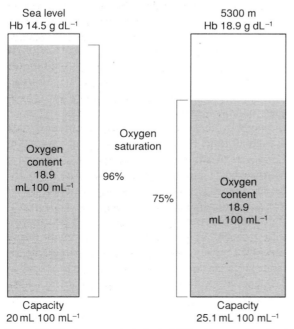

Figure 8.1 *The oxygen content of arterial blood in an acclimatized subject at 5300 m and at sea level.*

8.2 REGULATION OF HEMOGLOBIN CONCENTRATION

The hemoglobin concentration and packed cell volume (PCV) depend upon the ratio of the RCM to plasma volume (PV). These two variables are regulated by different mechanisms. The rate of formation of red cells (erythropoiesis) and their rate of loss determine the RCM.

Red blood cells are lost by death (their natural length of survival is about 120 days), or by hemorrhage. Their death can be hastened by a variety of pathological states such as hemolytic anemia. Erythropoiesis can be impaired by various deficiencies, such as iron or vitamin B_{12} (needed for hemoglobin synthesis), or by disorders of the bone marrow. In the absence of these, erythropoiesis is controlled by the level of the hormone EPO.

8.2.1 EPO and its regulation

EPO is produced mainly in the kidney, though 10–15 per cent of total production is in the liver (Erslev 1987). The gene coding for the hormone has been cloned and expressed in cultured cells, allowing for sufficient material to be produced for clinical studies. It has been shown to stimulate erythropoiesis in patients anemic with end-stage renal failure (Winearls *et al.* 1986).

The two classical stimuli for EPO secretion are hypoxia and blood loss, both of which result in tissue hypoxia. Of the two, blood loss is probably more important in evolutionary terms of survival of the organism. Blood loss is a far more common danger than is chronic hypoxia, and of course this system is no defense against acute hypoxia. The stimulus to EPO secretion is hypoxia at some tissue site, probably in the kidney, possibly identical with the site of production of the hormone. It is instructive to compare this system with another hypoxia-sensitive system in the body, the hypoxic ventilatory response (HVR), mediated mainly via the carotid body:

- The HVR appears in seconds after a step change in arterial P_{O_2} whereas there is no detectable rise in EPO concentration for over an hour, 114 min when exposed suddenly to 3000 m or 84 min at 4000 m (Eckardt *et al.* 1989).

- The carotid body is sensitive to reduction in P_{O_2} rather than oxygen content of the blood. Therefore it does not respond to anemia, whereas anemia stimulates EPO secretion.

From these observations it is assumed that, whereas the carotid body response is to arterial P_{O_2}, the sensing of P_{O_2} for EPO secretion is at the venous or tissue level. In patients with a reversed flow through a patent ductus arteriosus, there is cyanosis (hypoxia) in the lower half of the body only. These patients have high hemoglobin concentration, indicating that the P_{O_2} sensor is in the lower half of the body, presumably in the kidney. Fisher and Langston (1967) showed that EPO was produced in the juxtaglomerular apparatus in the kidney and that hypoxia was sensed there, since the isolated dog kidney increased its output of EPO when perfused with hypoxic blood.

8.2.2   Regulation of plasma volume

The central control of PV is probably by a feedback loop involving atrial natriuretic peptide (ANP) and the right atrium (Laragh 1985). ANP is released in response to stretching of the right atrium. Physiologically, this is produced by increased right atrial pressure. This in turn may be due to shifts of blood volume from the periphery, mainly the lower body, or by increase in the total blood volume (i.e. PV). ANP causes the kidney to excrete sodium and with it water, thus reducing the PV. This simple feedback loop is shown in Figure 8.2.

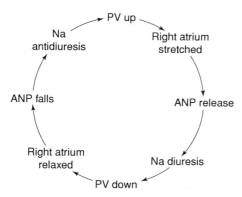

Figure 8.2 *The regulation of plasma volume (PV) by atrial natriuretic peptide (ANP).*

We can add on to this simple system a host of other factors which affect PV (Figure 8.3):

- Hydration and dehydration will obviously affect PV, along with all other body fluid compartments.
- The vascular capacity is determined by the tone of the vessels, especially the venous capacitance vessels and vessels in the skin. Vessel tone, in turn, depends on a number of factors, such as temperature and catecholamine levels. Peripheral vasoconstriction shifts blood from the periphery to the center, raising right atrial pressure and stimulating ANP release. Vasodilatation has the opposite effect. A change in vascular capacity also has a more direct effect on PV by shifting the balance of forces in the Starling equation. Vasodilatation will tend to reduce the intravascular pressure, favoring inward movement of fluid at the tissue level; vasoconstriction has the opposite effect. It is this direct effect that is depicted in Figure 8.3.
- Other factors that cause a shift of blood volume to the center include lying down, lower body immersion and G-suits. Zero gravity experienced by astronauts has a similar effect. Right atrial pressure is raised and ANP excretion is increased. Conversely, the upright position tends to shift volume away from the center to the lower body, reducing right atrial pressure and inhibiting ANP release.
- Antidiuretic hormone (ADH) secretion will result in increased PV by retaining water, but there is another feedback loop involving plasma osmolality and ADH. If plasma volume increase is caused by hydration, osmolality falls and secretion of ADH is inhibited. A water diuresis then follows which restores the osmolality and ADH levels rise again. This loop is not shown in Figure 8.3, to avoid overloading the diagram.
- The sodium status is important in determining the PV. A high sodium intake will tend to cause water retention and increase PV. Increase in ANP will then compensate for this. Stimulation of the renin–angiotensin–aldosterone system causes sodium retention with the same result. Renin is stimulated by posture (the upright position) and by exercise, though posture and exercise have effects on PV via other mechanisms (section 8.2.3).

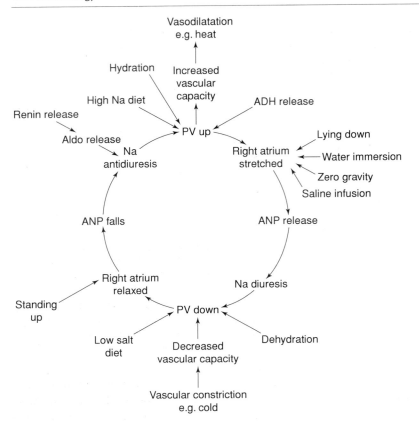

Figure 8.3 *Some of the factors affecting plasma volume (PV) and its regulation by atrial natriuretic peptide (ANP), antidiuretic hormone (ADH), aldosterone (Aldo) and vascular capacity.*

8.2.3   Posture and plasma volume

Seventy per cent of the blood volume is below the heart in the upright position and, of this, 75 per cent is in the distensible veins. On standing up, 500 mL of additional blood enters the legs, so that reflex tachycardia and vasoconstriction are essential to prevent fainting. Vasoconstriction maintains the blood pressure and reduces flow, especially to the skin, muscles, kidneys and viscera. The capillaries are exposed to the hydrostatic pressure of the column of venous blood. This will tend to increase filtration of fluid out of the vascular compartment, and hemoconcentration would be expected. Numerous investigators from Thompson *et al.* (1928) onwards have confirmed these theoretical expectations. Thompson *et al.* found a reduction of plasma volume of 15 per cent on assuming the upright position, but the magnitude of this effect is variable and is influenced by many factors, including environmental and subject temperature, state of hydration, etc.

The effect of posture is therefore significant and needs to be taken into account when considering the effect of other variables such as hypoxia or exercise on plasma volume.

8.2.4   Exercise and plasma volume

Exercise can have an important effect on plasma volume and hence on hemoglobin concentration and PCV, but the effect varies according to the intensity, duration and type of exercise. The temperatures of the environment and the subject modify the effect. It is also modified by posture (section 8.2.3). This is because temperature and posture affect the skin blood flow and hence the distribution of cardiac output to skin, working muscles, kidneys, splanchnic area, etc. This, in turn, affects the capillary and venous pressures in these areas and hence the balance of forces in the Starling equation. Many studies on the effect of exercise have ignored the effect of posture and have taken control samples in a different posture from exercise samples.

Harrison (1985) has reviewed the literature and, with a number of reservations, comes to the conclusion that, for bicycle ergometer exercise, there is a reduction in the PV soon after starting exercise. This reduction is proportional to the intensity of exercise or, more precisely, to the rise in atrial pressure. Thereafter there is little change with continued exercise at normal room temperature but in high temperatures there is a further reduction in PV with time. However, these laboratory studies tend to look at fairly high intensity exercise (greater than 50 per cent $V_{O_2 max}$) for periods of up to an hour or two.

Exercise on mountains is taken over periods of many hours and may go on day after day. The availability of fluid for drinking will obviously make a difference. If this is not available, dehydration will certainly reduce PV, but usually fluid is available to climbers and exercise heat stress can usually be avoided. Under these circumstances of exercise of 8 h or more at normal climbing rates (i.e. up to about 50 per cent $V_{O_2 max}$ but averaging much less) an increase in PV is found. Pugh (1969) found an increase in blood volume of 7 per cent after a 28 mile hill walk. Williams *et al.* (1979) found PV increased progressively for 5 days of strenuous daily hill walking to reach a 22 per cent expansion. Both these studies were carried out under cold conditions and subjects avoided both overheating and cold stress. The changes in PV, interstitial and intracellular volumes are shown in Figure 8.4.

The mechanism is probably via activation of the renin–angiotensin–aldosterone system, which results in sodium retention and thus a general expansion of the extracellular fluid (ECF) volume including the PV (Milledge *et al.* 1982). Under these circumstances the PCV decreased from a mean of 43.5 per cent to 37.9 per cent after 5 days of exercise.

8.3 EFFECT OF ALTITUDE ON PLASMA VOLUME

During the first few hours of altitude exposure the effect on PV is variable and data are scanty. In the field, the effect of hypoxia may be overshadowed by that of cold, dehydration and exercise but it seems that those subjects free from acute mountain sickness (AMS) have a diuresis and contract their PV. Singh *et*

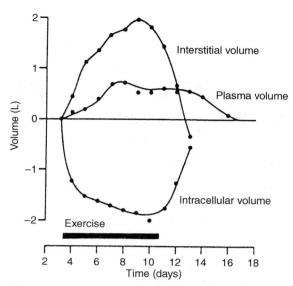

Figure 8.4 *The effect of five consecutive days' strenuous hill walking on body fluid compartments. The changes are calculated from changes in packed cell volume, and sodium and water balances. (Reproduced with permission from Williams et al. 1979.)*

al. (1990) found a reduction in PV from 40.4 mL kg^{-1} at sea level to 37.7 mL kg^{-1} on day 2 at 3500 m, and 37.0 mL kg^{-1} on day 12. Wolfel *et al.* (1991) reported similar changes in PV on ascent to 4300 m; PV fell from 48.8 mL kg^{-1} to 42.5 mL kg^{-1} on arrival at altitude and to 40.2 mL kg^{-1} by day 21. Some caution must be exercised in the interpretation of these studies in the light of a recent study by Poulson *et al.* (1998). They measured the change in PV of 10 subjects on being airlifted to the Vallot observatory (4350 m) using both the Evans' blue and the carbon monoxide methods. Twenty-four hours after arrival at altitude they found the expected reduction in PV with the carbon monoxide method (350 mL reduction) but not with the Evans' blue method (30 mL reduction). A possible explanation is that hypoxia induced an increase in capillary permeability to albumin so that the Evans' blue method, which would have included this extravascular pool of albumin, gave a falsely high result.

Subjects with AMS have an antidiuresis and probably expand their PV. Vigorous exercise taken on getting up to altitude or on arrival will also result in expansion of the PV, via the renin–aldosterone system (Milledge *et al.* 1983d).

Honig (1983) has reviewed the effect of acute hypoxia on body fluid volumes, especially in animal experiments. With exposure to moderate hypoxia equivalent to altitudes of 3000–6000 m there is a diuresis and natriuresis. After reviewing possible mechanisms via effects on the cardiovascular system, Honig presents evidence, from his own work, that the carotid body, stimulated by hypoxia, reduces the reabsorption of sodium by the kidney via neural pathways. This mechanism has not been demonstrated in humans. (This comprehensive review antedates the recognition of the importance of atrial natriuretic peptide.)

After this early phase of altitude exposure, there is a definite reduction in PV over the next few weeks. Pugh (1964b) found a 21 per cent reduction in PV after 18 weeks at altitudes above 4000 m in four members of the 1960–1 Silver Hut Expedition (Figure 8.5). During the following 7–14 weeks the PV returned towards control levels, values being on average 10 per cent less than control when corrected for changes in body weight.

Sanchez et al. (1970) found altitude residents at Cerro de Pasco (4370 m) in Peru to have a mean PV two-thirds that of a group of students at Lima (sea level). When allowance was made for the weight difference of the groups they still had a PV 27 per cent less in a blood volume that was 14 per cent greater.

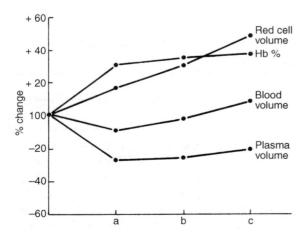

Figure 8.5 *Changes in hemoglobin concentration (Hb%), red cell volume, blood volume and plasma volume in four subjects during the Silver Hut Expedition: (a) after 18 weeks at between 4000 and 5800 m; (b) after a further 3–6 weeks at 5800 m; (c) after a further 9–14 weeks at or above 5800 m. (After Pugh 1964b.)*

8.4 ALTITUDE AND ERYTHROPOIESIS

8.4.1 EPO, HIF-1 and hypoxia

EPO is a hormone secreted by peritubular cells in the kidney. It is one of a number of gene products whose transcription is stimulated by hypoxia. These include aldolase A, enolase-1 glucose transporter-1, lactate dehydrogenase and phosphofructokinase, all involved with glycolysis; inducible nitric oxide synthase and heme oxygenase, involved with vasodilatation; and vascular endothelial growth factor which promotes angiogenesis. The link between hypoxia and the induction of the genes for all these proteins involves the recently discovered HIF-1. HIF-1 is a nuclear factor induced by hypoxia which binds to the promoter part of these genes. It was first identified as a nuclear factor that bound to the hypoxia response element of the EPO gene (Semenza et al. 1998). The other hypoxia-induced genes all have similar core binding sites for HIF-1.

8.4.2 Altitude and serum EPO concentration

Until about 1980, measurements of EPO in blood were by bioassays which could not detect the hormone until its concentration was above normal sea level values. Therefore, earlier work often relied on more indirect indices of erythropoietic activity such as intestinal iron absorption or reticulocyte counts. The latter is a rather late effect. Intestinal iron absorption has been shown to be independent of EPO and to be promoted as a direct effect of hypoxia rather than secondary to plasma iron turnover or erythropoietic activity (Raja et al. 1986). On going to altitude there is an elevation of EPO concentration in the first 24–48 h (Siri et al. 1966, Albrecht and Little 1972). Newer methods of EPO estimation using radioimmunoassays are sensitive to levels of EPO well below the normal range (13–37 mIU mL^{-1}). Using this type of assay it has been found that serum immunoreactive EPO concentration (SiEp) begins to rise within 2 h of hypoxic exposure, depending on the altitude (Eckardt et al. 1989), and reaches a maximum at about 24–48 h. Thereafter, it declines to reach values not measurably different from controls after about 3 weeks (Milledge and Cotes 1985). This is shown in Figure 8.6, which also shows the rise in

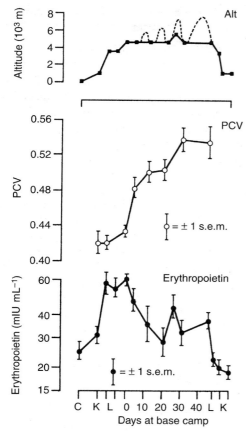

Figure 8.6 *The effect of going to altitude on the serum erythropoietin concentration. The top panel shows the altitude/time profile for the eight subjects. The dotted line indicates ascent above base camp between blood samples. Note, the samples at 30 days were taken at 5500 m after four sample times at base camp (4500 m). Mean packed cell volume (PCV) is shown in the center panel and mean erythropoietin concentration in the lower panel. C, control, sea level; K, Kashgar (1200 m); L, Karakol lakes (3500 m). (Reproduced with permission from Milledge and Cotes 1985.)*

PCV on going to altitude. A similar rapid rise and decline was found by Gunga *et al.* (1994) at the modest altitude of 2315 m.

The rise in SiEp with altitude shows great individual variability. In a study in the Andes, Richalet *et al.* (1994) found the increase to range from threefold to 134-fold in their group of subjects 1 week after arrival at 6540 m.

Figure 8.6 also shows that, even after 3 weeks above 4500 m, a rise in altitude to 5500 m caused another rise in SiEp. Quite a short pulse of hypoxia initiates a rise in SiEp, which continues after

normoxia is restored. For instance, 120 min breathing 10 per cent oxygen caused SiEp to rise just after normoxia was restored and the rise continued for a further 120 min (Knaupp *et al.* 1992).

It will be seen from Figure 8.6 that PCV continues to rise after SiEp falls to near control values. The rise in RCM continues even longer (section 8.4.3). In patients with polycythemia secondary to hypoxic lung disease the SiEp was found to be within the normal range in over 50 per cent of patients (Wedzicha *et al.* 1985). A continued erythropoiesis when levels of SiEp have fallen to near control values is unexplained.

8.4.3 Altitude and red cell mass

The result of increased erythropoiesis at altitude is an increase in RCM since the life span of the red cell is unchanged (Berlin *et al.* 1954). Figure 8.5 shows the rise in RCM, which is quite slow at first but continues for a long time. After about 6 months at altitudes above 4000 m it had increased by a mean of 50 per cent in absolute terms or 67.5 per cent when corrected for loss of body weight. By this time the blood volume had increased over control by 7.3 per cent or 22.8 per cent corrected for body weight (Pugh 1964a) (Figure 8.5). Sanchez *et al.* (1970) found altitude residents in the Andes to have a RCM 83 per cent greater than sea level residents when corrected for weight difference.

8.5 ALTITUDE AND HEMOGLOBIN CONCENTRATION

8.5.1 Lowlanders going from sea level to altitude

The combined effect of changes in PV and RCM results in an increase in hemoglobin concentration. This increase allows more oxygen to be carried per liter of blood at any given oxygen saturation. The price paid for this gain in oxygen capacity, however, is an increase in viscosity of the blood with the attendant increased risk of thrombosis (Chapter 22).

As discussed in section 8.3, the initial rise in hemoglobin concentration during the first few days and weeks at altitude is largely a result of reduction in PV. The hemoglobin concentration rise is roughly exponential, leveling out at about 6 weeks at a given altitude. However, after that, the RCM continues to rise but so does the PV so that hemoglobin concentration remains approximately constant (Figure 8.5).

Pugh (1964c) reviewed results from five expeditions (51 observations in 40 subjects) and concluded that the hemoglobin concentration after about 6 weeks at altitude averaged 20.5 g dL⁻¹. It was independent of altitude above 5500 m. Winslow *et al.* (1984), reviewing hemoglobin concentration values from the 1981 American Everest expeditions and two previous Everest expeditions, found the range of mean values was 17.8–20.6 g dL⁻¹ at altitudes of 5350–6300 m, with no correlation between altitude and hemoglobin concentration within this altitude range.

8.5.2   Residents at altitude

Figure 8.7 shows the rise in hemoglobin concentration with altitude in residents of high altitude from North and South America and Asia. Andean subjects have been reported to have values in the region of 22 g dL⁻¹ at altitudes of 4300–4500 m (Talbott and Dill 1936, Dill *et al.* 1937, Merino 1950). However,

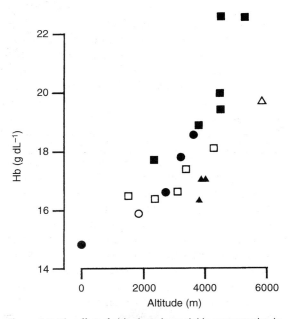

Figure 8.7 *The effect of altitude on hemoglobin concentration in male residents at altitude:* ●*, from the Tien Shan;* □*, from Colorado mining camps;* ○*, from south Indian hill towns;* ■*, from the Andes;* ▲ *from Nepal (Sherpas);* △*, climbers after 3 months or more at altitude.*

these studies may include subjects who would now be considered to have chronic mountain sickness. More recent publications from South America give mean values nearer 20 g dL⁻¹ (Peñaloza *et al.* 1971).

In Sherpa subjects hemoglobin concentration is lower, a mean of 17 g dL⁻¹ at 4000 m is given by Adams and Strang (1975) and of 16.2 g dL⁻¹ by Morpurgo *et al.* (1976). In this case the possibility that some subjects may be iron deficient cannot be ruled out. Morpurgo *et al.* argue that it represents greater adaptation. It is estimated that Tibetans have been resident at high altitude for perhaps 100 000 years, compared with about 20 000 years for Andean highlanders. However, results in residents of the Tien Shan and Pamirs by Son (1979) give values closer to those from South America (Figure 8.7) and would seem not to support this hypothesis. A possible explanation for the difference between Andean residents on the one hand and Sherpas and Tien Shan/Pamir residents on the other is that the latter move up and down in altitude more frequently than do Andean altitude dwellers on the altiplano. However, recent studies showing Tibetan populations to have lower hemoglobin concentration than Andean populations suggest there may be a genetic explanation.

A study from Tibet (Beall *et al.* 1987) demonstrated a hemoglobin concentration of 18.2 g dL⁻¹ in male and 16.7 g dL⁻¹ in female subjects resident at an altitude of 4850–5450 m, a value substantially lower than most results from the Andes at comparable altitude. More recent work by the same group (Beall *et al.* 1998) confirms this impression. In this study the same investigators using the same methods studied highland populations at altitude in Tibet and Bolivia. They found Tibetans had significantly lower hemoglobin concentration than the Bolivian highlanders (15.6 compared to 19.2 g dL⁻¹). They found that genetic factors accounted for a very high proportion of the phenotypic variance in hemoglobin concentration in both samples. This recent study is in line with that of Winslow *et al.* (1989) who compared Himalayan natives (Sherpas) to high altitude Andean natives at similar altitudes in Khundi, Nepal and Ollague (Chile) at 3700 m. Mean hematocrit values in Nepal were significantly lower than in Chile (48.4 compared with 52.2 g dL⁻¹). They also found SiEp concentrations to be higher in the Andean population, indicating that they were functionally anemic even with the higher hematocrit!

White people resident in high altitude towns in Colorado and acclimatized climbers tend to have lower hemoglobin concentration than Andeans but higher than Central Asian residents (Figure 8.7).

8.5.3 Polycythemia of high altitude

Excessive rise of hemoglobin concentration (i.e. above 22 g dL^{-1}) is generally considered to be pathological and diagnostic of chronic mountain sickness (Chapter 21). Both people native to high altitude and lowlanders resident at high altitude for some years are at risk of developing this condition. Huang *et al.* (1984) report that Han Chinese lowlanders resident on the Tibetan plateau have a higher incidence of this polycythemia than Tibetans.

8.5.4 Optimum hemoglobin concentration

An increase in hemoglobin concentration increases the oxygen-carrying capacity of blood since each gram of hemoglobin can carry 1.31 mL of oxygen (Gregory 1974). The oxygen content of the blood is the product of capacity and saturation (Sa_{O_2}) plus the dissolved oxygen. Thus the increase in hemoglobin concentration with altitude compensates for a reduction in arterial Sa_{O_2}. At altitudes up to about 5300 m this compensation results in an arterial oxygen content approximately equal to that at sea level in those who are acclimatized (Figure 8.1). However, increasing hemoglobin concentration results in increasing viscosity (Guyton *et al.* 1973). This increase in viscosity is curvilinear so that, with hemoglobin concentration above about 18 g dL^{-1}, viscosity increases rapidly. Eventually, this increased viscosity increases resistance in both systemic and pulmonary circulation, so impeding blood flow, and cardiac output falls. Oxygen supply to the tissues depends upon oxygen delivery, which is the product of arterial oxygen content and cardiac output.

These considerations result in the concept of an optimum hemoglobin concentration below which oxygen delivery is reduced because of reduction in oxygen content, and above which it is reduced because the great increase in viscosity causes a reduction in cardiac output which more than offsets the increase in content. The major problem in calculating what should be the value of this optimum hemo-

globin concentration is the viscosity of blood and its effect on cardiac output. Since blood is a non-Newtonian fluid, a single value for viscosity cannot be assigned to it at any given hemoglobin concentration. The value will vary according to the way it is measured *in vitro*. *In vivo* the effect on resistance will vary according to the diameter of the vessel under consideration as well as to whether flow is streamlined or turbulent. Apparent resistance will also vary with flow. If we ignore the physics and just look at the effect of changing hemoglobin concentration on cardiac output in acute animal experiments, these may not reflect the human situation at altitude where the vascular system has time to adapt to the polycythemia. The situation is so complex that it is clearly impossible, on theoretical grounds, to predict an optimum hemoglobin concentration. Another factor affecting the apparent viscosity is the deformability, or filterability, of the red cells. A study by Simon-Schnass and Korniszewski (1990) addressed this and concluded that altitude exposure resulted in an impaired filterability of red cells which was prevented by the administration of vitamin E.

From clinical experience, it seems that the extremely high hemoglobin concentration concentration found in chronic mountain sickness (Chapter 21) and in some patients with chronic hypoxic lung disease is deleterious. Hemodilution by venesection alone or with intravenous fluid replacement results in clinical improvement. In such patients reduction of PCV from 61 per cent to 50 per cent resulted in a decrease in pulmonary artery pressure and resistance (Weisse *et al.* 1975). Similarly, Winslow *et al.* (1985) found in Andean high altitude residents that reduction of PCV from 62 per cent to 42 per cent resulted in increased cardiac output and mixed venous P_{O_2}. Willison *et al.* (1980) found that reducing the PCV from 54 per cent to 48 per cent in patients resulted in an increase of cerebral blood flow from 44 to 57 mL min^{-1} per 100 g brain tissue. This would increase oxygen delivery to the brain by 15 per cent and was accompanied by an increase in alertness.

In a study of climbers at altitude by Sarnquist *et al.* (1986) it was found that hemodilution produced no improvement or deterioration in measured physical performance, though there was a small, significant improvement in psychomotor tests. However, the subjects studied, though having the highest PCV in the expedition, were not very polycythemic. Their

PCV ranged from 57 per cent to 60 per cent before hemodilution.

There is no obvious correlation between climbing performance and hemoglobin concentration within the range of values common on an expedition, at about 17–22 g dL^{-1} (Pugh 1964c). Indeed it is usual to find that climbers who perform best are at the lower end of this range, suggesting that the optimum hemoglobin concentration at altitudes above about 5000 m is in the region of 18 g dL^{-1}. Winslow and Monge (1987, p. 203) conclude that

> Excessive polycythemia serves no useful purpose. Indeed, it is doubtful whether there is any physiologic value in 'normal' polycythemia.

8.5.5 Effect of blood reinfusion on performance at altitude

At sea level there is no doubt that blood reinfusion (doping) has a significant effect in improving performance, as measured by $V_{O_2 max}$, and endurance (Buick et al. 1980). However, at altitude the situation is less clear. Young et al. (1996) found no significant benefit from reinfusion of 700 mL of autologous blood in subjects at 4300 m, though mean values for $V_{O_2 max}$ were slightly higher on day 1 at altitude in the test subjects. In a further study by Pandolf et al. (1998) they found no significant improvement in time for a 3.2 km run in subjects infused with 700 mL of autologous blood. They suggest that the effect diminishes with increasing altitude and quote earlier work supporting that concept.

8.5.6 Hemoglobin concentration on descent from altitude

On descent from altitude arterial oxygen saturation will return to the normal 96–98 per cent and this,

together with the now raised hemoglobin concentration, might be expected to inhibit EPO secretion. However, Milledge and Cotes (1985) reported that levels were 66 per cent of control values 8 h and 20 h after descent following 2 months at or above 4500 m. This reduced EPO level presumably is sufficient to reduce erythropoiesis since hemoglobin concentration declines after descent and reaches normal sea level values after about 6 weeks (Heath and Williams 1995, pp. 61–3).

8.6 PLATELETS AND CLOTTING AT ALTITUDE

These topics are discussed more fully in Chapter 22.

In summary, it seems that the physiological response to hypoxia does not involve any important changes in platelet count or adhesiveness, or in clotting factors. However, there may be changes associated with AMS. If there are changes in clotting factors, they may represent an effect or a complication of AMS rather than being essential in its genesis.

8.7 WHITE BLOOD CELLS

There seem to be variable changes in total white cell and differential count on going to altitude. One study reported a rise in granulocyte count on ascent to 4300 m (Simon-Schnass and Korniszewski 1990) and another an increase in certain lymphocyte subsets. CD16+ or natural killer cells were particularly increased in seven subjects in a decompression chamber at 380 mm Hg (Klokker et al. 1993). There is anecdotal evidence that infections in the skin and subcutaneous tissues are slow to clear at altitude. One could speculate that the above finding might have a bearing on this.

9

Blood gas transport and acid–base balance

SUMMARY

Alterations of the oxygen affinity of hemoglobin can alter the oxygen dissociation curve at high altitude and therefore affect oxygen transport by the blood. Many animals that live in oxygen deprived environments have high oxygen affinities of their hemoglobin. This is the case in the human fetus. It is interesting that climbers at extreme altitude increase their oxygen affinity by extreme hyperventilation which causes a marked respiratory alkalosis. The effect of the alkalosis overwhelms the small decrease in oxygen affinity caused by the increased concentration of 2,3-diphosphoglycerate in the red blood cells. The P_{50} of high altitude natives is essentially the same as the sea level value according to most studies. However, lowlanders living at high altitude for weeks tend to have a reduced P_{50}, indicating an increased oxygen affinity of hemoglobin. An increased oxygen affinity is advantageous at high altitude because it assists in the loading of oxygen by the pulmonary capillaries. The acid–base status of high altitude natives is a little controversial but many studies have found a normal arterial pH, indicating a fully compensated respiratory alkalosis. However, acclimatized lowlanders usually have an alkaline pH, indicating that metabolic compensation is not complete. There is evidence that at extreme altitude, metabolic compensation for the respiratory alkalosis is slow, possibly because of chronic volume depletion caused by dehydration.

9.1 INTRODUCTION

Physiological changes in the blood play an important role in acclimatization and adaptation to high altitude. In this chapter, the main topics considered are the changes in oxygen affinity of hemoglobin, and the alterations of the acid–base status of the blood. The increase in red cell concentration of the blood was discussed in Chapter 8, where the regulation of erythropoiesis was described. Some of the consequences of an altered oxygen affinity of hemoglobin are alluded to in other chapters, especially Chapter 6 on diffusion of oxygen across the blood–gas barrier, and Chapter 12 on limiting factors at extreme altitude.

9.2 HISTORICAL

The honor of first plotting the oxygen and carbon dioxide dissociation curves apparently belongs to Paul Bert. In his monumental book *La Pression Barométrique* he showed the relationships between partial pressure and blood gas concentration for both oxygen and carbon dioxide as experimental animals were exposed to lower and lower barometric pressures, or as they were gradually asphyxiated by rebreathing in a closed space (Bert 1878, pp. 135–8 in the 1943 translation). However, he did not discover the S-shaped curve for oxygen because he did not reduce the P_{O_2} far enough.

The first oxygen dissociation curve over its whole range was published by Christian Bohr in 1885. The measurements were made on dilute solutions of hemoglobin and showed precise hyperbolas (Bohr 1885). They were obviously not compatible with the data obtained by Bert in experimental animals, although Bohr did not comment on this. Hüfner (1890) published similar curves for hemoglobin solutions and argued that a hyperbolic shape would be expected from the simple equation

$$Hb + O_2 \rightarrow HbO_2$$

An important advance was made by Bohr when he used whole blood rather than hemoglobin solutions and this led him to the discovery of the now familiar S-shaped curve. In the following year he showed, in collaboration with Hasselbalch and Krogh, that the dissociation curve was shifted to the right when the P_{CO_2} of the blood was increased, a phenomenon which came to be known as the Bohr effect (Bohr et al. 1904). A few years later, Barcroft found that the addition of acid displaced the dissociation curve to the right (Barcroft and Orbeli 1910), and also that an increase in temperature had the same effect (Barcroft and King 1909). Astrup and Severinghaus (1986) wrote a valuable historical review of blood gases and acid–base balance.

It was not long after these important modulators of the oxygen affinity of hemoglobin were discovered that physiologists wondered about their importance at high altitude. For example, when Barcroft accompanied the first international high altitude expedition to Tenerife in 1910 he made a special study of the position of the oxygen dissociation curve, expecting it to be displaced to the left by the low arterial P_{CO_2}. In the event, he found that the oxygen dissociation curves of some members of the expedition at 2130 and 3000 m were shifted to the right when measured at the normal sea level P_{CO_2} of 40 mm Hg. However, when he repeated the equilibrations at the subjects' actual P_{CO_2} at altitude, the positions of the curves were essentially the same as at sea level (Barcroft 1911). He concluded that the decrease in carbonic acid in the blood was compensated for by an increase in some other acid, possibly lactic acid. One year later Barcroft went to Mosso's laboratory, the Capanna Regina Margherita on Monte Rosa (4559 m), and reported a slight excess acidity at that altitude (Barcroft et al. 1914).

Some 10 years later, during the 1921–2 Anglo-American Expedition to Cerro de Pasco in Peru, Barcroft and his colleagues found an increased oxygen affinity in acclimatized lowlanders as a result of the increased alkalinity of the blood. It also appeared that the increase in affinity was greater than could be explained by the change in acid–base status (Barcroft et al. 1923).

The question of hemoglobin–oxygen affinity was examined again on the International High Altitude Expedition to Chile in 1935. It was found that the 'physiological' dissociation curves (that is, measured at a subject's own P_{CO_2}) were displaced slightly to the left of the sea level values up to about 4270 m, but that above that altitude, the curves were displaced increasingly to the right of the sea level positions (Keys et al. 1936). Measurements of oxygen affinity of the hemoglobin were also made at constant pH and these showed a uniform tendency to a decreased affinity. The investigators argued that this rightward shift of the curve might be advantageous at high altitude because it would facilitate oxygen unloading to the tissues.

An important discovery was made in 1967 by two groups working independently (Benesch and Benesch 1967, Chanutin and Curnish 1967) that a fourth factor (in addition to P_{CO_2}, pH and temperature) had an important effect on the oxygen affinity of hemoglobin. This was the concentration of 2,3-diphosphoglycerate (2,3-DPG) within the red cells. This unexpected development raised doubts about much of the earlier work in which this important factor had not been controlled. It was subsequently shown that 2,3-DPG increased at high altitude (Lenfant et al. 1968) and it was argued that the resulting decrease in oxygen affinity, which facilitated unloading of oxygen in the tissues, was an important part of the adaptation process (Lenfant and Sullivan 1971).

Until recently relatively little information was available on the oxygen affinity of hemoglobin at extreme altitude. A few measurements from the Himalayan Scientific and Mountaineering Expedition for 1960–1 showed that lowlanders who were well acclimatized to 5800 m had an almost fully compensated respiratory alkalosis (West et al. 1962). Data above this altitude did not exist.

It was therefore astonishing to find on the 1981 American Medical Research Expedition to Everest that climbers near the summit apparently had an extreme degree of respiratory alkalosis which greatly increased the oxygen affinity of their hemoglobin. The arterial pH of Pizzo on the Everest summit exceeded 7.7 as determined from the alveolar P_{CO_2} and base excess, both of which were measured (section 9.4.4).

Turning now to the early history of acid–base balance at high altitude, it is clear from the above that it overlaps considerably with a discussion of oxygen affinity of hemoglobin. However, the reaction of the blood (as it was called) at high altitude created a great deal of interest in its own right. Indeed, the acid–base status of the blood played an important role in early theories of the control of breathing at high altitude (Kellogg 1980). As long ago as 1903, Galeotti found that, in various experimental animals taken to Mosso's Capanna Regina Margherita laboratory on Monte Rosa, the amount of acid needed to bring their hemolyzed blood to a standard pH (determined from litmus paper) was decreased compared with sea level (Galeotti 1904). He interpreted this decrease in titratable alkalinity to mean that there was an increase in some acid substance in the blood. It was known that hypoxia caused lactic acid production (Araki, 1891) and that acid blood stimulated breathing (Zuntz et al. 1906). It was therefore natural to conclude that this explained the hyperventilation of high altitude, and that the P_{CO_2} fell as a consequence (Boycott and Haldane 1908). Winterstein (1911) formulated what became known as the 'reaction theory' of breathing, which stated that the effects of both hypoxia and carbon dioxide as stimulants of ventilation could be explained by the fact that they both acidified the blood.

The correct explanation of how hypoxia stimulates ventilation at high altitude had to wait for discovery of the peripheral chemoreceptors by Heymans and Heymans (1925). Meanwhile Winterstein (1915) provided evidence against his own theory when he showed that, in acute hypoxia, the blood becomes alkaline rather than acid. A few years later, Henderson (1919) and Haldane et al. (1919) correctly explained the alkalinity as being secondary to the lowered P_{CO_2} caused by hyperventilation. Nevertheless, it is true that even today the control of ventilation during chronic hypoxia is a subject of intense research (Chapter 5) and interest still remains in the acid–base status of the extracellular fluid (ECF) which forms the environment of the central chemoreceptors.

9.3 OXYGEN AFFINITY OF HEMOGLOBIN

9.3.1 Basic physiology

Figure 9.1 shows the oxygen dissociation curve of human whole blood and the four factors that shift the curve to the right, that is decrease the affinity of hemoglobin for oxygen. These four factors are increases in: P_{CO_2}, hydrogen ion concentration, temperature, and the concentration of 2,3-DPG in the red cells. Increasing the ionic concentration of the plasma also reduces oxygen affinity.

Almost all of the change in oxygen affinity caused by P_{CO_2} can be ascribed to its effect on hydrogen ion concentration, although a change in P_{CO_2} has a small effect in its own right (Margaria 1957). The mechanism of the alteration of oxygen affinity through hydrogen ion concentration (Bohr effect) is through a change in configuration of the hemoglobin molecule which makes the binding site less accessible to molecular oxygen as the hydrogen ion concentration is raised. The molecule exists in two forms:

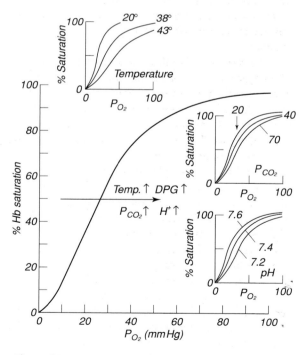

Figure 9.1 Normal oxygen dissociation curve and its displacement by increases in H⁺, P_CO₂, temperature and 2,3-diphosphoglycerate (DPG). (From West 1994.)

one in which the chemical subunits are maximally chemically bonded (T form), and another in which some bonds are ruptured and the structure is relaxed (R form). The R form has a higher affinity for oxygen because the molecule can more easily enter the region of the heme. The approximate magnitudes of the effects of change in P_{CO_2} and pH on the oxygen dissociation curve are shown in the right insets of Figure 9.1.

Increase in temperature has a large effect on the oxygen affinity of hemoglobin, as shown in the top inset of Figure 9.1. The temperature effect follows from thermodynamic considerations: the combination of oxygen with hemoglobin is exothermic so that an increase in temperature favors the reverse reaction, that is dissociation of the oxyhemoglobin.

The compound 2,3-DPG is a product of red cell metabolism, as shown in Figure 9.2. An increased concentration of this material within the red cell reduces the oxygen affinity of the hemoglobin by increasing the chemical binding of the subunits and converting more hemoglobin to the low affinity T form.

A useful number to describe the oxygen affinity of hemoglobin is the P_{50}, that is the P_{O_2} for 50 per cent saturation of the hemoglobin with oxygen. The normal value for adult whole blood at a P_{CO_2} of 40 mm Hg, pH 7.4, temperature 37 °C, and normal 2,3-DPG concentration is 26–27 mm Hg. Human fetal blood has a P_{50} of about 19 mm Hg because of the different chemical structure of fetal hemoglobin.

An increase of 2,3-DPG within the red cell increases the P_{50} by about 0.5 mm Hg mol^{-1} of 2,3-DPG. The magnitude of the Bohr effect is usually given in terms of the increase in log P_{50} per pH unit. The normal value for human blood is 0.4 at constant P_{CO_2}. Note that although historically the 'Bohr effect' referred to the change in affinity caused by P_{CO_2}, in modern usage the term is restricted to the effect of pH. The temperature effect is 0.24 for the change in log P_{50} (mm Hg °C^{-1}).

Much can be learned about the effect of changes in the oxygen affinity of hemoglobin on the physiology of high altitude by modeling the oxygen transport system using computer subroutines for the oxygen and carbon dioxide dissociation curves (Bencowitz *et al.* 1982). Kelman described useful subroutines for the oxygen dissociation curve (Kelman 1966a,b) and the carbon dioxide dissociation curve (Kelman 1967). The practical use of these procedures has been described (West and Wagner 1977). These procedures are able to accommodate changes in P_{CO_2}, pH, temperature and 2,3-DPG concentration, and allow the investigator to answer questions about the interactions of these variables which would otherwise be impossibly complicated.

9.3.2   Animals native to high altitude

It has been known for many years that animals that live at high altitude tend to have an increased oxygen

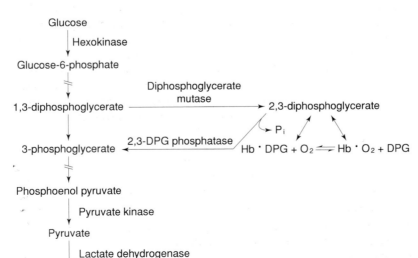

Figure 9.2 *Formation of 2,3-DPG in erythrocytes. The vertical chain at the left shows the glycolytic pathway in cells other than red blood cells. In red cells the enzyme DPG mutase catalyses the conversion of much of the 1,3-DPG to 2,3-DPG. (Modified from Mines 1981.)*

affinity of their hemoglobin. Figure 6.6 shows part of the oxygen dissociation curves of the vicuna and llama which are native to high altitude in the South American Andes (Hall *et al.* 1936). The diagram also shows the range of dissociation curves for eight lowland animals including humans, horse, dog, rabbit, pig, peccary, ox and sheep. It can be seen that the hemoglobin of high altitude native animals has a substantially increased oxygen affinity. This adaptation to high altitude is of genetic origin, as is shown by the fact that a llama brought up in a zoo at sea level has the same high oxygen affinity.

High altitude birds also show these phenomena. Hall and his colleagues (1936), during the 1935 International High Altitude Expedition to Chile, reported that the high altitude ostrich and huallata have higher oxygen affinities than a group of six lowland birds including the pigeon, muscovy duck, domestic goose, domestic duck, Chinese pheasant and domestic fowl. A particularly interesting example is the bar-headed goose which is known to fly over the Himalayan ranges as it migrates between its breeding grounds in Siberia and its wintering grounds in India. This remarkable animal has a blood P_{50} about 10 mm Hg lower than its close relatives from moderate altitudes (Black and Tenney 1980).

Deer mice, *Peromyscus maniculatus,* show the same relationships. A study was carried out on 10 subspecies that live at altitudes from below sea level in Death Valley in California to the high mountains of the nearby Sierra Nevada (4350 m), and it was found that there was a strong correlation between the habitat altitude and the oxygen affinity of the blood. The genetic source of this relationship was proved by moving one subspecies to another location and showing that the oxygen affinity was unchanged. Moreover, the relationship persisted in second generation animals (Snyder *et al.* 1982).

9.3.3 Animals in oxygen deprived environments

High altitude is just one of the oxygen deprived environments in which animals are found, and it is interesting to consider the variety of strategies that have been adopted to mitigate the problems posed by oxygen deficiency. Table 6.1 shows examples of some of the strategies that have been adopted through

genetic adaptation. The most familiar to most of us is the change in amino acid sequence in the globin chain of hemoglobin in the human fetus. This is also seen in the bar-headed goose. The next two groups increase the oxygen affinity of their hemoglobin by decreasing the concentration of organic phosphates. This is done with 2,3-DPG in the fetus of the dog, horse and pig, and by decreasing the concentration of ATP in the trout and eel.

Some species of tadpoles which frequently live in stagnant pools have a high oxygen affinity hemoglobin, whereas the adult frogs produce a different type of hemoglobin with a lower affinity that fits their higher oxygen environment. Note also that the tadpole blood shows a smaller Bohr effect. This is useful because low oxygen and high carbon dioxide pressures are likely to occur together in stagnant water, and a large Bohr effect would be disadvantageous because it would decrease the oxygen affinity of the blood when a high affinity was most needed.

As indicated earlier, the human fetus also has a high oxygen affinity by virtue of its fetal hemoglobin. This is essential because the arterial P_{O_2} of the fetus is less than 30 mm Hg. Indeed the human fetus and the adult climber on the summit of Mount Everest have some similar features in that in both cases the arterial P_{O_2} is extremely low, and the P_{50} of the arterial blood (at the prevailing pH) is also very low (section 9.4.4).

A particularly interesting example of an unusual human hemoglobin was described by Hebbel *et al.* (1978). The authors studied a family in which two of the siblings had a mutant hemoglobin (Andrew-Minneapolis) with a P_{50} of 17.1 mm Hg. They showed that the siblings with the abnormal hemoglobin tolerated exercise at an altitude of 3100 m better than the normal siblings.

The last row in Table 6.1 refers to the climber at extreme altitude who has a marked respiratory alkalosis which greatly increases the oxygen affinity of the hemoglobin. This is discussed in detail below.

9.3.4 High altitude natives

Barcroft *et al.* (1923) measured the oxygen dissociation curves of three natives of Cerro de Pasco (4330 m) in Peru at the prevailing P_{CO_2} (25–30 mm Hg) and showed that the curves were displaced to the left, i.e. there was an increased oxygen affinity. A similar result was found in acclimatized members of the expedition. Barcroft (1925) believed that part of the leftward shift was caused by increased alkalinity of the blood but part was also due to an intrinsic change in the affinity of hemoglobin.

During the International High Altitude Expedition to Chile in 1935, a number of measurements were made on high altitude natives who were living at 5340 m (P_B 401 mm Hg). Some of the men were accustomed to working each day at 5700 m. The dissociation curves were found to be within normal limits for men at sea level, or perhaps shifted slightly to the right (Keys *et al.* 1936). Measurements were also made on dilute solutions of hemoglobin taken both from high altitude residents and from acclimatized lowlanders (Hall 1936). The results were very similar to those obtained at sea level but the high altitude residents seemed to have a slightly reduced oxygen affinity.

Aste-Salazar and Hurtado (1944) measured the oxygen dissociation curves of 17 healthy Peruvians in Lima at sea level and 12 other permanent residents of Morococha (4550 m). These studies were subsequently extended to a total of 40 subjects in Lima and 30 in Morococha (Hurtado 1964). The mean value of the P_{50} at pH 7.4 was 24.7 mm Hg at sea level and 26.9 mm Hg at high altitude (Figure 9.3). It was

argued that the rightward displacement of the curve would enhance the unloading of oxygen from the peripheral capillaries.

More recently Winslow and his colleagues (1981) reported oxygen dissociation curves on 46 native Peruvians in Morococha (4550 m, P_B 432 mm Hg) and confirmed that at pH 7.4 the P_{50} was significantly higher in the high altitude population than in the sea level controls (31.2 mm Hg as opposed to 29.2 mm Hg, $p < 0.001$). However, these investigators also found that the acid–base status of the high altitude subjects was that of partially compensated respiratory alkalosis with a mean plasma pH of 7.44. When the P_{50} values were corrected to the subjects' actual plasma pH, the mean value of 30.1 mm Hg could no longer be distinguished from that of the sea level controls (Figure 9.4). The conclusion was that the small increase in P_{50} resulting from the increased

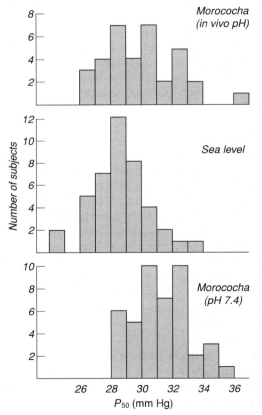

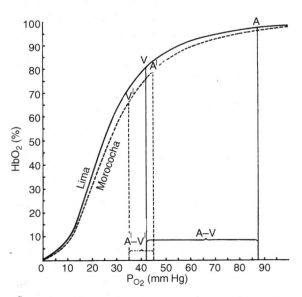

Figure 9.3 *Mean positions of the oxygen dissociation curves of Peruvians in Lima (sea level) and Morococha (4540 m). Note that the high altitude natives have a slightly reduced oxygen affinity. Mean values of the P_{O_2} in arterial (A) and mixed venous (V) blood for the two groups are also shown. (From Hurtado 1964.)*

Figure 9.4 *Distribution of P_{50} values at sea level and high altitude. In the top panel, values are expressed at the in vivo pH; in the bottom at pH 7.4. When corrected for the subjects' plasma pH, the in vivo P_{50} at high altitude falls in the sea level range in all but one subject. (From Winslow et al. 1981.)*

concentration of 2,3-DPG in the red cells was offset by the mild degree of respiratory alkalosis, with the net result that the position of the oxygen dissociation curve was essentially the same as that in sea level controls.

In a controversial study Morpurgo et al. (1976) reported that Sherpas living permanently at an altitude of 4000 m in the Nepalese Himalayas had a substantially increased oxygen affinity at standard pH. The P_{50} value of the high altitude Sherpas was 22.6 mm Hg, compared with 27.1 mm Hg in low altitude white people. The Sherpa blood was also reported to have an unusually large Bohr effect. Interestingly, Sherpas living at low altitude appeared to have an increased P_{50} value of 36.7 mm Hg. A weakness of this study was that the oxygen dissociation curves were determined 5–6 days after the blood was taken. A subsequent study by Samaja et al. (1979) failed to confirm these provocative findings. Samaja et al. also showed that the oxygen affinity could be completely accounted for by the known effectors of hemoglobin function: pH, P_{CO_2}, 2,3-DPG and temperature.

9.3.5 Acclimatized lowlanders

As discussed in section 9.2, Barcroft (1911) was perhaps the first person to measure the position of the oxygen dissociation curve in acclimatized lowlanders. This was done at altitudes of 2130 and 3000 m on Tenerife, and he reported that the curve was shifted to the right if measured at the normal P_{CO_2} of 40 mm Hg, but if the P_{CO_2} for those altitudes was used, the curves had the same position as at sea level. Barcroft made additional measurements on Monte Rosa in 1911 (Barcroft et al. 1914) and reported a slight rightward shift of the curves at the prevailing P_{CO_2}. However, during the expedition to Cerro de Pasco in 1922, a leftward shift was observed at the prevailing arterial P_{CO_2} of 25–30 mm Hg (Barcroft et al. 1923). They made the point that this might be beneficial because of enhanced oxygen uptake in the lung owing to the increased oxygen affinity of the hemoglobin.

During the International High Altitude Expedition to Chile 1935, three ways of measuring the oxygen affinity of the hemoglobin were employed: whole blood at normal pH, whole blood at the prevailing pH and dilute solutions of hemo-

globin. At constant pH, Keys et al. (1936) reported that the oxygen affinity of the hemoglobin was apparently slightly reduced with a change in P_{50} of approximately 3.5 mm Hg. However, the 'physiological' dissociation curves were displaced to the left from sea level up to an altitude of approximately 4270 m, though above that they were displaced increasingly to the right of the sea level positions. On dilute hemoglobin solutions, Hall (1936) showed that the oxygen affinity of the hemoglobin was essentially unchanged compared with sea level.

These somewhat confusing results were substantially clarified when the role of 2,3-DPG in the red cell was appreciated (Benesch and Benesch 1967, Chanutin and Curnish 1967). It was shown that this normal product of red cell metabolism reduced the oxygen affinity of hemoglobin, and it was then clear that many previous measurements were unreliable because of ignorance of this factor. Lenfant and his colleagues (Lenfant et al. 1968, 1969, 1971) showed that the concentration of 2,3-DPG was increased in lowlanders when they became acclimatized to high altitude. The primary cause of the increase in 2,3-DPG was the increase in plasma pH above the normal sea level value as a result of the respiratory alkalosis. When subjects were made acidotic with acetazolamide there was no increase in plasma pH or red cell 2,3-DPG concentration at high altitude, and the oxygen dissociation curve did not shift to the right. It was argued that the increase in 2,3-DPG was an important feature of the acclimatization process of lowlanders and of the adaptation to high altitude of highlanders (Lenfant and Sullivan 1971).

Subsequent measurements on lowlanders at high altitude have confirmed these changes, although there is still some uncertainty about whether acclimatized lowlanders develop complete metabolic compensation for their respiratory alkalosis (that is, whether the pH returns to 7.4). Certainly this does not happen at extremely high altitudes. During the 1981 American Medical Research Expedition to Everest, Winslow et al. (1984) made an extensive series of measurements on acclimatized lowlanders at an altitude of 6300 m. They also obtained data on two subjects who reached the summit (8848 m). These measurements were made on venous blood samples taken at an altitude of 8050 m the morning after the summit climb. Winslow and his colleagues found that the red cell concentration of 2,3-DPG increased with altitude (Figure 9.5) and that this was

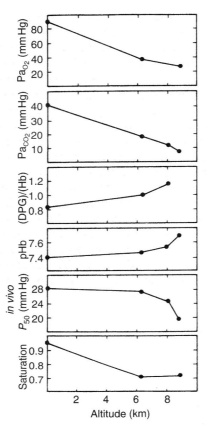

Figure 9.5 *Blood variables measured on the 1981 American Medical Research Expedition to Everest at sea level, 6300 m, 8050 m and 8848 m (summit). pHb, pH blood. (From Winslow* et al. *1984.)*

associated with a slightly increased P_{50} value when expressed at pH 7.4. However, because the respiratory alkalosis was not fully compensated, the subjects' *in vivo* P_{50} at 6300 m (27.6 mm Hg) was slightly less than at sea level (28.1 mm Hg). The estimated *in vivo* P_{50} was found to become progressively lower at 8050 m (24.9 mm Hg), and on the summit at 8848 m it was as low as 19.4 mm Hg in one subject. Thus these data show that, at extreme altitudes, the blood oxygen dissociation curve shifts progressively leftward (increased oxygen affinity of hemoglobin) primarily because of the respiratory alkalosis. Indeed this effect completely overwhelms the relatively small tendency for the curve to shift to the right because of the increase in red cell 2,3-DPG.

The results obtained on Operation Everest II were generally in agreement with these (Sutton *et al.* 1988) except that the P_{CO_2} values at extreme altitude were higher, and the blood pH values therefore lower.

These differences can probably be explained by the smaller degree of acclimatization because of the limited time available in the low pressure chamber.

9.3.6   Physiological effects of changes in oxygen affinity

As indicated above, there have been differences of opinion on whether a decreased or an increased oxygen affinity is beneficial at high altitude. Barcroft *et al.* (1923) found a slightly increased affinity and argued that this would enhance oxygen loading in the lung. However, Aste-Salazar and Hurtado (1944) reported a slight decrease in oxygen affinity in high altitude natives at Morococha and reasoned that this would enhance oxygen unloading in peripheral capillaries. The same argument was used by Lenfant and Sullivan (1971) when the influence of the increased red cell concentration of 2,3-DPG on the oxygen dissociation curve was appreciated. They stated that the decreased oxygen affinity would help the peripheral unloading of oxygen, and that this was one of the many features both of acclimatization of lowlanders to high altitude and of the genetic adaptation of highlanders.

However, there is now strong evidence that an increased oxygen affinity (left-shifted oxygen dissociation curve) is beneficial, especially at higher altitudes, and particularly on exercise (Bencowitz *et al.* 1982). Indeed this should not come as a surprise when it is appreciated that many animals increase the oxygen affinity of their blood in oxygen-deprived environments by a variety of strategies (section 9.3.3; Table 6.1). In addition, Eaton *et al.* (1974) reported that rats whose oxygen dissociation curve had been left-shifted by cyanate administration showed an increased survival when they were decompressed to a barometric pressure of 233 mm Hg. The controls were rats with a normal oxygen affinity. Turek *et al.* (1978) also studied cyanate-treated rats and found that they maintained better oxygen transfer to tissues during severe hypoxia than normal animals. In addition, we have already referred to the studies of Hebbel *et al.* (1978) who found a family with two members who had a hemoglobin with a very high affinity (Hb Andrew-Minneapolis, P_{50} 17.1 mm Hg). These two members performed better during exercise at an altitude of 3100 m than two siblings with normal blood.

Theoretical studies show that a high oxygen affinity is beneficial at high altitude, especially on exercise (Turek *et al.* 1973, Bencowitz *et al.* 1982). In one study, oxygen transfer from air to tissues was modeled for a variety of altitudes and a range of oxygen uptakes (Bencowitz *et al.* 1982). The oxygen dissociation curve was shifted both to the left and right with P_{50} of 16.8 mm Hg (left-shifted), 26.8 mm Hg (normal) and 36.8 mm Hg (right-shifted). The pulmonary diffusing capacity for oxygen was varied over a wide range and all the determinants of oxygen transport, including temperature, base excess, hemoglobin concentration and hematocrit, were taken into account.

The results showed that in the presence of diffusion limitation of oxygen transfer across the blood–gas barrier in the lung, a left-shifted curve resulted in the highest P_{O_2} of mixed venous blood (which was taken as an index of tissue P_{O_2}) (Figure 9.6). In other words, in the presence of diffusion limitation, an increased oxygen affinity of hemoglobin results in a higher tissue P_{O_2}. The explanation is that the increased affinity enhances the loading of oxygen in the lung more than it interferes with unloading in peripheral capillaries. This appears to be the physiological justification for the increased oxygen affinity so frequently seen among animals that live in low oxygen environments (Table 6.1).

The role of an increased oxygen affinity is seen dramatically in a climber on the summit of Mount Everest. Despite some increase of 2,3-DPG concentration within the red cell, the extremely low P_{CO_2} of 7–8 mm Hg as a result of the enormous increase in ventilation causes a dramatic degree of respiratory alkalosis with an arterial pH calculated to exceed 7.7 (West *et al.* 1983b). As a result, the *in vivo*

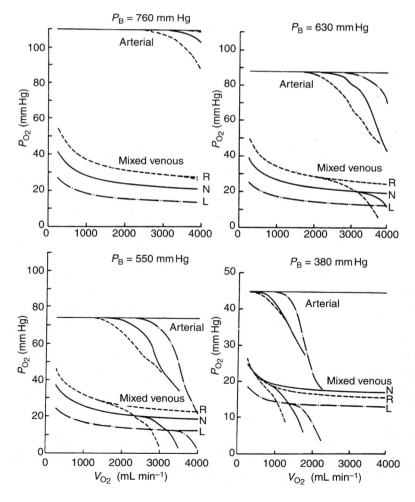

Figure 9.6 *Results of a theoretical study showing changes in calculated arterial and mixed venous P_{O_2} with increasing oxygen uptake at four altitudes for three values of P_{50}. The P_{50} values are normal (N, 26.8 mm Hg), right-shifted (R, 36.8 mm Hg), and left-shifted (L, 16.8 mm Hg). The nearly horizontal lines labeled 'mixed venous' show the P_{O_2} values for an infinitely high pulmonary oxygen diffusing capacity. The curved lines peeling away from these lines show the results of diffusion limitation. In this example, the diffusing capacity of the membrane for oxygen (DM_{O_2}) is 80 mL min^{-1} mm Hg^{-1}. Note that at the highest level of exercise, and especially at high altitude, the left-shifted curve gives the highest values of P_{O_2} in mixed venous blood and therefore the tissues. (From Bencowitz et al. 1982.)*

P_{50} is about 19 mm Hg, which is very similar to that of the human fetus *in utero*. The resulting striking increase in oxygen affinity of hemoglobin plays a major role in allowing the climber to survive this extremely hypoxic environment (Chapter 12).

9.4 ACID–BASE BALANCE

9.4.1 Introduction

This topic overlaps with that of the previous section, oxygen affinity of hemoglobin, because the affinity at high altitude is primarily determined by the pH of the blood together with the concentration of 2,3-DPG in the red cells. However, for convenience, available information on acid–base status is set out here.

9.4.2 During acclimatization

When a lowlander goes to high altitude, hyperventilation occurs as a result of stimulation of the peripheral chemoreceptors by the hypoxemia (Chapter 4), the arterial P_{CO_2} falls, and the arterial pH rises in accordance with the Henderson–Hasselbalch equation:

$$pH = pK + \log \frac{[HCO_3^-]}{0.03 P_{CO_2}}$$

where $[HCO_3^-]$ is the bicarbonate concentration in millimoles per liter and the P_{CO_2} is in mm Hg. However, the kidney responds by eliminating bicarbonate ion, being prompted to do this by the decreased P_{CO_2} in the renal tubular cells. The result is a more alkaline urine because of decreased reabsorption of bicarbonate ions. The resulting decrease in plasma bicarbonate then moves the bicarbonate/P_{CO_2} ratio back towards its normal level. This is known as metabolic compensation for the respiratory alkalosis. The compensation may be complete, in which case the arterial pH returns to 7.4 or, more usually, incomplete with a steady-state pH that exceeds 7.4.

The time course of the changes in arterial pH when normal subjects are taken abruptly to high altitude has been studied by several investigators (Severinghaus *et al.* 1963, Lenfant *et al.* 1971,

Dempsey *et al.* 1978). In one study, lowlanders were taken from sea level to an altitude of 4509 m (P_B 446 mm Hg) in less than 5 h, and remained there for 4 days. The arterial pH rose to a mean of about 7.47 within 24 h and then apparently slowly declined but was still about 7.45 at the end of the 4-day period. On return to sea level the pH fell steadily to reach the normal value of 7.4 after about 48 h (Lenfant *et al.* 1971).

In another study, four normal subjects were taken abruptly to 3800 m for 8 days. The arterial pH rapidly rose from a mean of 7.424 at sea level to 7.485 after 2 days, and remained essentially constant, being 7.484 at the end of 8 days (Severinghaus *et al.* 1963). In a further study, 11 lowlanders moved to 3200 m altitude where they remained for 10 days (Dempsey *et al.* 1978). The arterial pH rose by 0.03 to 0.04 units within 2 days and then remained essentially unchanged. In all instances, the arterial P_{CO_2} continued to fall as did the plasma bicarbonate concentration. However, it appears that the return of the arterial pH to (or near to) its sea level value is very slow.

9.4.3 High altitude natives

Most authors have reported a fully compensated respiratory alkalosis in high altitude natives with arterial pH values close to 7.4. Table 9.1 shows a summary of a number of published papers prepared by Winslow and Monge (1987). This is perhaps the expected finding. The body generally maintains the arterial pH within very narrow limits in health, and it seems reasonable that people who are born and live at high altitude would fully compensate for their reduced P_{CO_2} by eliminating bicarbonate and restoring the pH to the normal sea level value.

However, Winslow *et al.* (1981) measured the arterial pH in 46 high altitude natives of Morococha (4550 m, P_B 432 mm Hg) and reported that the mean plasma pH was 7.439 ± 0.065. In other words these highlanders did not have a fully compensated respiratory alkalosis but their blood lay slightly on the alkaline side of normal. As pointed out in section 9.3.4, the result of this mild respiratory alkalosis was to restore the oxygen dissociation curve to the normal sea level position because there was an increase in red cell 2,3-DPG concentration which tended to move the curve to the right.

Table 9.1 *Blood–gas and pH values in high altitude natives*

Altitude (m)	n	Hb[a]	Pa_{O_2} (mm Hg)	Sa_{O_2} (per cent)	Pa_{CO_2} (mm Hg)	pH	Source
4300	3	—	46.7	84.6	—	—	Barcroft et al. (1923)
4300	12	—	—	—	—	7.360	Aste-Salazar and Hurtado (1944)
4500	40	20.6[a]	45.1	80.1	33.3	7.370	Hurtado et al. (1956)
4515	22	19.5[a]	—	82.8	33.8	7.400	Chiodi (1957)
4300	6	56.0	—	—	32.5	7.431[b]	Monge et al. (1964)
4300	5	73.8	—	—	39.0	7.429[b]	Monge et al. (1964)
3700	—	—	—	—	3.0	7.431[b]	Monge et al. (1964)
4545	—	—	—	—	—	7.424[b]	Monge et al. (1964)
4820	—	—	—	—	—	7.426[b]	Monge et al. (1964)
3960	3	—	—	—	—	—	Lahiri et al. (1967)
4880	4	—	—	—	—	7.399	Lahiri et al. (1967)
4500	6	73.4	—	—	—	—	Lenfant et al. (1969)
4500	10	65.5	—	—	—	—	Lenfant et al. (1969)
4300	6	54.4	45.2	74.7	31.6	7.414	Torrance (1970)[c]
4500	4	63.3	44.1	73.3	32.2	7.405	Torrance (1970)[c]
4300	4	—	50.8	—	32.9	7.405	Rennie (1971)
4500	35	61.0	51.7	85.7	34.0	7.395	Winslow et al. (1981)

See Winslow and Monge (1987) for details and sources.
–, no data available.
[a] Hemoglobin concentration (g dL^{-1}).
[b] Plasma pH.
[c] Himalayan subjects.

The interpretation of these results is complicated by the fact that Winslow et al. (1981) believed that the increased red cell concentration that is seen at high altitude had an effect on the glass electrode for measuring pH (Whittembury et al. 1968). If the observed pH is corrected for this effect of increased red cell concentration, the calculated plasma pH becomes 7.395, as shown in the bottom row of Table 9.1. However, no other investigators have corrected the pH in this way and the conclusion from the work of Winslow and his colleagues is that high altitude natives have a mildly uncompensated respiratory alkalosis with an arterial pH that exceeds 7.4.

9.4.4 Acclimatized lowlanders

When sufficient time is allowed for extended acclimatization to high altitude, the arterial pH returns close to the normal value of 7.4, at least up to altitudes of 3000 m. For example, during the 1935 International High Altitude Expedition to Chile, Dill and his colleagues (1937) found that the arterial pH increased little if at all up to this altitude, but above 3000 m higher values of pH were found, with a mean of about 7.45 at an altitude of 5340 m. A few measurements on acclimatized subjects at an altitude of 5800 m during the 1960–1 Himalayan Scientific and Mountaineering Expedition indicated values of between 7.41 and 7.46 (West et al. 1962).

Extensive measurements were made by Winslow et al. (1984) during the 1981 American Medical Research Expedition to Everest. The mean arterial pH of acclimatized lowlanders living at an altitude of 6300 m was 7.47 (Figure 9.7). It was also possible to calculate the arterial pH at an altitude of 8050 m (Camp 5) and the Everest summit (8848 m). The calculations were made from the base excess measured on venous blood samples taken at 8050 m and measurements of alveolar P_{CO_2} on sealed samples of alveolar gas brought back to the USA. It was assumed that the arterial and alveolar P_{CO_2} values were the same, and also that base excess did not change over the 24 h between the summit and Camp 5. As discussed in section 9.4.5, there is evidence that base excess was changing very slowly at this great altitude. The mean arterial pH of two climbers at 8050 m was 7.55, and the one subject whose alveolar

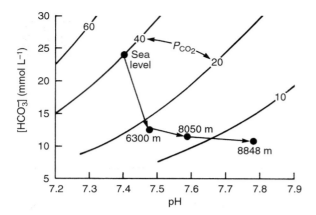

Figure 9.7 *Davenport diagram showing the pH, P_{CO_2} and plasma bicarbonate concentration of arterial blood during the 1981 American Medical Research Expedition to Everest at altitudes of 6300 m, 8050 m and 8848 m (summit). Note the increasingly severe respiratory alkalosis at the extreme altitudes. The points for 8050 and 8848 m are from Pizzo. (Data from Winslow* et al. *1984.)*

P_{CO_2} was measured as 7.5 mm Hg on the summit gave a calculated arterial pH of over 7.7.

These climbers were not 'acclimatized' to 8050 or 8848 m in the sense that they had spent long periods at these great altitudes. However, it is not possible to spend an extended time at an altitude such as 8000 m because high altitude deterioration occurs so rapidly. Thus the values probably represent the inevitable respiratory alkalosis which occurs in climbers who go so high.

9.4.5 Metabolic compensation for respiratory alkalosis

An interesting feature of the studies at extreme altitude referred to above is that metabolic compensation for the respiratory alkalosis appears to be extremely slow. The mean base excess measured on three subjects who were living at an altitude of 6300 m was −7.9 mmol L⁻¹. The measurements made on venous blood taken from two climbers at 8050 m gave a mean value of −7.2 mmol L⁻¹, essentially the same. The 8050 m measurements were taken several days after the climbers had left Camp 2 at 6300 m, and the

data therefore suggest that metabolic compensation was proceeding extremely slowly despite the fact that the P_{CO_2} had fallen considerably. For example, the mean P_{CO_2} at 6300 m was 18.4 mm Hg, at 8050 m 11.0 mm Hg, and at 8848 m (summit) 7.5 mm Hg. The last value was obtained from only one subject.

The reason for the very slow change in bicarbonate concentration at these great altitudes is unclear. One possible factor is chronic dehydration. Blume *et al.* (1984) measured serum osmolality at sea level, 5400 m and 6300 m in 13 subjects of the expedition and showed that the mean value rose from 290 ± 1 mmol kg⁻¹ at sea level to 295 ± 2 at 5400 m, and to 302 ± 4 at 6300 m. This volume depletion occurred despite adequate fluids to drink and a reasonably normal lifestyle. An interesting feature of the fluid balance studies was that plasma arginine vasopressin (AVP) concentrations remained unchanged from sea level to 6300 m despite the hyperosmolality. A possible factor in the volume depletion was the large insensible loss of fluid at these great altitudes as a result of hyperventilation. However, the failure of the vasopressin levels to change suggests that there is some abnormality of body fluid regulation.

It is known that the kidney is slow to correct an alkalosis in the presence of volume depletion. It appears that when given the option of correcting fluid balance or correcting acid–base balance, the kidney gives a higher priority to fluid balance. In order to correct the respiratory alkalosis, bicarbonate ion excretion must be increased (or reabsorption decreased) and this entails the loss of a cation which inevitably aggravates the hyperosmolality. This would explain the reluctance of the kidney to correct a respiratory alkalosis in the presence of volume depletion.

A different explanation was offered by Gonzalez *et al.* (1990) when they studied the slow metabolic compensation of respiratory alkalosis in a chronically hypoxic rat model. They found that the rate of metabolic compensation was indeed slower than in acute hypoxia, and they attributed this to the lower plasma bicarbonate concentration resulting from chronic hypoxia. They argued that, because proton secretion and reabsorption of bicarbonate are functions of the bicarbonate load offered to the renal proximal tubule, it is probable that the slower increase in bicarbonate excretion of the chronically hypoxic animals was ultimately the result of the lower plasma bicarbonate concentration.

Peripheral tissues

SUMMARY

The movement of oxygen from the peripheral capillaries to the mitochondria is the final link in the oxygen cascade. In muscle cells, the diffusion of oxygen may be facilitated by the presence of myoglobin, and it is possible that some convection also occurs in the cytoplasm of some cells. There is good evidence that the P_{O_2} in the immediate vicinity of the mitochondria of many cells is very low, of the order of 1 mm Hg. Many investigators believe that much of the pressure drop from the capillary to the mitochondria occurs very close to the capillary wall because of the limited surface area available for diffusion. This leads to the conclusion that the diffusion distance from the capillary wall to the mitochondria is relatively unimportant as a barrier to oxygen transport. This diffusion distance is decreased at high altitude, mainly because of the reduction in diameter of the muscle fibers. There is also an increase in myoglobin concentration and mitochondrial density at moderate altitudes. At extreme altitudes, mitochondrial volume in human skeletal muscle is decreased. Increases in the concentration of oxidative enzymes are seen at moderate altitudes, as is the case following training at sea level. The reverse occurs at extreme altitudes, where oxidative enzymes are decreased.

10.1 INTRODUCTION

The diffusion of oxygen from the peripheral capillaries to the mitochondria, and its consequent utilization by these organelles, constitutes the final link of the oxygen cascade which begins with the inspiration of air. Despite its critical importance, many uncertainties remain concerning the changes that occur in peripheral tissues both in acclimatized lowlanders and in the adaptation of high altitude natives. An obvious reason for this paucity of knowledge is the difficulty of studying peripheral tissues in intact humans. Much of our information necessarily comes from measurements on experimental animals exposed to low barometric pressures, though some additional studies have been made on tissue biopsies in humans.

It is probable that tissue factors play a very important role in the remarkable tolerance of high altitude natives to exercise at high altitude. As was pointed out in Chapter 5, people born at high altitude often have a reduced ('blunted') ventilatory response to hypoxia. At first sight this is counterproductive because it will result in a lower alveolar P_{O_2}, and therefore a lower arterial P_{O_2}, other things being equal. However, Samaja et al. (1997) found that the arterial P_{O_2} and oxygen saturation (estimated from earlobe blood) were the same in a group of Caucasians and Sherpas at altitudes of 3400 m, 5050 m and 6450 m, despite the fact that the Sherpas had a higher arterial P_{CO_2}. This suggests an improved efficiency of oxygen transfer in the lung, and may be linked to the higher pulmonary diffusing capacity of high altitude natives. However, even if the arterial P_{O_2} is the same in highlanders as lowlanders, the better exercise performance of the former at high altitude suggests that there are important adaptations within the tissues of which we are so far ignorant.

The present chapter overlaps with others to some extent. The principles of diffusion of gases through tissues were dealt with in Chapter 6, and there is a discussion in Chapter 11 of how diffusion limitation in peripheral tissues may limit oxygen delivery during exercise. This topic is also alluded to in Chapter 12 in the discussion of limiting factors at extreme altitudes.

10.2   HISTORICAL

Early physiologists interested in high altitude did not attach much importance to tissue changes. For example, Paul Bert in *La Pression Barométrique* hardly refers to the possibility of tissue acclimatization, although he deals at some length with changes in respiration and circulation. At one point he wonders whether the metabolism of high altitude natives is different from that of lowlanders:

> . . . just as a Basque mountaineer furnished with a piece of bread and a few onions makes expeditions which require of the member of the Alpine Club who accompanies him the absorption of a pound of meat, so it may be that the dwellers in high places finally lessen the consumption of oxygen in their organism, while keeping at their disposal the same quantity of vital force, either for the equilibrium of temperature, or the production of work. Thus we could explain the acclimatization of individuals, of generations, of races. (Bert 1878, p. 1004 in the 1943 translation)

Incidentally, we now know that the oxygen requirements of a given amount of work are no different at high altitude compared with sea level, or in high altitude natives compared with lowlanders. Bert goes on,

> But we should consider not only the acts of nutrition, but also the stimulation, perhaps less, which an insufficiently oxygenated blood causes in the muscles, the nerves, and the nervous centers. . . .

However, he does not carry his speculations any further.

There is a delightful section where Bert suggests that there may be changes in the blood at high altitude:

> We might ask first whether, by a harmonious compensation of which general natural history gives us many examples, either by a modification in the nature or the quantity of hemoglobin or by an increase in the number of red corpuscles, his blood has become qualified to absorb more oxygen under the same volume, and thus to return to the usual standard of the seashore (Bert 1878, p. 1000 in the 1943 translation).

He goes on to say that this hypothesis would be very easy to test. Since it had recently been shown:

> that the capacity of the blood to absorb oxygen does not change after putrefaction, nothing would be easier than to collect the venous blood of a healthy vigorous man (an acclimated European or an Indian) or of an animal, defibrinate it, and send it in a well-corked flask; it would then be sufficient to shake it vigorously in the air to judge its capacity of absorption during life (Bert 1878, p. 1008 in the 1943 translation).

This beautiful research project handed to the research community on a silver plate was taken up by Viault (1890) with exactly the results predicted by Bert. However, this project studied a change in the blood compartment of the body rather than in the peripheral tissues with which this chapter is chiefly concerned.

Following the work of Krogh (1919, 1929) on the increase in the number of open capillaries in muscle when the oxygen demands were raised by exercise, it was natural to wonder whether increased capillarization was a feature of tissue acclimatization in response to chronic hypoxia. It was subsequently reported that capillaries in the brain, heart and liver were significantly dilated and that their number was apparently increased after hypoxic exposure (Mercker and Schneider 1949, Opitz 1951). As we shall see later, some more recent measurements confirm these findings. However, other studies show that in some situations the actual number of capillaries in muscle tissue does not increase as a result of chronic hypoxia, but the intercapillary diffusion distance lessens because the muscle fibers become smaller.

Hurtado and his co-workers (1937) reported an increase in the intracellular concentration of the oxygen-carrying pigment, myoglobin, in high altitude animals. The measurements were made on dogs born and raised in Morococha (4550 m) and the increased concentrations were found in the diaphragm, myocardium and muscles of the chest wall and leg. The controls were dogs from Lima at sea level. Since then a number of other investigators have reported increased tissue myoglobin levels at high altitude.

An increase in mitochondrial density was shown in the myocardium of cattle born and raised at high altitude by Ou and Tenney (1970). Changes in mitochondrial enzymes in muscle of high altitude natives were reported by Reynafarje (1962). He found alterations in the enzyme systems NADH-oxidase, NADPH-cytochrome c-reductase, NAD[P]$^+$ transhydrogenase and others. These measurements were made on muscle biopsies taken from permanent residents of Cerro de Pasco in Peru at an altitude of 4400 m. The sea level controls were residents of Lima.

10.3 DIFFUSION IN PERIPHERAL TISSUES

10.3.1 Principles

Oxygen moves from the peripheral capillaries to the mitochondria, and carbon dioxide moves in the opposite direction by the process of diffusion. Fick's law of diffusion was discussed in section 6.3.2. It states that the rate of transfer of a gas through a sheet of tissue is proportional to the area of the tissue and to the difference in gas partial pressure between the two sides, and inversely proportional to the tissue thickness.

In discussing the lung, it was pointed out that the blood–gas barrier of the human lung is extremely thin, being only 0.2–0.3 μm in many places. By contrast, the diffusion distances in peripheral tissues are typically much greater. For example, the distance between open capillaries in resting muscle is of the order of 50 μm. However, during exercise, when the

oxygen consumption of the muscle increases, additional capillaries open up, thus reducing the diffusion distance and increasing the capillary surface area available for diffusion. As discussed in section 6.3.2, carbon dioxide diffuses about 20 times faster than oxygen through tissues because of its much higher solubility, and therefore the elimination of carbon dioxide poses less of a problem than oxygen delivery.

Early workers believed that the movement of oxygen through tissues was by simple passive diffusion. However, it is now believed that facilitated diffusion of oxygen probably occurs in muscle cells as a result of the presence of myoglobin. This heme-protein has a structure which resembles hemoglobin but the dissociation curve is a hyperbola, as opposed to the S-shape of the oxygen dissociation curve of whole blood (Figure 10.1). Another major difference is that myoglobin takes up oxygen at a much lower P_{O_2} than hemoglobin, that is, it has a very low P_{50} of about 5 mm Hg. This is a necessary property if the myoglobin is to be of any use in muscle cells where the tissue P_{O_2} is very low. Scholander (1960) and Wittenberg (1959) have shown experimentally that myoglobin can facilitate oxygen diffusion.

Other modes of oxygen transport are possible within cells. Streaming movements of cytoplasm have been observed and it is conceivable that such movements, known as 'stirring', enhance the transport of oxygen by convection. Another hypothesis is that oxygen moves into some cells along

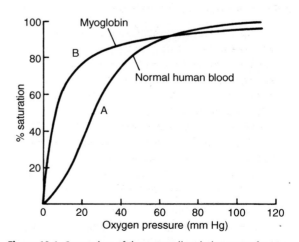

Figure 10.1 *Comparison of the oxygen dissociation curves for normal human blood (curve A) and myoglobin (curve B). The P_{50} values are approximately 27 and 5 mm Hg respectively. (From Roughton 1964.)*

invaginations of the lipid cell membrane in which it has a high solubility (Longmuir and Betts 1987).

There is good evidence that the P_{O_2} in the immediate vicinity of the mitochondria is very low, being of the order of 1 mm Hg. In fact many models of oxygen transfer in tissues assume that the mitochondrial P_{O_2} is so low that it can be neglected in the context of the P_{O_2} of the capillary blood, which is of the order of 30–50 mm Hg. In measurements of suspensions of liver mitochondria *in vitro*, oxygen consumption has been shown to continue at the same rate until the P_{O_2} of the surrounding fluid falls to the region of 3 mm Hg. Measurements of P_{O_2} at the sites of oxygen utilization based on the spectral characteristics of cytochromes also indicate that the P_{O_2} is probably less than 1 mm Hg (Chance 1957, Chance *et al.* 1962). Thus it appears that the purpose of the much higher P_{O_2} of capillary blood is to ensure an adequate pressure for diffusion of oxygen to the mitochondria and that, at the actual sites of oxygen utilization, the P_{O_2} is extremely low.

10.3.2   Tissue partial pressures

A classical model to analyze the distribution of P_{O_2} values in tissue was described by August Krogh (1919). He considered a hypothetical cylinder of tissue around a straight, thin capillary into which blood entered with a known P_{O_2}. As oxygen diffuses away from the capillary, oxygen is consumed by the tissue and the P_{O_2} falls. If simplifying assumptions are made, such as uniform consumption rate of oxygen in every part of the tissue, an equation can be written to describe the P_{O_2} profile (Krogh 1919, Piiper and Scheid 1986).

Another model is shown in Figure 10.2 (Hill 1928). In (a) we see a cylinder of tissue which is supplied with oxygen by capillaries at its periphery: in (1) the balance between oxygen consumption and delivery (determined by the capillary P_{O_2}, the inter-capillary distance R_C, and the oxygen consumption rate of the tissue) results in an adequate P_{O_2} throughout the cylinder; in (2) the intercapillary distance or the oxygen consumption has been increased until the P_{O_2} at one point in the tissue falls to zero. This is referred to as a critical situation. In (3) there is an anoxic region where aerobic (that is, oxygen-utilizing) metabolism is impossible. Under anoxic conditions the tissue energy requirements must be

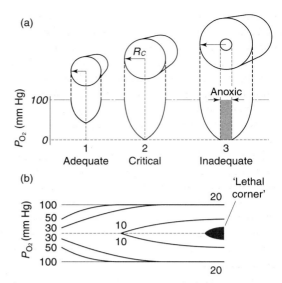

Figure 10.2 *Fall in* P_{O_2} *between adjacent capillaries. In (a) three hypothetical cylinders of tissue are shown and oxygen is diffusing into these cylinders from capillaries at the periphery. In (2) the cylinder had a critical radius (R_c), and in (3) the radius of the cylinder is so large that there is an anoxic zone in the middle of the cylinder. (b) shows a section along the hypothetical cylinder of tissue. The* P_{O_2} *in the blood adjacent to the tissue is assumed to fall from 100 to 20 mm Hg along the capillary. Lines of equal* P_{O_2} *are shown. Note the possibility of a 'lethal corner' in the middle of the cylinder at the venous end. (From West 1985.)*

met by obligatory anaerobic glycolysis with the consequent formation of lactic acid.

The situation *along* the tissue cylinder is shown in (b). It is assumed that the P_{O_2} in the capillaries at the periphery of the tissue cylinder falls from 100 to 20 mm Hg as shown from left to right. As a consequence the P_{O_2} in the center of the tissue cylinder falls towards the venous end of the capillary. It is clear that, on the basis of this model, the most vulnerable tissue is that furthest from the capillary at its downstream end. This was referred to as the 'lethal corner'. It is possible that this pattern of focal anoxia is responsible for some tissue damage at high altitude. For example, it may explain how some nerve cells of the brain are damaged at great altitudes causing the residual impairment of central nervous system function. This is discussed in Chapter 16.

The concept of a cylinder of tissue surrounded by a network of capillaries is supported by studies emphasizing the tortuosity of capillaries around skeletal muscle cells (Potter and Groom 1983, Mathieu-Costello 1987). Although in many histological sections the capillaries of skeletal muscle appear at first sight to run chiefly parallel to the muscle fibers, this is an oversimplification because of the connections between adjacent capillaries and also the tortuosity, which increases considerably as a result of muscle shortening (Mathieu-Costello 1987). Thus a reasonable model of oxygen delivery to muscle is a syncytium of capillaries surrounding a tubular muscle cell.

Recent studies by Honig and his associates (1991) have indicated that the P_{O_2} profiles shown in Figure 10.2 may be misleading in skeletal muscle. These investigators rapidly froze working muscles of experimental animals and then measured the degree of oxygen saturation of the intracellular myoglobin using a spectrometer with a narrow light beam. The intracellular P_{O_2} was inferred from the myoglobin oxygen saturation. These data and theoretical work by the same group suggest that the major resistance to oxygen diffusion from capillary to muscle fiber mitochondria is at the capillary–fiber interface, i.e. the thin carrier-free region including plasma, endothelium and interstitium. This in turn necessitates a large driving force (P_{O_2} difference) at that site to deliver oxygen to the muscle fibers. Some of the theoretical results of this group are shown in Figure 10.3 where it can be seen that most of the fall of P_{O_2} apparently occurs in the immediate vicinity of the peripheral capillary and that, throughout the muscle cell, the P_{O_2} is remarkably uniform and very low (of the order of 1–3 mm Hg). This pattern results chiefly from the presence of myoglobin which facilitates the diffusion of oxygen within the muscle fibers.

10.4   CAPILLARY DENSITY

One way to improve tissue diffusion under conditions of oxygen deprivation such as high altitude is to reduce the intercapillary distance. The technical name for the number of capillaries per unit volume of tissue is capillary density. It has been known since the time of Krogh (1919) that the number of open capillaries in a muscle depends on the degree of metabolic activity. During exercise additional capillaries open up, thus reducing the diffusing distance and increasing the diffusing surface area. Exercise training is known to increase the number of capillaries in skeletal muscle (Saltin and Gollnick 1983).

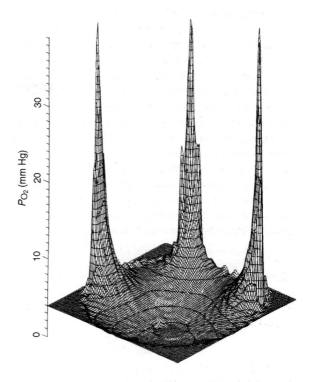

Figure 10.3 *Calculated distribution of P$_{O_2}$ around three capillaries in a heavily working red fiber of skeletal muscle. P$_{O_2}$ contours are at intervals of 1 mm Hg. There is a rapid fall of P$_{O_2}$ in the immediate vicinity of the capillary, and within the muscle cell the P$_{O_2}$ is relatively uniform and very low. (From Honig et al. 1991.)*

Early studies apparently showed increased vascularization of the brain, retina, skeletal muscle and liver of experimental animals exposed to low barometric pressures over several weeks (Mercker and Schneider 1949, Opitz 1951, Valdivia 1958, Cassin et al. 1971). Tenney and Ou (1970) measured the rate of loss of carbon monoxide from subcutaneous gas pockets in rats after 3 weeks of simulated exposure to 5600 m and concluded that there was a 50 per cent increase in capillary number.

However, some of these studies were questioned by Banchero (1982) who argued that the results obtained by Valdivia (1958) and Cassin et al. (1971) might be influenced by technical errors. Many investigators now believe that, although capillary density increases in skeletal muscles with exposure to high altitude, this is generally not caused by the formation of new capillaries, but by a reduction in size of the muscle fibers. This result has been found in guinea-pigs (Figure 10.4) which were studied at sea level, in Denver at 1610 m, at 3900 m (in a species native to the Andes) and at a simulated altitude of 5100 m (Banchero 1982).

The same pattern has been described in acclimatized humans where muscle samples were obtained by biopsy. For example, Cerretelli and his co-workers obtained muscle biopsies on climbers immediately after they had spent several weeks attempting to climb Lhotse Shar (8398 m) in Nepal and showed that, although the capillary density was somewhat raised, the increase could be wholly accounted for by a reduction of muscle fiber size (Boutellier *et al.* 1983, Cerretelli *et al.* 1984). A similar result was found in Operation Everest II in six volunteers who

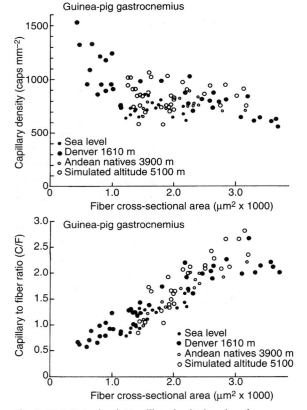

Figure 10.4 *Data showing capillary density (number of capillaries per square millimeter of cross-section) and capillary/fiber ratio (number of capillaries per muscle fiber) in gastrocnemius muscle of four groups of guinea-pigs. These were studied at sea level, in Denver at 1610 m, at 3900 m (Andean natives) and at simulated altitude of 5100 m. The data are consistent with the increase in capillary/fiber ratio being explained by a decrease in cross-sectional area of the muscle fibers. (From Banchero 1982.)*

were gradually decompressed to the simulated altitude of Mount Everest over a period of 40 days. Needle biopsies from the vastus lateralis showed a significant (25 per cent) decrease in cross-sectional area of type I fibers, and a 26 per cent decrease (nonsignificant) for type II fibers. Capillary to fiber ratios were unchanged and there was a trend (nonsignificant) towards an increase in capillary density (MacDougall *et al.* 1991).

In contrast to the studies showing that new capillaries in skeletal muscle do not develop as a result of exposure to high altitude, some recent reports do find increased capillarization. For example, Mathieu-Costello *et al.* (1998) reported increases in the number of capillaries in flight muscles of finches at high altitude, and increased capillarity was also found in leg muscles of finches living at high altitude (Hepple *et al.* 1998). These investigators believe that whether increased capillary number (and mitochondrial density) occur at high altitude depends on the level of metabolic stress on the muscle, and this links with the issue of training at altitude where similar changes are seen.

Although many studies show that the number of new capillaries in skeletal muscle does not increase as a result of exposure to prolonged hypoxia, it has been suggested that there are changes in the configuration of the capillaries with increased tortuosity that would effectively increase capillary surface area and enhance gas diffusion (Appell 1978). However, this result has not been confirmed by Mathieu-Costello and Poole (Mathieu-Costello 1989, Poole and Mathieu-Costello 1990), who showed that muscle capillary tortuosity does not increase with chronic exposure to hypoxia when account is taken of sarcomere length. These investigators believe that Appell's results may be explained by failure to control the state of contraction of the muscle. It is known that the degree of capillary tortuosity increases during muscle shortening (Mathieu-Costello 1987).

This lack of increase in the number of capillaries per muscle fiber at high altitude found in some studies should be contrasted with the increase in muscle capillarity which occurs with training. Longitudinal studies in humans have shown that exercise training increases muscle capillarity including both the capillary/fiber ratio and number of capillaries per square millimeter within several weeks (Andersen and Henricksson 1977, Brodal *et al.* 1977, Ingjer and Brodal 1978). Furthermore, it has been demon-

Table 10.1 *Comparison of tissue changes caused by training and those associated with exposure to high altitude*

Tissue changes	Endurance training	High altitude
Capillary density in skeletal muscle	Increased due to new capillaries	Increased due to reduction in diameter of muscle fibers
Fiber diameter of skeletal muscle	May be increased	Decreased
Myoglobin concentration	No change in humans	Increased in skeletal, heart muscle
Muscle enzymes	No change in glycolytic, increase in oxidative	Similar changes at moderate altitudes; at extreme altitudes, increase in glycolytic and decrease in oxidative
Mitochondria	Increased volume density	Increased volume density in some animals at moderate altitude but reduced density in humans at extreme altitude Different intracellular distribution, e.g. loss of subsarcolemmal mitochondria in comparison to training

strated that the increased capillary supply is proportional to the increased maximum oxygen uptake (Andersen and Henricksson 1977). The increase in capillaries is found in all fiber types provided that they are recruited during training (Andersen and Henricksson 1977, Nygaard and Nielsen 1978). If studies of acclimatization to high altitude involve increased levels of exercise, it is important to take account of this effect. Table 10.1 compares some of the tissue changes caused by training with those resulting from exposure to high altitude.

10.5   MUSCLE FIBER SIZE

As indicated above, one way to increase capillary density and thus reduce diffusion distance within skeletal muscle is to reduce the size of the muscle fibers. There is now good evidence that this occurs during high altitude acclimatization (Boutellier *et al.* 1983, Cerretelli *et al.* 1984, MacDougall *et al.* 1991). This topic is discussed further in Chapter 14.

The mechanism of muscle atrophy at high altitude is not well understood. It has been suggested that one contributing factor is lack of muscular activity. Certainly lowlanders who go to very high altitudes easily become fatigued and often spend much of their time at a reduced level of physical activity.

Indeed Tilman (1952, p. 79) once remarked that a hazard of Himalayan expeditions was bedsores!

However, reduced physical activity is unlikely to be the whole story as evidenced by the experience obtained on the 1960–1 Himalayan Scientific and Mountaineering Expedition. During several months at 5800 m, the level of physical activity was well maintained with opportunities for daily skiing and yet the expedition members suffered a relentless and progressive loss of weight which averaged 0.5–1.5 kg per week (Pugh 1964b). Moreover, estimates of energy intake were made and these were apparently more than adequate for the level of activity. It is true that appetite is reduced, and it may be that gastrointestinal absorption is impaired at high altitude (Chapter 14). However, it seems possible that there is some change in protein metabolism which results in extensive breakdown of muscle protein.

10.6   VOLUME OF MITOCHONDRIA

The muscle mitochondria are the primary sites of oxygen utilization by the body and thus constitute the final link of the oxygen cascade. In general, mitochondrial volume density (volume of mitochondria per unit volume of tissue) in skeletal muscle is related to maximal oxygen uptake and, for example, is greater in highly aerobic animals such as the horse compared with less active animals such as the cow (Hoppeler *et al.* 1987). It is also known that physical training increases mitochondrial volume density (Holloszy and Coyle 1984).

We might therefore expect that at high altitude where maximal oxygen uptake is reduced (Chapter 11) mitochondrial density would decrease. However, Ou and Tenney (1970) showed that the number of mitochondria in samples of myocardium was 40 per cent greater in cattle born and raised at 4250 m compared with cattle at sea level (Figure 10.5). The size of individual mitochondria was found to be the same and it was argued that the increase in mitochondrial number was advantageous because it reduced the diffusion distance of the intracellular oxygen. However, these interesting results may not apply to all species. Another investigation of the mitochondrial density of the myocardium of rabbits and guinea-pigs from Cerro de Pasco (4330 m) in Peru compared with those at sea level showed no increase in density (Kearney 1973).

Recent work indicates that the mitochondrial volume in human skeletal muscle decreases with exposure to very high altitude. In a study on muscle biopsies of climbers returning from two Swiss Himalayan expeditions, mitochondrial volume decreased by 20 per cent. This was associated with a decrease of 10 per cent in muscle mass. The net result was a decrease in absolute mitochondrial volume of nearly 30 per cent (Hoppeler *et al.* 1990). There was no significant increase in mitochondrial volume density in biopsies of vastus lateralis in subjects of Operation Everest II (MacDougall *et al.* 1991).

It may be that these discordant results can be explained by the differences between exposure to moderate and very high altitude. The increase in mitochondrial number found by Ou and Tenney (1970) was at an altitude of 4500 m, whereas the decrease in mitochondrial volume reported by Hoppeler *et al.* (1990) was in climbers who had been to altitudes over 6000 m. This is relevant to the discussion of high altitude acclimatization which occurs at moderate altitudes, and high altitude deterioration which occurs at extremely high altitudes, as discussed in Chapter 4.

There is an interesting difference between the mitochondrial density following exposure to high altitude on the one hand, and endurance training at sea level on the other, in their differential effects on subsarcolemmal and interfibrillar mitochondria. There is a greater loss of subsarcolemmal mitochondria at altitude, while subsarcolemmal mitochondria show a greater increase with training at sea level (Desplanches *et al.* 1993, Cerretelli and Hoppeler 1996).

10.7 MYOGLOBIN CONCENTRATION

As stated above, early studies by Hurtado and his colleagues (1937) showed increased concentrations of myoglobin in several muscles of dogs born and raised in Morococha (4550 m) in Peru. The controls were dogs in Lima at sea level. Increased myoglobin concentrations were found in the diaphragm, adductor muscles of the leg, pectoral muscles of the chest and the myocardium (Figure 10.6).

Reynafarje (1962) measured myoglobin concentrations in the sartorius muscle of healthy humans native to Cerro de Pasco (4400 m) and in other Peruvians native to sea level. Higher concentrations of myoglobin were found in the high altitude natives (7.03 mg g^{-1} tissue) than in the sea level controls (6.07 mg g^{-1}). The result was interpreted as a true high altitude effect because it was accompanied by an increased nitrogen content of the muscle, whereas

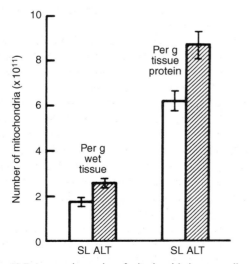

Figure 10.5 *Increase in number of mitochondria in myocardium of cattle born and raised at 4250 m (ALT) compared with another group born and raised at sea level (SL). The left-hand columns show the number of mitochondria (×10^{11}) per gram of wet tissue; the right hand columns show the number (×10^{11}) per gram of tissue protein. (Data from Ou and Tenney 1970.)*

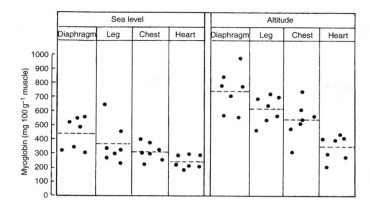

Figure 10.6 *Myoglobin concentration (mg 100 g⁻¹ of muscle) from seven sea level dogs compared with seven born and raised at 4540 m. (From Hurtado et al. 1937.)*

the lean body mass and body water content were the same as at sea level. This point was important because in another study (Anthony *et al.* 1959), a reported increase in myoglobin content of skeletal muscle in rats could possibly have been caused by a decrease in body weight as a result of dehydration. Other studies which have shown an increase in myoglobin as a result of acclimatization to hypoxia include those of hamster heart muscle (Clark *et al.* 1952), rat heart and diaphragm (Vaughan and Pace 1956) and various guinea-pig tissues (Tappan and Reynafarje 1957).

As discussed above, the chief value of myoglobin may be that it facilitates oxygen diffusion through muscle cells. However, it may also serve to buffer regional differences of P_{O_2} (Figure 10.3) and act as an oxygen store for short periods of very severe oxygen deprivation. It has been shown that increased levels of exercise raise the myoglobin content of muscles in experimental animals (Lawrie 1953, Pattengale and Holloszy 1967). Animals that exhibit large oxygen uptakes in conditions of reduced oxygen availability, such as seals, typically have very large amounts of myoglobin (Castellini and Somero 1981). However, a study comparing trained and untrained human subjects (Jansson *et al.* 1982) and another study of short-term training in humans (Svedenhag *et al.* 1983) both failed to show any effect of training on muscle myoglobin concentration.

10.8   INTRACELLULAR ENZYMES

Enzymes are essential to all aspects of the metabolic pathways involved in energy production. Figure 10.7

summarizes the three main stages in energy metabolism:

- the conversion of glucose units (from either glucose or glycogen, known as glycolysis), amino acids and fatty acids to acetyl CoA
- the citric acid or Krebs cycle
- the electron transport chain.

Because oxygen is not required for the glycolytic breakdown of glucose or glycogen, glycolysis represents an important though temporary source of energy under conditions of oxygen shortage or absence. By contrast, neither the Krebs cycle nor the electron transport chain can produce energy in the absence of oxygen.

There is evidence that chronic hypoxia caused by moderate or high altitude increases the concentration or activities of certain important enzymes involved in oxidative metabolism, but hypoxia does not appear to affect enzymes in the glycolytic pathway. However, it must be stressed that endurance exercise training also causes profound changes in the oxidative enzyme systems and it is difficult to maintain a given level of physical activity during exposure to chronic hypoxia. Similarly, it is also difficult to match sea level residents with residents at altitude with respect to physical activity.

Perhaps the first study of the enzymatic activity of human muscle at high altitude was that by Reynafarje (1962). The measurements were made on biopsies taken from the sartorius muscles of natives of Cerro de Pasco (4400 m) and these were compared with biopsies from residents of Lima at sea level. Reynafarje measured the activities of enzymes of glycolysis (lactate dehydrogenase), Krebs cycle

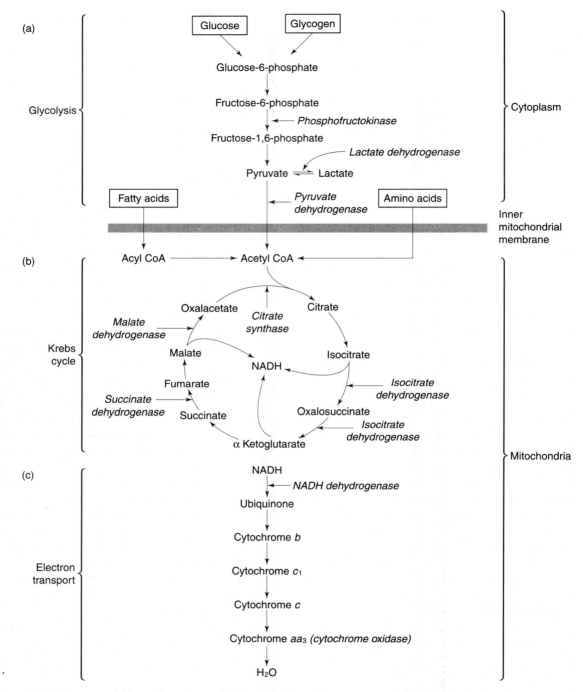

Figure 10.7 *Major energy-yielding pathways in muscle. The principal controlling enzymes are indicated. Altitude or hypoxic exposure and exercise training do not affect glycolytic capacity appreciably but cause substantial increases in oxidative capacity as demonstrated by augmented mitochondrial volume in some species and activity of major enzymes of the citric acid cycle and the electron transport chain.*

(isocitrate dehydrogenase), and the electron transport chain (NADH and NADPH-cytochrome c-reductase and NAD[P]$^+$ transhydrogenase). In this study Reynafarje found that the activities of NADH-oxidase, NADPH-cytochrome c-reductase and NAD[P]$^+$ transhydrogenase were significantly increased in the altitude residents.

Harris *et al.* (1970) reported on the levels of succinate dehydrogenase (Krebs cycle) and lactate dehydrogenase (glycolysis) activity in myocardial homogenates from guinea-pigs, rabbits and dogs indigenous to high altitude (4380 m) and compared the measurements with those made on the same species at sea level. They found a consistent increase in the activity of succinate dehydrogenase in the high altitude animals but no significant difference in lactate dehydrogenase. Ou and Tenney (1970) also found increased levels of succinate dehydrogenase and several enzymes of the electron transport chain including cytochrome oxidase, NADH-oxidase and NADH-cytochrome c-reductase in high altitude cattle.

In contrast to the effects of moderately high altitude (4000–5000 m), it appears that extreme altitude (above 6000 m) may cause a reduction in the activity of certain enzymes. The effect of exposure to extreme altitude on muscle enzyme systems has been studied by taking muscle biopsies from climbers before and after the Swiss expeditions to Lhotse Shar in 1981 (Cerretelli 1987) and Mount Everest in 1986 (Howald *et al.* 1990) and also from experimental subjects before and after prolonged decompression during Operation Everest II (Green *et al.* 1989). All of these studies reported decreased activities of oxidative enzymes. Results on three subjects from the Lhotse Shar expedition suggest that extreme altitude reduces the activity of both Krebs cycle (succinate dehydrogenase) and glycolytic (phosphofructokinase and lactate dehydrogenase) enzymes (Cerretelli 1987). In a more comprehensive study of seven climbers from the Swiss 1986 expedition, reduced activity of enzymes of the Krebs cycle (citrate synthase, malate dehydrogenase) and electron

transport chain (cytochrome oxidase) were reported (Howald *et al.* 1990). In contrast to the Lhotse Shar study, this latter study found increases in enzyme activities of glycolysis. In Operation Everest II, significant reductions were found in succinate dehydrogenase (21 per cent), citrate synthase (37 per cent) and hexokinase (53 per cent) at extreme altitudes (Green *et al.* 1989).

Interestingly, the enhanced capacity for oxidative metabolism found in the face of an unchanged glycolytic potential after high altitude (below 5000 m) exposure is qualitatively similar to the changes found in skeletal muscle after endurance exercise training (Holloszy and Coyle 1984). This observation supports the notion that tissue hypoxia may be responsible for the changes in mitochondrial density and oxidative enzyme capacity under both conditions. However, as pointed out earlier, there are differences between the two stresses, for example in the intracellular distribution of mitochondria.

It has been argued that the primary importance of an augmented oxidative capacity of skeletal muscle lies not in the ability to achieve a higher maximum oxygen uptake but, rather, to sustain a given submaximal oxygen uptake with less intracellular metabolic disturbance (i.e. change of ADP and inorganic phosphate (P_i), both potent stimulators of glycolysis) (Gollnick and Saltin 1982, Holloszy and Coyle 1984, Dudley *et al.* 1987). Thus, for strenuous exercise where fatigue is associated with depletion of muscle glycogen stores, an augmented muscle oxidative capacity enables a given oxygen uptake to be sustained at lower intracellular ADP and P_i concentrations. Consequently, muscle glycogen stores would be conserved and fat oxidation would contribute proportionally more to the energetic output of the muscle, resulting in an enhanced endurance capacity (Holloszy and Coyle 1984, Dudley *et al.* 1987). In conclusion, these changes in tissue enzymes (with the exception of those at extreme altitudes) are consistent with the assumption that the muscles are improving their ability for oxidative metabolism in the face of oxygen deprivation or deficiency.

11

Exercise

SUMMARY

Exercise at high altitude makes enormous demands on the oxygen transfer system of the body because of the increased oxygen uptake in the face of the reduced inspired P_{O_2}. Consequently, reduced exercise tolerance is one of the most obvious features of exposure to high altitude. Maximal exercise is accompanied by extremely high ventilations (measured at body temperature and pressure); these can approach 200 L min^{-1} at extreme altitudes, which is close to the maximum voluntary ventilation. Diffusion limitation of oxygen transfer across the blood–gas barrier is an important limiting factor. As a result, arterial P_{O_2} levels typically fall greatly as the work rate is increased. Some additional ventilation/perfusion inequality also often develops, possibly because of subclinical pulmonary edema. Maximal cardiac output is reduced at high altitude, although, in acclimatized subjects, the relationship between cardiac output and work rate is the same as at sea level. Maximal oxygen consumption in acclimatized subjects falls from about 4–5 L min^{-1} at sea level to just over 1 L min^{-1} at the Everest summit. Part of the reduction in $\dot{V}_{O_2\,max}$ can be ascribed to diffusion limitation within the exercising muscle. The oxygen consumption for a given work rate is independent of altitude. Although aerobic performance is greatly impaired at high altitude, there is no change in maximal anaerobic peak power (for example as measured by a standing jump) unless muscle mass is reduced.

11.1 INTRODUCTION

The hypoxia of high altitude puts stress on the oxygen transfer system of the body even at rest. If the oxygen requirements are further increased by exercise, the problems of oxygen delivery to the mitochondria of the working muscles are correspondingly exaggerated. Indeed, one of the most obvious consequences of going to high altitude is a reduced exercise tolerance.

In this chapter we examine the physiology of oxygen transfer from the air to the mitochondria in the face of the reduced inspired P_{O_2}. The steps in the oxygen cascade include getting the oxygen to the alveoli via pulmonary ventilation, diffusion of oxygen across the blood–gas barrier, uptake by the pulmonary capillary blood, removal from the lung by the cardiac output, transport to the tissues via the arterial blood, diffusion of oxygen to the mitochondria and utilization of oxygen by the cellular biochemical reactions. The present chapter synthesizes information, some of which occurs in other chapters. The subject of limitation of oxygen uptake under the conditions of extreme altitude is dealt with in Chapter 12. The literature on exercise at altitude is very extensive and the present chapter is necessarily selective. Many monographs and reviews have been published including Margaria (1967), Cerretelli and Whipp (1980), Sutton et al. (1983 1987), Cerretelli (1992) and Wagner (1996).

11.2 HISTORICAL

A reduced exercise tolerance at high altitude has been recognized since humans began to climb high mountains. For example, extreme fatigue was often reported in the early climbs of the European Alps and in fact this led to one of the popular theories of mountain sickness. The argument ran that the normal barometric pressure was necessary to maintain the proper articulation of the head of the femur in the acetabulum of the pelvis, and that at high altitude, when the reduced barometric pressure did not assist this as it should, the muscles became fatigued as a result (Bert 1878, pp. 343–6).

Some of the earliest measurements of exercise at high altitude were made by Zuntz, Durig and their colleagues in the first few years of the twentieth century (Zuntz et al. 1906, Durig 1911). For example, Zuntz showed that there was a decline in oxygen consumption but increase in ventilation at high altitude when trekkers walked at the speed that they normally adopted in an Alpine setting. Douglas, Haldane and their colleagues (1913) studied muscular exercise during walking uphill on Pikes Peak during the Anglo-American Expedition of 1911. They made the important observation that a given amount of work required the same amount of oxygen at 4300 m altitude as at sea level.

Colorful descriptions of the great difficulties of exercise at very high altitudes were common in the early Everest expeditions. Indeed, the accounts of the 1921 reconnaissance expedition (Howard-Bury 1922), and the expeditions of 1922 (Bruce 1923) and 1924 (Norton 1925) make graphic reading even today. Typical is E. F. Norton's account of his climb to nearly 8600 m without supplementary oxygen in 1924 (Norton 1925, pp. 90–119). He wrote

> ... our pace was wretched. My ambition was to do twenty consecutive paces uphill without a pause to rest and pant, elbow on bent knee, yet I never remember achieving it – thirteen was nearer the mark. (Norton 1925, p. 111)

Norton was accompanied to just below that altitude by the surgeon T.H. Somervell who subsequently wrote 'for every step forward and upward, 7 to 10 complete respirations were required' (Somervell 1936).

Of course, these were observations by lowlanders who were at extreme altitudes after relatively short periods of time for acclimatization. It is interesting to compare the observations of Barcroft who led an expedition at about the same time (winter of 1921–2) to Cerro de Pasco at an altitude of 4330 m in the Peruvian Andes (Barcroft et al. 1923). Naturally this was at a considerably lower altitude than near the summit of Mount Everest. Nevertheless, the lowlanders were amazed at the capacity of the high altitude residents for physical work, and they were astonished at the popularity of energetic sports such as soccer. The contrast between poorly acclimatized lowlanders and native high altitude dwellers, who had been at the same altitude for perhaps generations, was very clear.

Valuable findings on exercise at high altitude were made during the 1935 International High Altitude Expedition to Chile (Keys 1936). The expedition members studied their own maximal working capacity and showed how this fell as the altitude increased despite acclimatization. Christensen (1937) made measurements up to an altitude of 5340 m using a bicycle ergometer and confirmed the findings of Douglas et al. (1913) that the efficiency of muscle exercise was independent of altitude, that is that the oxygen consumption for a given work level was the same. In addition he showed that although exercise ventilation measured at BTPS (body temperature, ambient pressure, saturated with water vapor) was greatly increased at high altitudes, ventilation expressed at STPD (standard temperature and pressure, dry gas) was essentially independent of altitude over a wide range of altitudes and work rates.

An interesting observation was made by Edwards who documented a curious paradox about lactate levels in the blood on exercise. Generally, exhaustive exercise is accompanied by relatively high blood lactate levels, especially in unfit subjects, as the muscles outstrip their capacity for aerobic work and resort to anaerobic glycolysis. It would be natural to expect this to occur to an extreme extent at high altitude, as it does in acute hypoxia, but Edwards found the opposite. Exhaustive work at very high altitude was associated with very low levels of blood lactate (Edwards 1936). Dill and colleagues (1931) had previously seen the same phenomenon in a similar series of measurements.

The expedition members were also surprised by the tolerance of the miners for energetic physical activity at the Aucanquilcha mine, which they believed was at an altitude of 5800 m. We now know that the mine is actually higher, the altitude being 5950 m. The exercise level of the miners is indeed astonishing as they break large pieces of sulfur ore (caliche) with sledgehammers (McIntyre 1987). The miners are predominantly Bolivians who were born at moderately high altitudes and since most of them live at Amincha (altitude 4200 m) they have a considerable degree of high altitude acclimatization.

In preparation for the British Mount Everest expedition of 1953, Pugh measured oxygen uptakes on climbers in the field near Cho Oyu in the Nepal Himalayas in 1952. These data were then used to determine the amount of oxygen to be carried by the 1953 expedition during which Pugh made further measurements of exercise physiology (Pugh 1958). He subsequently greatly extended this programme in the ambitious Himalayan Scientific and Mountaineering Expedition (Silver Hut) of 1960–1 in which several physiologists spent the winter in a prefabricated hut at an altitude of 5800 m (Pugh 1962a). Further measurements of maximal oxygen consumption were carried out in the spring when the expedition moved to Mount Makalu (8481 m) and a bicycle ergometer was erected on the Makalu Col (altitude 7440 m) (Figure 1.8). Those measurements of maximal work remain the highest ever made (Pugh *et al.* 1964). The data assembled by Pugh and his co-workers (Figure 11.1) were of great interest because they predicted that, near the summit of Mount Everest, the maximal oxygen uptake would be very close to the basal oxygen requirements, and therefore it seemed problematic whether humans could ever reach the summit without supplementary oxygen (West and Wagner 1980).

Additional measurements of maximal oxygen consumption were made by Cerretelli during an Italian expedition to Mount Everest in 1973 (Cerretelli 1976a). All the data were obtained at Base Camp (altitude 5350 m) but they included measurements on climbers who had been above 8000 m. One of the many interesting observations was the failure of the maximal oxygen uptake of acclimatized subjects at 5350 m to return to the sea level value when pure oxygen was breathed. The explanation of

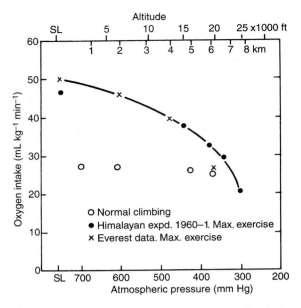

Figure 11.1 $\dot{V}_{O_2\,max}$ against barometric pressure in acclimatized subjects (●, ×) as reported by Pugh et al. (1964). Data from normal climbing rates are also shown (○).

this finding, also made by Pugh and others, is still controversial.

The issue of whether the partial pressure of oxygen at the summit of Mount Everest was sufficient for humans to reach it without supplementary oxygen was finally answered in 1978 by Reinhold Messner and Peter Habeler. However, their accounts make it clear that neither had much in reserve (Habeler 1979, Messner 1979). The intriguing question of how the body is just able to transport sufficient oxygen to the exercising muscles under these conditions of profound hypoxia is considered in detail in Chapter 12.

During the 1981 American Medical Research Expedition to Everest (AMREE), extensive measurements of maximal oxygen uptake were made in the main laboratory camp, altitude 6300 m. However, data were also obtained for exercise at higher altitudes by giving the well acclimatized subjects inspired mixtures containing low concentrations of oxygen. For example, when the inspired P_{O_2} was only 42.5 mm Hg, corresponding to that on the summit of Mount Everest, the measured maximal oxygen consumption was just over 1 L min^{-1} (West *et al.* 1983c). Although this is very low, being equivalent to that of someone walking slowly on the level, it is apparently just sufficient to explain how a climber can reach the summit without supplementary oxygen (Chapter 12).

A further extensive series of exercise measurements was made during Operation Everest II in the autumn of 1985 (Houston *et al.* 1987). The eight subjects spent 40 days in a large low pressure chamber being gradually decompressed to the barometric pressure existing at the summit of Mount Everest, and a series of measurements of maximal exercise was made using a bicycle ergometer. The measured oxygen consumptions agreed well with those found in the field by the 1981 expedition (Sutton *et al.* 1988), but Operation Everest II had the great additional advantage that many invasive measurements could be made which were impracticable in the field. These included extensive measurements of pulmonary vascular pressures, muscle volume and muscle biopsies (Sutton *et al.* 1987).

11.3   VENTILATION

Exercise at high altitude is accompanied by very high levels of ventilation. Indeed, this was one of the most obvious features of climbing at extreme altitudes in the early Everest expeditions, as evidenced by the quotations from Norton and Somervell in the preceding section.

Ventilation is normally expressed at body temperature, ambient pressure and with the gas saturated with water vapor (BTPS). This is because the volumes of gas moved then correspond to the volume excursions of the chest and lungs. Ventilation can also be expressed at standard temperature and pressure for dry gas (STPD). These volumes are very much smaller at high altitude and bear no obvious relationship to the actual chest movements. However, the oxygen consumption and carbon dioxide output are traditionally expressed in these units so that the values are independent of altitude.

For a given work level, the ventilation expressed as BTPS increases at high altitude. Typical results are shown in Figure 11.2b, which shows data obtained during the 1960–1 Silver Hut expedition (Pugh *et al.* 1964). Figure 11.2c shows ventilations expressed as STPD. Here the values also tend to be somewhat higher than those measured at sea level, especially at

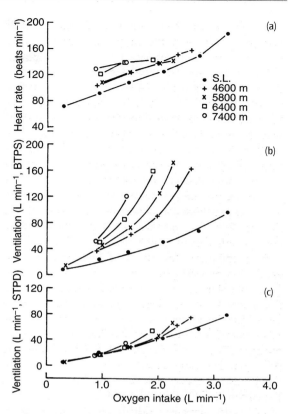

Figure 11.2 *Relationship between ventilation, both BTPS and STPD, and oxygen uptake at various altitudes. Heart rate is also shown. (From Pugh et al. 1964.)*

work levels approaching the maximum for the altitude, but the differences are clearly much less than for ventilation expressed as BTPS.

Ventilation (BTPS) can reach extremely high levels, as evidenced by data obtained during the 1981 AMREE expedition at an altitude of 6300 m (P_B 351 mm Hg). In eight subjects who exercised at a work rate of 1200 kg min⁻¹, the mean ventilation (BTPS) was 207 L min⁻¹ with a mean respiratory frequency of 62 breaths min⁻¹. These values were for a mean oxygen consumption of 2.31 L min⁻¹. These levels of ventilation far exceed anything ever seen at sea level and are approaching the maximal voluntary ventilation (MVV), that is the maximal amount of air that can be moved per minute by breathing in and out as rapidly and deeply as possible, usually measured over 15 s.

It is interesting that these extremely high levels of ventilation are not seen at the highest altitudes. For example, when two subjects on the 1981 expedition were given a 14 per cent oxygen mixture to breathe at an altitude of 6300 m (inspired P_{O_2} 42.5 mm Hg), the maximal exercise ventilation was only 162 L min⁻¹. This inspired P_{O_2} corresponded to that at the Everest summit. A reasonable explanation for the lower exercise ventilation is that the work rate was very much lower, being only 450 kgm min⁻¹ as opposed to 1200 kgm min⁻¹ at the altitude of 6300 m while breathing air. Another possibility is that the respiratory muscles were limited by the severe hypoxemia. Figure 11.3 shows maximal exercise ventilation plotted against inspired P_{O_2} (dashed line) and the fact that there is a maximal value is clearly seen, although there are only four points on the curve. A similar pattern was found during the 1960–1 expedition. For example, the maximal exercise ventilation at 5800 m had a mean value of 173 L min⁻¹. At the higher altitude of 6400 m this had fallen to 161 L min⁻¹, while at the highest altitude of 7440 m, the value was only 122 L min⁻¹. Corresponding to the fall in maximal exercise ventilation, the work rate decreased from 1200 kgm min⁻¹ at 5800 m, to 900 kgm min⁻¹ at 6400 m, to 600 kgm min⁻¹ at 7400 m.

These extremely high exercise ventilations are facilitated by the reduced work of breathing as a result of the lowered density of the air at high altitude. The reduced density also results in an increased MVV (or maximum breathing capacity) as altitude is increased (Cotes 1954). For example, Cotes showed that the MVV (BTPS) increased from 158 L min⁻¹ at sea level to 197 L min⁻¹ at a simulated altitude of 5180 m in a low pressure chamber. In a further study, a mean value of 203 L min⁻¹ was observed at a simulated altitude of 8250 m (Cotes 1954). The increase in MVV was compatible with the hypothesis that the work of maximum breathing remains constant at high altitude. The reduction in the work of breathing at high altitude caused by the change in gas density was also analyzed by Petit et al. (1963).

Oxygen breathing reduces exercise ventilation for a given work rate at high altitude. However, as Figure 11.4 shows, the ventilations do not return to the sea level values but are intermediate between the high altitude and sea level values for ambient air.

The pattern of breathing during exercise at high altitude is characterized by very high frequencies and relatively small tidal volumes. Somervell's observation, referred to in section 11.2, of 7–10 complete respirations per step is evidence for that. The highest measurements of respiratory frequency and tidal

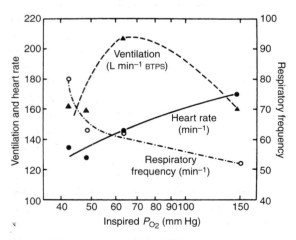

Figure 11.3 Maximal ventilation (BTPS), maximal respiratory frequency, and maximal heart rate plotted against inspired P_{O_2} on a log scale. This scale was chosen only because otherwise the high altitude points fall very close together. Note that both maximal ventilation and heart rate fall at extreme altitudes because work levels become so low. However, respiratory frequency continues to increase. (From West et al. 1983a.)

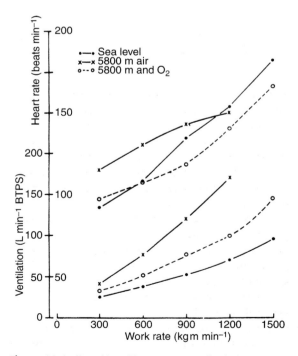

Figure 11.4 Effect of breathing oxygen at sea level pressure on ventilation and heart rate in acclimatized subjects at 5800 m. The points are mean values from two subjects. (From Pugh et al. 1964.)

volume yet made were those on Pizzo during the 1981 Everest expedition (West *et al.* 1983c). Pizzo climbed for about 7 min at an altitude of 8300 m (P_B 271 mm Hg) while measuring his ventilation with a turbine flow meter, and the output was registered on a slow-running tape recorder. During the middle 4 min of this period, his mean respiratory frequency was 86 ± 2.8 (SD) breaths min^{-1}, mean tidal volume was 1.26 L, and mean ventilation was 107 L min^{-1} at BTPS. Thus his breathing was shallow and extremely rapid. Reference has already been made to the measurements of maximal exercise at an inspired P_{O_2} of 42.5 mm Hg corresponding to that on the Everest summit which was obtained by making the subjects inspire 14 per cent oxygen at an altitude of 6300 m. For two subjects, the mean respiratory frequency was 80 breaths min^{-1}.

This pattern of breathing is consistent with the very powerful hypoxic drive via the peripheral chemoreceptors. As pointed out in Chapter 5, it is remarkable that the hypoxic drive is so strong under these conditions because the arterial P_{CO_2} is less than 10 mm Hg and the arterial pH is over 7.7. A very low P_{CO_2} and high pH normally inhibit ventilation.

11.4 DIFFUSION

As discussed in Chapter 6, there is strong evidence that diffusion limitation of oxygen transfer in the lung occurs during exercise at high altitude. This is the primary reason for the progressive fall in arterial P_{O_2} and arterial oxygen saturation which has been consistently observed. Analysis of the situation at extreme altitude indicates that the diffusing capacity of the blood–gas barrier is one of the chief limiting factors for maximal exercise (Chapter 12).

There is no evidence that the diffusing capacity of the blood–gas barrier increases during acclimatization to high altitude in normal subjects. Measurements from the 1960–1 Silver Hut Expedition showed that the diffusing capacity of the blood–gas barrier for a given level of exercise was the same as at sea level (West 1962a). Overall pulmonary diffusing capacity for carbon monoxide increased by 19 per cent at an altitude of 5800 m, but this could be attributed to the more rapid rate of combination of carbon monoxide with oxygen because of the low prevailing P_{O_2}. The volume of blood in the

pulmonary capillaries as determined by measuring the diffusing capacity at two values of alveolar P_{O_2} showed no change or possibly a slight fall. This may have been due to hypoxic pulmonary vasoconstriction.

These results also imply that, in acclimatized subjects, the transit time for red cells in the pulmonary capillaries at a given work level is approximately the same as at sea level. The transit time of the pulmonary capillary blood is given by the pulmonary capillary blood volume divided by the cardiac output (Roughton 1945). As discussed in Chapter 7, there is good evidence that, in acclimatized lowlanders at high altitude, the cardiac output for a given work level is the same as at sea level (Pugh 1964c, Reeves *et al.* 1987). Thus, since both the pulmonary capillary blood volume and the cardiac output are essentially unchanged, this indicates that the transit time through the pulmonary capillaries will also be the same as at sea level.

11.5 VENTILATION/PERFUSION RELATIONSHIPS

Until recently it was believed that the only change in ventilation/perfusion relationships at high altitude was a more uniform topographical distribution of blood flow. This is caused by the increased pulmonary arterial pressure as a result of hypoxic pulmonary vasoconstriction (Chapter 7). For example, measurements with radioactive xenon have shown that the topographical differences of blood flow between apex and base of the upright lung are reduced at an altitude of 3100 m (Dawson 1972). As discussed in Chapter 12, measurements by Wagner and his co-workers show a broadening of the distribution of ventilation/perfusion ratios during severe exercise at high altitude, the cause of which is still uncertain. The change in the distribution takes the form of a shoulder on the left of the blood flow distribution (plotted against ventilation/perfusion ratio), that is, an increase in blood flow to poorly ventilated lung units.

These changes have now been seen in normal subjects who are exercising while acutely exposed to hypoxia in a low pressure chamber (Gale *et al.* 1985), exercising normal subjects who are inhaling low oxygen mixtures (Hammond *et al.* 1986) and normal subjects during a 40-day exposure to low pressure in a chamber during Operation Everest II (Wagner *et al.* 1988a). Evidence from this last study suggests that the ventilation/perfusion abnormalities are most likely to be seen in poorly acclimatized subjects after a rapid ascent. In general, the abnormalities were most marked at the most severe levels of hypoxia, and at the heaviest exercise levels.

A reasonable hypothesis is that these changes are caused in some way by subclinical pulmonary edema which results in inequality of ventilation. As discussed in Chapter 19, high altitude pulmonary edema (HAPE) is a well known complication of going to high altitude. The likely mechanism is uneven hypoxic pulmonary vasoconstriction, which allows some capillaries to be exposed to high pressure with subsequent damage to their walls (West and Mathieu-Costello 1992a). The increase in pulmonary artery pressure is exaggerated during heavy exercise (Groves *et al.* 1987).

11.6 CARDIOVASCULAR RESPONSES

The cardiovascular effects of altitude are discussed in Chapter 7. In nonacclimatized and poorly acclimatized lowlanders who go to high altitude, cardiac output at rest and during exercise for a given work level is increased compared with sea level values. The same is true of heart rate.

In acclimatized lowlanders, cardiac output for a given work level returns to its sea level value, as shown by Pugh (1964c) during the 1960–1 Silver Hut Expedition, and more recently during Operation Everest II (Reeves *et al.* 1987). However, heart rate for a given level of exercise remains higher at altitude and therefore stroke volume is less. Measurements of contractile function of the heart during Operation Everest II in exercising subjects at all altitudes showed remarkable preservation despite the very severe hypoxemia (Reeves *et al.* 1987).

Pulmonary artery pressures are increased during exercise at altitude compared with sea level values at the same work level. The elevated pressures are seen in both unacclimatized (Kronenberg *et al.* 1971) and acclimatized (Groves *et al.* 1987) lowlanders, and in native highlanders (Peñaloza *et al.* 1963, Lockhart *et al.* 1976). The basic cause of the pulmonary hypertension is presumably hypoxic pulmonary vaso-

constriction. However, it is of considerable interest that in the subjects of Operation Everest II the pulmonary vascular pressures did not return to normal when 100 per cent oxygen was breathed, even though the subjects had been at high altitude for only 2–3 weeks (Groves *et al.* 1987). This indicates some structural changes (remodeling) in the pulmonary arteries in addition to hypoxic vasoconstriction.

11.7 ARTERIAL BLOOD GASES

At high altitude, the resting pattern of a low arterial P_{O_2} and P_{CO_2} is also seen during exercise. Arterial P_{O_2} typically falls further on exercise because of diffusion limitation. In addition, at high work levels, the arterial P_{CO_2} often falls below the resting value, indicating that alveolar ventilation increases more than carbon dioxide production. The falling P_{CO_2} is associated with an increased respiratory exchange ratio, which may rise to values over 1.2 at the highest work loads at very high altitudes (West *et al.* 1983c). This represents an unsteady state since the respiratory quotient of the metabolizing tissues cannot exceed 1.0. At sea level, such an increase in respiratory exchange ratio is often associated with lactate production from exercising muscles as a result of anaerobic glycolysis. However, at very high altitude, blood lactate levels remain surprisingly low even following exhausting exercise (Edwards 1936, Cerretelli 1980, West 1986c).

Arterial pH is near normal in well acclimatized subjects up to altitudes of about 5400 m, though Winslow obtained evidence that there is often a small degree of uncompensated respiratory alkalosis, even in native highlanders (Winslow *et al.* 1981, Winslow and Monge 1987). At higher altitudes the arterial pH at rest tends to increase and it exceeds 7.7 on the Everest summit (West *et al.* 1983b). The respiratory alkalosis is exaggerated on exercise because the arterial P_{CO_2} tends to fall and levels of blood lactate are low.

As stated in section 11.2, extensive observations that blood lactate is low in acclimatized subjects at high altitude, even during maximal work, were first made by Edwards (1936) during the 1935 International High Altitude Expedition to Chile, although Dill *et al.* (1931) had obtained some data

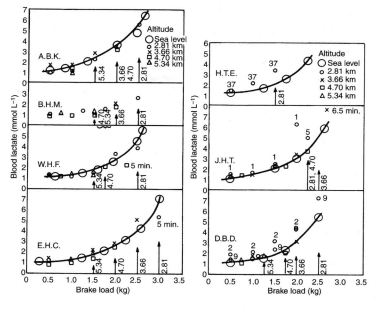

Figure 11.5 *Venous blood lactate after exercise as reported by Edwards from the 1935 International High Altitude Expedition to Chile. The lines are drawn through the sea level values. In general, lactate levels at high altitude lie on the same line, the only obvious exceptions being measurements made at the lowest altitude of 2.81 km. The small figures above these points indicate the number of days spent at that altitude and in most instances this was insufficient for acclimatization. (From Edwards 1936.)*

prior to that. Figure 11.5 is redrawn from Edward's paper and shows that the levels of blood lactate during exercise at high altitude (up to 5340 m) were essentially the same as at sea level. This means that the blood lactate levels for a given work level were apparently independent of tissue P_{O_2}. The only clear exceptions to this were the points shown by the open circles which were obtained at the lowest altitude of 2810 m. The small numbers over these points indicate the number of days that the subject had spent at this lowest altitude when the measurement was made, and it is clear that in most instances these data were obtained before the subject had had time to become fully acclimatized. Since maximal work capacity declines markedly with increasing altitude, the data of Figure 11.5 imply that maximal blood lactate falls in acclimatized subjects as altitude increases.

These results have been extended by Cerretelli (1976a,b, 1980) with additional measurements made at an altitude of 6300 m on the 1981 AMREE expedition (West *et al.* 1983c). Figure 12.5 summarizes the data on resting and maximal blood lactate (West 1986c) and suggests the surprising conclusion that, after maximal exercise at altitudes exceeding 7500 m, there will be no increase in lactate in the blood at all despite the extreme oxygen deprivation. Possible reasons for this are discussed in more detail in Chapter 12.

11.8 PERIPHERAL TISSUES

The changes that occur in peripheral tissues at high altitude were discussed in Chapter 10. Animal studies indicate an increase in capillary density in some tissues as a result of chronic hypoxia. However, data available from human muscle biopsies indicate that the number of capillaries remains constant in acclimatized lowlanders, but the average distance over which oxygen diffuses is reduced because the muscle fibers become smaller. There are changes in intracellular enzymes, and some studies show an increase in muscle myoglobin which may enhance oxygen diffusion. All these factors will play an important role in oxygen delivery and utilization during exercise.

Recently there has been considerable interest in the possible role of oxygen diffusion from capillaries to mitochondria as a factor-limiting exercise at high altitude. Traditionally, many physiologists have argued that the power of working muscles at high altitude is determined by the amount of oxygen reaching them via the arterial blood. Oxygen delivery, defined as the arterial oxygen concentration multiplied by the blood flow to the muscle, has often been regarded as the critical variable.

Wagner and his co-workers have analyzed the relationship between oxygen uptake and the P_{O_2} of

(a)

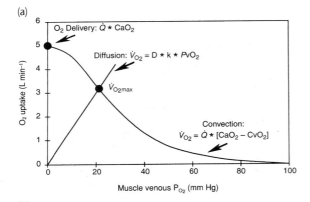

(b)

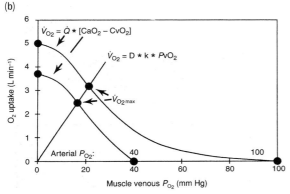

Figure 11.6 *(a) How $\dot{V}_{O_2\,max}$ is determined, assuming that oxygen diffusion from the peripheral capillary to the mitochondria is the limiting factor. The two lines show the oxygen uptake available from the Fick principle on the one hand, and Fick's law of diffusion on the other. The $\dot{V}_{O_2\,max}$ is given by the intersection of the two lines. See text for details. (From Wagner) (b) As (a) except an additional line has been added to represent the Fick equation at high altitude. This reduces the $\dot{V}_{O_2\,max}$ as shown. See text for details. (From Wagner.)*

muscle capillary blood on the assumption that the uptake is limited by oxygen diffusion from the capillaries to the mitochondria (Hogan *et al.* 1988a). Figure 11.6a shows the relation of oxygen uptake to the P_{O_2} of muscle venous blood, taken as an index of muscle capillary P_{O_2}. The line sloping from top left to bottom right shows the amount of oxygen being delivered to the muscle by the capillaries (Fick principle). The line from bottom left to top right shows the pressure gradient available to cause oxygen diffusion from the red cells to the mitochondria (Fick's law) assuming that the mitochondrial P_{O_2} is

nearly zero. The slope of this line is the lumped 'diffusing capacity for oxygen' of the tissues. The point where the two diagonal lines cross represents the $\dot{V}_{O_2\,max}$. Regions to the left of this indicate situations where ample oxygen is available in the blood but the diffusing head of pressure is inadequate. Regions to the right indicate a more than adequate diffusing head of pressure but inadequate amounts of oxygen in the blood.

Figure 11.6b shows the same diagram with another line added indicating the presumed situation at high altitude. Because the oxygen concentration of the arterial blood is low, the line representing the Fick principle is displaced downwards and to the left. The $\dot{V}_{O_2\,max}$ is therefore lower. The diagram assumes that the 'diffusing capacity for oxygen' of the tissue is the same at sea level and at altitude. It could be argued that this is not the case if the diffusing distance is reduced by the appearance of more capillaries, or the size of muscle fibers is reduced. However, experimental evidence indicates that these factors are relatively unimportant and that the diffusing capacity is essentially determined by the number of open capillaries (Hepple *et al.* 2000). This is in line with the fact that most of the fall in P_{O_2} is believed to be at the capillary wall (see Chapter 10), and that the myoglobin or other mechanisms of enhanced intracellular transport make the diffusion distance unimportant.

Several pieces of evidence now support this concept. For example, a retrospective analysis of data from Operation Everest II showed that the points relating the P_{O_2} of mixed venous blood to oxygen uptake tend to lie on a straight line passing through the origin. On the assumption that the P_{O_2} of mixed venous blood reflects the P_{O_2} of the blood in the capillaries of the exercising muscles, this relationship supports the notion. Indeed, it was this observation that prompted the hypothesis.

More direct evidence comes from a prospective study in which normal subjects exercised at high work loads breathing hypoxic mixtures, and samples of femoral venous blood were taken via an indwelling catheter (Roca *et al.* 1989). Again a plot of the P_{O_2} of femoral venous blood against oxygen uptake for different inspired oxygen concentrations showed the points lying close to a straight line passing near to the origin. A similar plot was found when the calculated mean capillary P_{O_2} was substituted for femoral venous P_{O_2}.

Additional studies have been carried out on an isolated dog gastrocnemius preparation where the muscle was supplied with hypoxic blood and stimulated maximally. Again a good relationship was found between the P_{O_2} of the effluent blood and the maximal oxygen uptake at different levels of hypoxia (Hogan *et al.* 1988a). This preparation allowed a test of two competing hypotheses, that referred to above, and an alternative hypothesis that $\dot{V}_{O_2 max}$ is determined by the amount of oxygen delivered to the muscle via the blood. The test was made by supplying the isolated muscle with the same amounts of oxygen (arterial oxygen concentration × blood flow) but using different blood flows (and therefore oxygen concentrations). The results showed that $\dot{V}_{O_2 max}$ was more closely related to the P_{O_2} of muscle venous blood than to the oxygen delivered via the arterial blood, and therefore the results support the hypothesis of diffusion limitation (Hogan *et al.* 1988b).

The diffusion limitation hypothesis has also been tested in more recent studies. In one, the oxygen affinity of hemoglobin was increased by feeding dogs sodium cyanate and it was shown that for the same convective oxygen delivery (cardiac output × arterial oxygen concentration) the maximal oxygen concentration of dog muscle was reduced compared with animals in which the oxygen affinity was normal (Hogan *et al.* 1991). The converse experiment was also carried out by reducing the oxygen affinity of hemoglobin using the allosteric modifier methylpropionic acid. In this case, the dog muscle showed an increased maximal oxygen consumption at a constant blood oxygen delivery compared with an animal with a normal oxygen affinity of hemoglobin (Richardson *et al.* 1998). There therefore are considerable experimental data supporting the analysis shown in Figure 11.6.

11.9 MAXIMAL OXYGEN UPTAKE AT HIGH ALTITUDE

Many investigators have documented the fall in maximal oxygen uptake at high altitude since the early studies of Zuntz *et al.* (1906), and the results of Pugh and his co-workers are shown in Figure 11.1. Figure 11.7a shows data from a number of studies collated by Cerretelli (1980). Note that, even at the

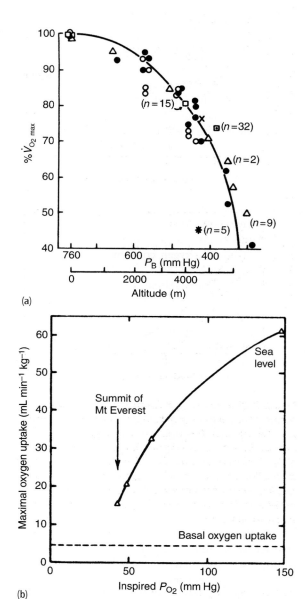

(a)

(b)

Figure 11.7 *(a)* $\dot{V}_{O_2 max}$ *as a percentage of the sea level value plotted against barometric pressure and altitude. (○, △), acute hypoxia; (●), chronic hypoxia; (×), high altitude natives. See original text for complete explanation of symbols. (From Cerretelli 1980.) (b) Maximal oxygen uptake against inspired P_{O_2} as measured on the 1981 American Medical Research Expedition to Everest. The lowest point was obtained by giving well acclimatized subjects at an altitude of 6300 m an inspired gas mixture containing 14 per cent oxygen. The inspired P_{O_2} was 42.5 mm Hg, which is equivalent to that on the Everest summit. Compare Figure 11.1. (Modified from West* et al. *1983a.)*

very modest altitude of 2500 m, there is already an average decrease of $\dot{V}_{O_2\,max}$ of 5–10 per cent as compared to sea level. Cerretelli pointed out that these data do not show any consistent differences between subjects exposed to acute hypoxia and those who have had the advantage of acclimatization to high altitude. This conclusion goes against the experience of many climbers who feel that they can work harder at high altitude after acclimatization, and the conclusion cannot presumably be true at the most extreme altitudes where acute exposure to the prevailing barometric pressure (for example on the summit of Mount Everest) results in loss of consciousness within a few minutes in most un-acclimatized individuals. It is of interest that elite high altitude climbers have only moderately high levels of maximal oxygen consumption at sea level (Oelz et al. 1986).

These data on maximal oxygen uptake were extended by the 1981 AMREE studies, where measurements were made at an altitude of 6300 m on subjects breathing ambient air, but also breathing 16 and 14 per cent oxygen (West et al. 1983c). The last gave an inspired P_{O_2} of 42.5 mm Hg, equivalent to that on the Everest summit. The results are shown in Figure 11.7b, where it can be seen that in these subjects who were well acclimatized to very high altitude, the $\dot{V}_{O_2\,max}$ fell to 15.3 mL min^{-1} kg^{-1} O_2, which was equivalent to 1.07 L min^{-1}. Thus at the highest point on Earth, the maximal oxygen uptake is reduced to between 20 per cent and 25 per cent of the sea level value. As pointed out in Chapter 12, this oxygen uptake is equivalent to that seen when a subject walks slowly on the level but nevertheless is apparently sufficient to explain how Messner and Habeler were able to reach the Everest summit without supplementary oxygen in 1978. Indeed, Messner's statement that the last 100 m took more than an hour to climb fits with this measured oxygen uptake (Messner 1979).

Measurements of $\dot{V}_{O_2\,max}$ at various altitudes were also made during Operation Everest II and the data are almost superimposable on those shown in Figure 11.7b at the highest altitudes (Sutton et al. 1987). This is interesting because the subjects of Operation Everest II were probably not as well acclimatized to the extreme altitudes as the members of the 1981 expedition, as judged from their alveolar gas composition and other measurements (West 1993b). The values for $\dot{V}_{O_2\,max}$ at any given altitude as

determined by the 1981 Everest expedition (Figure 11.7b) are higher than those earlier reported by Pugh et al. (1964) based on measurements made during the Silver Hut Expedition and previous measurements on Mount Everest. This can be explained by the higher level of fitness of subjects on the 1981 expedition. For example, several of the AMREE members were competitive marathon runners.

Several studies since the early measurements of Douglas et al. (1913) have shown that the relationship between oxygen uptake and work rate (or power) is independent of altitude. Figure 11.8a shows a comparison of data from the 1960–1 Himalayan Scientific and Mountaineering Expedition, and Figure 11.8b from the 1981 Everest expedition. The message of the two plots is the same, but note the much higher work rates at sea level recorded prior to the 1981 expedition which provide further evidence of the high level of athletic ability of these subjects.

As indicated earlier, breathing pure oxygen at high altitude does not return the $\dot{V}_{O_2\,max}$ to the sea level value, as shown by Cerretelli (1976a) and others. The reason is unclear; the opposite might be expected since the subjects acclimatized to high altitude have higher blood hemoglobin levels. However, against this are the results of a more recent study showing that when erythrocytes were infused into lowlanders after 1 or 9 days at an altitude of 4300 m, there was no improvement in the decreased $\dot{V}_{O_2\,max}$ (Young et al. 1996). It has been suggested that the reduced $\dot{V}_{O_2\,max}$ is caused by the loss of muscle mass at high altitude, and that if $\dot{V}_{O_2\,max}$ were related to lean body mass, the reduction would not be found. As discussed in Chapter 10, the diameter of muscle fibers decreases during acclimatization. Another possibility is that the increased red cell concentration causes uneven blood flow and sludging in peripheral capillaries and this interferes with oxygen unloading.

Does a period of acclimatization at high altitude improve $\dot{V}_{O_2\,max}$ at sea level? Again the answer is not clear. Cerretelli (1976a) measured $\dot{V}_{O_2\,max}$ in a group of subjects at sea level shortly before they were exposed to an altitude of 5350 m for 10–12 weeks, and again at sea level about 4 weeks after return from altitude. Although there was an approximately 11 per cent increase in hemoglobin concentration, this was not accompanied by a statistically significant rise in $\dot{V}_{O_2\,max}$. On the other hand, more recent studies involving the reinjection of a subject's own red cells in order

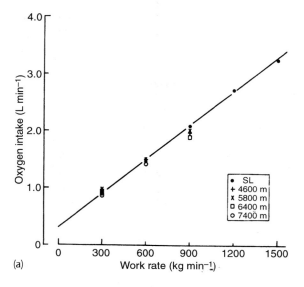

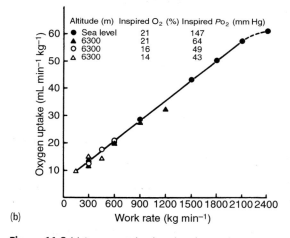

Figure 11.8 *(a) Oxygen uptake plotted against work rate at various altitudes during the Silver Hut Expedition showing that the relationship remains essentially the same as at sea level. (From Pugh* et al. *1964.) (b) Similar plot as in (a) but showing the much higher work rates at sea level obtained during the 1981 AMREE. (From West* et al. *1983a.)*

to raise the hematocrit have shown a small but significant increase in $\dot{V}_{O_2 max}$ at sea level (Spriet *et al.* 1986). This result would suggest that a period at medium altitude (certainly lower than 5350 m) may improve exercise tolerance at sea level. Perhaps the reduction of muscle fiber size at very high altitudes is the explanation for the failure to see an increase in $\dot{V}_{O_2 max}$ after acclimatization at very high altitude. As noted above, red cell infusions into lowlanders exposed to an altitude of 4300 m for 1 or 9 days did not improve the $\dot{V}_{O_2 max}$ at that altitude (Young *et al.* 1996).

It should be pointed out that the $\dot{V}_{O_2 max}$ determined at any particular altitude is something of an artificial measurement because climbers, for example, do not ordinarily exercise at that intensity. Pugh (1958) showed that climbers typically select an oxygen uptake of one-half to three-quarters of their maximum for normal climbing at altitudes up to 6000 m. Actual values of oxygen uptake measured by Pugh during normal climbing are included in Figure 11.1.

11.10   ANAEROBIC PERFORMANCE AT HIGH ALTITUDE

Reference has already been made to the paradoxically low levels of blood lactate following exhaustive exercise at extreme altitude (section 11.7, Figure 11.5). This phenomenon may be related to the reduced plasma bicarbonate concentration which interferes with buffering of hydrogen ion, as discussed in Chapter 12. Cerretelli (1992) has shown that the rate of increase of $\dot{V}_{O_2}$ when exercise is suddenly begun was slower in subjects after return from the 1981 Swiss Lhotse Expedition compared with before departure. This finding may be related to changes in anaerobic performance. However, it was also shown that maximal anaerobic (alactic) 'peak' power as measured by a standing jump was not affected by exposure of up to 3 weeks at 5200 m. Thereafter it tended to fall along with the reduction of muscle mass.

12

Limiting factors at extreme altitude

SUMMARY

The fact that a well acclimatized human can just reach the highest point on Earth without breathing supplementary oxygen is an extraordinary coincidence. Several experimental and theoretical studies in the early part of the twentieth century predicted that this would not be possible, and therefore it was of great interest when Messner and Habeler realized the feat in 1978. A critical factor is the higher barometric pressure in the great mountain ranges at latitudes near the equator than that predicted by the standard atmosphere. Another critical factor is the extreme hyperventilation that the successful climber generates, thus forcing his alveolar P_{CO_2} below 10 mm Hg and consequently defending his alveolar P_{O_2} at viable levels. Also important is the extreme respiratory alkalosis that increases the oxygen affinity of hemoglobin and thus assists in the loading of oxygen by the pulmonary capillary. Even so, the maximal oxygen consumption on the summit of Everest is only just above 1 L min^{-1}, and the arterial P_{O_2} is less than 30 mm Hg during physical work. The analysis of the physiological conditions near the Everest summit explains why tragedies occur when unexpected circumstances arise, such as deterioration of the weather. The fact that normal humans can survive the extreme derangement of blood gases which is necessary for these climbs to extreme altitudes is a graphic reminder of the resilience of the human organism.

12.1 INTRODUCTION

It is a remarkable coincidence that when humans are well acclimatized to high altitude, they can just reach the highest point on Earth without breathing supplementary oxygen. This feat was only realized in 1978 and many physiologists and physicians interested in high altitude had previously predicted that it would not be possible (West 1998). It was truly the end of an era when Messner and Habeler stood on the summit of Mount Everest on 8 May 1978.

This chapter examines the profound physiological changes that are necessary for humans to survive and do small amounts of work at extreme altitudes like the summit of Mount Everest. It includes an analysis of the factors that limit performance at these great altitudes and shows that such ascents are possible only if both the physiological make-up of the climber and physical factors such as barometric pressure are right.

12.2   HISTORICAL

12.2.1   Sixteenth to nineteenth centuries

It has been known for many centuries that very high altitude has a deleterious effect on the human body and that the amount of work that a person can do becomes more and more limited as the altitude increases. One of the first descriptions of the disabling effects of high altitude was given by the Jesuit missionary Joseph de Acosta who accompanied the early Spanish conquistadores to Peru in the sixteenth century. He described how, as he traveled over a high mountain, he 'was suddenly surprised with so mortall and strange a pang, that I was ready to fall from the top to the ground.' His dramatic description was first published in 1590 (Acosta 1590).

In the eighteenth century, climbers in the European Alps reported a variety of disagreeable sensations which now seem to us greatly exaggerated. For example, the physicist De Saussure, who was the third person to reach the summit of Mont Blanc, reported during the climb:

> When I began this ascent, I was quite out of breath from the rarity of the air . . . The kind of fatigue which results from the rarity of the air is absolutely unconquerable; when it is at its height, the most terrible danger would not make you take a single step further.

When he was near the summit he complained of extreme exhaustion:

> This need of rest was absolutely unconquerable; if I tried to overcome it, my legs refused to move, I felt the beginning of a faint, and was seized by dizziness. . .

On the summit itself he reported:

> When I had to get to work to set out the instruments and observe them, I was constantly forced to interrupt my work and devote myself to breathing (de Saussure, 1786–7).

These dramatic complaints at an altitude of only 4807 m or less reflect a combination of an almost complete lack of acclimatization and the fear of the unknown.

In the nineteenth century numerous ascents were made of higher mountains, including those in the Andes, and there were abundant accounts of the disabling effects of extreme altitude. In 1879, Whymper made the first ascent of Chimborazo and described how, at an altitude of 16 664 ft (5079 m), he was incapacitated by the thin air:

> . . . in about an hour I found myself lying on my back, along with both the Carrels [his guides], placed *hors de combat,* and incapable of making the least exertion . . . We were unable to satisfy our desire for air, except by breathing with open mouths . . . Besides having our normal rate of breathing largely accelerated, we found it impossible to sustain life without every now and then giving spasmodic gulps, just like fishes when taken out of water (Whymper 1892).

However, Whymper and his two guides gradually recovered their strength and in fact his lively account shows that he was aware of the beneficial effects of high altitude acclimatization.

In the latter part of the nineteenth century, there was considerable interest in the highest altitude that could be tolerated by climbers. Thomas W. Hinchliff, President of the (British) Alpine Club (1875–7), wrote an account of his travels around the world and described his feelings as he looked at the view from Santiago in Chile.

> Lover of mountains as I am, and familiar with such summits as those of Mont Blanc, Monte Rosa, and other Alpine heights, I could not repress a strange feeling as I looked at Tupungato and Aconcagua, and reflected that endless successions of men must in all probability be forever debarred from their lofty crests . . . Those who, like Major Godwin Austen, have had all the advantages of experience and acclimatization to aid them in attacks upon the higher Himalayas, agree that 21 500 ft [6553 m] is near the limit at which man ceases to be capable of the slightest further exertion (Hinchliff 1876).

12.2.2   Twentieth century

In 1909, the Duke of Abruzzi attempted an ascent of K2 in the Karakoram Mountains, and although his party was unsuccessful in reaching the summit, they reached the remarkable altitude of 7500 m without supplementary oxygen. According to the Duke's biographer, one of the reasons given for this expedition was 'to see how high man can go' (de Fillippi 1912), and certainly the climb had a dramatic effect on both the mountaineering and the medical communities interested in high altitude tolerance. In contrast to the florid accounts of paralyzing fatigue and breathlessness given by De Saussure, Whymper and others at much lower altitudes, the Duke made light of the physiological problems associated with this great altitude. However, as we saw earlier (Chapter 6), his feat prompted heated arguments among physiologists about whether the lungs actively secreted oxygen at this previously unheard of altitude.

Ten years later, a milestone in the history of the physiology of extreme altitude was provided by the British physiologist, Alexander M. Kellas, whose contributions have been almost completely overlooked. Kellas was lecturer in chemistry at the Middlesex Hospital Medical School in London during the first two decades of the century, but, despite this fulltime faculty position, managed to make eight expeditions to the Himalayas, and probably spent more time above 20 000 ft (6100 m) than anyone else. In 1919 he wrote an extensive paper entitled 'A consideration of the possibility of ascending Mount Everest', which unfortunately was only published in French in a very obscure place (Kellas 1921). In this he analyzed the physiology of a climber near the Everest summit, including a discussion of the summit altitude, barometric pressure, alveolar P_{O_2}, arterial oxygen saturation, maximal oxygen consumption and maximal ascent rate. On the basis of his study he concluded that

> Mount Everest could be ascended by a man of excellent physical and mental constitution in first-rate training, without adventitious aids [supplementary oxygen] if the physical difficulties of the mountain are not too great.

The importance of this study was not so much that he reached the correct conclusion. He had so few data that many of his calculations were incorrect. However, Kellas asked all the right questions and he can claim the distinction of being the first physiologist to seriously analyze the limiting factors at the highest point on Earth. It was not until almost 60 years later that all his predictions were fulfilled.

Kellas was a member of the first official reconnaissance expedition to Everest in 1921, but tragically he

died during the approach march just as the expedition had its first view of the mountain they came to climb. Three years later, E. F. Norton, who was a member of the third Everest expedition, reached a height of about 8589 m (28 150 ft) on the north side of Everest without supplementary oxygen. He was accompanied to just below that altitude by Dr T. H. Somervell, who collected alveolar gas samples at an altitude of 7010 m, though unfortunately these were stored in rubber bladders through which the carbon dioxide rapidly diffused (Somervell 1925). Somervell also referred to the extreme breathlessness at that altitude, stating that 'for every step forward and upward, 7 to 10 complete respirations were required'.

The summit of Everest was finally attained in 1953 by Hillary and Tensing (Hunt 1953). Naturally, this was a landmark event in the physiology of extreme altitude, but the fact that the two climbers used supplementary oxygen still did not answer the question of whether it was possible to reach the summit breathing air. Hillary did remove his oxygen mask on the summit for about 10 min and at the end of the time reported

> I realized that I was becoming rather clumsy-fingered and slow-moving, so I quickly replaced my oxygen set and experienced once more the stimulating effect of even a few litres of oxygen.

Nevertheless, the fact that he could survive for a few minutes without additional oxygen came as a surprise to some physicians who had predicted that he would lose consciousness.

However, there was a precedent for surviving for this period on the summit in the experiment Operation Everest I, carried out by Houston and Riley in 1945. As briefly described in Chapter 1, four volunteers spent 34 days in a low pressure chamber and two were able to tolerate 20 min without supplementary oxygen on the 'summit'. In fact, the equivalent altitude was even higher because the standard atmosphere pressure was inadvertently used (section 12.3.2).

Additional information on whether there was enough oxygen in the air to allow a climber to reach the Everest summit while breathing air was obtained by Pugh and his colleagues during the 1960–1 Himalayan Scientific and Mountaineering (Silver Hut) Expedition (Pugh et al. 1964). Measurements of maximal oxygen consumption were made using a bicycle ergometer on a group of physiologists who wintered at an altitude of 5800 m and who were therefore extremely well acclimatized to this altitude. Figure 12.1 (lower curve) shows the results of measurements made up to an altitude of 7440 m. Note that extrapolation of the line to a barometric pressure of 250 mm Hg on the Everest summit suggested that almost all the oxygen available would be required for the basal oxygen uptake. (For details of the extrapolation procedure, refer to West and Wagner 1980.) Thus these results strongly suggested that a climber who could reach the Everest summit without supplementary oxygen would be very near the limit of human tolerance.

This ultimate climbing achievement occurred when Reinhold Messner and Peter Habeler reached the summit of Everest without supplementary oxygen in May 1978. Messner's account (Messner 1979) makes it clear that he had very little in reserve:

> After every few steps, we huddle over our ice axes, mouths agape, struggling for sufficient breath . . . As we get higher it becomes necessary to lie down to recover our breath . . . Breathing becomes such a strenuous business that we scarcely have strength to go on.

And when he eventually reaches the summit:

> In my state of spiritual abstraction, I no longer belong to myself and to my eyesight. I am nothing more than a single, narrow gasping lung, floating over the mists and the summits.

The long period of 25 years between the first ascent of Everest in 1953 and this first 'oxygenless' ascent also suggests that we are near the limit of human tolerance. Again, as indicated earlier, Norton and Somervell ascended to within 300 m of the Everest summit as early as 1924, but it was not until 1978 that climbers reached the top without supplementary oxygen. Thus the last 300 m took 54 years!

Since that historic climb, Messner has further confirmed his outstanding tolerance to the extreme hypoxia of great altitudes. In 1980, he became the first man to ascend Everest alone without supplementary oxygen (Messner 1981), and in 1986 he became the first man to climb all 14 of the 8000 m peaks without supplementary oxygen. These accomplishments assure him a place not only in the history of mountaineering but also in the history of the physiology of extreme altitude.

12.3 PHYSIOLOGY OF EXTREME ALTITUDE

12.3.1 Introduction

This section is devoted to human performance at altitudes over 8000 m. There has been a renewed interest in this topic since Messner and Habeler climbed Everest without supplementary oxygen in 1978 but, as indicated above, the issue of whether humans would be able to tolerate the highest altitude on Earth was raised early in this century, notably by Kellas in 1919.

The following analysis is based primarily on data from three studies. The first was the 1960–1 Silver Hut Expedition during which data were obtained on maximal oxygen consumptions as high as 7440 m (P_B 300 mm Hg) and alveolar gas samples were taken as high as 7830 m (P_B 288 mm Hg). These measurements were extended to the Everest summit by the 1981 American Medical Research Expedition to Everest (AMREE), where measurements on the summit included barometric pressure, alveolar gas sam-

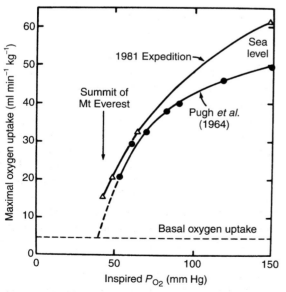

Figure 12.1 *Maximal oxygen uptake against inspired* P_{O_2}. *The lower line shows data from Pugh* et al. *(1964) suggesting that all the oxygen available at the Everest summit would be required for basal oxygen uptake. However, as the upper line shows, the 1981 AMREE measured an oxygen uptake of just over 1 L min^{-1} for an inspired* P_{O_2} *of 43 mm Hg. (From West* et al. *1983a.)*

ples and electrocardiograms, with additional measurements made between the summit and the highest camp situated at 8050 m (P_B 284 mm Hg). The third study was Operation Everest II in 1985 when eight volunteers were gradually decompressed to a barometric pressure of 240 mm Hg over a period of 40 days in a low pressure chamber. Although the rate of simulated ascent was too fast for optimal acclimatization, many valuable data were obtained, particularly in the areas of cardiopulmonary and muscle physiology.

12.3.2 Barometric pressure

Barometric pressure is a critical variable in physiological performance at extreme altitude because it determines the inspired P_{O_2}. This is the first link in the chain of the oxygen cascade from the atmosphere to the mitochondria. As pointed out in Chapter 2, there has been considerable confusion in the past about the relationships between barometric pressure and altitude on high mountains such as the Himalayan chain. The resulting errors are particularly important at extreme altitude because it can be shown that maximal oxygen consumption is exquisitely sensitive to barometric pressure. It is remarkable that Paul Bert gave essentially the correct value of barometric pressure for the Everest summit in Appendix I of his classic book *La Pression Barométrique* (Bert 1878). His figure of 248 mm Hg was based on an extrapolation of measurements made by Jourdanet at various locations including the Andes (Jourdanet 1875).

However, when the standard atmosphere was introduced and used extensively by aviation physiologists in the 1930s and 1940s, it was erroneously applied to Mount Everest, giving a value of 236 mm Hg, which was much too low. Nevertheless, this figure was used by several high altitude physiologists. For example, during Operation Everest I when four naval recruits were gradually decompressed to what was thought to be the simulated altitude of Mount Everest, they were exposed to a pressure of 236 mm Hg and their alveolar P_{O_2} fell to as low as 21 mm Hg (Riley and Houston 1950–1)! As the next section shows, this is about 14 mm Hg less than that of a well acclimatized climber on the summit of Mount Everest.

As described in Chapter 2, Dr Christopher Pizzo measured a barometric pressure of 253 mm Hg on the Everest summit on 24 October 1981. This was about 2 mm Hg higher than that expected from the mean barometric pressure for that month based on extensive weather balloon data (Figure 2.4). The discrepancy can be accounted for by normal variation and the high pressure system which made the weather ideal for climbing. The reading of 253 mm Hg was within 1 mm Hg of the pressure predicted for an altitude of 8848 m from radiosonde balloons released in New Delhi, India, on the same day (West *et al.* 1983a).

As section 12.4 shows, exercise performance at these extreme altitudes is exquisitely sensitive to barometric pressure. This is chiefly because the lung is working very low on the oxygen dissociation curve where the slope is steep. As a consequence, a fall of barometric pressure of as little as 3 mm Hg (less than twice the daily standard deviation) will apparently cause a reduction of maximal oxygen uptake of over 5 per cent. This means that even the daily variations of barometric pressure caused by weather can affect physical performance.

Seasonal variations of barometric pressure can be expected to have a marked effect on maximal oxygen uptake. As Figure 2.2 shows, mean barometric pressure falls from nearly 255 mm Hg in the summer months to only 243 mm Hg in mid-winter. This decrease is predicted to reduce maximal oxygen uptake by some 25 per cent. It is noteworthy that Mount Everest has only once been climbed during winter without supplementary oxygen (in December 1987), despite several attempts, and although the very cold temperatures and high winds are naturally a factor, the reduced barometric pressure must certainly contribute (section 2.2.8).

As pointed out in Chapter 2, the location of Mount Everest at 28°N latitude is fortunate because the barometric pressure at its summit is considerably higher than would be the case if it were at a higher latitude. As an example, if Mount McKinley were 8848 m high, its barometric pressure for May and October (preferred climbing months for Everest) would be only 223 mm Hg. It would apparently be impossible to reach the summit without supplementary oxygen under these conditions.

A similar argument would apply if the barometric pressure on the Everest summit were only 236 mm Hg, as predicted from the standard atmosphere model. The reduction of pressure by

17 mm Hg below that measured by Pizzo would reduce the maximal oxygen consumption by over 30 per cent, according to the analysis presented in the present chapter. It seems very probable that climbing Everest without supplementary oxygen under these conditions would be impossible. Thus the higher pressure that Everest enjoys because of its near equatorial latitude makes it just possible for humans to reach the highest point on Earth.

12.3.3 Alveolar gas composition

On ascent to high altitude, the alveolar P_{O_2} falls because of the reduction in the inspired P_{O_2}. At the same time, alveolar P_{CO_2} falls because of increasing hyperventilation. As described in Chapter 5, Rahn and Otis (1949) clarified the differences between unacclimatized and fully acclimatized subjects at high altitude by plotting their alveolar gas P_{O_2} and P_{CO_2} values on an oxygen–carbon dioxide diagram (Figure 5.4).

Figure 12.2 shows alveolar P_{CO_2} plotted against barometric pressure at extreme altitude. The closed circles show data reported by Greene (1934), Warren (1939), Pugh (1957) and Gill et al. (1962). The triangles show data obtained on the AMREE (West et al. 1983b). It can be seen that alveolar P_{CO_2} declines approximately linearly as barometric pressure falls and that the pressure on the summit of Mount Everest is about 7–8 mm Hg. The measurements

made on the summit itself had high respiratory exchange ratio (R) values, for reasons which are not clear. However, the data obtained at the slightly lower altitude of 8400 m (P_B 267 mm Hg) had a mean R value of 0.82 with a P_{CO_2} of 8.0 mm Hg, which means we can be confident of the very low values at this great altitude.

Figure 12.3 shows the line drawn by Rahn and Otis (1949) for fully acclimatized subjects (lower line on Figure 5.4) together with additional data obtained at barometric pressures below 350 mm Hg (Table 12.1). Note that the AMREE data (triangles) fit well with the extrapolation of the line. This method of plotting the data shows that, as well acclimatized humans go to higher and higher altitudes, the P_{O_2} falls because of the decreasing inspired P_{O_2}, and the P_{CO_2} falls because of the increasing hyperventilation. However, above an altitude of about 7000 m (P_B 325 mm Hg) the alveolar P_{O_2} becomes essentially constant at a value of about 35 mm Hg. More recent measurements of alveolar P_{O_2} up to an altitude of 8000 m by Peacock and Jones (1997) are in good agreement with these data. This means that successful climbers are able to defend their alveolar P_{O_2} by the process of extreme hyperventilation. In other words, they insulate the P_{O_2} of their alveolar gas from the falling value in the atmosphere around them. This appears to be the most important feature of acclimatization at extreme altitude.

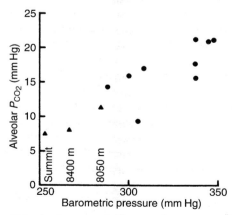

Figure 12.2 Alveolar P_{CO_2} against barometric pressure at extreme altitudes. Triangles show the means of measurements on the AMREE. Circles are results from previous investigators at barometric pressures below 350 mm Hg (Table 12.1). (From West et al. 1983b.)

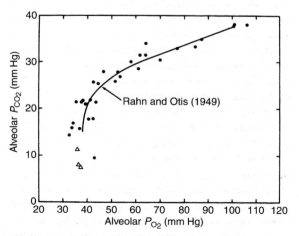

Figure 12.3 Oxygen–carbon dioxide diagram showing alveolar gas values collated by Rahn and Otis (1949) (circles) together with values obtained at extreme altitudes by the AMREE (triangles) (From West et al. 1983b.)

Table 12.1 *Alveolar P_{O_2} and P_{CO_2} in acclimatized subjects at barometric pressures below 350 mm Hg*

Source	Barometric pressure	P_{O_2}	P_{CO_2}	Respiratory exchange ratio (R)
Greene (1934)	337	40.7	17.7	0.87
	305	43.0	9.2	0.79
Warren (1939)	337[a]	37.0	15.6	0.60
Pugh (1957)	347	39.3	21.0	0.87
	337	35.5	21.3	0.87
	308	34.1	16.9	0.77
Gill *et al.* (1962)	344	38.1	20.7	0.82
	300	33.7	15.8	0.78
	288	32.8	14.3	0.77
West *et al.* (1983b)	284	36.1	11.0	0.78
	267	36.7	8.0	0.82
	253	37.6	7.5	1.49

All pressure values are given in mm Hg.
[a] Barometric pressure estimated from curve of Zuntz *et al.* (1906).

Not everyone can generate the enormous increase in ventilation required for the very low P_{CO_2} values shown in Figures 12.2 and 12.3. This explains why climbers with a large hypoxic ventilatory response usually tolerate extreme altitude better than those with a more modest response (Schoene *et al.* 1984). Indeed, experience on the AMREE showed that individuals who had an unusually low hypoxic ventilatory response were not able to remain at the higher camps (West 1985a).

The pattern of alveolar gas values shown in Figure 12.3 is only obtained if sufficient time is allowed for full respiratory acclimatization. Figure 12.4 compares the results found in unacclimatized and fully acclimatized subjects at high altitude (Figures 5.4, 12.3) with alveolar gas data reported from two low pressure chamber experiments in which the simulated rate of ascent was much faster. It can be seen that in Operation Everest I (Riley and Houston 1950–1) the subjects reached the simulated summit after only 31 days and at the extreme altitudes the data fell close to the region predicted by the line for unacclimatized humans. In Operation Everest II (Malconian *et al.* 1993) the ascent was a little slower, with the first simulated summit excursion occurring after 36 days. However, the alveolar gas values at extreme altitudes still deviated considerably from those found in fully acclimatized subjects. Little information is available about the time required for full respiratory acclimatization at extreme altitudes, say over 8000 m, but Figure 12.4 suggests that 36 days is inadequate whereas 77 days is apparently sufficient. However, it may be that other factors such as the level of physical activity are also important.

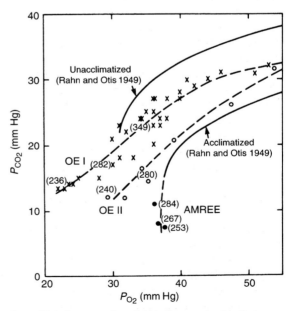

Figure 12.4 *Oxygen–carbon dioxide diagram showing the two lines described by Rahn and Otis (1949) for unacclimatized and acclimatized subjects at high altitude (compare Figure 5.4). In addition, data from Operation Everest I (OE I) and Operation Everest II (OE II) are included. Note that the OE I subjects were poorly acclimatized at extreme altitudes whereas the OE II had intermediate values. (From West 1998.)*

12.3.4 Acid–base status

Relatively little is known about acid–base changes at extreme altitude, despite the importance of this topic. Some data are available from two well acclimatized subjects of the AMREE, based on blood samples removed during the morning after they had reached the summit. Venous blood samples taken at the highest camp (8050 m; P_B 267 mm Hg) showed a mean base excess of −7.2 mmol L^{-1}. This was a considerably higher base excess than expected (in other words the base deficit was less than predicted) and the result was an extremely high arterial pH of over 7.7 calculated for the Everest summit (West *et al.* 1983b). This calculation assumes that there was no change in base excess in the previous 24 h and that a climber resting on the summit had a negligible blood lactate concentration (see below). In addition, the measured alveolar P_{CO_2} of 7.5 mm Hg is assumed to apply to the arterial blood.

A remarkable feature of these base excess values is that they were essentially unchanged from those measured in 14 subjects living for several weeks at Camp 2 (6300 m, P_B 351 mm Hg) where the mean value was −8.7 ± 1.7 mmol L^{-1} (Winslow *et al.* 1984). This suggests that base excess was changing extremely slowly above an altitude of 6300 m. The reason for this is not known but may be related to the chronic volume depletion which was observed in climbers living at 6300 m. At this altitude the serum osmolality was 302 ± 4 mmol kg^{-1}, which was significantly higher ($p < 0.01$) than in the same subjects at sea level, where the value was 290 ± 1 mmol kg^{-1} (Blume *et al.* 1984). It is known that the kidney gives a higher priority to correcting dehydration than acid–base disturbances, and in order to excrete more bicarbonate to reduce the base excess, it would be necessary to lose corresponding cations, which would aggravate the volume depletion. This may be the basis for the slow renal bicarbonate excretion.

These acid–base changes may be part of the explanation of why climbers can spend only a relatively short time at extreme altitudes, say above 8000 m. It was pointed out in Chapter 6 that the marked respiratory alkalosis which increases the oxygen affinity of the hemoglobin at extreme altitude is beneficial because it accelerates the loading of oxygen by the pulmonary capillaries. If a climber remains at extreme altitude for several days, presumably there is some renal excretion of bicarbonate (though this appears to be slow) and the resulting metabolic compensation would move the pH back towards 7.4. Thus the advantage of a left-shifted dissociation curve would tend to be lost.

One way to counter this disadvantage during a climb of Mount Everest would be to put in the high camps and then return to Base Camp at a lower altitude for several days. This period at medium altitude would then allow the body to adjust again to this more moderate oxygen deprivation and enable the blood pH to stabilize nearer its normal value. The final summit assault would then be as rapid as possible to take advantage of the nearly uncompensated respiratory alkalosis. In fact this was the pattern adopted by Messner and Habeler in their first ascent of Mount Everest without supplementary oxygen in 1978.

Blood lactate is known to be very low in acclimatized subjects at high altitude even during maximal work, an observation made by Edwards (1936) during the International High Altitude Expedition to Chile in 1935. Figure 12.5 shows data on resting and maximal blood lactate obtained by Cerretelli (1980). Also shown are measurements made at 6300 m after maximal exercise at the rate of 900 kg min^{-1}, that is, an oxygen uptake of 1.75 L min^{-1} (West 1986c). The mean value after exercise at 6300 m was only 3.0 mmol L^{-1} despite arterial P_{O_2} of less than 35 mm Hg and, presumably, extreme tissue hypoxia.

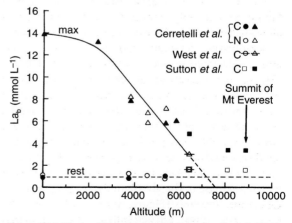

Figure 12.5 *Maximal blood lactate (La_b) as a function of altitude. Most of the data are redrawn from Cerretelli (1980). The filled circles and triangles show data for acclimatized Caucasians (C); the open circles and triangles are for high altitude natives (N). The data for 6300 m are from the AMREE for acclimatized lowlanders. (From West 1986.) The points marked Sutton* et al. *are from Operation Everest II (Sutton* et al. *1988).*

Note that extrapolation of the line relating maximal blood lactate concentration to altitude suggests that, after maximal exercise at altitudes exceeding 7500 m, there will be no increase in lactate in the blood at all despite the extreme oxygen deprivation. This is indeed a paradox.

The blood lactate concentrations after maximal exercise were appreciably higher on Operation Everest II (Sutton *et al.* 1988). For example, at an inspired P_{O_2} of 63 mm Hg, the mean lactate concentration following maximal exercise was 4.7 mmol L^{-1}, that is about 56 per cent higher than on the AMREE for the same inspired P_{O_2}. Moreover, the 'summit' measurements on Operation Everest II gave a blood lactate concentration of 3.4 mmol L^{-1}, a higher value than that found at only 6300 m on the AMREE (Figure 12.5). It is known that the low lactate concentrations following maximal exercise at high altitude come about as a result of high altitude acclimatization, because acute hypoxia causes very high lactate levels. Presumably therefore the higher values seen on Operation Everest II compared with the AMREE and other field studies can be explained by the limited degree of acclimatization.

The reasons for the low blood lactate levels following maximal exercise in well acclimatized subjects as opposed to poorly acclimatized subjects at high altitude are still unclear. One hypothesis is that on acute exposure to hypoxia, sympathetic stimulation leads to augmented muscle lactate production and blood lactate concentration through a beta-adrenergic mechanism. By contrast, chronic hypoxia causes beta-adrenergic adaptation and the result is a reduced lactate response after acclimatization. However, studies on unacclimatized and acclimatized subjects at 4300 m altitude have not supported this hypothesis (Brooks *et al.* 1998). Another hypothesis is that the bicarbonate depletion that occurs as a result of acclimatization interferes with the buffering of released lactate and hydrogen ions, and the consequent fall in local pH inhibits the enzyme phosphofructokinase in the glycolytic cycle and thus puts a brake on glycolysis (Figure 10.7). It is known that the activity of phosphofructokinase is reduced as the pH is lowered. Certainly Cerretelli has shown that the changes in blood hydrogen ion concentration as a result of increases in blood lactate are higher in acclimatized than unacclimatized subjects (Cerretelli 1980). However, many other factors affect blood lactate and the issue is far from settled.

12.3.5 Cardiac output

Intuitively, it would be reasonable to expect an increased cardiac output for a given work level at extreme altitude compared with sea level. It is known that cardiac output increases as a result of acute hypoxia (Chapter 7). Furthermore, the oxygen concentration of the arterial blood is extremely low at very high altitude, and an increase in cardiac output would be expected to help to compensate for the reduced oxygen delivery. Paradoxically, however, the relationship between cardiac output and oxygen uptake in acclimatized subjects at an altitude of 5800 m is essentially the same as at sea level (Figure 7.2) and this apparently holds true even at extreme altitudes, although data are sparse. Reeves *et al.* (1987) showed that the sea level relationship was maintained down to a barometric pressure of 282 mm Hg, and almost maintained at an inspired P_{O_2} equivalent to the summit of Mount Everest, though at that extreme altitude the cardiac output appeared to be slightly higher (Figure 7.3). Possibly this apparent paradox can be explained by the fact that, as the cardiac output is increased under these very hypoxic conditions, there is increasing diffusion limitation of oxygen transfer, both in the lung and in the muscle. In a theoretical study, Wagner (1996) showed that increasing cardiac output for the conditions on the Everest summit did not improve calculated $\dot{V}_{O_2 \, max}$ because of diffusion limitation (Figure 7.5).

12.3.6 Pulmonary diffusing capacity

As discussed in Chapter 6, oxygen transfer during exercise at high altitude is, in part, diffusion limited, and all calculations suggest that this limitation will be exaggerated at the extreme altitudes near the summit of Mount Everest. However, very few data on diffusing capacity at high altitude are available. Available measurements at an altitude of 5800 m (P_B 380 mm Hg) indicate that the diffusing capacity for carbon monoxide during exercise is essentially unchanged from the sea level value except for the expected increase caused by the faster rate of combination of carbon monoxide with hemoglobin under the prevailing hypoxic conditions (West 1962a). These data suggest that the diffusing capacity of the pulmonary membrane itself is unaltered by acclimatization.

Measurements of the diffusing capacity for carbon monoxide at different alveolar P_{O_2} values allow calculation of the pulmonary capillary blood volume. Again, in measurements made at 5800 m, there appeared to be little change in capillary blood volume, although there was a suggestion that it was slightly lower, possibly as a result of hypoxic pulmonary vasoconstriction (West 1962a). If we accept the conclusion that capillary blood volume is unchanged, and that the cardiac output/oxygen consumption relationship is the same as at sea level (section 12.3.5), this implies that capillary transit time in the lung is normal since this is given by capillary blood volume divided by cardiac output (Roughton 1945).

Using these data it is possible to calculate the changes in P_{O_2} along the pulmonary capillary for a climber at rest on the summit of Mount Everest (Figure 6.4). This shows that the rate of oxygenation is extremely slow and that the end-capillary P_{O_2} is much lower than the alveolar value, indicating severe diffusion limitation of oxygen transfer.

12.3.7 P_{O_2} of venous blood

During maximal exercise at extreme altitude, the extraction of oxygen by the peripheral tissues results in very low values of venous P_{O_2} in the exercising muscles. This in turn reduces the P_{O_2} of mixed venous blood. In order to analyze the relationships between the many variables and determine what limits exercise performance at extreme altitude, one possible assumption is that the body will not tolerate a P_{O_2} of mixed venous blood below a certain value, for example 15 mm Hg (West and Wagner 1980, West 1983). This assumption received strong support from Operation Everest II, where direct measurements of the P_{O_2} in mixed venous blood gave very similar values (Sutton et al. 1988). For example, on the 'summit' during 60 W of exercise, the P_{O_2} of mixed venous blood had a mean value of 14.8 mm Hg, and at 120 W, which was the highest work level, the mean P_{O_2} was 13.8 mm Hg.

12.3.8 Heat loss by hyperventilation

Matthews (1932) argued that tolerance to extreme altitude might be limited by the high rate of heat loss from the lungs as a result of the extreme hyperventilation. However, subsequent experience has not borne this out. Calculations of net heat loss are complex because the upper respiratory tract acts as a heat exchanger. During expiration, expired gas warms the respiratory tract, and this heat is then available to warm the cold inspired gas. Climbers who have reached the summit of Mount Everest without supplementary oxygen have not been affected by cold beyond the extent expected from the very low temperatures of the environment. When Pizzo reached the summit to take his alveolar gas samples during the course of the AMREE, he became overheated during the climb and photographs taken on the summit when he was breathing air show that he was not even wearing his down jacket, which he carried with him in his backpack (West 1985a, facing p. 51).

12.3.9 Oxygen cost of ventilation

A climber at extreme altitude has considerable hyperventilation at rest, and even more during moderate exercise. An alveolar P_{CO_2} of 7–8 mm Hg was measured on the Everest summit and, since it is known that the carbon dioxide production both at rest and for a given work level is independent of altitude, we can conclude that the alveolar ventilation on the summit was at least five times the resting value. Even small amounts of physical activity will greatly increase this. If we take the normal resting ventilation to be 7–8 L min^{-1}, this means that the resting ventilation on the summit is at least 40 L min^{-1}.

Cibella et al. (1999) studied the oxygen cost of ventilation in four normal subjects during exercise at sea level and after a 1-month sojourn at 5050 m. From simultaneous measurements of esophageal pressure and lung volume, the mechanical power (work rate) of breathing was determined. As expected, maximal exercise ventilation and maximal power of breathing were higher at high altitude than at sea level, whereas maximal oxygen uptake was reduced in all subjects at high altitude. Interestingly, in three subjects the relationship between mechanical power of breathing and minute ventilation was the same at sea level and high altitude, whereas in only one individual was it lower at high altitude for a given ventilation. It might have been expected that the mechanical power of breathing would be reduced at high altitude in all subjects because of the reduced density of the air.

Assuming a mechanical efficiency of 5 per cent, the oxygen cost of breathing at high altitude and sea level amounted to 26 and 5.5 per cent of $\dot{V}_{O_2\,max}$, respectively. The authors concluded that, at high altitude, the mechanical power of breathing may substantially limit the ability to do external work. They also calculated what they called the 'critical ventilation', that is the ventilation at which the mechanical power of breathing was so high that increasing ventilation above this level did not provide additional oxygen for external work. At the altitude of 5050 m the maximal exercise ventilation exceeded the critical

ventilation even when the efficiency was assumed to be as high as 20 per cent (Figure 12.6).

12.4 WHAT LIMITS EXERCISE PERFORMANCE AT EXTREME ALTITUDE?

12.4.1 Concept of limitation

The oxygen cascade from the atmosphere to the mitochondria includes the processes of convective ventilation of oxygen to the alveoli, diffusion of oxygen across the blood–gas barrier, uptake of oxygen by the hemoglobin in the pulmonary capillaries,

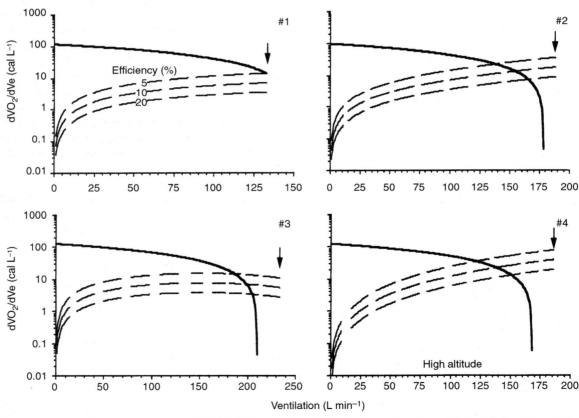

Figure 12.6 *Increase in oxygen consumption divided by the increase in ventilation for four subjects at an altitude of 5050 m. The solid line shows the relationship for total oxygen consumption; the dashed lines show the relationship for the oxygen consumption of the respiratory muscles, assuming mechanical efficiencies of 5, 10 and 20 per cent. Arrows show the maximal exercise ventilation. The intersection of the solid and dashed lines shows the critical ventilation above which no increase in external work was possible because the oxygen consumption of the respiratory muscles was so high. In three of the subjects, the maximum ventilation exceeded the critical ventilation for all assumed mechanical efficiencies, though in one of the subjects this was only the case for an efficiency of 5 per cent. (From Cibella et al. 1999.)*

convective flow of the blood to the peripheral capillaries, unloading of the oxygen from the hemoglobin, diffusion to the mitochondria and utilization of oxygen by the electron transport system. How can we determine to what extent each of these factors is limiting exercise at extreme altitude?

One approach is to use the analogy of a turbine that is fed by water flowing through a pipe which has a series of constrictions in it (Figure 12.7). Clearly, all sections of the pipe limit the flow of water to some extent. However, a useful description of the extent to which flow is limited by any particular section of the pipe can be found by calculating the percentage change in total flow for a given (say 5 per cent) change in diameter at that point. In carrying out this calculation, we assume that all other factors remain unchanged. Clearly, such an analysis can only be carried out if the whole system is modeled using a computer.

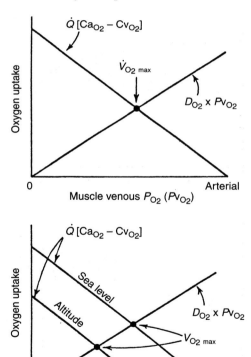

Figure 12.7 *Hydraulic analogy to clarify the concept of limitation of oxygen transfer. Each part of the pipe limits the flow of water to some extent. However, the extent of the limitation can be determined by noting the change in flow for a given (say 5 per cent) change in diameter (D) at a particular point. P is pressure at turbine.*

12.4.2   Limitations to oxygen uptake on the summit of Mount Everest

The model analysis described above has been carried out for a hypothetical subject exercising on the summit of Mount Everest (West 1983). Some assumptions and extrapolations are necessary because so few data have yet been obtained at these great altitudes. In general, the physiological variables were those set out in section 12.3. Table 12.2 summarizes some of the key variables. The whole oxygen transport system was modeled using numerical procedures previously described (West and Wagner 1977, 1980).

Figure 12.8 shows the calculated changes in the P_{O_2} of alveolar gas, arterial blood, and mixed venous blood as the oxygen uptake is increased for a climber on the summit of Mount Everest. For clarity, a maximum membrane oxygen diffusing capacity of 100 mL min^{-1} mm Hg^{-1} has been used for all values of oxygen uptake, though in practice the diffusing capacity would presumably be smaller at the lower work levels. Note the relentless fall in the P_{O_2} of the arterial and mixed venous bloods as the oxygen demand is increased. The decrease in arterial P_{O_2} in the face of a constant or rising alveolar P_{O_2} is the hallmark of diffusion-limited oxygen transfer. The slight rise in alveolar P_{O_2} at low work levels reflects the assumed increase in respiratory exchange ratio (R) from 0.8 at rest to 1.0 on moderate exercise.

To calculate maximal oxygen uptake ($\dot{V}_{O_2 max}$) it was assumed that the P_{O_2} of mixed venous blood could not fall below 15 mm Hg. As discussed in section 12.3.7, direct measurements of the P_{O_2} of mixed

Table 12.2 *Key variables for analysis factors limiting oxygen uptake on the summit of Mount Everest*

Measured	
Barometric pressure	253 mm Hg
Alveolar P_{CO_2}	7.5 mm Hg
Hemoglobin concentration	18.4 g dL^{-1}
P_{50} at pH 7.4	29.6 mm Hg
Base excess	−7.2 mmol L^{-1}
Assumed	
Respiratory exchange ratio	1.0
Cardiac output/oxygen uptake	Same as sea level
Maximal DM_{O_2}[a]	100 mL min^{-1} mm Hg^{-1}
Capillary transit time	0.75 s

[a] DM_{O_2}, diffusing capacity of the membrane for oxygen.

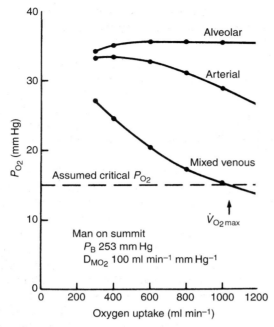

Figure 12.8 *Predicted changes in the* P_{O_2} *of alveolar gas and arterial and mixed venous blood as oxygen uptake is increased for a climber on the summit of Mount Everest. It is assumed that* $\dot{V}_{O_2 max}$ *will occur when* P_{O_2} *of venous blood falls to 15 mm Hg. Lower values of venous* P_{O_2} *may allow higher values of* $\dot{V}_{O_2}$. *(From West 1983.)*

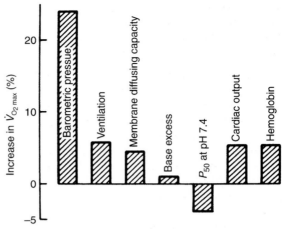

Figure 12.9 *Sensitivity of calculated maximal oxygen consumption* $(\dot{V}_{O_2 max})$ *to changes in variables for a climber on the summit of Mount Everest. The initial conditions are those shown in Table 12.2, and each variable was increased by 5 per cent leaving all the others constant. See text for details. (From West 1983.)*

venous blood during Operation Everest II support this assumption. The calculated $\dot{V}_{O_2 max}$ shown in Figure 12.9 of just over 1 L min^{-1} agrees well with results obtained on the AMREE when well acclimatized subjects performed maximal exercise with an inspired P_{O_2} of 42.5 mm Hg, equivalent to that on the Everest summit (West *et al.* 1983c). In addition, essentially the same value for $\dot{V}_{O_2 max}$ was reported by Sutton *et al.* (1988) in their measurements during Operation Everest II when the subjects had an inspired P_{O_2} of 43 mm Hg.

Figure 12.9 shows the sensitivity of $\dot{V}_{O_2 max}$ to the variables in this theoretical study using the type of analysis shown in Figure 12.7. Note that the calculated $\dot{V}_{O_2 max}$ is exquisitely sensitive to barometric pressure, a 5 per cent increase in this variable resulting in a 25 per cent increase in $\dot{V}_{O_2 max}$ when all the other variables were held constant. This is the basis for the assertion made in section 12.3.2 that even day-by-day variations of barometric pressure at these extreme altitudes may measurably affect exercise performance.

Figure 12.9 also shows that $\dot{V}_{O_2 max}$ is very sensitive

to the level of alveolar ventilation and the magnitude of the membrane oxygen diffusing capacity. The ventilation is important because any increase raises the alveolar P_{O_2}. The diffusing capacity is important because oxygen transfer under these conditions is diffusion limited (Chapter 6).

An increase in base excess results in a small rise in calculated $\dot{V}_{O_2 max}$. The reason is that for a given level of ventilation, and therefore arterial P_{CO_2}, a rise in base excess causes an increase in pH which moves the oxygen dissociation curve further to the left and increases the oxygen affinity of the hemoglobin. This assists in the loading of oxygen in the pulmonary capillaries (section 6.3.7).

By the same token, an increase in P_{50} of the oxygen dissociation curve reduces the calculated $\dot{V}_{O_2 max}$. The reason is the same: a reduced oxygen affinity of hemoglobin slows down the loading of oxygen in the pulmonary capillaries. This is an interesting point because it has often been claimed that the increase in 2,3-diphosphoglycerate (2,3-DPG) which is seen in the red cells at high altitude is a useful feature of acclimatization (Lenfant *et al.* 1971). In this analysis, increases of cardiac output and hemoglobin also improve the $\dot{V}_{O_2 max}$. However, in another theoretical analysis which takes account of diffusion limitation of oxygen transfer in the exercising muscles, this improvement is not seen (Figure 7.5). In fact, in practice, as discussed in Chapter 6, the relationship between cardiac output and $\dot{V}_{O_2 max}$ in acclimatized subjects at high altitude appears to be the same as at sea level. The chief conclusions from the analysis shown in Figure 12.9 are as follows:

- A climber attempting an ascent of Mount Everest without supplementary oxygen should ideally choose a day with a relatively high barometric pressure. Indeed, this appears to be the most critical variable. Fortunately, climbers generally try to make a summit assault when the weather is fine and usually this means a high pressure. Note, however, that this factor makes a winter ascent of Mount Everest without supplementary oxygen particularly difficult.
- The climber should not have a low hypoxic ventilatory response because this is critical in maintaining an adequate alveolar P_{O_2}.
- It is advantageous to have a high oxygen diffusing capacity at a moderate work level.
- The climber should have as high a base excess as possible. Presumably one way to ensure this is to avoid prolonged stays at extreme altitudes.
- Any rise in the level of 2,3-DPG in the red cell is apparently a liability because it increases the P_{50} and interferes with the loading of oxygen by the pulmonary capillaries.

12.4.3 How high can humans climb without supplementary oxygen?

We have seen that the $\dot{V}_{O_2 max}$ in acclimatized subjects with an inspired P_{O_2} of 43 mm Hg, equivalent to that on the Everest summit, is only a little over 1 L min^{-1}. This oxygen uptake is equivalent to walking slowly on level ground. Clearly, humans at the highest point on Earth are very close to the limit of hypoxic tolerance.

Nevertheless, it is interesting to speculate on how much higher humans could climb wihtout supplementary oxygen. The answer from Figure 12.8 seems to be very little. For example, only a 5 per cent decrease in barometric pressure from 253 to 240 mm Hg is calculated to reduce the $\dot{V}_{O_2 max}$ by 25 per cent, or to less than 800 ml min^{-1}. This would occur at an altitude of about 9250 m at the latitude of Everest, that is 400 m above the summit. Note also that the pressure of 240 mm Hg is still above that predicted for the summit of Mount Everest by the standard atmosphere (Chapter 2), indicating again that it is only the equatorial bulge in barometric pressure (Figures 2.3 and 2.5) which allows humans to reach the highest mountain top without supplementary oxygen.

13

Sleep

SUMMARY

Sleep is very commonly impaired at high altitude. Typically, people complain that they wake frequently, have unpleasant dreams and do not feel refreshed in the morning. Polysomnographic studies confirm the increased frequency of arousals. Electrencephalograms show changes in the architecture of sleep, with a great reduction in time spent in rapid eye movement (REM) sleep. Periodic breathing is almost universal at high altitude, and is accompanied by apneic periods which may be as much as 10–15 s long. The mechanism of the periodic breathing may be related to the strong hypoxic ventilatory drive. High altitude natives who have a blunted ventilatory response to hypoxia show less or no periodic breathing compared with lowlanders at high altitude. The severe arterial hypoxemia which follows the long apneic periods may reduce the arterial P_{O_2} to its lowest levels of the 24-h period. Acetazolamide stimulates ventilation at high altitude, reduces the time spent in periodic breathing and improves the arterial oxygen saturation during sleep. Oxygen enrichment of room air at high altitude results in fewer apneas, less time spent in periodic breathing and an improved subjective assessment of sleep quality.

13.1 INTRODUCTION

Everyone who has been to high altitude knows that sleeping is often impaired. This ubiquitous problem affects the skier or trekker who sleeps at altitudes of 2500–3000 m, as well as the well acclimatized climber who spends a night as high as 8000 m. The altitude of many modern skiing resorts is over 2700 m and many people who move rapidly from sea level to that altitude have difficulties with sleep for the first 2 or 3 nights. Often they cannot get to sleep for a long period, or they wake frequently, and often they complain that they do not awake refreshed in the morning. This last comment is also frequently heard from climbers at great altitudes on expeditions (Pugh and Ward 1956). Some people trying to sleep at high altitude complain that the mind races with a kaleidoscope of thoughts tumbling through it; this is certainly the case with the writer, who recognizes this as a very characteristic feature of the first night or two at high altitude.

Climbers at high altitude are often urged to climb high during the day but sleep low during the night. This advice acknowledges the increased incidence of difficulties during sleep. Many climbers over an altitude of about 7000 m find that a very low flow of supplementary oxygen of perhaps 1 L min^{-1} greatly improves the quality of sleep.

Periodic breathing during sleep at high altitude has been recognized since the nineteenth century. It is extremely common and may pose a hazard at extreme altitude because of the severe arterial hypoxemia which follows the apneic periods (West et al. 1986). Indeed, this may be one of the factors that influences tolerance to very great altitudes. From a scientific point of view, periodic breathing during sleep at high altitude throws light on the control of breathing under these special conditions.

The present chapter overlaps the material of Chapter 5 on the control of ventilation, and also has some links with Chapter 7 on cardiovascular responses because of the alterations in heart rate that occur with periodic breathing.

13.2   HISTORICAL

13.2.1   Quality of sleep

There have been a number of anecdotal references to the poor quality of sleep at high altitude. A particularly colorful description was given by Barcroft when he recounted his experiences during the glass chamber experiment carried out at Cambridge (Barcroft *et al.* 1920). On that occasion he spent 6 days in a closed chamber in which the concentration of oxygen was regulated so that the initial equivalent altitude was 10 000 ft (3048 m) and the final altitude 16 000 ft (4877 m). He wrote:

> In the glass case experiment I had the opportunity of judging a little more exactly of anoxaemic sleeplessness than is usually the case. A committee of undergraduate pupils of mine made up their minds that I was never to be left alone, two of them therefore sat up each night outside the case lest help of any sort should be required. I used to ask them in the morning how I had slept, and each morning except perhaps the last they said I had slept well. My own view of the matter was quite otherwise. I thought I had been awake half the night and was unrefreshed in the morning. I was conscious of their moving about and looking in through the glass to see whether or not I was awake. I used to count my pulse at intervals. The two opinions can only be reconciled on the hypothesis that whilst I spent most of the night in sleep, the slumber was very light and fitful with incessant dreams. Even some low degree of consciousness which fell short of wakefulness. At Cerro it was the same: measured in hours we slept well, but the quality of the sleep in most cases was of an inferior order. The night seemed long and we woke unrefreshed (Barcroft 1925, p. 166).

13.2.2   Periodic breathing

Various references to the uneven pattern of breathing during sleep at high altitude were made during the nineteenth century. One was by the eminent English physicist Tyndall who was one of the most ardent Alpine mountaineers in the middle of the century. Paul Bert commented that 'every year sees him planting his alpenstock on some new summit' (Bert 1878). During Tyndall's first ascent of Mont Blanc in 1857, he became very fatigued. 'I stretched myself upon a composite couch of snow and granite, and immediately fell asleep. My friend, however, soon aroused me "You quite frighten me" he said, "I listened for some minutes and have not heard you breathe once".' On renewing the ascent, Tyndall complained of palpitations. 'At each pause my heart throbbed audibly, as I leaned upon my staff, and the subsidence of this action was always the signal for further advance' (Tyndall 1860).

Another early comment on periodic breathing was made by Egli-Sinclair (1894) in an article on mountain sickness. He noted that, at an altitude of 4400 m, respiration 'had the Stokes character, that is, it seemed regular during a certain time, after which a few rapid and profound breaths were drawn, a total suspension of a few seconds then following.' Here he was referring to the Irish physician, Dr. William Stokes, who described the pattern of breathing which 'consists in the occurrence of a series of inspirations, increasing to a maximum and then declining in force and length until a state of apparent apnoea is established' (Stokes 1854). Another Irish physician, John Cheyne, had described the same pattern in 1818 (Cheyne 1818) and so the breathing pattern is often known as Cheyne–Stokes breathing. However, Ward (1973) pointed out that John Hunter had given a lucid and succinct description of the same condition in 1781 (Hunter 1781).

The first extensive studies of periodic breathing at high altitude were made by Angelo Mosso, Professor of Physiology at the University of Turin, Italy. As mentioned earlier, he was one of the first people to use the Capanna Regina Margherita on the Monte Rosa at an altitude of 4559 m for scientific work. He measured the breathing movements by means of a lever which rested on the chest. An example of one of his measurements on his brother, Ugolino Mosso, is shown in Figure 13.1a. The periods of apnea lasted about 12 s. Note that in this instance,

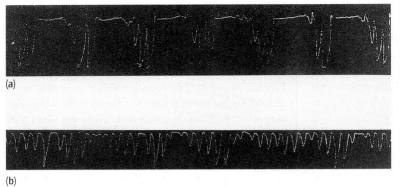

(a)

(b)

Figure 13.1 *Earliest tracings showing periodic breathing at an altitude of 4560 m: (a) a record from Ugolino Mosso, brother of Angelo Mosso. Note the apneic periods of approximately 12 s; (b) a tracing from Francioli, keeper of the Regina Margherita hut. Note the waxing and waning of respiration. (From Mosso 1898.)*

the first breath after the apneic period was the largest. A more typical pattern is that shown in Figure 13.1b which was measured on Francioli, keeper of the Regina Margherita hut. In this instance the waxing and waning of breathing movements are clearly seen and the periods of apnea are shorter (Mosso 1898, pp. 42–7).

A curious feature of Mosso's measurements was that he concluded that ventilation was actually decreased at high altitude, apparently because he converted his readings to standard conditions (0 °C and 1000 mm Hg in his case) rather than BTPS (body temperature and pressure saturated). Interestingly, Paul Bert also believed that hyperventilation did not occur at high altitude (Bert 1878, p. 106 in the 1943 translation). He wrote, 'What is really certain is that . . . a dweller in lofty altitudes, does not even try to struggle against the decrease of oxygen in his arterial blood by speeding up his respirations excessively, as was first supposed. The observations of Dr. Jourdanet are conclusive.' Bert probably reached this conclusion because he worked exclusively with low pressure chambers that only allowed short-term observations. It was not until Mosso could work in the Capanna Regina Margherita a few years later that measurements were easily made on subjects exposed to high altitude for several days although, as indicated above, he thought that ventilation was decreased.

Mosso realized that the alveolar P_{CO_2} was reduced in people living in the Capanna Regina Margherita at 4559 m, but instead of attributing this to an increased ventilation, he argued that the low pressure at high altitude extracted carbon dioxide from the blood just as does a mercury pump in a blood–gas analysis apparatus. Barcroft (1925) could not follow

Mosso's argument and remarked: 'I speak with all deference, but Mosso seems to me to have overlooked the fact that the body is exposed to what is practically a vacuum of carbon dioxide, whether it be at the Capanna Margherita or in his own laboratory at Turin.' Mosso introduced the term 'acapnia' to refer to the reduction of P_{CO_2} and believed that this was an important factor in the development of acute mountain sickness (AMS). Indeed, it may well be that the symptoms of this condition are related in part to the respiratory alkalosis. However, Barcroft (1925) pointed out that Mosso's theory was not supported by the experience at the Alta Vista hut (3350 m) on Tenerife during the First International High Altitude Expedition of 1910. Barcroft had an almost normal alveolar P_{CO_2} (38 mm Hg) but was incapacitated by the altitude, whereas Douglas, whose P_{CO_2} was only 32 mm Hg, was 'perfectly free from all symptoms'. Thus hypoxia (which was more severe in Barcroft because he did not increase his ventilation) rather than the low P_{CO_2} was implicated in the etiology of mountain sickness.

13.3 PHYSIOLOGY OF SLEEP

Despite the fact that we spend up to one-third of our lives in the sleeping state, the physiology is not completely understood. Sleep can be defined as a state of unconsciousness from which the subject can be aroused by sensory or other stimuli. As such it can be distinguished from deep anesthesia and diseased states which cause coma, though these have some features in common with true sleep.

Two major types of sleep are recognized.

13.3.1   Slow wave sleep (SWS)

This is often called non-REM or NREM sleep, or sometimes normal sleep. It is characterized by decreased activity of the reticular activating system, and is called slow wave sleep (SWS) because of the predominance of slow delta waves in the electroencephalogram (EEG). These slow waves have a high voltage and occur at a rate of 1 or 2 s^{-1}. In the early stages of sleep, the alpha rhythm (8–13 Hz), which is always present during wakefulness, becomes more obvious. In addition, sleep spindles (14–16 Hz) may appear. These features can be used to divide SWS into four stages (I–IV). The delta waves probably originate in the cortex of the brain when it is not driven from below because of the reduced level of activity of the reticular activating system. SWS is dreamless, very restful and associated with a decreased peripheral vascular tone, blood pressure, respiratory rate and basal metabolic rate.

13.3.2   Paradoxical or REM sleep

This is called REM sleep because, although the eyes remain closed, there are rapid horizontal eye movements. In a normal night of sleep, bouts of REM sleep lasting 5–20 min usually appear on the average about every 90 min. Often the first such period occurs 80–100 min after the subject falls asleep. The EEG tracing resembles the waking state, but the person is actually more difficult to arouse than during NREM sleep. REM sleep is usually associated with active dreaming; the muscle tone throughout the body is greatly depressed, but there may be occasional muscular twitching and limb jerking. The heart rate and respiration usually become irregular. Thus, in this type of sleep, the brain is quite active but the activity is not channeled in the proper direction for the person to be aware of his or her surroundings.

In experimental animals, sleep can be produced by electrically stimulating the raphe nuclei in the pons and medulla. There are extensive nerve fiber connections between these nuclei and the reticular formation. These nerve fibers secrete serotonin and some physiologists believe that this is a major transmitter substance associated with the production of sleep. However, other possible transmitter substances may play a role in the onset of sleep.

Sleep deprivation impairs mental function, the higher brain functions being the most susceptible. There are similarities between the behavior of sleep-deprived subjects and people at high altitude whose brains are affected by hypoxia. In both instances, mental activities which are 'mechanical' in nature, such as tabulating a set of data, can be accurately accomplished, whereas activities that require problem solving and initiative are seriously affected (Chapter 16). It may be that some of the impairment of CNS function in individuals living at high altitude can be ascribed to the poor quality of sleep, but the direct effects of hypoxia on the brain also clearly play a role.

13.4   CHARACTERISTICS OF SLEEP AT HIGH ALTITUDE

13.4.1   Increased frequency of arousals

People at high altitude often report that they wake more frequently during the night than at sea level, and this has been confirmed by careful studies (Reite et al. 1975, Weil et al. 1978, Salvaggio et al. 1998). The subjects had continuous recordings of the EEG, electromyogram (EMG) and eye movements, and an arousal was recognized by the occurrence of EMG activation, eye movements and alpha wave activity on the EEG. In one study an average of 36 arousals per night occurred at an altitude of 4300 m compared with 20 at sea level (Weil et al. 1978). Administration of the drug acetazolamide, which is known to stimulate ventilation at high altitude, reduced the frequency of arousals.

Some investigators believe that the arousals are caused in some way by periodic breathing. There is some evidence that arousals are more frequent when the strength of periodic breathing is high. It is easy to imagine that the strenuous muscular activity required to generate large breaths after a prolonged period of apnea could contribute to an arousal. A common nightmare at high altitude is that the tent has been covered with snow by an avalanche and the subject wakes violently feeling suffocated and very short of breath. This may be associated with the air hunger caused by a long apneic period as part of periodic breathing. However, arousals are more frequent at high altitude, even in individuals who do not have periodic breathing (Reite et al. 1975).

13.4.2   Changes of sleep state

EEG studies confirm that there is a deterioration in the quality of sleep at high altitude. Light sleep (stages I and II of NREM) is increased, whereas there are decreases both in deep sleep (stages III and IV of NREM) and in REM sleep. In some studies, REM sleep is virtually abolished (Pappenheimer 1977, Megirian *et al.* 1980). These studies of the electrical activity of the brain support the subjective conclusions of climbers that sleep at high altitude is often of poor quality, and not as refreshing as sleep at sea level.

Studies on rats by Pappenheimer (1977, 1984) have clarified the alterations in sleep at high altitude. In one study rats were exposed to 10 per cent oxygen, equivalent to an altitude of approximately 5490 m. The proportion of time spent in slow wave (NREM) sleep was measured from EEG recordings via chronically implanted cortical electrodes. Rats typically sleep on and off during the day, and during this period the proportion of time spent in SWS was 45 per cent when the rats breathed air, but only 27 per cent when they breathed the low oxygen mixture. Adding carbon dioxide to the inspired gas failed to prevent the reduction of SWS during hypoxia. This indicated that the effects of hypoxia on sleep depended on the changes in P_{O_2} rather than on the changes in P_{CO_2}.

The effect of sleep and hypoxia on the pattern of breathing was also studied. SWS decreased breathing frequency and minute volume by 10–20 per cent. However, when the animals inhaled the hypoxic mixture, the frequency increased markedly when the animals entered SWS, though the minute volume was not significantly changed. It was concluded that stimulation of breathing by hypoxia was greater during SWS than during wakefulness.

In a subsequent study (Pappenheimer 1984), the amplitudes of the cortical slow waves were measured during NREM sleep, and the relative amounts of REM and NREM sleep were also assessed. It was found that acute exposure of rats to 10.5 per cent oxygen (5030 m altitude equivalent) during daylight hours virtually abolished REM sleep. In addition, the distribution of amplitudes of the EEG of SWS shifted towards the values seen in awake animals. Adding carbon monoxide to the inspired gas sufficient to increase the concentration of carboxyhemoglobin to 35 per cent did not alter respiration rate and alveolar ventilation. It was therefore inferred that hypoxic stimulation of sleep was not mediated by peripheral chemoreceptors regulating breathing.

Pappenheimer also measured the amplitude of the cortical slow waves during sleep and showed that this was greatly reduced at the simulated high altitude (Figure 13.2). In fact, the primary effects of hypoxia were to reduce the amplitude of the EEG slow waves, and to shift the distribution of amplitudes towards the awake values, as shown in Figure 13.2. Pappenheimer suggested that this reduction in amplitude reflected the poor quality of the NREM sleep. In other words, even if the duration of NREM sleep as determined by conventional EEG recordings is not greatly reduced at high altitude, the quality of the NREM sleep may be greatly impaired. This conclusion fits with the assessments of the poor quality of sleep at high altitude given by many climbers, and Barcroft's colorful description quoted in section 13.2.1.

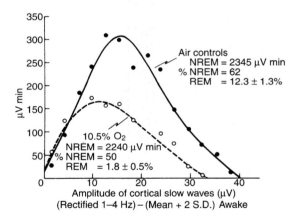

Figure 13.2 *Effects of acute hypoxia on the EEG pattern of sleeping rats. The ordinate shows the product of EEG amplitude and time. Hypoxia shifts the distribution of slow waves to lower amplitudes (light sleep), and reduces the amount of both NREM and REM sleep. (From Pappenheimer 1984.)*

13.5   PERIODIC BREATHING

13.5.1   Characteristics

Early records of chest movements during periodic breathing are shown in Figure 13.1. This pattern has

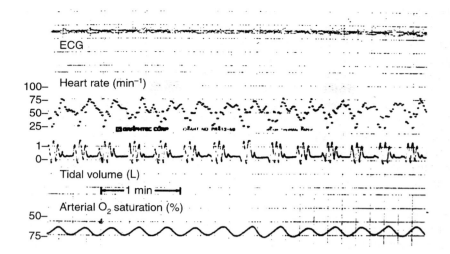

Figure 13.3 *Example of periodic breathing at altitude 6300 m (P_B 351 mm Hg). (From West* et al. *1986.)*

now been confirmed in many studies carried out at various altitudes from sea level up to 8050 m (Douglas and Haldane 1909, Douglas *et al.* 1913, Weil *et al.* 1978, Sutton *et al.* 1979, Berssenbrugge *et al.* 1983, Lahiri *et al.* 1983, West *et al.* 1986).

A typical pattern recorded at an altitude of 6300 m (P_B 351 mm Hg) in a well acclimatized lowlander using modern equipment is shown in Figure 13.3 (West *et al.* 1986). Note that the tidal volume waxed and waned during each burst of breathing, with apneic periods of about 8 s. Arterial oxygen saturation as measured by ear oximeter fluctuated with the same frequency as the periodic breathing. Note the

phase difference; the highest arterial oxygen saturation (inverted scale) occurred at approximately the end of the apneic period. This can be accounted for by the circulation time from the lung capillaries to the ear where the oxygen saturation was measured. Heart rate was measured from the electrocardiogram (ECG) and showed marked fluctuations with the same frequency as the periodic breathing. Note that the highest heart rate appeared at the end of the burst of ventilation.

Nocturnal periodic breathing is extremely common in lowlanders who ascend to high altitude. In the study from which Figure 13.3 is taken, all eight

Table 13.1 *Features of periodic breathing at 6300 m altitude*

Subject	Age (yr)	Duration of study (min)	% of time definite periodic breathing	% of time uncertain periodic breathing	No. of periodic breathing cycles analyzed	Cycle length of periodic breathing (s)	Apneic cycle ratio	Duration of apnea (s)
RP	25	94	85.3	0	80	17.9	0.42	7.5
DG	30	97	61.3	12.5	61	23.4	0.38	8.8
CP	31	62	90.0	2.6	59	19.5	0.36[a]	7.0
DK	33	133	71.3	17.7	78	19.7	0.40	7.9
PH	33	170	57.2	13.2	54	20.1	0.38	7.6
DJ	33	210	77.7	15.8	66	24.3	0.38	9.2
FS	38	138	76.1	5.5	84	21.4	0.40	8.6
JM	51	123	61.0	15.3	79	17.7	0.35	6.2
Mean	34.3	128	72.5	10.3	70.1	20.5	0.38	7.9
SD	±7.7	±46	±12.0	±6.7	±11.4	±2.4	±0.02	±1.0

Source: West *et al.* (1986).
[a] Apneic periods were only seen in a small proportion of cycles in this subject.

subjects who were living at an altitude of 6300 m showed obvious periodic breathing during the several weeks over which the measurements were made.

Table 13.1 shows some of the features of periodic breathing during this study. Measurements were made over a period of about 1–3.5 h late at night and the proportion of the study period during which periodic breathing was seen varied between 57 per cent and 90 per cent. In general, the percentage of time occupied by periodic breathing increases with altitude. For example, Waggener *et al.* (1984) reported that periodic breathing with apnea occupied 24 per cent of the time at 2440 m, and that the percentage increased to 40 per cent at 4270 m. This increase in proportion of time is consistent with a theoretical model discussed below (Khoo *et al.* 1982) and with the fact that periodic breathing is

occasionally observed during sleep at sea level but the proportion of time spent in periodic breathing is small (Priban 1963, Goodman 1964, Lenfant 1967).

In the American Medical Research Expedition to Mount Everest (AMREE) study from which Figure 13.3 is taken, we were not able to determine how much of the time the subjects were actually asleep. However, other studies have shown that periodic breathing is very common during NREM sleep at high altitude, but that it is uncommon during REM periods (Reite *et al.* 1975, Berssenbrugge *et al.* 1983). Of course, as indicated above, REM sleep itself is uncommon at high altitude.

Table 13.1 shows that the duration of the periodic breathing cycle had a mean of 20.5 s. This was the same as the cycle length measured in a companion study at 5400 m (Lahiri *et al.* 1983). There is evidence that cycle length decreases with increasing altitude (Waggener *et al.* 1984) and studies at sea level indicate a cycle period of about 30 s (Douglas and Haldane 1909, Specht and Fruhmann 1972, Lugaresi *et al.* 1978). Figure 13.4 shows a plot of cycle time against altitude for several experimental studies and the theoretical model developed by Khoo *et al.* (1982). It can be seen that the cycle times from the AMREE studies were somewhat greater than predicted by the model.

There is evidence that the apneic periods are of central nervous origin rather than being caused by airway obstruction. This is supported by the absence of rib cage and abdominal movements as determined from an inductance plethysmograph, a device used for detecting changes in circumference of the chest and abdomen. There was no evidence that the percentage of time during which periodic breathing was observed was altered by the duration of acclimatization. All subjects showed obvious periodic breathing but all were well acclimatized.

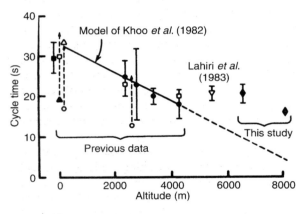

Figure 13.4 *Variation of cycle time of periodic breathing with altitude. Points marked 'Previous data' were originally published as Figure 8 in the paper by Khoo* et al. *(1982), the solid line being results predicted by their model (●). Vertical broken lines indicate differences caused by scaling between neonates and adults. For sources of data see Khoo* et al. *(1982). 'This study' refers to West* et al. *(1986). (From West* et al. *1986.)*

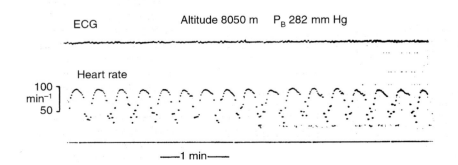

Figure 13.5 *Cyclic variation of heart rate caused by periodic breathing in a climber at 8050 m altitude. P_B = 282 mm Hg. (From West* et al. *1986.)*

Changes of heart rate during the periodic breathing cycle were seen in all subjects and Figure 13.3 is a good example. In general, the maximum heart rate appeared shortly after the peak of the hyperpnea. Cardiac rhythm abnormalities were infrequent. In one subject, ventricular premature contractions occurred mainly during the apneic periods. However, this subject had a history of occasional ventricular premature contractions at sea level. There were no other observable changes in ECG pattern except for minor alterations that could be attributed to changes in the position of the heart caused by breathing movements.

In four subjects, evidence of periodic breathing was obtained at an altitude of 8050 m (P_B 282 mm Hg). In these studies, breathing movements were not recorded directly because of the very remote location of the camp. However, continuous ECG tracings were obtained during the night using a Holter-type monitor, and the occurrence of periodic breathing was inferred from the variations in heart rate as described by Guilleminault et al. (1984). An example is shown in Figure 13.5. This particular subject showed extremely regular cyclic regulation of heart rate over long periods of time (up to 40 min). It was easy to distinguish between this type of cyclic variation caused by periodic breathing and sinus arrhythmia.

13.5.2 Control of breathing

The control of breathing during sleep has been extensively studied: for a review see Phillipson et al. (1978). The ventilatory response to carbon dioxide is reduced, at least in NREM sleep (Bulow 1963). However, there is more uncertainty about the hypoxic ventilatory response; some studies indicate that it is increased in NREM sleep (Pappenheimer 1977, Phillipson et al. 1978). Responses to pulmonary stretch receptor stimulation appear to be intact during NREM sleep but may be decreased in REM sleep (Phillipson et al. 1978).

The control of ventilation during hypoxic sleep has been less well studied and there are many unanswered questions (Dempsey 1983). Lahiri et al. (1983) studied the role of added oxygen and carbon dioxide, and the importance of the hypoxic ventilatory response to periodic breathing in both well acclimatized lowlanders and native Sherpas at an altitude of 5400 m.

Figure 13.6 shows the effect of adding oxygen to the inspired air. It can be seen that there was an immediate increase in the apneic period from about 10 s to 17 s. Subsequently, the apneic period shortened and shallow rhythmic breathing resumed as the arterial P_{CO_2} increased because of the fall in alveolar ventilation. In most subjects, the periodicity of breathing did not totally disappear following the addition of oxygen, but the strength of the periodic breathing was clearly greatly diminished. The changes can be partly explained by the reduction in respiratory drive from the peripheral chemoreceptors when the arterial P_{O_2} was raised.

Adding carbon dioxide to the inspired gas did not abolish the periodic breathing, although it did eliminate the periods of apnea. Withdrawal of carbon dioxide from the inspired air was followed by a prompt reappearance of apnea, and the rapidity of the response suggested a dominant role for the peripheral chemoreceptors.

An important finding was that, although the lowlanders showed marked periodic breathing at 5400 m, the Sherpas generally did not. The only

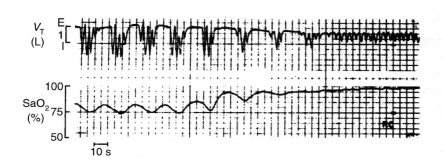

Figure 13.6 *Effect of increasing the inspired P_{O_2} on periodic breathing in a lowlander during sleep at 5400 m. Note that adding oxygen to the inspired gas raised the arterial oxygen saturation, eliminated the apneic periods, and reduced the strength of periodic breathing. V_T, tidal volume; Sa_{O_2}, arterial oxygen saturation; E, expiration, I, inspiration. (From Lahiri and Barnard 1983.)*

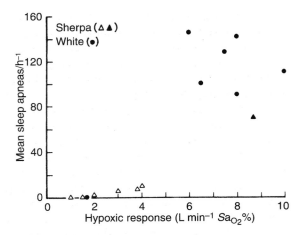

Figure 13.7 *Relationship between frequency of sleep apnea and ventilatory response to hypoxia (awake).* ●, *acclimatized lowlanders;* △, *high altitude Sherpas;* ▲, *lower altitude Sherpa. One lowlander did not have periods of apnea, and the low altitude Sherpa showed periodic breathing. (From Lahiri* et al. *1983.)*

exception was one Sherpa who had spent long periods of time at low altitudes. As discussed in Chapter 5, the Sherpas generally show low ventilatory responses to hypoxia, although the low altitude Sherpa had an intermediate value. Figure 13.7 shows the relationship between the frequency of apnea during sleep at 5400 m and the hypoxic ventilatory response. It is clear that a high hypoxic ventilatory response predisposes to periodic breathing.

13.5.3 Mechanism

It is profitable to discuss the mechanism of periodic breathing in terms of control theory, and a particularly useful analysis was presented by Khoo *et al.* (1982). They pointed out that two factors are necessary for self-sustained oscillatory behavior in a control system. In such a system we can identify a 'disturbance', for example a change in alveolar ventilation caused by some adventitious factor such as a sigh or alteration of body position. This is followed by a 'corrective action' which tends to suppress the disturbance. In the case of an increase in alveolar ventilation (caused by a sigh, for example) the corrective action would be a lowering of P_{CO_2}, which would tend to reduce ventilation by its action on central and peripheral chemoreceptors and thus

constitute negative feedback. The first necessary requirement for sustained oscillatory behavior is that the magnitude of the corrective action exceeds that of the disturbance, this ratio being known as the loop gain.

The second necessary condition is that the corrective action be presented 180° out of phase with the disturbance, so that what would otherwise inhibit the change in ventilation now augments it. This sustained oscillatory behavior occurs when the loop gain exceeds unity at a phase difference of 180°.

This theory predicts that the higher the loop gain at a phase angle of 180°, the more likely periodic breathing is to occur, the more marked the pattern of periodic breathing, and the shorter the cycle length of the periodic breathing. The main factor increasing loop gain in acclimatized lowlanders at high altitude is the increased chemoreceptor gain, particularly the response to severe hypoxia (Chapter 5). Other contributing factors may be the hyperventilation, which increases the rate of wash out of carbon dioxide and wash in of oxygen in the lungs, and the reduction of functional residual capacity in supine subjects.

This analysis explains why there is a difference between acclimatized lowlanders and Sherpas in periodic breathing. Because native highlanders have a blunted hypoxic ventilatory response (Severinghaus *et al.* 1966a, Milledge and Lahiri 1967), the loop gain of the control system is reduced and the factors promoting periodicity are weak. Lahiri *et al.* (1983) have argued that this represents an important feature of the true adaptation of native highlanders such as Sherpas to high altitude. Periodic breathing is disadvantageous because of the very low levels of arterial P_{O_2} following the apneic periods (section 13.5.4). In addition, the reduced ventilation at high altitude lowers the oxygen cost of ventilation.

In the analysis discussed above, a disturbance, for example an arousal, is postulated to play an important role in the genesis of periodic breathing. However, Khoo *et al.* (1996) looked at the relationship between arousals and the initiation of periodic breathing in healthy volunteers at simulated altitudes of 4572, 6100 and 7620 m. They found that although arousals promoted the development of periodic breathing with apnea in some instances, arousals were not necessary for the initiation of periodic breathing in all circumstances.

In another study of periodic breathing at high

altitude, measurements were made on nine Japanese climbers who participated in an expedition to the Kunlun mountains (7167 m) in China (Matsuyama *et al.* 1989). There was a significant correlation between the degree of periodic breathing during sleep and both the hypoxic ventilatory response and hypercapnic ventilatory response measured at sea level ($p < 0.05$). Although all climbers showed desaturation during sleep, there was a negative correlation between the degree of desaturation and the hypoxic ventilation response (HVR) ($p < 0.05$). The authors concluded that the high HVR helped to maintain the arterial oxygenation during sleep, and that it was therefore advantageous.

In a further study, subjects with early high altitude pulmonary edema (HAPE) showed a trend towards more periodic breathing than subjects without HAPE, probably because of lower values of arterial oxygen saturation (Eichenberger *et al.* 1996). In a study of patients with chronic mountain sickness at 3658 m altitude, sleep-disordered breathing was more common than in a control group (Sun *et al.* 1996).

13.5.4   Gas exchange

Periodic breathing causes marked fluctuations in the arterial P_{O_2}, which is not surprising considering the long periods of apnea that sometimes occur. Figure 13.3 shows a typical record of fluctuations in arterial oxygen saturation as recorded by ear oximeter. Another example is seen in Figure 13.6.

In the study of nocturnal periodic breathing carried out at an altitude of 6300 m during the 1981 AMREE, the mean fluctuation in arterial oxygen saturation between subjects was approximately 10 per cent (West *et al.* 1986). In order to determine the proportion of the time during which the arterial oxygen saturation fell below a particular value, the analysis described by Slutsky and Strohl (1980) was carried out. This showed that the arterial oxygen saturation below which the subjects spent 50 per cent of their time varied from a minimal value of 64.5 per cent to a maximum of 74.5 per cent with a mean of 68.8 per cent.

Since it is not usually feasible to sample arterial blood over prolonged periods of time, most investigators of periodic breathing have relied on the arterial oxygen saturation measured by ear oximetry.

However, based on spot measurements of arterial P_{O_2} it was calculated that the maximum and minimum values of saturation of 73.0 per cent and 63.4 per cent from the AMREE study corresponded to arterial P_{O_2} values of approximately 39 and 33 mm Hg respectively. The conclusion was that the minimal arterial P_{O_2} during sleep was approximately 6 mm Hg lower than the resting daytime value, a substantial difference on this very steep part of the oxygen dissociation curve. It should be pointed out that, at high work rates, the arterial P_{O_2} falls considerably below the resting value. However, climbers during their normal activity do not generally work at more than two-thirds of their maximal power (Pugh 1958; section 11.9) so it was concluded that the most severe arterial hypoxemia over the course of the 24 h probably occurred during sleep as a result of the periodic breathing.

Another factor which may exaggerate the effects of this arterial hypoxemia is the augmented cardiac output during the periods when the arterial P_{O_2} is near its lowest value. As Figures 13.3 and 13.6 show, the lowest arterial oxygen saturation typically occurs just after the peak of ventilation during the periodic breathing cycle. If venous return and thus cardiac output are enhanced during this hyperpneic phase, this would lead to enhanced delivery of this poorly oxygenated blood. Thus it may be that the phasing of arterial P_{O_2} and cardiac output aggravate the resulting impairment of oxygen delivery.

It is possible that the severe arterial hypoxemia during periodic breathing affects tolerance to extreme altitude. This leads to a paradox. As Figure 13.7 shows, there is a correlation between hypoxic ventilatory response and the strength of the periodic breathing, as would be expected from the control theory discussed in section 13.5.3. This would suggest that climbers with a high hypoxic ventilatory response would tolerate altitude poorly. However, the opposite is generally found to be the case (Schoene *et al.* 1984; Chapter 5). This can be explained by the better ability of these climbers to defend their alveolar P_{O_2} against the low inspired value by hyperventilation (Chapter 12). However, it is clear that some elite mountain climbers have, in fact, a relatively low hypoxic ventilatory response (Milledge *et al.* 1983c, Schoene *et al.* 1987). One possible explanation is that these climbers maintain a higher arterial P_{O_2} during the night, and this is a factor in their tolerance to extreme altitude.

13.5.5 Effects of drugs

Because of the poor quality of sleep at high altitude and the suspicion that this is sometimes related to periodic breathing, there has been considerable interest in the use of drugs to promote a normal breathing pattern. Sutton *et al.* (1979) showed that the administration of acetazolamide at a dose of 250 mg three times per day decreased the time spent in periodic breathing from 80 per cent to 35 per cent at an altitude of 5360 m. This was associated with an improvement in arterial P_{O_2} as judged by the arterial oxygen saturation measured by ear oximetry. Weil *et al.* (1978) used acetazolamide at an altitude of 4400 m and found that the duration of periodic breathing decreased from 35 per cent to 18 per cent. Hackett *et al.* (1987a) found a decrease from 41 per cent to 17 per cent at 4400 m in four subjects with the same drug.

The mode of action of acetazolamide is not fully understood, but it stimulates ventilation possibly

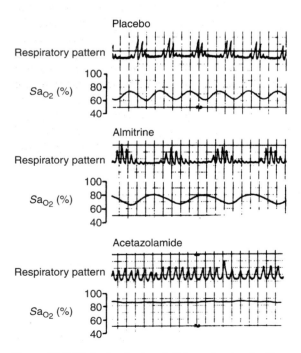

Figure 13.8 *Effects of a placebo, almitrine and acetazolamide on periodic breathing and arterial oxygen saturation (Sa_{O_2}) at an altitude of 4400 m. Note that acetazolamide abolished the apneic periods whereas almitrine exaggerated them. (From Hackett* et al. *1987.)*

because it induces a metabolic acidosis. At any event, its value at high altitude is now generally accepted in that it reduces the incidence of acute mountain sickness (Hackett and Rennie 1976), maintains a higher alveolar P_{O_2} and lower P_{CO_2}, and may even prevent some of the weight loss which normally occurs as a result of muscle protein breakdown (Birmingham study 1981).

Almitrine is another drug that stimulates ventilation, apparently through its effect on peripheral chemoreceptors. It has been shown to improve the arterial oxygenation of patients with chronic bronchitis and emphysema during sleep at sea level (Connaughton *et al.* 1985). Hackett *et al.* (1987a) compared the effects of almitrine and acetazolamide on the respiratory pattern of four subjects at an altitude of 4400 m on Mount McKinley in Alaska in a double-blind, randomized, three-way crossover trial. Both almitrine and acetazolamide increased the arterial oxygen saturation during sleep but, whereas acetazolamide decreased periodic breathing, almitrine increased it (Figure 13.8). This result is consistent with the data of Figure 13.7 and the discussion in section 13.5.3 where it was pointed out that the strength of periodic breathing is related to the hypoxic ventilatory response. Since almitrine increases this response by stimulating peripheral chemoreceptors, it is not surprising that it exaggerates the periodic breathing. It should also be pointed out that almitrine tends to increase pulmonary vascular resistance by enhancing hypoxic pulmonary vasoconstriction (section 7.5.1), and since pulmonary hypertension occurs at high altitude through this mechanism, this is an undesirable side effect. Thus the use of almitrine is probably contraindicated at high altitude.

Other drugs have also been studied in an attempt to improve the quality of sleep at high altitude. There have been several studies of the benzodiazepine family. Dubowitz (1998) reported that the number and severity of changes in arterial oxygen saturation during sleep were decreased, and the quality of sleep was improved following administration of temazepam at an altitude of 5300 m. He found no significant drop in mean oxygen saturation values during sleep. However, Röggla *et al.* (1994) found that low dose sedation with diazepam reduced the ventilatory response at moderate altitude. In a subsequent study of temazepam, Röggla *et al.* (2000) showed that, at an altitude of 3000 m, the arterial

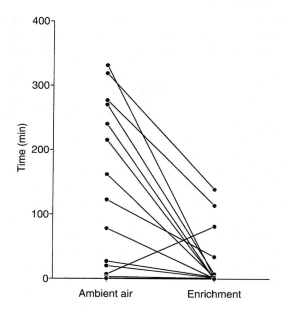

Figure 13.9 *Comparison of the time spent by 18 subjects in periodic breathing with apneas during sleep in ambient air, compared with an atmosphere of 24 per cent oxygen at an altitude of 3800 m. The paired differences were significant (*p < 0.01*). (From Luks et al. 1998.)*

ber, Beaumont *et al.* (1996) reported improved sleep quality at high altitude without adverse effects on respiration. Blood gases were not looked at in this study.

13.5.6 Effect of oxygen enrichment of room air

Adding oxygen to the ventilation of a room shows promise as a way of combating the hypoxia of high altitude, particularly for people who commute to high altitude to work (see Chapter 29). Luks *et al.* (1998) carried out a randomized, double-blind trial at an altitude of 3800 m to determine whether oxygen enrichment of room air to 24 per cent at night improved sleep quality and performance and well being the following day. They found that, with oxygen enrichment, the subjects had significantly fewer apneas and spent significantly less time in periodic breathing with apneas than when they slept in ambient air (Figure 13.9). Subjective assessments of sleep quality were also significantly improved. There was a lower acute mountain sickness score in the morning after oxygen-enriched sleep, using the Lake Louise criteria. Of particular interest, subjects who slept in the oxygen-enriched atmosphere had a significantly greater increase in arterial oxygen saturation from evening to morning compared with subjects who slept in ambient air. This latter finding suggested either that the control of breathing may have been altered by sleeping in an oxygen-enriched atmosphere, or that there was less subclinical pulmonary edema.

P_{CO_2} (determined from earlobe blood) was significantly increased and the arterial P_{O_2} significantly decreased after 10 mg of temazepam.

In a study of zolpidem, an imidazopyridine hypnotic drug, on sleep and respiratory patterns at a simulated altitude of 4000 m in a low pressure cham-

Nutrition and intestinal function

SUMMARY

Loss of appetite and loss of weight are common at altitude. Initially these may be due to acute mountain sickness (AMS). At heights below about 4500 m appetite returns after a few days but at more extreme altitudes anorexia persists and may get worse. Weight loss on an altitude trip can have many causes. On trek, initial weight loss may be the shedding of excess fat due to a sedentary lifestyle. Intestinal infections can cause diarrhea and weight loss. High on the mountain unavailability of food and liquid can be the cause but even in the absence of these factors weight loss is seen, as in long-term chamber studies.

In considering energy balance at altitude, basal metabolic rate is increased 10–17 per cent at 4000–6000 m and possibly more at extreme altitudes. Exercise increases energy needs, though the reduction in maximum work rate would be expected to reduce the energy requirement of climbing. However, the use of new techniques has given values of energy expenditure when climbing at extreme altitudes that are at least as high as in the Alps, if not higher. So daily energy needs are high while intake is often reduced because of anorexia. Recent research suggests that the cause of this anorexia may be mediated by the hormone leptin or by cholecystokinin.

Weight loss results in a change of body composition; fat tends to be lost at low elevations but muscle at higher altitudes.

Apart from calorie imbalance, there is some evidence that at altitude above about 5500 m there is malabsorption of food and an increase in intestinal permeability. This effect of hypoxia on the gut will increase the weight loss.

Diet is important on treks and expeditions. There are good physiological reasons to advise a high carbohydrate, low fat diet and most climbers seem to favor this. However, palatability is probably more important than composition in combating the loss of appetite. Taste is dulled and most find that they want more highly flavored, spicy foods. A craving for fresh rather than preserved food develops. Fluids remain acceptable and many calories can be taken in sweet milky drinks. Supplements such as vitamins and minerals are probably not necessary if a balanced diet is taken, with the possible exception of iron supplements for pre-menopausal women.

14.1 INTRODUCTION

Anorexia and weight loss are well known features of life at high altitude, especially extreme altitudes. The mechanism of this anorexia is not known. During the first few days after a rapid ascent, anorexia may be part of the symptomatology of AMS, but after this, when all other symptoms of AMS are gone, anorexia may remain. Recent studies have suggested that the anorexia of AMS may be mediated by the hormone leptin (Tschop *et al.* 1998) or by increased levels of cholecystokinin (Bailey *et al.* 2000). This continuing anorexia is not common below about 5000 m but is almost universal above 6000 m and becomes worse at even higher altitudes, though the severity varies considerably between individuals.

Weight loss is also common, though not inevitable, even at extreme altitudes (see below) and is partly due to the reduced energy intake consequent on the anorexia, but the possibility that it might be due also to other factors, such as malabsorption, is reviewed in this chapter. This chapter also considers diet at altitude and the evidence for the value of a high carbohydrate diet.

14.2   ENERGY BALANCE AT ALTITUDE

14.2.1   Energy output

BASAL METABOLIC RATE (BMR)

Nair *et al.* (1971) found that after a week at 3300 m the basal metabolic rate (BMR) was elevated by about 12 per cent. Exposure to cold as well as hypoxia (in a second group of subjects) made no difference to this effect compared with hypoxia alone. By week 2, BMR was back to control values and was below control by week 3. Cold exposure at this time resulted in elevation of BMR to above sea level values by week 5 and it remained elevated a week after return to sea level. Butterfield *et al.* (1992) found BMR to be elevated by 27 per cent on day 2 at Pikes Peak (4300 m) in Colorado. The BMR then decreased over the next few days to plateau at +17 per cent compared with sea level by day 10.

After acclimatization, BMR measured at 5800 m was found to be elevated by about 10 per cent in subjects who had been at altitude for 82–113 days (Gill and Pugh 1964). It is likely that BMR rises again if subjects climb to altitudes to which they are not acclimatized and we have no data on BMR at altitudes above 6000 m when weight loss becomes even more rapid, but its elevation might well be a factor.

BMR was found to be high at altitude in altitude residents (Ladakhis and Sherpas) compared with lowlanders and with predicted values (Gill and Pugh 1964, Nair *et al.* 1971). This elevation of BMR remained even when allowance was made for the fact that these people generally have less fat in their body composition. Picon-Reategui (1961) also reported elevated BMR in Andean miners at 4540 m. The mechanism for this rise in BMR is uncertain. Fecal and urinary excretion of energy nitrogen and volatile acids are not altered in the early days at altitude (Butterfield *et al.* 1992). There is increase in sympathetic activity at this time (section 15.6) and the finding that this increase in metabolic rate can be inhibited by a beta-blocker (Moore *et al.* 1987) suggests it is a likely factor. Increased thyroid activity may also play a part, especially in the longer-term elevation of BMR (section 15.7).

ENERGY EXPENDITURE DUE TO EXERCISE

Work in absolute terms requires the same oxygen intake at altitude as at sea level until near-maximum work rate is reached (Pugh *et al.* 1964, West *et al.* 1983c, Wolfel *et al.* 1991). At altitude the maximum work rate is reduced (Chapter 11) and all activity seems disproportionately fatiguing. At 8000 m, even rolling over in a sleeping bag demands a great effort. Thus, energy expenditure for normal activities of daily living must be reduced at extreme altitude. Another fact of life at extreme altitudes is that often the only warm place is a sleeping bag and much of the 24 h of the day is spent lying down. The increased work of breathing has a small opposite effect, as does the increase in BMR, so that the daily energy expenditure is probably about the same as at sea level (see below). At intermediate altitudes (2500–4500 m), although maximum work rate is reduced, energy expenditure on normal daily activities of short duration is probably not much altered. For longer-term work such as hill climbing, much will depend upon the degree of acclimatization and fitness. Pugh *et al.* (1964) found $\dot{V}_{O_2}$ intake on climbers climbing at their 'preferred' rate to decline very little up to about 5000 m (Figure 11.1), whereas Butterfield *et al.* (1992) found a 37 per cent reduction in energy expenditure for exercise 'more strenuous than walking'. But the overall requirement for energy to maintain body weight increased from 13.22 MJ at sea level to 14.64 MJ a day at 4300 m due to the increase in BMR.

Until recently it has been impossible to measure energy expenditure over long periods, but a doubly labeled water technique has now been developed which makes this possible. Water is labeled with both deuterium and oxygen-18. The deuterium is eliminated as water while the oxygen is eliminated as both water and carbon dioxide. Thus carbon dioxide production can be calculated from the different elimination rates (Schoeller and van Santen 1982, Coward 1991). Using this technique, Westerterp et al. (1992) found average daily energy expenditure in the Alps (2500–4800 m) to be 14.7 MJ and on Mount Everest (5300–8848 m) it was not significantly different at 13.6 MJ. Very similar daily results were obtained in the 1992 British Winter Everest Expedition of 11.7–15.4 MJ (Travis et al. 1993). Pulfrey and Jones (1996), using the same technique at altitudes of 5900–8046 m, found the very high mean values of 19.4 MJ day^{-1} and a negative energy balance of 5.1 MJ day^{-1}. More recently Reynolds et al. (1999) found an even higher mean value of 20.6 MJ day^{-1} above Base Camp with a dietary intake of only 10.5 MJ, giving a deficit of 10 MJ day^{-1}!

14.2.2 Energy intake and caloric balance

Up to about 4500 m, once acclimatized, people have normal appetites and normal food intake (Consolazio et al. 1968). Above 6000 m most climbers experience anorexia. This tends to become more pronounced the longer one stays at these altitudes. Climbers complain about the food available and feel that the preserved nature of food increases the anorexia and reduces their intake. There are few data on actual calorie intake under these circumstances. Those that there are rely on diary cards and estimates of portion size. On Cho Oyu in Nepal in 1952 food eaten at between 5250 and 6750 m was only about 13.4 MJ a day compared with 17.6 MJ on the march out, and on Everest in 1953, above 7250 m, the intake was only about 6.3 MJ (Pugh and Band 1953). On the Silver Hut Expedition (1960–1), in four climbers at 5800 m whose living conditions were excellent and where a good variety and quantity of food was available, a daily intake of 12.6–13.4 MJ day^{-1} was estimated (Pugh 1962a). Boyer and Blume (1984) reported that on the American Medical Expedition to Everest (AMREE) in 1981, over 3 days

four subjects had a mean intake of 9.34 MJ at 6300 m compared with 12.5 MJ at sea level. Dinmore et al. (1994) found intakes similar during the march in (1500–2000 m) and above 5500 m (10.8 and 10.3 MJ). However, Westerterp et al. (1992) and Travis et al. (1993) estimated intakes high on Everest of 7.5 MJ and 8.6 MJ respectively, indicating the expected reduction in intake above 6300 m.

Clearly, high on major mountains (above 6000 m), when actively climbing, it is not possible to maintain caloric balance even when acclimatized. Westerterp et al. (1994) on Mount Sajama (6542 m) in Bolivia found an energy deficit of 3.5 MJ day^{-1} in 10 subjects camped on the summit for 21 days. The average weight loss was 4.9 kg (1.6 kg week^{-1}), 74 per cent of it being due to loss of fat. In Everest climbers studied by Westerterp et al. (1992) there was a daily negative balance of 5.7 MJ. Clearly, more studies using this new technique are needed to answer the question of whether acclimatized subjects can maintain energy balance at intermediate altitudes (4500–6000 m) when semi-sedentary.

14.3 WEIGHT LOSS ON ALTITUDE EXPEDITIONS

14.3.1 Weight loss on the march out

Most climbing and trekking groups experience weight loss in the initial 1–3 weeks of an expedition, even when walking below 3000 m. This is probably due to the change in lifestyle for most subjects from an urban semi-sedentary existence to the more active lifestyle of marching 16 km (10 miles) a day with some considerable ascents and descents. In addition, gastrointestinal infections are common.

Boyer and Blume (1984) found that 13 AMREE members, during the march out to the Everest region, lost an average of 2 kg (range 0–6 kg). Those with the highest percentage of body fat to start with lost most weight, the correlation being significant; 70 per cent of this weight loss was due to loss of fat. Two subjects with less than 13 per cent of body fat lost no weight. Dinmore et al. (1994) similarly found an average loss of 1.3 kg during the first week of trekking but only a further 0.5 kg in the next week.

Weight loss during this phase of an expedition or trek can be considered as shedding unnecessary fat.

14.3.2   Weight loss at altitude

On first arrival at altitude, AMS may cause anorexia and vomiting with resultant weight loss, though usually the duration is not long enough to do this. Also, fluid may be retained and subjects with AMS often gain weight (Hackett *et al.* 1982). Consolazio *et al.* (1972) found a small gain in weight on the first day at altitude followed by a loss of weight of about 1 kg over the next 5 days at 4300 m. Recently leptin has been discovered as a hormone which influences appetite. In subjects taken to 4559 m by helicopter, Tschop *et al.* (1998) found that the leptin levels in those who complained of anorexia were higher than those with no loss of appetite. Leptin is secreted in a pulsatile manner with normal diurnal fluctuations so it is necessary to measure it on a number of occasions over some hours. This they did, as shown in Figure 14.1. This work suggests that leptin may be involved in the mechanism of appetite loss at altitude but needs confirmation.

After acclimatization, weight loss is usually seen only above about 5000 m. Dinmore *et al.* (1994) found an average loss of 3.9 kg during two weeks' climbing above 5000 m; on the 1992 British Winter Everest Expedition a mean weight loss of 5 kg was observed

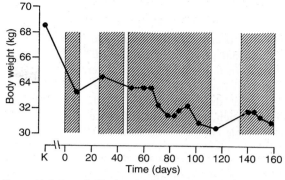

Figure 14.2 *Record of body weight of one subject during the Silver Hut Expedition 1960–1. After the march out from Kathmandu (K) and the initial period of preparation, he was in residence at 5800 m (hatched areas) or at Base Camp at 4500 m. Note the loss of weight at 5800 m but weight gain during two breaks at 4500 m.*

above 5400 m out of a total loss of 7.8 kg (Travis *et al.* 1993). Figure 14.2 shows the crucial effect of altitude on body weight on one well acclimatized subject. The combined effects of the march out and early residence at the Silver Hut, at 5800 m, produced a weight loss of 5.3 kg. Thereafter, during time spent at the Silver Hut the subject lost weight steadily at a weekly rate of just under 400 g, but, on two occasions, on descent to altitudes of 4000–4500 m, he began to gain weight. Most subjects in the Silver Hut lost between 0.5 and 1.5 kg a week (Pugh 1962a).

Rai *et al.* (1975) found no weight loss in their subjects living at 3500–4700 m, even though they were working quite hard at road building and digging. Indeed, on a high fat diet (232 g daily) they actually gained an average of 1.4 kg during 3 weeks at 4700 m. Butterfield *et al.* (1992) also found that it was possible to attenuate weight loss at 4300 m by increasing dietary intake in proportion to the increase in BMR. However, at Advanced Base Camp (6300 m) in the Western Cwm on Everest most subjects lost weight. Boyer and Blume (1984) document this weight loss as an average of 4 kg (range 0–8 kg) over a mean of 47 days in 13 subjects. Again, there was considerable individual variation in the amount of weight lost which correlated with initial percentage of body fat. Boyer and Blume also found that Sherpas, who averaged only half as much body fat as the white climbers, lost no weight during the time spent above Base Camp, mostly at or above 6300 m (see also section 14.9).

Women seem to lose less weight than men do. Hannon *et al.* (1976) found their female subjects lost

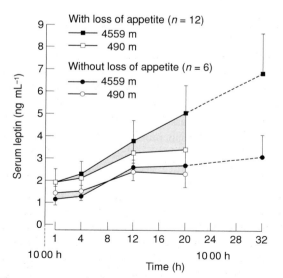

Figure 14.1 *Serum leptin concentrations at 490 and 4559 m (Capanna Margherita) in 18 subjects with and without loss of appetite. The increase in leptin from low to high altitude (area between curves) was significant for subjects with loss of appetite (p = 0.008) but not for those with no appetite loss (p = 0.35). From Tschop* et al. *(1998) with permission.*

an average of only 1.8 per cent of body weight during 7 days at 4300 m whereas studies, previously reported, of men at this altitude had found losses of 3.5 and 5.0 per cent. Collier *et al.* (1997b) found changes in body mass index at Everest Base Camp (5340 m) over a median of 15 days: 22 men lost 0.11 kg m^{-2} day^{-1} compared with 0.02 kg m^{-2} day^{-1} in eight women, a significant difference ($p = 0.03$). The seven male climbers who climbed to between 7100 and 8848 m, using oxygen at extreme altitude, all lost weight, averaging 0.15 kg m^{-2} day^{-1}. The one female climber who spent 4 nights above 8000 m without supplementary oxygen lost no weight between leaving and arriving back at Base Camp!

14.3.3 Weight loss in chamber experiments

It could be argued that some of the weight loss on expeditions is due to cold, limited food supplies, and the increased energy expenditure of climbing. This may often be the case, although not so in a number of the studies quoted above. Chamber studies avoid this potential criticism; most are of too short a duration to be relevant, but the two Operation Everest studies of 40 days' duration showed that, despite good environmental conditions of temperature, humidity and diet *ad lib.*, subjects lost weight (Rose *et al.* 1988). In Operation Everest II the six subjects lost an average of 7.4 kg during the 38 days of observations as they ascended the simulated height of the summit of Everest. Energy intake fell by 43 per cent and, interestingly, the subjects chose a diet that resulted in a reduction of carbohydrate from 62 per cent to 53 per cent of the total diet. The authors considered that the weight loss could not be accounted for totally by the reduction in intake and considered that malabsorption or increase in energy expenditure due to increased BMR must be invoked (section 14.2.1). The exercise taken in this chamber study would probably be less than on a climbing expedition.

14.4 BODY COMPOSITION AND WEIGHT LOSS

Assuming much of the weight loss is due to negative energy balance, a simplistic view would be that the body would use up fat stores first and then start using protein from the lean body mass, principally the muscles. However, even with a most carefully controlled diet aimed at fat reduction, it is never possible to lose fat exclusively and retain all the lean body mass (Garrow 1987). The best that can be achieved is that, of the weight lost, 75 per cent is fat and 25 per cent lean body tissue. This compares with the situation during a complete fast when fat and lean body tissues are lost in roughly equal proportions (Forbes and Drenick 1979).

Boyer and Blume (1984) used skinfold measurements to estimate body fat. There are uncertainties about the absolute results of this method, but relative changes probably can be reliable. They found that, of the average 2 kg loss during the march out to Base Camp, 70 per cent was due to loss of fat, which is a figure close to the most efficient muscle sparing regimen available. However, above 5400 m, mainly at or above 6300 m, of the 4 kg average weight loss only 27 per cent was due to loss of fat and 73 per cent due to loss of lean body tissue, despite the fact that subjects still had at least 10 per cent of their body weight as fat. This percentage loss of muscle, greater than that seen in starvation, suggests that at this altitude hypoxia may be interfering with protein metabolism (section 14.5).

In the Operation Everest II study (Rose *et al.* 1988) there was loss of 2.5 kg of fat (1.6 per cent body weight) and 4.9 kg of lean body tissue. Computerized tomographic examination of the thigh showed a 17 per cent loss of muscle and a 34 per cent loss of subcutaneous fat. Although loss of muscle mass must be a disadvantage, one beneficial effect is to increase the density of muscle capillaries. This is because the loss of muscle mass is achieved by reducing fiber diameter rather than number, with the number of capillaries per fiber remaining constant. Thus the intercapillary distance decreases with an improvement in oxygenation of the muscles (Chapter 10). Evidence in support of this speculation is found in the work of Oelz *et al.* (1986), who studied muscle biopsies from six elite climbers at sea level some months after return from altitude. It was found that their muscle fibers were smaller and the capillary density greater than controls. Another explanation for the loss of muscle mass is that with decreased overall activity at altitude there is some disuse atrophy which would similarly reduce muscle fiber diameter. These two explanations are not mutually exclusive. Results of muscle biopsy studies during

Operation Everest II (MacDougall *et al.* 1991) showed similar histological changes in muscle fiber size (Chapter 10 contains a fuller discussion of changes in muscle histology).

14.5   INTESTINAL ABSORPTION AND HYPOXIA

In view of the continued weight loss at altitudes above 5000 m with, in some cases, adequate intake and reduced energy output, the possibility of malabsorption and malutilization of food must be considered. Pugh (1962a) reported that members of the Silver Hut Expedition noted that stools tended to be greasy and bulky, suggesting possible steatorrhea due to malabsorption of fat.

As mentioned in section 14.3, weight loss is not a feature of living at altitudes below about 5000 m, and the fact that most altitude research is conducted below this level may explain why so little work has been carried out on the topic of intestinal absorption. Other reasons for the neglect of this field may be that the methods involved are either too sophisticated for easy use in the field (e.g. absorption of radioactive materials), or are unattractive to investigators (e.g. fecal collection, liquidization and aliquot sampling, etc.). Finally, few altitude physiologists have a background in gastroenterology.

14.5.1   Carbohydrate absorption and hypoxia

Milledge (1972) studied patients who were hypoxic either because of congenital heart disease or chronic obstructive lung disease. Xylose absorption decreased with decreasing arterial oxygen saturation (Figure 14.3).

On relieving the hypoxia by surgery in the cardiac cases, or by 13 h of supplementary oxygen breathing in the respiratory cases, there was improvement in xylose absorption in all patients. The xylose absorption test has a rather uncertain lower normal limit, especially in a population in which intestinal parasitic infection is common (the study was carried out in South India). However, the results suggest that, below an arterial saturation of about 70 per cent, absorption was impaired (Figure 14.3); improvement on relief of hypoxia supports this view.

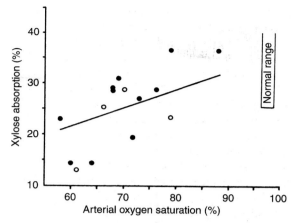

Figure 14.3 *Xylose absorption in patients hypoxic because of either congenital cyanotic heart disease (○), or chronic respiratory disease (●), plotted against their arterial oxygen saturation.*

Pritchard and Lane (1974) did not find malabsorption in 26 patients with chronic obstructive lung disease. However, the lowest arterial P_{O_2} was 48 mm Hg, equivalent to about 78 per cent saturation. Chesner *et al.* (1987) found no malabsorption of xylose in 11 subjects up to 4846 m. However, 60-min plasma xylose concentrations were reduced in subjects who ascended to 5600 m, confirming that absorption is not affected until hypoxia is severe. Boyer and Blume (1984), who studied subjects at 6300 m, found xylose absorption decreased by 24 per cent in six out of seven subjects, compared with sea level controls.

However, absorption measured by xylose has the drawback that the result is influenced by factors such as gastric emptying time, absorption area, intestinal transit and renal function. Dinmore *et al.* (1994) used a double carbohydrate test; the two nonmetabolized carbohydrates used undergo different forms of mediated absorption but are otherwise subject to the same external influences which cancel out when results are expressed as a ratio (Menzies 1984). D-xylose is absorbed by passive mediated transport, whereas 3-*o*-methyl-D-glucose is absorbed by active mediated, sodium-dependent transport. Dinmore *et al.* found that at 6300 m there was 34 per cent decrease in D-xylose (Figure 14.4) and a 15 per cent decrease in 3-*o*-methyl-D-glucose absorption. The ratio was consistently decreased at altitude and in a subsequent study the 60-min serum xylose/3-*o*-methyl-D-glucose ratio was 17 per cent lower at 5400 m than at sea level (Travis *et al.* 1993). These more sophisticated studies

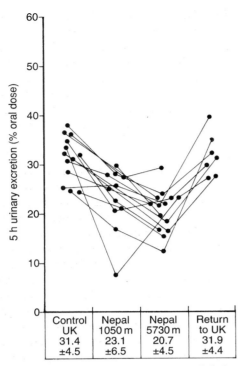

Figure 14.4 *D-xylose absorption tested in a group of climbers at sea level (UK), at altitudes indicated in Nepal and after return to UK (with mean and S.D. values at each location). (Data from* Dinmore et al. *1994.)*

therefore support the hypothesis that at these high altitudes carbohydrate absorption is impaired.

14.5.2   Fat absorption and hypoxia

Rai *et al.* (1975) found no malabsorption for fat at 4700 m; neither did Chesner *et al.* (1987) at 3100 m and 4800 m. Imray *et al.* (1992), using the [14C]-tri-olein breath test, found no malabsorption of fat at 5500 m on Aconcagua in Argentina, and Butterfield *et al.* (1992) found no increase in fecal excretion of volatile fatty acids at 4300 m. However, Boyer and Blume (1984) found fat absorption decreased by 49 per cent at 6300 m compared with sea level results in three acclimatized subjects.

14.5.3   Protein absorption and hypoxia

Kayser *et al.* (1992) measured protein absorption using urinary and fecal nitrogen-15 excretion after ingestion of nitrogen-15 labeled soya protein. They found no reduction in absorption in subjects after

3 weeks at 5000 m. Westerterp *et al.* (1994) on Mount Sajama (6542 m) found that gross energy digestibility decreased to 85 per cent, indicating some malabsorption, though most of the weight loss was attributable to low food intake.

14.5.4   Summary: malabsorption at altitude

There is no evidence of malabsorption up to an altitude of about 5000 m and this has been confirmed by measurements of fecal energy excretion which have shown that 96 per cent of energy intake is assimilated (Kayser *et al.* 1992). Above 5000 m, however, there may be malabsorption of carbohydrate, fat and protein. The mechanism of this hypoxic malabsorption is unknown. It might be due to bowel wall hypoxia, or the fat malabsorption could be due to pancreatic insufficiency and the xylose malabsorption secondary to fat malabsorption.

14.6   INTESTINAL PERMEABILITY

Pappenheimer (1988) showed that the space between adjacent epithelial cells in the small intestine (zona occludens) became less with hypoxia. This may be by contraction of the actin–myosin cytoskeletal system (myoepithelial cells) which control the caliber of these pores. This would reduce sodium-coupled transport of material across the luminal cell wall.

Intestinal permeability is the facility with which molecules pass through the intestinal epithelium by passive, nonmediated transport. It can be measured by the ratio of urinary lactulose and L-rhamnose after ingestion of these test carbohydrates (Travis and Menzies 1992). Lactulose is thought to permeate through paracellular pores of low frequency and L-rhamnose through transcellular pores at a much higher rate (Menzies 1984). Permeability increases if the integrity of the intestinal mucosa is compromised by, for instance, mucosal damage. Dinmore *et al.* (1994) measured intestinal permeability in this way in 11 climbers. After arrival in Nepal there was an increase in permeability due possibly to 'tropical enteropathy' because of changes in gut flora. This is normally a transient phenomenon in travelers to the tropics. When the climbers ascended to altitude, studies at 5730 m showed that the ratio returned to sea level values (Figure 14.5).

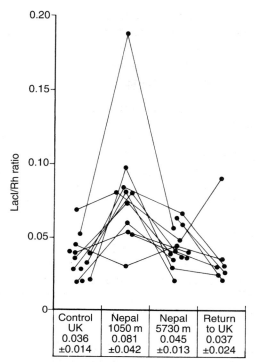

Figure 14.5 *Intestinal permeability (lactose/ʟ-rhamnose ratio) in a group of climbers tested at sea level (UK), at altitudes indicated in Nepal and after return to the UK (with mean and S.D. values at each location). Results show an increase in permeability after arrival in Nepal, possibly due to a change in gut flora, but a return to sea level values at 5730 m. (Data from Dinmore* et al. *1994.)*

However, the transcellular permeation of the monosaccharide ʟ-rhamnose showed a 45 per cent decrease at 5730 m, which is a change unique to high altitude. These findings suggest that at these high altitudes the 'porosity' of the gut is unchanged but that changes may be occurring in the epithelial membranes, perhaps through a change in membrane fluidity (Travis and Menzies 1992).

14.7 PROTEIN METABOLISM AT ALTITUDE

The obvious muscle wasting seen especially in climbers returning from extreme altitude prompts the question of whether hypoxia affects protein metabolism directly. There are very few data on this topic in humans.

Consolazio *et al.* (1968) studied protein balance at altitude and found no difference between subjects there and at sea level, but the altitude station was

Pikes Peak (4300 m), below the crucial height at which continued weight loss is observed.

Rennie *et al.* (1983) studied the effect of acute hypoxia in a chamber (equivalent altitude 4550 m) on leucine metabolism in forearm muscles. They found that acute hypoxia resulted in a net loss of amino acids from the muscles, probably due to a fall in muscle protein synthesis. If this finding can be extrapolated to the situation of chronic hypoxia at altitudes of above 5000–6000 m (where hypoxia in acclimatized subjects would be similar to that in the above study), then it provides a further contributing factor to the loss of muscle mass described above. It has been suggested that protein or branched-chain amino acid (BCAA) supplementation might be helpful in reducing the muscle loss. Bigard and colleagues (1996b) gave one group of skiers BCAA supplementation while participating in six sessions of ski mountaineering at altitudes of 2500–4100 m. They found that they did no better than a control group given 98 per cent carbohydrate supplement with respect to changes in body composition or performance of isometric contraction. However, body weight loss was possibly less in the BCAA group. In another study (Bigard *et al.* 1996a) they found that adding protein to the diet of growing rats did not affect the depression of muscle growth caused by altitude.

14.8 DIET FOR HIGH ALTITUDE

Views on diets (not only at altitude) are strongly held, often the strength of opinion being inversely related to the strength of scientific evidence.

14.8.1 High carbohydrate diet

There is a preference amongst climbers for a high carbohydrate, low fat diet at altitude and there are good physiological reasons for this. Figure 14.6 shows the basis for advising a high carbohydrate diet, which moves the respiratory quotient (RQ) from 0.7, if one uses fat exclusively for energy, to 1.0 when carbohydrate (or protein) is used.

The result of such a change of RQ is that for any given PA_{CO_2} the PA_{O_2} is increased. In the case illustrated in Figure 14.6, the subject is considered to be at 5800 m in the Himalayas or Andes when the barometric pressure is half that at sea level and the PI_{O_2} is

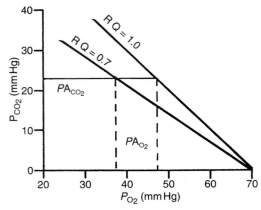

Figure 14.6 *Oxygen–carbon dioxide diagram showing the effect of the respiratory quotient (RQ) on alveolar P_{O_2} at a given PA_{CO_2}. By changing from an RQ of 0.7 (the RQ when utilizing fat) to 1.0 (the RQ when using carbohydrate) the PA_{O_2} is increased from 37.2 to 47.0 mm Hg.*

70 mm Hg. PA_{CO_2} is assumed to be 23 mm Hg. With an RQ of 0.7 the PA_{O_2} would be 37.2 mm Hg, whereas with an RQ of 1.0 it would be 47 mm Hg; this is a very important gain in arterial oxygen saturation. This represents the extreme case of a switch from pure fat to pure carbohydrate utilization, but even a partial switch in this direction would be helpful to the climber at extreme altitudes.

Consolazio *et al.* (1969) compared a normal with a high carbohydrate diet in two groups of subjects at 4300 m. The performance of the group on a high carbohydrate diet was superior in that they had a greater endurance for heavy work, though $V_{O_2 max}$ was not significantly better. Also, the symptoms of AMS were less in the high carbohydrate group.

Another reason for recommending a high carbohydrate diet is that the body becomes more dependent upon blood glucose as a fuel both at rest and on exercise after acclimatization (Brooks *et al.* 1991, Roberts *et al.* 1996). However, Reynolds *et al.* (1998) in a study on Everest found that subjects did not shift their food selections from high fat towards high carbohydrate items as they ascended from Base Camp to camps higher up the mountain.

14.8.2 Low fat diet

Most climbers find fatty foods become distasteful at altitude, in contrast to the preference shown by Arctic and Antarctic travelers. Tilman, who was experienced in both Arctic and mountain travel, writes:

If you do succeed in getting outside a richly concentrated food like pemmican a great effort of will is required to keep it down – absolute quiescence in a prone position and a little sugar are useful aids. Eating a large mug of pemmican soup at 27 200 feet as Peter Lloyd and I did in '38 is, I think, an unparalleled feat and shows what can be done by dogged greed (Tilman 1975).

There are good physiological reasons for a low fat diet at altitude: the effect of fat as an energy source on the RQ (as discussed above) and the possible effect of fat malabsorption on the absorption of sugars and amino acids. This fat intolerance is unfortunate because fat provides more calories weight for weight than carbohydrate or proteins.

14.8.3 Other dietary constituents

IRON

Since the red cell mass is increased at altitude it has been suggested that extra iron should be taken. Unless there is pre-existing iron deficiency the iron stores of the body and the iron content of a normal diet will be adequate. However, in premenopausal women there may be a degree of deficient iron stores and the addition of iron may be indicated (Richalet *et al.* 1994). A rapid response to hypoxia is an increase in intestinal iron absorption from the gut before any change in plasma iron turnover, at least in rats and mice (Hathorn 1971, Raja *et al.* 1986). Thus the iron stores of the body are replenished even before they begin to be depleted.

VITAMINS

It is common for expedition and trekking parties to take added vitamins, but although such dietary supplements probably do no harm, there is no evidence that they are needed provided that a normal, balanced diet is taken.

14.8.4 Fresh food, flavor, variety

The appetite becomes jaded at high altitude and the most common complaints on expeditions are about the drab sameness of the flavor of preserved foods. More experienced climbers tend to adopt a policy of eating local fresh foods, supplemented by the minimum of imported preserved foods. The sense of taste seems to be dulled at altitude, and western food tastes insipid. The addition of strong flavors such as curries and herbs is increasingly appreciated. There is great individual variation in likes and dislikes, even more than at sea level. The wise quartermaster of an expedition will attempt to meet this by providing as wide a variety of foods and flavors as possible. However, the task is unenviable since, whatever the quartermaster provides, fellow expedition members will yearn for what is unavailable.

14.9 NUTRITION AND METABOLISM IN HIGH ALTITUDE NATIVES

Little work has been done on nutrition in peoples native to high altitude. There is the impression that Sherpas do better than lowland climbers with respect to weight loss, and Boyer and Blume (1984), as mentioned in section 14.3.2, documented this. There are caretakers who live at the Aucanquilcha mine in Chile (5950 m) for 1–2 years. Presumably they do not lose weight in the relentless way we did in the Silver Hut (5800 m), though it must be added that only a subset of miners is able to stay at this altitude indefinitely (West 1998, p. 227).

Hochachka *et al.* (1996) studied the metabolism of Sherpas under normoxic and hypoxic conditions. They found that, compared to lowlanders, the Sherpas made greater use of carbohydrate substrates for cardiac function and less use of free fatty acids. This metabolic organization is advantageous in hypoxic conditions because the ATP yield per molecule of oxygen is 25–60 per cent greater with glucose than with free fatty acids.

15

Endocrine and renal systems at altitude

SUMMARY

The chronic hypoxia of altitude has an effect on many endocrine systems. Among those most studied are hormones that affect the salt and water balance of the body and are involved in cardiovascular function. Exercise affects many hormonal systems and is an important activity at altitude; the effect of altitude and exercise therefore needs to be considered. The possible role of certain hormones in the mechanism of acute mountain sickness (AMS) has to be addressed by comparing levels in subjects with and without AMS.

Levels of antidiuretic hormone (ADH) are not affected by altitude, exercise or AMS except in cases with severe nausea when levels are elevated. After full acclimatization and at more extreme altitudes there is high osmolality with inappropriately low levels of ADH.

The renin–angiotensin–aldosterone system is activated by exercise and, in the case of the long continued exercise involved in mountaineering, can produce sodium and some water retention. Altitude in the absence of exercise results in lower levels of aldosterone, but exercise involved with ascent to altitude results in raised levels of aldosterone.

On first arrival at altitude, corticosteroids are elevated by ACTH then decline to baseline levels over 5–7 days. Even in subjects who had spent some weeks above 6000 m, corticosteroid levels were normal, but one report of subjects who spent months at this altitude did show high levels.

The adrenosympathetic system is stimulated during the first few days at altitude with high levels of urinary catecholamines. These decline with acclimatization in line with the changes in resting heart rate.

Thyroid function is enhanced in humans at altitude, unlike in animals in which it is depressed by hypoxia. Because of this and the increased sympathetic activity, basal metabolic rate (BMR) is increased on going to altitude and remains elevated after acclimatization.

Insulin and glucose levels tend to be lower at altitude, indicating increased insulin sensitivity.

Plasma endothelin levels are raised by hypoxia in line with the raised pulmonary artery pressure and are high in high altitude pulmonary edema (HAPE) patients and subjects susceptible to HAPE.

Glucagon, growth hormone, bradykinin and the sex hormones are little affected by hypoxia except that the exercise response to growth hormone is enhanced and sex hormones tend to be decreased.

Renal function is remarkably little affected by altitude. At extreme altitude, above 6500 m, renal compensation for further respiratory alkalosis seems to be incomplete. There is an increase in microproteinuria, especially on first going to altitude, which is greater in subjects with AMS.

15.1   INTRODUCTION

Endocrinology comprises many systems controlling a great variety of bodily functions and the effect of altitude has been studied on only a fraction of these. The areas studied reflect the interests of scientists going to altitude. Thus hormones that play a part in fluid and electrolyte balance have been widely studied because of their possible relevance to AMS and its complications, as have thyroid hormones because of their effect on metabolic rate. Another factor in the selection of systems for study has, of course, been the availability and ease of relevant assays. This chapter surveys the principal systems studied to date but clearly there are great areas of endocrinology in which the effects of acute and chronic hypoxia have yet to be explored.

The study of endocrinology at altitude is perfectly feasible, but attention to details of sampling, such as time of day, subject's posture, diet and exercise is required, as it is in studies at sea level. Practical aspects of collection and storage of samples are discussed in Chapter 32.

15.2   ANTIDIURETIC HORMONE

There is considerable evidence that ascent to altitude is associated with changes in body fluid compartments both in those with AMS and in asymptomatic subjects. Not surprisingly, therefore, investigators have studied the role of ADH in both the normal (healthy) response to hypoxia and AMS. Reports on the effect of hypoxia on ADH have given conflicting results.

15.2.1   Exercise and ADH

Williams *et al.* (1979) studied exercise in the absence of hypoxia. They studied the effect of daylong hill walking over 7 consecutive days and found no alteration in ADH concentration, despite the fact that their subjects developed peripheral (exercise) edema associated with sodium retention (section 15.3.3).

15.2.2   Acute hypoxia and ADH

Forsling and Milledge (1977) found that breathing 10–10.5 per cent oxygen for 4 h had no effect on ADH levels in samples taken at intervals of from 3 min to 4 h of hypoxia. In a chamber experiment, where subjects were taken to an equivalent altitude of 4000 m for 14 h, there was no significant change in ADH plasma concentration until subjects began to feel nauseated, when levels rose markedly (Forsling and Milledge 1980). Claybaugh *et al.* (1982) took subjects to various equivalent altitudes in a chamber and found an initial increase of urinary ADH at 8–12 h of hypoxia with subsequent return to sea level values. In two subjects with AMS there was a rise in urinary excretion of ADH at 2–4 h of hypoxia. De Angelis *et al.* (1996) studied 26 young pilots in a chamber at an altitude of 5000 m equivalent for 3 h. They found a significant increase in ADH as a result of this quite severe hypoxic stress. It would seem, therefore, that acute hypoxia alone has very little effect but nausea due to AMS is associated with a rise in ADH, analogous to that seen in motion sickness (Eversman *et al.* 1978).

15.2.3   Chronic hypoxia and ADH

Studies conducted in the field include one by Singh *et al.* (1974), who measured a number of hormones in a group of subjects who had a history of HAPE. In those who remained free of symptoms on going to altitude, there was no change in ADH concentration. In subjects who became sick there was a tendency to higher levels but this was mainly seen after a few days at altitude and was not statistically significant. Harber *et al.* (1981) found no significant change in urinary ADH concentration on going to altitudes up to 5400 m; nor was there any relationship with AMS. Even in a fatal case of high altitude cerebral edema there was no significant rise in ADH. Cosby *et al.* (1988) found higher levels of ADH in five skiers with HAPE compared with controls at the same altitude, but the difference did not reach statistical significance. Ramirez *et al.* (1992) found no change in ADH with altitude.

Hackett *et al.* (1978) found normal levels in trekkers at 4300 m, including those with and without symptoms of AMS; the only exceptions were higher concentrations in two cases of HAPE.

The conclusion from this work would seem to be that hypoxia *per se* has no significant effect on ADH concentration. High values may be associated with AMS but not all cases have high values (Claybaugh *et al.* 1982). Where high concentrations are found they may be an effect of AMS rather than its cause.

15.2.4   Inappropriate ADH secretion at altitude

Blume *et al.* (1984) presented evidence of inappropriately low excretion of ADH at altitude. They studied 13 subjects after some weeks at 5400 m and 6300 m on Everest during the American Medical Research Expedition to Everest (AMREE) in 1981 and found ADH concentration unchanged from sea level despite a significant increase in plasma osmolality with increasing altitude. At 6300 m the serum osmolality was 302 mosm kg^{-1} compared with 290 mOsm kg^{-1} at sea level (normal value 280–295 mOsm kg^{-1}). An overnight dehydration test at sea level which might produce this degree of hyperosmolality would result in ADH concentrations of about 7 µU mL^{-1}, whereas subjects on Everest had a mean value of only 0.9 µU mL^{-1}; 12-h urinary ADH showed the same lack of response. Sodium, potassium, calcium and phosphate concentrations were all modestly increased compared with sea level values. A study by Ramirez *et al.* (1992) confirmed these observations. They increased osmolality by intravenous sodium, loading a group of subjects at sea level and at altitude (3000 m). At sea level there was the expected rise in ADH but at altitude there was no significant rise. Thus, at altitude, there seems to be a failure of the osmoregulatory mechanism. This is the converse of the clinical syndrome of inappropriate ADH secretion often associated with small cell carcinoma of the lung (Bayliss 1987). In such cases serum sodium concentration and osmolality are low but ADH secretion is inappropriately high. A more recent study (Ramirez *et al.* 1998) found evidence of reduced sensitivity of the kidney to ADH in acclimatized individuals and that infusion of exogenous ADH caused an increase of urinary arginine vasopressin (AVP) sensitive water channel (aquaporin-2).

15.3   RENIN–ANGIOTENSIN–ALDOSTERONE SYSTEM

This system is depicted in Figure 15.1. Renin is released in response to a number of stimuli, including posture, exercise and, possibly, hypoxia. The mechanism common to these stimuli is sympathetic activation, and both circulating catecholamine and direct sympathetic nervous stimulation result in release of renin from the juxtaglomerular apparatus of the kidney.

Renin has no biological activity but acts on its circulating substrate (angiotensinogen), cleaving it to produce the octapeptide angiotensin I, which is also devoid of activity. Angiotensin converting enzyme (ACE), found on the luminal surface of endothelial cells, converts angiotensin I to angiotensin II by cleaving the final two amino acids. The principal site of conversion is in the rich capillary network of the lung where nearly 90 per cent of angiotensin I is converted to angiotensin II in a single passage. Angiotensin II is a powerful vasopressor and also acts on the cells of the adrenal cortex via a receptor mechanism to release aldosterone. Aldosterone acts on the renal tubules, promoting the reabsorption of sodium. In this way the system is important in the salt and water economy of the body, which is why it has been quite intensively studied at altitude.

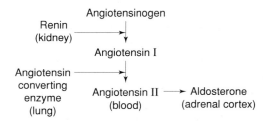

Figure 15.1 *Renin–angiotensin–aldosterone system. Renin and angiotensin converting enzyme (ACE) act as enzymes hydrolyzing angiotensinogen and angiotensin I to angiotensin II. The latter stimulates release of aldosterone from adrenocortical cells by a receptor mechanism.*

15.3.1   Aldosterone and altitude

Indirect evidence of the effect of altitude on aldosterone activity was first provided by Williams (1961), who brought back samples of saliva from the

Karakoram. The ratio of sodium to potassium in these samples indicated suppression of aldosterone at altitude. This has been confirmed by direct measurements of either plasma aldosterone concentration or urinary metabolites (Tuffley *et al.* 1970, Hogan *et al.* 1973, Frayser *et al.* 1975, Pines *et al.* 1977, Sutton *et al.* 1977, Keynes *et al.* 1982, Ramirez *et al.* 1992, Antezana *et al.* 1995, Zaccaria *et al.* 1998). In one study the secretion rate was shown to be reduced (Slater *et al.* 1969). Milledge *et al.* (1983a) studied the time course of the effect of altitude over a 6-week stay at or above 4500 m. After initial suppression, aldosterone concentration rose to control values after 12–20 days. All these studies were made on resting subjects. In subjects who had been above 6000 m for more than 10 weeks and had expanded fluid compartments (blood volume 85 per cent above normal) the aldosterone concentration was twice normal (Anand *et al.* 1993). These subjects were probably in incipient subacute mountain sickness (Chapter 21).

15.3.2 Renin activity and altitude

The effect of altitude on plasma renin activity (PRA) has been studied by a number of groups with conflicting results. Some have found a rise (Slater *et al.* 1969, Tuffley *et al.* 1970, Frayser *et al.* 1975) and others a fall (Hogan *et al.* 1973, Maher *et al.* 1975a, Keynes *et al.* 1982, Antezana *et al.* 1995, Zaccaria *et al.* 1998) and one group no change (Sutton *et al.* 1977). However, most studies have shown a reduced response of aldosterone to renin. This is obvious where PRA has increased and aldosterone has decreased but even where both have declined, the reduction in aldosterone has usually been greater.

It is not clear why these different studies produced different results. One possibility is that subjects, though sampled at rest, may have been more active in some studies, resulting in a rise in PRA. However, this is unlikely in view of the fact that one study showing a rise in PRA was conducted in a chamber (Tuffley *et al.* 1970) and in another, samples were taken before getting up in the morning after subjects had been flown to altitude in a helicopter (Slater *et al.* 1969). The main stimulus to renin release is thought to be sympathetic drive and this certainly occurs with exercise but is probably also induced by altitude hypoxia alone if sufficiently

severe (section 15.4), although with great individual variation.

15.3.3 Exercise and the renin–aldosterone system

Since exercise frequently accompanies ascent to altitude, the effect of exercise needs to be considered in relation to the effect of altitude. Exercise stimulates renin release via activation of the adreno-sympathetic system. The effect can be blocked by beta-blockers (Bonelli *et al.* 1977, Bouissou *et al.* 1989). After intense short-term exercise (3 × 300 m sprints in 10 min) PRA, angiotensin II and aldosterone concentration were elevated at 30 min but measurable elevation was still present up to 6 h later (Kosunen and Pakarinen 1976). The rise in PRA is also proportional to the intensity of the work, both at sea level and at altitude (Maher *et al.* 1975a).

Mountaineers are more concerned with daylong exercise, often continuing for a number of days. Williams *et al.* (1979) showed that this form of exercise resulted in marked sodium retention after 7 days and suggested that this was due to activation of the renin–aldosterone system. There was a mean cumulative retention of 358 mmol of sodium with a modest retention of 650 mL of water. Since plasma sodium concentration did not change significantly it was argued that the extracellular space must have been expanded by 2.68 L (of which 0.68 L was in the plasma volume), mainly at the expense of the intracellular volume. These calculated changes are shown in Figure 15.2. This increase in extracellular fluid (ECF) is the probable cause of the dependent edema frequently found after exercise of this sort.

The same group (Milledge *et al.* 1982) studied the effect of 5 consecutive days' hill walking on the renin–aldosterone system and on sodium and water balance, and confirmed the suggestion, from the previous study, that the sodium retention was due to activation of the renin–aldosterone system. There was elevation of PRA and aldosterone at the conclusion of each day's exercise. This was maximal on day 2 or 3 and less marked on days 4 and 5, perhaps reflecting a training effect. Values were back to control on day 2 after stopping exercise. The effect of exercise and altitude was studied by repeating the same protocol but on the first exercise day subjects climbed to 3100 m and stayed there for 5 days,

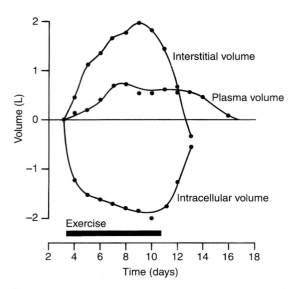

Figure 15.2 *Calculated changes in body fluid compartments with exercise at sea level. (From Williams et al. 1979.)*

exercising for 8 h each day. The results were very similar to sea level results in terms of changes in fluid and sodium balance and hematocrit. Renin and aldosterone also increased, but the aldosterone response to the renin rise was blunted (see section 15.3.5; Milledge *et al.* 1983b).

15.3.4   Control of aldosterone release

The control of aldosterone release via renin and angiotensin has been mentioned above and is shown in Figure 15.1, but ACTH and the sodium status of the subject also control aldosterone concentration. Salt depletion increases aldosterone release whereas salt loading inhibits it. Anderson *et al.* (1986) have shown that atrial natriuretic peptide (ANP) infusion inhibits the response of aldosterone to angiotensin II.

15.3.5   Effect of altitude on the aldosterone response to renin

Milledge and Catley (1982) showed that, if after 1 h of exercise the inspired oxygen was reduced, renin activity increased while aldosterone levels decreased, indicating that the aldosterone response to renin became blunted. In the chronic situation of hill walking or climbing at altitude compared with sea

level the same phenomenon is seen. This is shown in Figure 15.3, which shows data from three studies, at sea level, at 3100 m and on Mount Everest. This blunting has been confirmed by Shigeoka *et al.* (1985), who found the response completely abolished by hypoxia, by Lawrence *et al.* (1990), and, in acute hypoxia, by De Angelis *et al.* (1996). Antezana *et al.* (1995) also found the response in lowlanders to be blunted in La Paz (3600m). Andean highlanders with polycythemia showed a reduced response but highlanders without polycythemia had a normal response at this altitude.

The cause of this blunting is not entirely clear. It had been suggested that ACE activity was reduced by hypoxia, but most workers have found this not to be the case (Milledge and Catley 1987, Bouissou *et al.* 1988). However, Vonmoos *et al.* (1990) have found that, although angiotensin I levels were unchanged with acute hypoxia, levels of angiotensin II were reduced. The next stage in the promotion of aldosterone release is adrenal stimulation by angiotensin II. Colice and Ramirez (1986) studied the effect of angiotensin II infusion on aldosterone release and found that hypoxia had no effect, suggesting that it did not result in an increase of inhibitors of this part of the system. However, Raff and Kohandarvish (1990) found evidence that adrenocortical cells *in vitro* were less responsive to angiotensin II under hypoxic conditions. More recently Raff *et al.* (1996)

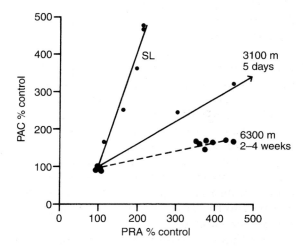

Figure 15.3 *Plasma aldosterone concentration (PAC) response to plasma renin activity (PRA) from a sea level (SL) study and from two separate altitude studies. (From Milledge et al. 1983b.)*

have shown that chronic hypoxia in rats (10 per cent oxygen for 3 days) results in a decrease in expression of the steroidogenic enzyme P-450c11AS in adreno-cortical cells. This enzyme is unique to the aldo-sterone pathway. However, with less severe hypoxia, 12 per cent oxygen for 3 days, there was no effect.

Aldosterone secretion is stimulated by ACTH as well as by angiotensin II. Ramirez et al. (1988) found this effect to be reduced in subjects at altitude whereas the ACTH-induced secretion of cortisol was unaffected. ANP has been found to inhibit aldo-sterone release (Elliott and Goodfriend 1986). It is therefore possible that the rise in ANP on going to altitude (section 15.4.4) may be a factor in blunting this response at rest (Lawrence et al. 1990) and on exercise (Lawrence and Shenker 1991).

15.4 ALTITUDE AND ATRIAL NATRIURETIC PEPTIDE

15.4.1 ANP release and actions

ANP is secreted by the atria of the heart in response to stretching. Atrial stretch is usually caused by an increase in atrial pressure. However, in the case of cardiac tamponade the pressure is high but the atrial wall is not stretched. As the tamponade is relieved the pressure falls and the atrium dilates. It has been found that relief of tamponade results in a rise in ANP plasma levels, indicating that stretch rather than pressure is the stimulus for ANP synthesis and release (Au et al. 1990).

Amongst its actions, ANP has the effect of increasing sodium excretion by the kidneys and thus of promoting a natriuresis and diuresis (Morice et al. 1988). This provides a homeostatic mechanism for salt and water. If the plasma volume is increased, the raised atrial pressure results in atrial stretch and secretion of ANP, diuresis follows and vascular pressures and volume return to normal. This system is further considered in relation to the regulation of plasma volume in Chapter 8 (section 8.2.2). ANP possibly also has a role as a vasodilator, countering the pressor effect of hypoxia on the pulmonary artery. It has been shown to have this effect in a dose-dependent manner in the isolated rat lung (Stewart et al. 1991) and in the pig (Adnot et al. 1988). Liu et al. (1989) infused ANP (20 mg min^{-1}

for 10 min) into four patients with HAPE and showed a reduction in pulmonary artery pressure for 1 h after the infusion.

15.4.2 ANP and hypoxia

In the last decade, since the first edition of this book, there have been numerous reports of the effect of hypoxia on the plasma levels of ANP at rest and on exercise.

Ten minutes of severe hypoxia on isolated rat and rabbit heart with constant flow perfusion caused a fourfold increase in ANP released (Baertschi et al. 1986). The same group found increases in ANP blood levels in the whole animal made hypoxic under anesthesia. There was great variability in the response, which correlated with the baseline central venous pressure, but not with any other measured variables. Winter et al. (1989) also found ANP levels to be increased by hypoxia in the rat after 24 h but not after only 2 h. In patients with chronic hypoxic lung disease, levels of ANP were elevated and varied inversely with the Pa_{O_2} (Winter et al. 1987b).

In healthy volunteers Kawashima et al. (1989) studied the effect of 10 min of hypoxia at two levels; 15 per cent oxygen breathing produced no change, but 10 per cent oxygen breathing increased ANP levels by 15 per cent accompanied by an increase in pulmonary artery pressure. Vonmoos et al. (1990) found that 60 min of 12 per cent oxygen breathing produced a small but significant elevation of ANP. Lawrence et al. (1990) found that the same hypoxic stimulus produced a 50 per cent increase in ANP levels in subjects on a low salt diet and whose endogenous cortisol was suppressed with dexa-methasone. Conversely, Ramirez et al. (1992) did not find a significant rise in ANP levels with either acute (60 min) or chronic hypoxia at 3000 m, although the ANP response to a sodium load was greater at altitude. Antezana et al. (1995) found a reduction in ANP levels in lowlanders at 3600 m compared with sea level and highlanders had significantly lower ANP than lowlanders at altitude.

15.4.3 Exercise and ANP: normoxia

Somers et al. (1986) found that a progressive exercise test to maximum exercise resulted in an almost fourfold increase in plasma ANP with a decline to baseline after 1 h at rest. Similar results have been found for short-term exercise by Schmidt *et al.* (1990) and by Lawrence and Shenker (1991). Hill walking exercise for 5 days also resulted in elevated ANP levels to about twice baseline values (Milledge *et al.* 1991b). It is interesting to note that during this type of exercise sodium is retained despite elevated ANP levels.

15.4.4   Exercise and ANP: hypoxia

Mountaineers and trekkers going to altitude normally have the double stimulus of exercise and hypoxia. Schmidt *et al.* (1990) studied exercise while breathing air or reduced oxygen (92 mm Hg). With both maximal and submaximal exercise the ANP response to exercise was reduced under hypoxic conditions. In contrast, Lawrence and Shenker (1991), using less severe hypoxia (16 per cent inspired oxygen) and exercise such as to give a heart rate of 70–75 per cent of maximum for 30 min, found that hypoxia enhanced the ANP response. A third study using a decompression chamber to give a simulated altitude of 3000 m and a progressive exercise test to maximum showed a reduced response (Vuolteenaho *et al.* 1992). The reasons for these differing results are not apparent.

Milledge *et al.* (1989) reported levels of plasma ANP in 15 subjects before and after ascent on foot from 3100 m to 4300 m. Values tended to be higher at altitude but were significantly so only in the 4 a.m. sample on the second altitude day, there being no difference on day 1 at altitude or in the 9 a.m. sample on either day. Bärtsch *et al.* (1991a) found, in blood samples taken on the morning after the ascent to 4559 m on foot, no increase in ANP levels in a group of nine climbers who did not have AMS. Five subjects who did become sick had elevated levels. These subjects had a history of HAPE and were shown by echocardiography to have increased atrial diameters at altitude. The increase in ANP is probably secondary to developing high pulmonary artery pressures. Kawashima *et al.* (1992) showed that, in subjects susceptible to high altitude pulmonary edema, breathing 10 per cent oxygen resulted in a greater rise in ANP levels than in controls, and that the rise correlated with the rise in pulmonary artery pressure.

15.4.5   ANP and AMS

An important motive for the study of the effect of altitude hypoxia on ANP has been the hypothesis that it may play a part in the genesis of AMS. Milledge *et al.* (1989) did not find any correlation between levels of ANP on the morning after arrival at altitude and the AMS symptom score. However, Bärtsch *et al.* (1988) and Cosby *et al.* (1988) found subjects with AMS or HAPE to have higher levels than subjects without AMS. If the rise in ANP in AMS sufferers is related to high pulmonary arterial pressure, elevation would be expected mainly in AMS with pulmonary edema and not in the milder, nonpulmonary cases. In the first-mentioned study there was no clinical evidence of pulmonary edema.

15.4.6   ANP and chronic mountain sickness

Antezana *et al.* (1995) have reported higher levels of ANP in patients with chronic mountain sickness (CMS) than in controls in Andean highlanders. In this study pulmonary artery pressure was assessed by Doppler ultrasound and found to be raised.

In conclusion, it seems that although both exercise and hypoxia cause an elevation of ANP, the combined stimulus does not result in very high levels at altitude. Despite its name, ANP is not a powerful natriuretic hormone. Levels of ANP are elevated in conditions where the pulmonary artery pressure is raised, including HAPE and polycythemia, and this rise is presumably secondary to the raised pressure causing some atrial enlargement. The rise in ANP is probably beneficial in that it tends to reduce the pressure by its vasodilatory function.

15.5   CORTICOSTEROIDS AND ALTITUDE

On ascent to altitude, there is stimulation of the adrenal cortex by ACTH and cortisol is secreted. Early work documented this as a rise in 17-hydroxy-corticosteroids (17-OHCS) during the first few days at altitude, which decreased to control values by days 5–7 (MacKinnon *et al.* 1963, Moncloa *et al.* 1965). This has been confirmed by measurement of plasma cortisol by Frayser *et al.* (1975) and Sutton *et al.* (1977), who showed that with the elevation of plasma cortisol there was a decrease in its normal diurnal variation on the first day of altitude exposure. Richalet *et al.* (1989), in a chamber experiment, also found elevation of plasma cortisol with re-establishment of the diurnal variation after the first altitude day. Many of the subjects of these studies, taken rapidly to an altitude of 4300–5300 m, suffered from AMS, but even those free of symptoms showed this transitory rise in cortisol or its urinary metabolite. It is assumed that this is a nonspecific stress response.

CASE REPORT

An interesting case report shows that there is a clinical lesson to be learnt. A 58-year-old man, who had had his pituitary removed 10 years earlier for an adenoma, went trekking in Nepal. On arrival at Menang (3535 m) he complained of fatigue, abdominal pain, nausea and vomiting, but no headache. He was on regular medication with cortisone 25 mg daily and had taken his treatment. Twenty-four hours later he had deteriorated and was unable to stand. He was treated with dexamethasone 5 mg i.v., 5 mg i.m. and oral rehydration, and his cortisone dose was quadrupled. Within 24 h all symptoms had disappeared, and the next day he successfully crossed the Thorong La (5450 m) (Westendorp *et al.* 1993). Clearly the lesson is that subjects on corticosteroid replacement therapy should increase their dosage on going to altitude. The authors point out that this does not apply to thyroid replacement therapy since thyroid stimulating hormone (TSH) is not increased by hypoxia.

The effect of prolonged stay at more extreme altitude was studied by Siri *et al.* (1969). They brought back urine samples from the 1963 Everest expedition from climbers staying at 5400 m and 6500 m. The 17-OHCS levels were not significantly different from sea level values. They also demonstrated a normal response to injected ACTH. Mordes *et al.* (1983) collected samples from subjects who had been at 5400 m and 6300 m for some weeks and found no change from sea level values in either morning or evening cortisol concentrations.

In animals studied after chronic hypoxia there was some hyperplasia of the adrenal cortex and of the corticotrophic cells in the pituitary. No such morphological changes have been found in humans with long-standing chronic bronchitis (Gosney

1986). However, in subjects who had spent more than 10 weeks above 6000 m, the cortisol level was found to be three times normal (Anand *et al.* 1993). Marinelli *et al.* (1994) studied athletes taking part in a marathon race from 3860 m to 5100 m and down to finish at 3400 m. Cortisol levels were similar at altitude before the race but were greatly elevated at the end.

In people resident at the moderate altitude of 2600 m in Columbia, Ramirez *et al.* (1995) found an enhanced response to corticotrophin releasing hormone, with higher levels of both ACTH and β-endorphin after stimulation than in sea level control subjects. This was true for a number of tropic hormones (sections 15.7.1 and 15.9.2).

15.6   ADRENOSYMPATHETIC SYSTEM

15.6.1   Acute hypoxia

Acute hypoxia increases heart rate at rest and on exercise (Maher *et al.* 1975b). This is presumed to be due to increased sympathetic activity stimulating the β-adrenergic receptors on heart muscle cell membrane. However, measurements of plasma, epinephrine and norepinephrine after 10 min of mild isocapnic hypoxia at rest showed no increase over control values despite a rise in heart rate from 70 to 83 beats/min^{-1} (Ind *et al.* 1984). On light exercise, plasma catecholamine levels are increased by acute hypoxia, but this is not seen after heavy exercise (75 per cent $V_{O_2 max}$) (Maher *et al.* 1975b). Bouissou *et al.* (1989) also found a 32 per cent increase in norepinephrine after 48 h at altitude but on maximal exercise the rise in catecholamines was no different from that seen at sea level. Mazzeo *et al.* (1991) found reduced norepinephrine and raised epinephrine levels at rest. On submaximal exercise, norepinephrine levels rose as they did at sea level. Epinephrine rose with exercise at altitude whereas it remained unchanged at sea level.

15.6.2   Chronic hypoxia

Cunningham *et al.* (1965) reported elevated plasma and 24-h urinary catecholamines during 17 days at 4559 m on Monte Rosa. There was no significant change in epinephrine but the increase in norepinephrine was greater on day 12 at altitude. Pace *et al.* (1964) found similar results at 3850 m, with urinary norepinephrine excretion rising slowly during 14 days at altitude without change in urinary epinephrine secretion. Maher *et al.* (1975b) found increased urinary catecholamines at 4300 m. Levels were increased on day 1 compared with sea level and further increased on day 11. On exercise, both light and severe, the effect of chronic hypoxia compared with acute was to increase levels still further. Hoon *et al.* (1977) found no significant change in urinary catecholamine secretion in a total of 76 subjects who had no symptoms of AMS. However, in 29 symptomatic subjects there was a small but significant rise on the first day at altitude, which was maintained through to day 10 at altitude. Mazzeo *et al.* (1991) found that, at rest, norepinephrine and epinephrine levels were higher at altitude than at sea level. With submaximal exercise, norepinephrine rose to higher values than expected at sea level, whereas epinephrine levels did not rise, though values remained above those at sea level. In Operation Everest II at extreme altitude (282 mm Hg) after 40 days in the chamber, resting plasma norepinephrine was raised but epinephrine was reduced. On maximum exercise, values for both catecholamines fell with increasing altitude (Young *et al.* 1989).

In subjects who had spent more than 10 weeks above 6000 m the plasma norepinephrine concentration was found to be almost three times normal (Anand *et al.* 1993). Gosney *et al.* (1991) studied the adrenal and pituitary glands of five lifelong residents of La Paz who had lived at 3600–3800 m, and compared their glands with those of controls from sea level. The adrenal glands were significantly bigger, by about 50 per cent. The pituitary glands were not larger but contained more corticotrophs. They surmised that greater amounts of ACTH were required to maintain adrenal function, perhaps because of hypoxic inhibition of adrenocortical sensitivity. However, Ramirez *et al.* (1988) found no such inhibition.

15.6.3 Adrenergic response and acclimatization

Acute hypoxia causes an increase in heart rate and cardiac output. However, after several days at altitude the heart rate and cardiac output fall back towards sea level values. On exercise the maximum heart rate is limited to well below the sea level maximum, being typically 140–150 beats min^{-1} compared with 180–200 beats min^{-1} at sea level (Chapter 7). This reduction in maximal heart rate and cardiac output takes place at a time when the plasma and urinary catecholamines are higher than at sea level.

Evidently, the heart's response to sympathetic stimulation becomes blunted. This has been demonstrated by Maher *et al.* (1975b), who showed in dogs that the cardio-acceleratory effect of an infusion of isoproterenol was reduced after 10 days' altitude acclimatization. Workers from the same institution (Maher *et al.* 1978) found in cardiac muscle of acclimatized goats that there was a twofold rise of the enzyme *o*-methyltransferase. This enzyme inactivates cardiac norepinephrine, and its induction during acclimatization may account for the blunting of the adrenergic response to exercise. Another possibility is that there may be downregulation, that is, a reduction in the density of adrenergic receptors on the heart muscle. Voelkel *et al.* (1981) have shown this to be the case in rats kept for 5 weeks at a simulated altitude of 4250 m. These two possible mechanisms are not mutually exclusive. Sherpa high altitude residents do not suffer this heart rate limitation on maximal exercise. Their heart rates can go up to 190–198 beats min^{-1} at 4880 m (Lahiri *et al.* 1967).

In summary, hypoxia has no effect on epinephrine levels in the blood or urine but there is a modest rise in norepinephrine levels. This may be more marked in subjects with AMS. The response of the heart to adrenergic stimulation becomes blunted after a week or 10 days at altitude and this is probably due to downregulation of receptors and induction of the enzyme responsible for catecholamine metabolism.

15.7 THYROID FUNCTION AND THE ALTITUDE ENVIRONMENT

Hypothalamic–pituitary–thyroid axis function is affected by hypoxia and possibly by cold. The effect of cold on thyroid function is considered in Chapter 24. Iodine is essential for synthesis of thyroid hormone and is deficient in the soil and water of some mountainous regions, so that thyroid function in residents of these regions is affected.

15.7.1   Thyroid function and hypoxia

The response of the hypophyseal–thyroid axis to hypoxia seems to be quite different in humans compared with animals. In animals, hypoxia results in depression of thyroid function (Heath and Williams 1995, pp. 265–6). In the pituitary gland the number of thyrotrophs – cells that secrete TSH – is reduced, suggesting a decreased output of TSH (Gosney 1986). In humans, however, thyroid activity is increased at altitude. Surks (1966) found elevated levels of thyroxine binding globulin (TBG) and free thyroxine (T_4) in the first 2 weeks at altitude (4300 m), with a peak at 9 days. Kotchen et al. (1973), in a 3-day chamber experiment (3650 m equivalent), found T_4 elevated (free and bound) but TSH to be unchanged, suggesting a shift of T_4 from extravascular to intravascular compartments rather than increased pituitary activity. Westendorp et al. (1993) also found no increase in TSH in response to a 1-h acute hypoxia equivalent of 4115 m.

These results have been confirmed in a number of field studies (Rastogi et al. 1977, Stock et al. 1978b) which showed levels returning towards control in the third week at altitude. Sawhney and Malhotra (1991) studied both acclimatized lowlanders and high altitude natives, and found levels of triiodothyronine (T_3) and T_4 to be higher than sea level residents. T_4 concentration in red cells was decreased at high altitude but there was no change in levels of reverse T_3 (rT_3), TBG, and T_4 binding capacity of TBG and thyroxine binding prealbumin. They also found no change in TSH. In L-eltroxine-treated men they still found a rise in T_3 and T_4, suggesting the rise to be independent of pituitary stimulation.

Exercise increases T_3 and T_4 to a greater extent at altitude than at sea level (Stock et al. 1978b). At higher altitudes of 5400 m and 6300 m, Mordes et al. (1983) showed elevated resting T_3, free T_4 and T_3 in subjects who had been at altitude for some weeks. In these subjects TSH was also elevated, in contrast to the finding at lower altitudes.

The basal metabolic rate is elevated during the first 2 weeks at moderate altitude and correlates with the free T_4 (Stock et al. 1978a). At higher altitudes (above 5500 m) it remains elevated for months (Gill and Pugh 1964), as does T_4 (Mordes et al. 1983). Mordes et al. (1983) also found evidence of impaired conversion of T_4 to T_3 at 6300 m. Perhaps there is a change in the set point for the pituitary negative feedback system, resulting in higher levels of TSH. They also found that the response of the pituitary to an injection of thyrotrophin releasing hormone was enhanced at 6300 m compared with sea level. Recently a similar finding has been reported (Ramirez et al. 1995) in resident highlanders at only 2600 m.

15.7.2   Iodine deficiency, goitre and altitude

The frequency of goitre in mountainous areas is well known and is discussed in Chapter 17. In England it was known as 'Derbyshire neck' and it was equally well known in the Pyrenees, the Alps, the Andes and the Himalayas, but it is not confined to the mountains.

The association of iodine deficiency and mountainous areas is mainly due to the geological factors (Chapter 17) but altitude hypoxia stimulates thyroid function (section 15.7.1). Thus the effect of iodine deficiency will result in more exaggerated hyperplasia, which contributes to the extremely high rate of goitre in resident populations at altitude.

15.8   CONTROL OF BLOOD GLUCOSE AT ALTITUDE

15.8.1   Acute hypoxia

On acute exposure to hypoxia there is a rise in fasting blood glucose of about 1.7 mmol L^{-1}, followed by a fall towards control values by the end of a week. At the same time insulin levels are elevated (Williams 1975). This is presumably part of the nonspecific stress response indicated by the concurrent rise in plasma cortisol levels (section 15.5).

15.8.2   Chronic hypoxia

In subjects acclimatized to high altitude, fasting blood glucose was found to be lower than at sea level by some workers (Blume and Pace 1967, Stock et al. 1978b, Blume 1984) but unchanged by others (Sawhney et al. 1986). Singh et al. (1974) found a persistently raised glucose level after 10 months at altitude. Resting insulin levels have also been found to be reduced (Stock *et al.* 1978b).

Glucose loading increases both blood glucose and insulin levels at altitude as it does at sea level, but the rise in both was found to be less than at sea level in two studies (Stock *et al.* 1978b, Blume 1984) but greater in one (Sawhney *et al.* 1986). There are a number of explanations for this blunted response. Glucose may be absorbed less rapidly, though this is probably only true above about 5500 m (section 14.5). Liver glycogen synthesis may be enhanced at altitude and some evidence for this has been found in rats injected with labeled glucose at altitude (Blume and Pace 1971). There may be increased target organ sensitivity to insulin, presumably by upregulation (increased density) of insulin receptors on target cells. This is a feature of athletic training and may well happen as part of altitude acclimatization.

Braun *et al.* (1998) studied the glucose response to a standard meal in women at sea level and at 4300 m in the presence of estrogen (E) and estrogen plus progesterone (E+P). The peak of glucose was lower and returned to baseline more slowly at altitude than at sea level although the insulin levels were the same. The response was also lower in E than E+P at sea level but the difference at altitude was not significant. It would seem that at altitude the relative concentration of ovarian hormones does not appear to be important in glucose control.

15.9 ENDOTHELIN

15.9.1 Endothelin family

The endothelins are a family of peptides produced by a wide variety of cells affecting mainly blood vessels. Endothelin-1 (ET-1), clinically the most important member of the family, is the most potent vasoconstrictor yet discovered with about 100 times the activity of norepinephrine. Other members of the family identified are ET-2 and ET-3, which are more localized to certain organs. All three peptides bind to the same two receptors, A and B, though with differing binding affinities. Synthetic inhibitors of these receptors are now available and their use has served to elucidate some of the actions of these peptides. ET-1 is produced by the endothelium and as much as 75 per cent of the production is exported from the side of the cell opposite to the vessel lumen, where it acts on the adjacent smooth muscle without contributing to the plasma pool. In this way it perhaps should be considered as mainly a paracrine, rather than an endocrine, hormone. However, plasma levels probably do reflect the output of ET-1 and parallel the severity of the condition in, for instance, congestive cardiac failure.

A good clinical review has been published by Levin (1995), and Holm (1997) has provided a more pharmacological review.

15.9.2 Altitude and endothelin

Horio *et al.* (1991) showed that ET-1 in rats increased with increasing hypoxia. Since then there have been a number of studies in humans at altitude. Cargill *et al.* (1995) found that 30 min of acute hypoxia (Sa_{O_2} 75–80 per cent) raised plasma ET-1 levels to about 2.5 times baseline. A group of hypoxic patients with cor pulmonale had similar levels. Similar results were found by Ferri *et al.* (1995) in patients with chronic obstructive lung disorder (COLD). They also found that ET-1 levels correlated with pulmonary artery pressure. Morganti *et al.* (1995) studied 10 subjects on a 2-day ascent of Monte Rosa (4559 m) and eight subjects in the Everest region at 5050 m. They found plasma ET-1 raised progressively with increasing altitude, the level correlating with the fall in Sa_{O_2}. There was no correlation with blood pressure or hematocrit. Richalet and colleagues (1995) studied 10 subjects on Sajama (6542 m) and found modest increases in ET-1 at both rest and exercise. Levels were highest after 1 week and decreased slightly after 3 weeks' altitude exposure. A Japanese group (Droma *et al.* 1996a) reported detailed findings on a single case of HAPE with pulmonary hypertension and found ET-1 levels elevated on admission. The levels reverted to normal as the patient recovered and pulmonary artery pressure fell. The same team (Droma 1996b) studied a group of HAPE-susceptible subjects. Their subjects had a greater hypoxic vascular response than controls but no significant change in ET-1 levels with a hypoxic challenge. However, the hypoxia was only of 5-min duration (10 per cent oxygen). Blauw *et al.* (1995) studied the effect of hypoxia and ET-1 infusion on forearm blood flow. Forearm blood flow was not changed by hypoxia, but the ET-1 plasma increased significantly. They conclude that hypoxia causes release of ET-1 from the pulmonary circulation but that this does not influence peripheral vascular tone. Cruden *et al.* (1998) measured both ET-1 and big ET-1 in a group of mountaineers. Both were increased on ascent to altitudes above 2500 m, indicating that the increase in ET-1 was due to increased production and not decreased elimination. After 3 weeks at altitude, levels had returned to baseline values. Exercise had no effect on endothelin levels. In a separate study, they also found increases in both ET-1 and big ET-1 with cold exposure (Cruden *et al.* 1999).

In conclusion, it seems likely that ET-1 plays a part in the mechanism of hypoxic pulmonary vaso-constriction, at least in the pig (Holm 1997). Whether it has a role in the mechanism of high altitude pulmonary edema remains to be determined.

15.9.3 Bradykinin

The levels of bradykinin, a potent vasodilator, are not changed by acute hypoxia (Ashack *et al.* 1985),

15.10 ALTITUDE AND OTHER HORMONES

15.10.1 Glucagon

Fasting glucagon levels are the same at altitude and at sea level and are slightly depressed after glucose loading (Blume 1984).

15.10.2 Growth hormone

Levels are unchanged in most subjects but were found to be increased fivefold in two subjects who had lost 15 kg in body weight (Blume 1984). Although acute hypoxia causes no change in growth hormone levels, exercise under acute hypoxic conditions causes a 20-fold increase in this hormone, whereas normoxic exercise causes only a modest rise (Sutton 1977, Raynaud *et al.* 1981). Ramirez *et al.* (1995) studied residents at Pasto, Columbia (2600 m), and found that response of growth hormone to stimulation with growth hormone releasing hormone was greatly enhanced compared with lowland control subjects.

15.10.3 Testosterone, luteinizing hormone, follicle stimulating hormone and prolactin

Sawhney *et al.* (1985) studied levels of testosterone, luteinizing hormone (LH), follicle stimulating hormone (FSH) and prolactin in lowland men after ascent to 3500 m. On day 1 at altitude there were no significant changes from sea level values, though LH and testosterone levels were already falling. By day 7, LH and testosterone levels were significantly reduced and remained so to day 18; by then prolactin levels were significantly elevated. After 7 days at sea level all values had reverted to control except for some residual depression in LH levels. These results are in accord with previous work (Guerra-Garcia 1971) which found urinary testosterone excretion to be reduced by 50 per cent on day 3 at 4300 m. Sawhney *et al.* (1985) also found a negative correlation between prolactin and testosterone levels at altitude but no correlation with LH levels. They suggested that the reduction in testosterone is due to increase in prolactin secretion rather than to a reduction in LH or a direct effect of hypoxia on the testes.

In a separate experiment at sea level Sawhney *et al.* (1985) showed a reduction in LH levels in response to daily cold exposure after 1 and 5 days, and suggested that the reduction in LH found at altitude might be due to cold rather than hypoxia. However, low levels of LH have been found in hypoxia due to chronic lung disease in hospital patients with no cold exposure (Semple 1986); these patients also had low testosterone levels which correlated with their Pa_{O_2}.

Semple (1986) found normal testosterone levels in patients who were hypoxic because of congenital cardiac defects, presumably because of lifelong adaptation to hypoxemia. He suggests that an alternative mechanism may be that testosterone depression is a response to dips in oxygen saturation at night, due to sleep apnea in patients with chronic obstructive lung disease, and a result of periodic breathing in lowlanders at altitude. In high altitude residents, Bangham and Hackett (1978) found reduced levels of LH after 10 days but no changes in levels of FSH, testosterone or prolactin.

Testosterone is increased in exercise and Bouissou *et al.* (1986) studied the effect of acute hypoxia (14 per cent oxygen, equivalent to 3000 m) on this response. They found that, when the exercise was expressed as a percentage of maximum exercise, there was no effect of acute hypoxia. This is also true for the acute hypoxic effect on the exercise-induced rises of lactate, epinephrine and norepinephrine.

15.11   RENAL FUNCTION AT ALTITUDE

15.11.1   General function

The kidney is remarkably resistant to altitude hypoxia. This is not surprising since it is designed to suffer quite severe reductions in blood flow, and therefore oxygen delivery, during exercise. At 5800 m, after 24-h dehydration, the kidney concentrates urine normally and eliminates a water load as well as it does at sea level. It also responds to ingestion of bicarbonate or ammonium chloride (metabolic alkalosis or acidosis) by producing appropriate changes in pH (Ward, reported by Pugh 1962a). Olsen *et al.* (1993) found a 10 per cent reduction in effective renal plasma flow (ERPF) but normal glomerular filtration rate and sodium clearance in eight normal subjects at 4350 m. Dopamine infusion had less effect on ERPF than at sea level, presumably because of increased adrenergic activity (norepinephrine was increased). The diuretic effect of dopamine was reduced, possibly because of an altitude effect on distal tubular function. High altitude residents at 4300 m showed no evidence of deficient renal oxygenation (Rennie *et al.* 1971a).

However (as discussed in section 9.4.5), at extreme altitude (above 6500 m) the renal compensation for respiratory alkalosis is slow and incomplete; that is, the blood bicarbonate is very little further reduced and the blood pH becomes very alkaline as the P_{CO_2} is reduced by extreme hyperventilation. Whether this represents a degree of renal failure is debatable, since it results in a shift of the oxygen dissociation curve to the left (because of the alkaline pH), which is beneficial for oxygen transport at extreme altitude (section 9.3.6).

15.11.2   Proteinuria at altitude

Rennie and Joseph (1970) showed that proteinuria became apparent on ascent to altitude. Values rose from 290 to 578 μg mmol^{-1} as their subjects climbed to 5800 m in 12 days. There was a time lag of 1–3 days between peak altitude and peak proteinuria. Figure

15.4 shows that there is a good correlation between the degree of proteinuria and altitude, provided allowance is made for a 24-h time lag between ascent and its effect on the kidney.

In another study, Rennie *et al.* (1972) found no effect of acclimatization on proteinuria but Pines (1978) found less proteinuria on repeat ascents to the same altitude, and also that subjects with AMS had the greatest proteinuria. High altitude residents excrete more protein in the urine than subjects of the same race at sea level (Rennie *et al.* 1971b).

Patients with cyanotic heart disease who are chronically hypoxic from birth also have increased proteinuria, the severity being directly related to the degree of polycythemia (and hypoxia) (Rennie 1973); it is also found in patients with chronic obstructive lung disease (Wilkinson *et al.* 1993).

Bradwell and Delamere (1982) studied the effect of acetazolamide on altitude proteinuria as part of a double blind trial of the drug as a prophylactic for AMS. They found that, at 5000 m, albuminuria was six times greater in subjects on placebo tablets than in those on acetazolamide. They found an inverse correlation between Pa_{O_2} and percentage increase in urine albumin. The eight subjects on acetazolamide were of course less hypoxic, with $Pa_{O_2} > 42$ mm Hg, than nine subjects on placebo with $Pa_{O_2} < 42$ mm Hg. The authors suggest that the effect of acetazolamide on albuminuria was due to this reduction in hypoxia. The mechanism for altitude proteinuria may be either a reduction in tubular reabsorption of protein or increased glomerular permeability to protein, or both.

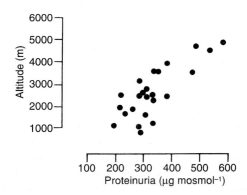

Figure 15.4 *Proteinuria at altitude, the altitude being that of the subjects 24 h before urine sampling. (After Rennie 1973.)*

16

Central nervous system

SUMMARY

The central nervous system (CNS) is exquisitely sensitive to hypoxia and so it is not surprising that impairment of neuropsychological function can be demonstrated at high altitude. Brain oxygenation is a function of both arterial P_{O_2} and cerebral blood flow. The latter is regulated in part by the arterial blood gases. Hypoxemia causes cerebral vasodilatation whereas a reduced arterial P_{CO_2} results in cerebral vasoconstriction: these are therefore conflicting factors at high altitude. Some impairment of neuropsychological function, for example slow learning of complex mental tasks, can be demonstrated at altitudes of less than 2000 m. At higher altitudes many aspects of neuropsychological function have been shown to be impaired, including reaction time, hand–eye coordination, and higher functions such as memory and language expression. Several studies have documented residual impairment of neuropsychological function after ascents to very high altitude. An interesting finding is that climbers with a high hypoxic ventilatory response tend to have the most severe residual impairment, possibly because the associated reduced arterial P_{CO_2} causes cerebral vasoconstriction and therefore more severe cerebral hypoxia. Oxygen enrichment of room air improves neuropsychological function at an altitude of 5000 m and may therefore improve performance in commuters to mines and telescopes.

16.1 INTRODUCTION

Of all the parts of the body, the CNS is one of the most vulnerable to hypoxia. It is not surprising, therefore, that people who go to high altitude often have changes in neuropsychological function, including special senses such as vision, higher functions such as memory and affective behavior such as mood. Such changes have been observed in individuals acutely exposed to hypoxia, in lowlanders sojourning at high altitude, and in high altitude natives.

In addition to the changes in neuropsychological function seen in individuals at high altitude, there is mounting evidence that there may be persistent defects of CNS function on return to sea level after periods of severe hypoxia at high altitude. These findings are of special interest now because increasing numbers of climbers choose to climb at great altitudes without supplementary oxygen. Many people are concerned about the increase in morbidity and mortality on expeditions to extreme altitude, and irrational decisions made by severely hypoxic climbers probably play an important role.

16.2 HISTORICAL

Changes in mood and behavior at high altitude have been recognized from the early days of climbing high mountains. However, the most extreme effects of hypoxia on the CNS were seen by the early balloonists where partial paralysis, difficulties with vision, mood changes and even loss of consciousness are well documented. For example, during the famous flight of the balloon 'Zenith' by Tissandier and his two companions (Tissandier 1875) we read,

> towards 7500 metres, the numbness one experiences is extraordinary. . . . One does not suffer at all; on the contrary. One experiences inner joy, as if it were an effect of the inundating flood of light. One becomes indifferent. . . .

This lack of appreciation of the dangers of acute hypoxia is well known to aircraft pilots and is the reason why there are stringent regulations on using oxygen above certain altitudes despite the fact that the pilot may not feel that he needs it.

The paralysing effects of hypoxia were vividly described during the balloon ascent by Glaisher and Coxwell in 1862 (Glaisher et al. 1871). At the highest altitude, Glaisher collapsed unconscious in the basket and it was left to Coxwell to vent the hydrogen from the balloon to bring it down. However, Coxwell had apparently lost the use of his hands and instead had to seize the cord that controlled the valve with his teeth and dip his head two or three times. Incidentally, this flight also underscored the rapid recovery from severe acute hypoxia. When the balloon landed, Glaisher stated that he felt 'no inconvenience' and they both walked between 7 and 8 miles to the nearest village because they had come down in a remote country area.

When climbers began to reach great altitudes, neuropsychological disturbances were frequently reported. For example, there were several descriptions of bizarre changes in perception and mood on the early expeditions to Mount Everest. During the 1933 Everest expedition, Smythe gave a dramatic description of a hallucination when he saw pulsating cloud-like objects in the sky (Ruttledge 1933). Smythe also reported a strong feeling that he was accompanied by a second person; he even divided food to give half to his nonexistent companion. On occasions, the changes in CNS function suggest attacks of transient cerebral ischemia. For example, the very experienced mountaineer, Shipton, had a remarkable period of aphasia at an altitude of about 7000 m on the same expedition (Shipton 1943). He reported that 'if I wished to say "give me a cup of tea", I would say something entirely different – maybe "tram-car, cat, put" . . . I was perfectly clear-headed . . . but my tongue just refused to perform the required movements. . . .'

In the last few years there has been increasing interest in the neuropsychological effects of high altitude. For example, the Polish climber and psychiatrist Ryn found a range of psychiatric disturbances in mountaineers who had ascended to over 5500 m (Ryn 1971). He also reported that symptoms similar to an organic brain syndrome persisted for several weeks after the expedition. Some climbers had electroencephalogram abnormalities after climbs to great altitudes. Studies made during the war between China and India in the early 1960s, when Indian troops were rapidly airlifted to high altitude, showed residual changes in psychomotor function on return to sea level (Sharma et al. 1975, 1976). Townes et al. (1984) made measurements on members of the American Medical Research Expedition to Everest (AMREE) after they had returned to sea level following about 3 months at altitudes of 5400–8848 m and found residual abnormalities of neuropsychological performance. Similar results were found on Operation Everest II, including the additional interesting observation that climbers with the highest hypoxic ventilatory response were more severely affected. There have been steady improvements in the techniques of neuropsychological testing and it is becoming clear that minor changes in function are extremely common at high altitude, and that some residual impairment often remains in some climbers who return to sea level from great altitudes.

16.3 MECHANISMS OF ACTION OF HYPOXIA

16.3.1 Hypoxia and nerve cells

Despite a great deal of research over the last few decades, a clear understanding of the effect of hypoxia on nerve cells remains elusive (Siesjo

1992a,b, Haddad and Jiang 1993, Hossmann 1999). Mild hypoxia accelerates glucose utilization by nerve cells, but utilization is depressed during severe hypoxia. Within the brain, the hippocampus, white matter, superior colliculus and lateral geniculates appear particularly sensitive to levels of oxygen. Brain lactate levels increase in early stages of hypoxia. Brain tissue concentrations of ATP, ADP and AMP apparently remain close to normal even during severe hypoxia.

Altered ion homeostasis during hypoxia clearly occurs, though whether the ionic changes are primary, or whether they are due to altered oxidative or neurotransmitter metabolism, is unclear. Hypoxia interferes with calcium homeostasis. For example, very low oxygen levels diminish calcium uptake at synapses. One hypothesis is that the decrease of calcium in the endoplasmic reticulum is a critical factor (Paschen 1966). Intracellular levels of potassium are increased during severe hypoxia. There is accumulation of free radicals which cause further injury, particularly to the capillaries. Neurotransmitter metabolism is thought to be sensitive to hypoxia although there is conflicting evidence about which transmitter or metabolic step is most sensitive. There is evidence that acetylcholine synthesis by brain is oxygen dependent, as is the biosynthesis of amino acid neurotransmitters. Brain catecholamine concentrations are apparently decreased by hypoxia though the mechanism is unclear. Much of the experimental work has been done on ischemia, and the relationship of the changes to those caused by pure hypoxia is controversial.

The effects of hypoxia on brain synapses and membrane polarization interfere with the normal electrical activity of the brain and alter the electroencephalogram (EEG). In cats in which the arterial P_{O_2} is gradually reduced from 80 to 20 mm Hg, the EEG amplitude initially increases slightly and then slow waves and sharp spikes appear. Subsequently the slow waves decrease in amplitude and then disappear. Later these small spikes become sporadic and finally the EEG flattens. The initial activation which is followed by depression may be due to the effect of hypoxia on the reticular activating system.

Evoked potentials are also altered by hypoxia. Brainstem auditory response is abolished by low levels of oxygen. Visually evoked potentials are initially increased and then abolished as the level of oxygen is reduced.

Histological changes in the brain result from severe hypoxia. The changes are indistinguishable from those due to hypotension and the greatest changes are seen in the cortex and basal ganglia. Microvacuolation of neuronal perikaryon occurs first, the H1 zone (Sommer sector) of the hippocampus being the most vulnerable region.

16.3.2 Cerebral blood flow

The levels of arterial P_{O_2} and P_{CO_2} have crucial effects on cerebral blood flow and since these levels are greatly altered by going to high altitude, the results are important. Arterial hypoxemia dilates cerebral blood vessels and greatly increases cerebral blood flow. Figure 16.1 shows typical results found in anesthetized normocapnic rats. It can be seen that cerebral blood flow was little changed until the arterial P_{O_2} fell below 60 mm Hg but with lower levels of P_{O_2} there was a dramatic increase in cerebral blood flow. Note that at an arterial P_{O_2} of 25 mm Hg, cerebral blood flow was approximately five times the normoxic level. As indicated in Chapter 12, the arterial P_{O_2} of a climber resting on the summit of Mount Everest is 25–30 mm Hg.

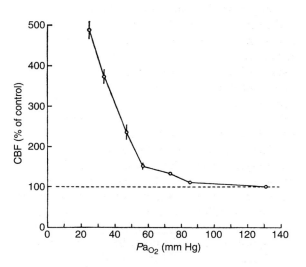

Figure 16.1 *Effect of changes of arterial* P_{O_2} *on cerebral blood flow (CBF) in anesthetized rats. The arterial* P_{CO_2} *was maintained normal. Note the very sharp rise in blood flow as the arterial* P_{O_2} *was reduced below 50 mm Hg. (From Borgström et al. 1975.)*

The results shown in Figure 16.1 were obtained in mechanically ventilated animals where P_{CO_2} was kept constant at the normoxic level. However, in conscious animals and humans, the hyperventilation caused by the hypoxemia will cause a reduction in arterial P_{CO_2} and an increase in pH which will cause cerebral vasoconstriction. Therefore the results shown in Figure 16.1 cannot be applied directly to the climber at extreme altitude.

A reduction in arterial P_{CO_2} has a strong vasoconstrictor effect on cerebral blood vessels and consequently reduces cerebral flood flow. Figure 16.2 shows typical results in mechanically ventilated anesthetized dogs which were made hypocapnic by increasing the ventilation, or hypercapnic by adding carbon dioxide to the inspired gas. In every instance the arterial P_{O_2} was maintained at approximately the normal level. Note that when the arterial P_{CO_2} fell to about 15 mm Hg, cerebral blood flow was reduced by about 40 per cent (Harper and Glass 1965).

In humans at high altitude, the two effects of hypoxemia and hypocapnia will clearly have opposing effects on the cerebral circulation. There have not been systematic studies of cerebral blood flow at various altitudes, partly because of the difficulties of measurement. However, Severinghaus et al. (1966b) measured cerebral blood flow in seven normal subjects by a nitrous oxide method at sea level and after

6–12 h and 3–5 days at an altitude of 3810 m. The blood flow increased by an average of 24 per cent at 6–12 h, and by 13 per cent at 3–5 days at altitude. Acute correction of the hypoxia restored the cerebral blood flow to normal. Extrapolation of additional data suggested that if the P_{CO_2} had not been reduced at high altitude, the cerebral blood flow would have been 60 per cent above the control. An interesting feature of the data obtained by Severinghaus et al. (1966b) is that a subsequent analysis shows that oxygen delivery to the brain (as calculated from cerebral blood flow multiplied by arterial oxygen concentration) was held essentially constant (Wolff 2000). However, there is no known receptor that responds to oxygen delivery.

Indirect evidence about cerebral blood flow in humans can be obtained by measuring blood flow velocity in the internal carotid artery by Doppler ultrasound. Huang et al. (1987) measured flow velocities in the internal carotid and vertebral arteries in six subjects within 2–4 h of arrival on Pikes Peak (4300 m) in Colorado, and found that the velocities in both arteries were slightly increased above sea level values; 18–44 h later, a peak increase of 20 per cent was observed. However, over days 4–12, velocities declined to values similar to those at sea level. In the further study by the same group (Huang et al. 1991) the effect of prolonged exercise (45 min at approximately 100 W) on blood flow velocity in the internal carotid artery was studied at sea level and at 4300 m. The velocities at sea level and high altitude were similar. In a low pressure chamber study, Reeves et al. (1985) measured blood flow velocity in the internal carotid artery of 12 subjects at Denver (1609 m) and repeatedly up to 7 h at a simulated altitude of 4800 m. Their hypothesis was that an increase in blood flow velocity might be associated with the development of high altitude headache, but no correlation was found. Other studies by Doppler ultrasound have shown no correlation between cerebral blood flow and acute mountain sickness (Baumgartner et al. 1999), or cerebral blood flow and susceptibility to high altitude pulmonary edema (HAPE) (Berre et al. 1999). On the other hand, Jansen et al. (1999) reported that subjects with acute mountain sickness (AMS) had higher cerebral blood flows than normals, and also a greater hemodynamic response to hyperventilation.

Huang et al. (1992) measured blood flow velocity in the internal carotid arteries of 15 native Tibetans and 11 Han Chinese residents of Lhasa (3658 m) both at rest and during exercise. There were no

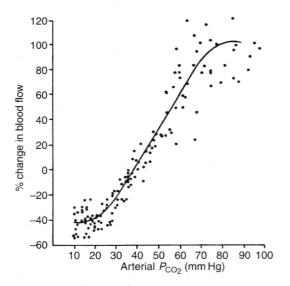

Figure 16.2 *Effect of alterations in arterial P_{CO_2} on cerebral cortical blood flow in anesthetized dogs. The zero reference line for blood flow is at an arterial P_{CO_2} of 40 mm Hg. Animals were normoxic and normotensive. (From Harper and Glass 1965.)*

differences at rest and during submaximal exercise. At peak exercise, the Tibetans showed an increase in flow velocity and cerebral oxygen delivery whereas the Hans did not. Frayser *et al.* (1970) measured the mean circulation time through the retina following fluorescein injection and found that the circulation time decreased from a mean of 4.9 s at base camp to 3.4 s at an altitude of 5330 m. This is consistent with an increase in cerebral blood flow.

Another possible factor at high altitude which could influence cerebral blood flow is an increased viscosity of the blood caused by polycythemia. Although this has not been specifically studied, it is known that a blood flow of less than half the normal value can occur in severe polycythemia vera (Kety 1950) and that cerebral blood flow is significantly increased in severe anemia (Heyman *et al.* 1952, Robin and Gardner 1953). Some drugs, including caffeine, reduce cerebral blood flow.

Recently, interesting observations on brain oxygenation at high altitude were obtained by Imray and colleagues (2000) who studied members of a climbing expedition in the Andes. They used near-infrared spectroscopy which allows measurements to be made through the skull. The signal comes from the hemoglobin in the brain blood, and although it includes some arterial blood, it is apparently heavily weighted towards the capillary and venous saturation, and therefore probably gives a useful measure of trends in the oxygenation of brain tissue. The most interesting results were found using voluntary hyperventilation. At sea level, hyperventilation caused a fall in oxygen saturation presumably because of the reduction in blood flow. However, at an altitude of 3560 m, there was no change in oxygen saturation by this technique, and at the higher altitude of 4680 m, the saturation increased. Presumably the explanation is that at the higher altitude, the increase in arterial oxygen saturation had more effect on brain oxygenation than the reduction of cerebral blood flow.

16.4 CENTRAL NERVOUS SYSTEM FUNCTION AT HIGH ALTITUDE

16.4.1 Moderate altitudes

There is general agreement that CNS function is impaired at altitudes over about 4500 m, but an interesting question concerns the lowest altitude at which minor alterations in function occur. This question frequently arises in the aviation industry because it is important in selecting the cabin pressure of commercial aircraft. Most high flying commercial aircraft are pressurized to maintain the cabin pressure at or below an equivalent altitude of about 2500 m. This ceiling was accepted after considering the penalty of extra weight and expense which would have to be paid in order to reduce it further.

However, there is some evidence that at a pressure equivalent to an altitude of 2440 m, subjects are slower to learn complex mental tasks than at sea level. Even at the considerably lower altitude of only 5000 ft (1524 m), eight subjects were slower to learn complex tasks than a matched group breathing an enriched oxygen mixture (Denison *et al.* 1966). The tests here involved recognizing the posture of human-like figures having different orientations and presented in random sequence on a screen. Thus it appears that even at the cabin altitudes of commercial aircraft, sensitive psychometric tests can pick up minor degrees of impairment.

Interesting problems concerning CNS function at moderate altitudes occur in relation to the operation of optical and infrared telescopes on mountain summits (see also Chapter 29). The reduction in the absorption of optical and infrared radiation because of the reduced thickness of the Earth's atmosphere at high altitude makes high mountains ideal locations for astronomical observatories. For example, several telescopes are located on the summit of Mauna Kea (4200 m), on the island of Hawaii.

The barometric pressure on the summit of Mauna Kea is only about 468 mm Hg, giving a moist inspired P_{O_2} of 88 mm Hg. The telescope operators frequently live at sea level and ascend rapidly by car to the summit. Forster (1986) measured arterial blood gases on 27 telescope personnel on the first day of reaching 4200 m and reported a mean arterial P_{O_2} of 42 mm Hg, P_{CO_2} 29 mm Hg and pH 7.49. After 5 days, during which time the nights were spent in dormitories at an altitude of 3000 m, the arterial blood gases at 4200 m showed a mean P_{O_2} of 44 mm Hg, P_{CO_2} 27 mm Hg and pH of 7.48.

A number of psychometric measurements showed no change on ascending to 4200 m, though performance of the digit symbol backwards test did deteriorate on the first day. At the end of 5 days, however, the scores had returned to sea level values. Numerate memory and psychomotor ability were also reported to be impaired in commuters to Mauna Kea. Several features of AMS were noted in shift workers, particularly on their first day at the summit. Headache was the most disabling symptom but others included insomnia, lethargy, poor concentration and poor memory.

16.4.2   High altitudes

A classical series of studies was carried out by McFarland (1937a,b, 1938a,b) in connection with the International High Altitude Expedition to Chile which took place in 1935. In his first study, McFarland reported on the psychophysiological effects of sudden ascents to 5000 m in unpressurized aircraft and compared the results with ascents by train and car to villages as high as 4700 m in Chile. The measurements showed that the rate of ascent was an important variable, with the rapid increase in altitude by aircraft being the most damaging. Both simple and complex psychological functions were significantly impaired at high altitudes including arithmetical tests, writing ability, and the appearance and disappearance time of after-images following exposure of the eye to a bright light. There were increased memory errors, errors in perseverance, and reductions in auditory threshold and words apprehended.

In a second study of sensory and motor responses during acclimatization, when measurements were obtained at altitudes as high as 5330 and 6100 m, significant reductions in audition, vision, and hand–eye coordination were seen. Measurements were made at several altitudes but in general, impairment of function was not significant below an altitude of 5330 m. Again members of the expedition with the longest periods of acclimatization appeared to suffer less deterioration.

In a further study, mental and psychosomatic tests were also administered at the same altitudes and these showed deterioration. Tests involving the quickness of recognizing the meaning of words, mental flexibility or tendency to perseveration, and immediate memory showed significant impairment. It was noted that complex mental work could be carried out if the subjects increased their concentration but in general there was increased distractibility and lethargy which tended to reduce the ability to concentrate.

In a final series of measurements, sensory and circulatory responses were measured on sulfur miners residing permanently at an altitude of 5330 m at Aucanquilcha in Chile. They were compared with a group of workmen at sea level who were similar in age and race, and also with members of the expedition. It was found that the miners at high altitude were slower in simple and choice reaction times and less acute in auditory sensitivity than the workmen at sea level. However, McFarland and his colleagues were impressed by the evidence for circulatory and respiratory adaptation in these permanent residents at an altitude of 5330 m.

More recently, additional studies on the deleterious effects of acute hypoxia on visual perception have been carried out, partly because of the importance of this topic in aviation. For example, Kobrick (1975) documented impaired response times in the detection of flash stimuli at equivalent altitudes of sea level, 4000 m, 4600 m and 5200 m during acute exposure in a low pressure chamber. The effects of hypoxia on other peripheral stimuli have also been studied (Kobrick 1972).

A special opportunity to study the CNS effects of high altitude occurred during the India–China border war in the early 1960s when large numbers of Indian troops were rapidly taken to an altitude of 4000 m and remained there for as long as 2 years. Sharma and his colleagues (1975) measured psychomotor efficiency in 25 young Indians ranging in age from 21 to 30 years. Psychomotor performance including speed and accuracy was determined by administering a hand–eye coordination test in which a stylus was moved in a narrow groove so that it did not touch the sides. The tests were performed at sea level and at an altitude of 4000 m after periods of 1, 10, 13, 18 and 24 months. Figure 16.3 shows how overall psychomotor efficiency declined over the first 10 months of altitude exposure but then recovered somewhat over the ensuing 13 months as a result of acclimatization.

Overall psychomotor efficiency as shown in Figure 16.3 includes both the speed and accuracy scores from the test. Figure 16.4 shows a breakdown of the accuracy and speed of this test of psychomotor performance. Note that the accuracy of the measurement increased substantially after the 10-month period but there was little improvement in speed. This result is consistent with the impression given by many people who have worked at high altitude: thought processes are slowed, but accurate procedures can be carried out if one concentrates hard enough.

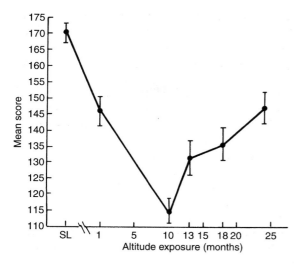

Figure 16.3 *Psychomotor efficiency in young adults rapidly taken to an altitude of 4000 m where they remained for 2 years. Psychomotor efficiency was calculated using a hand–eye coordination test which included speed and accuracy. Note the deterioration in psychomotor efficiency over the first 10 months, which then gradually improved. (From Sharma* et al. *1975.)*

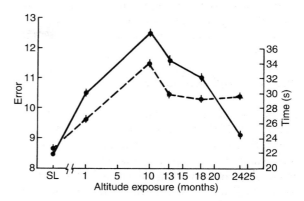

Figure 16.4 *Same data as in Figure 16.3 except that psychomotor efficiency is broken down into accuracy and speed of hand–eye coordination. Note that the accuracy of the measurement (solid line) increased after 10 months but there was relatively little improvement in speed (dashed line). (From Sharma* et al. *1975.)*

In a related study, Sharma and Malhotra (1976) compared the performance of three groups of Indians drawn from the Gurkha, Madrasi and Rajput areas after 10 months' stay at an altitude of 4000 m. There were no differences in the scores for hand–eye coordination and social interaction at altitudes for the three ethnic groups. However, the Gurkhas showed a better toleration of altitude stress as evidenced by the effects on concentration, anxiety and depression.

In a study of 20 male soldiers exposed to a simulated altitude of 4700 m for 5–7 h, the relationships between symptoms and signs of AMS, mood and psychometric performance were studied (Shukitt-Hale *et al.* 1991). It was found that evidence of AMS was best correlated with symptoms, then mood changes and least with performance.

An unusual opportunity for studying the effects of very high altitude on mental performance was offered by the 1960–11 Silver Hut Expedition when several normal subjects spent up to 3 months at an altitude of 5800 m. Mental efficiency was tested by asking the subjects to sort playing cards into bins using specially designed equipment which recorded events on magnetic tape (Gill *et al.* 1964). It was found that the efficiency of sorting cards was less at the high altitude than at sea level. The ineffi-

ciency took the form of a delay in placing the cards into the correct bins rather than errors of sorting. Again these results reinforce the common notion that accurate work can be done at high altitude, but it takes longer, and more effort in concentration is required. Cahoon (1972) also showed a reduced efficiency of card sorting in eight normal subjects exposed to a simulated altitude of 4600 m for 48 h.

During the 1981 AMREE, a series of psychometric tests was carried out prior to the expedition, at the Base Camp (5400 m), at the Main Laboratory Camp (6300 m) and immediately after and 1 year after the expedition (Townes *et al.* 1984). The main emphasis was on a comparison of CNS function before and after exposure to extreme altitude, and only a few of the measurements made at high altitude were reported. However, finger-tapping speed decreased significantly over the course of the expedition. Mean taps of the right hand were 53.7 (pretest), 52.6 (5400 m altitude), 50.8 (6300 m altitude), 48.1 (on subjects returning to 6300 m altitude from 8000 m) and 45.4 (immediately after the expedition). It is not clear from these results whether the reduction in finger-tapping speed was a function of altitude, time at high altitude, or both.

16.4.3   Electroencephalogram

Ryn (1970, 1971) reported EEG abnormalities in 11 of 30 climbers who had been over 5500 m altitude. The predominant abnormality was a decreased frequency of alpha waves and a diminution of their amplitude. He also reported paroxysmal and focal pathology in EEG records performed at high altitude.

Zhongyuan and his colleagues (1983) also reported changes in the EEG at altitudes above 5000 m in members of a Chinese expedition to Mount Everest. There was a reduced amplitude of the alpha rhythm but in this instance there was an increase in its frequency. The EEG changes were less than those observed during acute hypoxia of the same degree in a low pressure chamber before the expedition. Apparently members of the expedition who tolerated the acute hypoxia well tended to show fewer EEG changes on the mountain itself.

Nevison carried out an extensive series of EEG measurements during the Himalayan Scientific and Mountaineering Expedition of 1960–1. Although the results were not written up in the open literature, he apparently found no abnormalities in subjects living at 5800 m. Also the EEG appearances were not altered by hyperventilation or 100 per cent oxygen breathing.

16.5   RESIDUAL CENTRAL NERVOUS SYSTEM IMPAIRMENT FOLLOWING RETURN FROM HIGH ALTITUDE

In view of the known vulnerability of the CNS to hypoxia, it is hardly surprising that neurobehavioral abnormalities can be demonstrated at high altitudes. However, there has been great interest in the possibility of residual impairment of CNS function following return to sea level.

An extensive study was carried out by Townes *et al.* (1984), referred to in section 16.4.2. The subjects were 21 members of the 1981 AMREE, and all were males between 25 and 52 years of age with a mean age of 36.4 years. The general level of education was high, with 15 subjects having either an MD or PhD degree. Before the expedition, the following psychological tests were administered at the San Diego Veterans Administration Hospital: Halstead–Reitan battery (Reitan and Davison 1974), repeatable cognitive–perceptual–motor battery (Lewis and Rennick 1979),

selective reminding test (Buschke 1973) and Wechsler memory scale (Russell 1975). These same measurements were repeated immediately after the expedition in Kathmandu, Nepal. At an expedition meeting held in Colorado 1 year later, the following tests were readministered: Halstead–Wepman aphasia screening test, B trials and the finger-tapping test from the Halstead–Reitan battery, the digit vigilance task from the repeatable battery, and a verbal passage from the Wechsler memory scale.

Table 16.1 shows the significant changes found between pre-expedition, post-expedition and follow-up performance on the neuropsychological tests. It can be seen that verbal learning and memory declined significantly from the beginning to the end of the expedition as measured by the Wechsler memory scale. In the Halstead–Wepman aphasia screening test, the number of expressive language errors increased significantly between pre-test and post-test after the expedition. The number of aphasic errors was significantly related to the altitude attained by the subject.

As indicated in section 16.4.2, finger-tapping speed decreased significantly over the course of the expedition. This was measured by requiring the subject to tap a lever as rapidly as possible over a period of 10 s. For a test to be acceptable, five measurements on each hand gave a difference of fewer than five taps between trials. Before the expedition all subjects reached this criterion. However, at Kathmandu immediately after the expedition, 15 of 20 subjects could not sustain motor speed, and 13 of 16 subjects could not do so 1 year later.

These findings are of great interest because they provide strong objective evidence for CNS deterioration as a result of exposure to high altitude, a subject which has been debated vigorously in the past. However, other authors have reported similar or consistent findings. Ryn (1970, 1971) also found persistent abnormalities in a group of 20 male and 10 female Polish climbers several weeks after a Himalayan expedition. Half of the male climbers who ascended over 5500 m experienced symptoms similar to the acute organic brain syndrome, and for several weeks after the expedition they had changes in affect and impaired memory. Eleven of the 30 climbers had EEG abnormalities immediately after the climb. Psychological testing (Bender, Benton and Graham-Kendall tests) was reported to be normal in 13 subjects, borderline in 12 and indicative of organic pathology in 5 climbers.

Table 16.1 Wilcoxon signed-rank tests comparing performance before, immediately after (in Kathmandu), and 1 year after an expedition to Mount Everest

	Result, means ± SE			Paired responses, z values		
	Before	After	Follow-up	Before and after	After and follow-up	Before and follow-up
Improved performance						
Tactual performance test (right hand)	4.68 ± 1.56	3.86 ± 1.46		2.72*		
Category test	24.29 ± 15.46	11.05 ± 8.39		3.48+		
Decline in performance						
Finger-tapping test						
Right hand	53.71 ± 4.07	45.40 ± 6.18	48.40 ± 6.60	3.39+	1.32	2.20‡
Left hand	47.65 ± 4.60	42.45 ± 5.96	41.73 ± 5.23	2.30‡	0.66	2.93*
Criterion right	1.00 ± 0	0.14 ± 0.36	0.27 ± 0.46	3.06*	0.73	2.67*
Criterion left	1.00 ± 0	0.14 ± 0.36	0.13 ± 0.35	2.93‡	0.54	2.93*
Wechsler memory scale						
Short-term verbal recall	18.12 ± 1.90	15.90 ± 2.15	17.13 ± 2.20	2.60*	2.12‡	0.98
Trials to criterion	1.24 ± 0.44	2.40 ± 1.54	2.27 ± 0.70	2.37‡	0	2.67*
Long-term verbal recall	16.35 ± 2.91	12.70 ± 3.78	14.50 ± 2.85	2.32‡	2.75	0.94
Aphasia screening test	0.59 ± 0.79	1.25 ± 1.25	0.47 ± 0.52	2.22‡	2.31‡	0.47

Source: Townes *et al.* (1984).

* $p < 0.01$; + $p < 0.001$; ‡ $p < 0.05$.

Persistent cognitive impairment was described in five world-class climbers who had reached summits over 8500 m without supplementary oxygen (Regard *et al.* 1989). The abnormalities were in the ability to concentrate, short-term memory, and cognitive flexibility (the ability to shift from one learned concept to another).

In a brief report, Cavaletti *et al.* (1987) showed residual impairment of memory in seven climbers who returned to sea level after ascending to 7075 m on Mount Satopanth in India without supplementary oxygen. The measurements were made before leaving Italy, at the base camp after the ascent, and 75 days after the expedition. It was shown that memory performance decreased both at base camp and, to a lesser degree, at sea level 75 days after the climb. However, tests of fluency and 'idiomotor ability' were unaffected by altitude. In a more recent study, persistent changes in memory, reaction time and concentration were reported 75 days after a single ascent over 5000 m (Cavaletti and Tredici 1993).

One study reports cortical atrophy and brain magnetic resonance imaging (MRI) changes in 26 climbers who ascended to over 7000 m without supplementary oxygen (Garrido *et al.* 1993). No MRI studies were performed before the climbs; the measurements were made 26 days to 36 months after return to sea level. The controls were 21 normal subjects, and 46 per cent of the climbers showed MRI abnormalities.

Not everyone has found CNS abnormalities following return after ascent to very high altitude. For example, Clark *et al.* (1983) tested 22 mountaineers before and 16–221 days after Himalayan climbs above 5100 m with a battery of psychological and neurophysiological tests but found no evidence of cerebral dysfunction. This was a well designed study and it is not clear why these climbers showed no abnormalities. In another study, Anooshiravani *et al.* (1999) carried out brain MRI studies and performed neuropsychological testing on eight male climbers before and after ascents to over 6000 m without oxygen. Although they found increases in symptoms of AMS, there were no alterations in brain imaging or neuropsychological tests between 5 and 10 days after returning to sea level.

Measurements from the 1985 Operation Everest II confirmed the changes in psychometric function found on the 1981 AMREE, and extended the observations in an interesting and unexpected direction.

During Operation Everest II, eight normal subjects spent 40 days in a low pressure chamber and were gradually decompressed, ultimately being exposed to the simulated altitude of the Everest summit. Impairments in motor speed and persistence, memory, and verbal expressive abilities were found after the simulated ascent, just as with the 1981 Everest expedition (Hornbein et al. 1989).

The new finding was a significant negative correlation between hypoxic ventilatory response and neurobehavioral function measured after the expedition. In other words, those climbers with the largest hypoxic ventilatory response showed the greatest decrement in neurobehavioral function. This was unexpected; indeed, the prediction might have been that those who increased their ventilation most would protect their CNS function by preserving their alveolar and therefore arterial P_{O_2}.

A hypothesis to explain these unexpected findings was advanced by Hornbein et al. (1989). They argued that the subjects with the highest hypoxic ventilatory response would reduce their arterial P_{CO_2} the most and therefore develop the most cerebral vasoconstriction. This in turn would cause the most severe cerebral hypoxia even though their arterial P_{O_2} would actually be higher than that in the subjects with the smaller ventilatory responses to hypoxia.

Note that this hypothesis is not supported by the measurements of cerebral blood flow against arterial P_{CO_2} in anesthetized dogs shown in Figure 16.2. Those data show that cerebral blood flow apparently levels off at values of P_{CO_2} below approximately 15 mm Hg. However, the situation with acclimatization may be different because the arterial pH returns towards normal and this may improve cerebral blood flow. In addition, the scatter in the data is such that this result may not be reliable. It should also be pointed out that the relationship between cerebral blood flow and arterial P_{CO_2} is very sensitive to the systematic arterial pressure (Harper and Glass 1965). Hypotensive dogs show a much smaller change in cerebral blood flow for a given change in P_{CO_2} than normotensive animals. Whether changes in systemic blood pressure occur at extreme altitudes is not known, although there are no obvious alterations at 5800 m (Pugh 1964c).

The correlation between hypoxic ventilatory response and residual impairment of CNS function leads to an interesting paradox. On the one hand, a brisk hypoxic ventilatory response is advantageous for a climber to reach extreme altitudes because otherwise the alveolar P_{O_2} cannot be maintained at the required levels. However, the only way of maintaining the P_{O_2} is by extreme hyperventilation, which reduces the arterial P_{CO_2}, which in turn reduces cerebral blood flow. Thus such a climber is likely to suffer more residual central nervous impairment. In other words, the climber who is endowed by nature to go the highest is likely to suffer the most severe nervous system damage.

16.6 EFFECT OF OXYGEN ENRICHMENT OF ROOM AIR ON NEUROPSYCHOLOGICAL FUNCTION AT HIGH ALTITUDE

Increasing numbers of people are commuting to high altitude for commercial purposes such as mining, and scientific purposes such as astronomy (see Chapter 29). In order to reduce the neuropsychological impairment that occurs at high altitudes, oxygen enrichment of room air is now being tested. This is remarkably effective because every 1 per cent increase in oxygen concentration (for example from 21 to 22 per cent) reduces the equivalent altitude by about 300 m. Gerard et al. (2000) evaluated the effectiveness of enriching room air oxygen by 6 per cent at simulated 5000 m altitude. A randomized double-blind study was carried out on 24 subjects who underwent neuropsychological testing in a specially designed facility at 3800 m that could simulate both an ambient 5000 m atmosphere and an atmosphere of 6 per cent oxygen enrichment at 5000 m. The 2-h test battery of 16 tasks assessed various aspects of motor and cognitive performance. Compared with simulated breathing air at 5000 m, oxygen enrichment resulted in higher arterial oxygen saturations, quicker reaction times, improved hand–eye coordination, and a more positive sense of well being, each significant at the $p < 0.05$ level.

It is interesting that other aspects of neuropsychological function were not significantly improved by 6 per cent additional oxygen. One reason may be that short-term concentration may temporarily overcome real underlying deficits. The problem was succinctly stated by Barcroft et al. (1923) reporting on the 1921–2 International High Altitude Expedition to Cerro de Pasco, Peru (4330 m). Barcroft wrote:

Judged by the ordinary standards of efficiency in laboratory work, we were in an obviously lower category at Cerro than at the sea level. By a curious paradox this was most apparent when it was being least tested, for perhaps what we suffered from chiefly was the difficulty of maintaining concentration. When we knew we were undergoing a test, our concentration could by an effort be maintained over the length of time taken for the test, but under ordinary circumstances it would lapse. It is, perhaps, characteristic that, whilst each individual mental test was done as rapidly at Cerro as at the sea level, the performance of the series took nearly twice as long for its accomplishment. Time was wasted there in trivialities and 'bungling', which would not take place at sea level (Barcroft et al. 1923).

In view of the above, it would be very interesting to develop neuropsychological tests which were embedded in the normal daily activities of the subject. In other words, it would be valuable to be able to measure the mental efficiency of the subjects when they were unaware of being tested. A formal study along these lines has not yet been carried out at high altitude.

17

High altitude populations

SUMMARY

Many people live permanently at altitudes which have a significant effect on their physiology (see Chapter 3 for numbers and world distribution). Studies of such populations are hampered by the problem of appropriate comparison groups. Often a group of high altitude residents is compared with a group of lowlanders from a different ethnic, socioeconomic and genetic background so that it is difficult to know to what factors any differences may be attributed. Also it is becoming clear that not all high altitude residents are the same. Recent studies have found interesting differences between South American and central Asian high altitude residents.

Altitude residence does not seem to have important demographic effects; economic factors are of greater importance. Fertility, which is reduced in newcomers to altitude, seems to be normal in peoples resident for generations. Fetal growth in the last stages of pregnancy is retarded and birth weight falls with increasing altitude of residence. Growth in childhood has been claimed to be retarded but continues for longer, though again this could be due, in part at least, to economic or nutritional factors rather than altitude *per se*.

The physiology of high altitude residents differs from that of lowlanders at altitude in some respects. The former have lower total ventilation at rest and exercise and blunted hypoxic ventilatory response (though in Tibetans this is less so than in South American highlanders). Despite lower ventilation their oxygen saturation and P_{O_2} are similar to those of lowlanders at altitude. They have higher lung diffusing capacities than lowlanders, an important advantage at altitude where work rate is limited by diffusion. They have slightly larger lungs. Animals adapted to high altitude have very little pulmonary artery pressor response to hypoxia. Tibetans show a degree of this adaptation, but not South American high altitude residents. There are also differences in hemoglobin concentration and oxygen saturation between these populations, all suggesting that the Tibetans, with their longer lineage at altitude, have undergone a greater degree of altitude adaptation.

Certain diseases are found commonly among altitude residents. Again some are the result of socioeconomic factors and are common in poor populations at sea level. Cold and cold injury are more common at altitude but, of course, not confined to it. The commonest disease due to altitude hypoxia is chronic mountain sickness. This is covered in Chapter 21. Others include chemodectoma, a benign tumor of the carotid body, and a high incidence of patent ductus arteriosus in infants. Goiter, though strictly not confined to high altitude, is much more prevalent there since iodine-deficient soils are more common at high elevations and possibly the demands for iodine are greater at altitude. Finally sickle cell disease, though not caused by altitude, is more serious there.

17.1   INTRODUCTION

This chapter considers the characteristics of people born and raised at high altitude and whose ancestors have resided at high altitude for many generations. In Chapter 3 the locations of these populations have been discussed. In general the altitude considered is above 3000 m. The duration of residence of the population is impossible to determine; it ranges from perhaps 50 000 to 100 000 years in Tibet and 20 000–30 000 years in the Andes to a few generations in the high mining towns of Colorado, USA.

Our knowledge of the effect of lifelong residence at altitude has come from studies of particular peoples. A major problem in interpreting results is to decide whether the characteristics found to differ from lowland populations are really due to the high altitude environment (hypoxia or cold) or due to racial, nutritional or economic factors.

Some studies have sought to eliminate racial factors by using low altitude residents of the same ethnic background as controls. It is difficult to control for nutritional factors since high altitude residents may well be economically disadvantaged when compared with their low altitude controls. This seems to be the case in the Andes. The effects of poor nutrition and chronic hypoxia are similar on factors such as growth and development, thus confounding the interpretation of results. The economic advantage may be reversed, as in Ethiopia, where the highland regions are free from malaria and the residents more wealthy and better fed. The result is that studies from this part of the world do not show the differences between high and low altitude residents that are reported from the Andes. There are fewer studies from the Himalayas and Tibet than from the Andes, though this has been redressed in recent years with a number of studies from Lhasa.

However, if these reservations are kept in mind, some conclusions can be drawn from the many surveys about the effects of lifelong residence at high altitude, especially on birth weight and childhood

development. Recent studies have addressed the question of differences between South American and Tibetan high altitude residents and the related one of whether there has been natural selection for giving a biological advantage to either of these populations.

17.2   DEMOGRAPHIC ASPECTS

17.2.1   Population age and sex distribution

A few high altitude groups have been analyzed in some detail and the population of the Nunoa district (4000 m) of Peru showed some differences compared with the total Peruvian population (Baker and Dutt 1972). The high altitude population was somewhat younger and the ratio of females to males was larger during infancy and childhood, but in addition there appeared to be more elderly people among the high altitude than the general population.

The explanation seems to be that, in the high altitude population, there was a high birth rate and high adult emigration rate. Male mortality was higher than female in infancy, childhood and early adolescence. The larger number of older individuals may have been due to the prestige associated with telling observers that they were of a great age. Claims to longevity are hard to substantiate because birth certificates and baptismal registers are seldom kept and some individuals lie outrageously about their age. In north Bhutan the oldest individuals were over 80 but not above 90 years old (Jackson *et al.* 1966, p. 99) and some Tibetan lamas claim to have lived to a great age. There seems to be little concrete evidence for unusual longevity at high altitude.

In the Khumbu region of northeastern Nepal, male infant mortality was higher than female. There was little permanent emigration but a higher percentage of males was involved in accidents. In northwest Nepal the number of males born relative to females was higher but mortality in male infants was increased (Baker 1978).

17.2.2   Fertility

Adaptation to the environment must include the ability of the species to reproduce. The Spanish who occupied the high altitude regions of South America in the sixteenth and seventeenth centuries found that neither their animals nor their womenfolk had live offspring. This was in contrast to the indigenous animals and peoples. Clegg (1978) quotes two well-observed Spanish accounts of La Calancha (1639) and Cobo (1653). The former recounts the early history of the city of Potosí (4060 m) in present day Bolivia with a population of 20 000 Spaniards and 100 000 Indians. Children born to Spanish couples died either at birth or within 2 weeks. Pregnant Spanish women developed the habit of going down to low altitude for their pregnancy and delivery and keeping their babies there until a year old. Han Chinese women living in Tibet follow a similar pattern. The cause of failure to thrive in these infants may well have been subacute mountain sickness (Chapter 21). The Amerindians, of course, had no such problems nor do the indigenous Tibetans. It was not until 53 years after its foundation that the first Spanish child was born and reared in the city. Cobo says that Jauja (3500 m), the early capital of Peru, was considered 'a sterile place' where horses, pigs, or fowls could not be raised, whereas 100 years later it was a principal area producing pigs and poultry and supplying Lima with these products.

Cobo also pointed out that infant survival depended upon the proportion of Indian blood in the child, with pure-blooded Spanish children mostly dying, children of mixed blood faring rather better, and pure-blooded Indian children having the lowest mortality, despite much poorer living conditions.

What is the cause of this lack of fertility in lowlanders at altitude? Sperm counts in lowland men fall temporarily on going to altitude but then recover. Testosterone levels also fall and then recover after a week or two (section 15.9.4). In the female, on going to altitude, there may be temporary disturbances in menstruation (Sobrevilla *et al.* 1967). Conception rates are virtually impossible to measure, especially since chronic hypoxia may increase the frequency of early abortions. The reduced fertility may be due to a number of factors, possibly reduced conception, probably increased numbers of early abortions, stillbirths and neonatal deaths.

In altitude residents fertility was thought to be reduced. Hoff and Abelson (1976), using aggregate data from Peru, found that fertility, measured as the number of children under the age of 5 divided by the number of women aged 15–49 years, fell linearly with altitude ($p < 0.01$) but they were cautious when interpreting the data on which this was based. They also found that high altitude women who migrate to low altitude increase their fertility. However, more recently both Carrillo (1996) and Gonzales *et al.* (1996) found global fecundity rates higher than at sea level.

17.3 FETAL AND CHILDHOOD DEVELOPMENT

17.3.1 Pregnancy

ABORTION

Abortion rates are notoriously difficult to measure, but Clegg (1978) quotes a number of Andean studies giving incredibly low rates ranging from 0 to 1 per cent (compared with worldwide rates of about 15 per cent). He suggested this might be due to a high rate of very early abortions (before 2 weeks) which would be unrecognized and would help to account for the low fertility. In Ethiopian women, Harrison *et al.* (1969) reported a rather higher rate (9.1 per cent) at 3000 m compared with less than 1 per cent in an ethnically similar population at low altitude; however, both rates are low compared with rates in many populations.

PLACENTAL GROWTH

Placentas are not significantly heavier at high altitude but since birth weights are low the placental/birth weight ratio is significantly increased (McClung 1969, Mayhew 1986), clearly an adaptation which would benefit fetal oxygenation. The numbers of villi and capillaries are increased in the placentas from high altitude women; this increases the surface area for diffusion (Clegg 1978), although Mayhew (1986) found a smaller surface area of villi but a thinner diffusion barrier, thus preserving the membrane diffusing capacity. Placental infarcts are more common in altitude placentas and more frequent in women with a European admixture of genes (McClung 1969).

FETAL GROWTH

The evidence suggests that, after the hazards of the first few weeks of pregnancy, growth is probably normal until the last trimester, when it slows to produce a lighter baby at term. The cause of this growth retardation is not clear, since the evidence reviewed by Clegg (1978) suggests that the fetus at this altitude is not hypoxic compared with lowland fetuses. Possibly this is a genetic adaptive change with elimination, over generations, of genes which produce a larger baby. This would be advantageous since smaller babies are less likely to outgrow the placental capacity for oxygen transfer.

17.3.2 Birth weight and infant mortality

Results from a number of studies in the Andes and Tibet showed lower birth weight at altitude (Haas 1976, Li 1985). The mean weight declined from about 3.5 kg in Lima to 2.8 kg at Cerro de Pasco (4300 m) and, although there is the possibility that the nutritional status of mothers may be a factor, it is unlikely to account for more than a proportion of this difference. A similar effect of altitude has been reported from the USA (Lichty et al. 1957, Grahn and Kratchman 1963, Unger et al. 1988). Women native to high altitude who descend to low altitude have heavier babies at low altitude (Hoff and Abelson 1976). These studies include women from both indigenous high altitude populations and low altitude stock, and indicate that it is the high altitude environment rather than genetics which result in low birth weights. A recent study from Colorado also concludes that altitude is an independent factor in causing low birth weights. The authors obtained data from 3836 birth certificates and found that none of the characteristics associated with low birth weight – gestational age, maternal weight gain, parity, smoking, hypertension, etc. – interacted with the effect of altitude; the decline in birth weight averaged 102 g per 1000 m (Jensen and Moore 1997). However, genetic factors may play a role. In a study in Lhasa (3658 m) Niermeyer et al. (1995) reported that Han Chinese infants had lower birth weights than Tibetan babies born at the same altitude. They also had lower Sa_{O_2} and higher hemoglobin levels. Possibly the genetic factors work through giving better oxygenation to Tibetan mothers (see section 17.5.2).

Infant mortality depends heavily on living standards and medical facilities and the very high infant mortality rates reported probably reflect these factors more than the effect of altitude per se. In Ethiopia, Harrison et al. (1969) reported a rate of 200 per 1000 live births at high altitude and 176 per 1000 at low altitude, whereas in the Andes a rate of 180 per 1000 was found in the rural area of Nunoa (4000 m) but only 73 per 1000 in urban La Paz (Baker 1978). In Himalayan Sherpas, Lang and Lang (1971) gave a figure of 51 per 1000 at 4300 m, and in North Bhutan the rate was 189 per 1000 (Jackson et al. 1966, p. 99). In experimental animals under controlled conditions, hypoxia increases neonatal mortality, so probably the high rates found in mountain peoples are at least partly due to the altitude. Apart from the direct effect of hypoxia an important indirect effect may be through the reduced amount of liver glycogen present at birth, an important energy store until suckling becomes established (Clegg 1978).

17.3.3 Growth through childhood

The high altitude baby starts life smaller than the average low altitude baby does, and its early growth is slower. Milestones such as sitting and walking are slightly later but the differences between high and low altitude residents of the same race are less than those between different races or between urban and rural populations (Clegg 1978).

In Quechua Indians in Peru, throughout childhood the high altitude child lags behind his low altitude counterpart in height by about 2 years. The adolescent growth spurt is less pronounced in high altitude youths but their growth continues for about 2 years longer and their adult stature is not reached until 22 years of age (Frisancho 1978). In Ethiopia, there were no such differences. Indeed, high altitude males were taller and heavier for their age than lowlanders. In the Himalayas, a comparison of high altitude Sherpas (3075–5050 m) with Tibetans resident at 1400 m was made by Pawson (quoted by Frisancho 1978) who found no difference in the height of children in these populations, though other indices of maturation (skeletal and dental development and menarche) show the Sherpa children to lag behind the low altitude Tibetans. Recently a study from Ecuador found very little difference in rates of body weight increase in children at altitude compared with children from low altitude. There were some minor differences in rates of height increase but the authors conclude that hypoxia plays a relatively small role in shaping growth in the first 5 years after birth (Leonard *et al.* 1995).

On the other hand, investigations amongst the children of Kirghiz tribes of the Tien Shan mountains showed delayed growth in the high altitude children, equivalent to a lag of about 1 year. The altitude of residence was 2300–2800 m but in the summer months they go up to 3500 m to graze their cattle (Frisancho 1978).

Menarche is a milestone well documented in studies from various high altitude regions and, in girls living in the Andes, Himalayas and Tien Shan, it is 1–2 years later than in low altitude girls (Frisancho 1978, Jackson *et al.* 1966, pp. 40–4). The Ethiopian highlanders again are the exception as no difference was found (Harrison *et al.* 1969). Adrenarche, the increase in serum androgens, also occurs 1–2 years later in children at altitude compared with sea level in Peru (Goñez *et al.* 1993).

17.4 PHYSIOLOGY

17.4.1 Stature, lung development and function

Compared with Europeans and North Americans, most high altitude residents have a smaller stature and are lighter in weight, but when compared with people of similar race and living standards most of this difference disappears. The delayed growth (see above) is almost counteracted by the prolongation of active growth to beyond 20 years.

One of the most quoted aspects of lifelong adaptation to high altitude is the deep-chested development of the thorax in high altitude residents (Barcroft 1925). This has been documented by measurement of chest circumference and vital capacity in South American Indians living above 4500 m but is quite a small difference even in this population. Vital capacity was about 300 mL higher than predicted when corrected for body size (Velasquez 1976). However, at 3500 m these measurements were smaller and less than the values published in the USA. High altitude residents in the Himalayas do not have large circumference chests or bigger vital capacities than lowlanders (Frisancho 1978) nor do younger white residents of Leadville (3100 m), but those over 50 years of age did have significantly larger vital

capacities, by 440 mL, than predicted (DeGraff *et al.* 1970). Sun *et al.* (1990) compared Tibetans and Han Chinese residents of Lhasa. Their mean ages, heights and weights were similar, but, whereas the Tibetans were lifelong residents, the Han have been resident for a mean time of 8 years. The Tibetans had vital capacities significantly greater than the Han did: 5080 mL compared with 4280 mL.

In Andean residents at 4540 m, the total lung capacity is about 500 mL larger than at sea level, most of the increase being due to increased residual volume (Velasquez 1976). Infants born at high altitude have greater thoracic compliance than infants of the same ethnic background born at low altitude (Mortola *et al.* 1990). In adults the thoracic blood volume is increased and the residual volume/total lung capacity ratio increases from 21 per cent to 28 per cent in high altitude compared with low altitude residents. There may be some benefit from this since it would have the effect of reducing the breath-by-breath oscillations of P_{CO_2} and, hence, pH. At altitude these oscillations would otherwise be increased due to the reduction in plasma bicarbonate as part of the acclimatization process (Chapter 5). However, these changes in lung volumes, even when found, are quite small and probably have little effect on performance.

The increased lung capacity may allow for an increased area for gas diffusion which, together with the increased blood volume, results in increased lung diffusing capacity. Details of studies in Andean and Caucasian residents are given in section 6.4.2. This increase in gas transfer should give the altitude resident a distinct performance advantage over the newcomer to altitude. Recent work from Tibet by Chen *et al.* (1997) indicates that Tibetan highlanders also have higher lung diffusing capacities when compared with Han Chinese. Also Samaja *et al.* (1997), who studied Sherpas and Caucasian lowlanders at 3400 and 6450 m, found that the Sherpas were less alkalotic at the higher altitude due to a higher P_{CO_2}, although the P_{O_2} and Sa_{O_2} were the same as those of Caucasians. This indicates that their oxygen transport was more efficient.

Vital capacity decreases with age at sea level but this reduction is much greater at altitude, at least in Andean residents (Monge *et al.* 1990), which may account in part for the increasing incidence of chronic mountain sickness with age (Chapter 21).

17.4.2 Ventilatory control at rest and exercise

Newcomers to high altitude find, often to their surprise, that they have to hyperventilate on the slightest exertion. They may notice that high altitude residents seem to be relatively unaffected in this way.

Measurements of resting and exercise ventilation in high altitude residents confirmed this impression to be true. Chiodi (1957) showed that resting ventilation was higher in newcomers to altitude than in residents. At 3990 m the values were 5.3 and 4.5 L min^{-1} m^2, and at 4515 m, 5.6 and 4.9 L min^{-1} m^2 for newcomers and residents respectively. The Pa_{CO_2} values were in accordance with these differences. Santolaya et al. (1989) studied workers at the Aucanquilcha mine (5950 m) in Chile. Their mean Pa_{CO_2} was 27.5 mm Hg whereas lowlanders at that altitude would have a value about 5 mm Hg lower, indicating ventilation 22 per cent higher. They also showed no respiratory alkalosis (pH 7.4), which lowlanders would have at that altitude.

On exercise, Buskirk (1978) found a similar distinction in Andean high altitude residents as did Lahiri et al. (1967) in Sherpa subjects compared with lowlanders at altitude. It is likely that this lower ventilation in high altitude residents is due to their low hypoxic ventilatory response (HVR), which is well documented (Chapter 5), since HVR correlates with exercise hyperventilation. As discussed in Chapter 5 this blunting of the HVR appears to take place over decades at altitude. Children resident at high altitude have normal HVR and this blunting is seen in white subjects resident in Leadville (3100 m) in Colorado, so it does not seem to be genetically determined (Weil et al. 1971, Lahiri et al. 1976).

Work by Zhuang et al. (1993) showed some interesting differences between lowland born Han Chinese and highland born Tibetans studied in Lhasa (3658 m). The Han had migrated to altitude in childhood, adolescence or adulthood. They showed the decline in HVR with length of residence at altitude as seen in Colorado altitude residents, but the Tibetans, who had a higher HVR (parameter A) than the Han, showed very little decline with age. However, Tibetans showed a paradoxical increase in ventilation on breathing 70 per cent oxygen, a response not seen in Han subjects. Tibetan lifelong residents at 4400 m when studied at 3658 m and compared with Tibetans living there had blunted HVRs though their resting ventilation was similar (Curran et al. 1995). Recently the same team has looked at a group of men of mixed Han–Tibetan parentage. They found that HVR was decreased with time of residence at altitude but that resting ventilation did not reduce, as is the case with Han subjects. They exhibited the same paradoxical response to oxygen breathing as did Tibetan subjects (Curran et al. 1997).

Beall and colleagues have compared Tibetan and South American Aymara highlanders. They found resting ventilation was roughly 1.5 times higher in the Tibetans and HVR about double that of the Aymara. They also found that the contribution of genetic differences to the variance in ventilation was 35 per cent in the Tibetan population and nil in the Amayra. The figures for HVR were 31 and 21 per cent respectively (Beall et al. 1997a; see also section 17.5.2).

17.4.3 Hemoglobin concentration

The increase in hemoglobin concentration at altitude is one of the best known adaptations to altitude hypoxia. It is found in both acclimatized lowlanders and lifelong residents at altitude. This is discussed in detail in Chapter 8.

In the Andes, some workers have found very high hemoglobin concentration in residents (Talbott and Dill 1936, Dill et al. 1937, Merino 1950) and suggested that this is part of their long-term adaptation to altitude. However, subjects may have been included in these study populations who would now be considered to have chronic mountain sickness or Monge's disease (Chapter 21). More recent studies have not found such high levels or a significant difference between residents and acclimatized lowlanders (Peñaloza et al. 1971). Frisancho (1988) reviewed the published data and showed that hemoglobin concentration values from mining areas in the Andes were higher than from nonmining areas, and that if studies from nonmining areas were compared with those from the Himalayas there was no significant difference. However, Beall et al. (1998) found Aymara Andean high altitude natives to have hemoglobin concentration significantly higher, by 3–4 g/dL, than Tibetans at a similar altitude.

In the Himalayas and on the Tibetan plateau, residents tend to have rather lower hemoglobin concentration than acclimatized lowlanders. As discussed in Chapter 8, it is thought that, although a modest rise in hemoglobin concentration (to perhaps 18.0 g/dL) is advantageous, values much above this level are probably detrimental. So the Tibetans' lower hemoglobin concentration values are considered to be evidence of greater altitude adaptation.

17.4.4 The carotid body and chemodectoma

Chronic hypoxia causes an increase in the size and weight of the carotid body. This was first reported in high altitude Andean natives by Arias-Stella (1969). He found the weight of the two carotid bodies in residents of Lima to be just over 20 mg, whereas in altitude residents they totaled over 60 mg. Heath and co-workers found a similar increased weight of carotid bodies in patients with chronic hypoxic lung disease. They found a good correlation between carotid body and right ventricular weight, suggesting that a common correlation with hypoxia was the cause of the hyperplasia (Heath 1986).

The principal cell involved in this hyperplasia is the sustentacular (type II) cell with compression and obliteration of clusters of chief (type I) cells. This type of hyperplasia is similar to that seen in systemic hypertension (Heath 1986).

Chemodectoma, a tumor of the carotid body, is rare at sea level, but appears to be relatively common at high altitude. In 1973 Saldana et al. reported its occurrence in a higher proportion of Peruvian adults born and living at 4350 m than in those living at 3000 m. All were benign and the incidence was higher in women. An association between chemodectoma and thyroid carcinoma has been noted in two patients at 2380 m (Saldana et al. 1973). No cases of chemodectoma have yet been reported from the Tibetan plateau or the high Himalayan valleys.

17.4.5 Cardiovascular adaptations

Andean high altitude residents share with newcomers the raised pulmonary artery and right ventricular pressure due to the hypoxic pulmonary pressor response (Chapter 7), resulting in right ventricular hypertrophy (Recavarren and Arias-Stella 1964). Indeed, in Andean children at high altitude, the usual involution of the muscular coat of the pulmonary artery after birth does not take place, or does so only partially, so that the pulmonary arteries, both large and small, show far greater muscularization than is normal in sea level residents (Saldana and Arias-Stella 1963a,b,c).

This finding of right ventricular hypertrophy, continued muscularization of the pulmonary arteries and raised pulmonary artery pressure in residents at high altitude should be regarded as a response to high altitude rather than an adaptation, since there is no evidence that it has any physiological benefit. Indeed, it merely throws more strain on the right heart.

The purpose of the hypoxic pressor response in humans at sea level, apart from its vital role in prenatal life, is presumably to redistribute blood away from areas of the lung that are hypoxic because of, for instance, atelectasis, and thus improve matching of ventilation and blood flow in various clinical situations. It would probably be beneficial to lose this response at altitude, and the altitude adapted yak would seem to have done this (section 17.5).

Studies in Tibetan highlanders suggest that they have achieved a similar adaptation to the yak and do not have raised pulmonary artery pressures at altitude and little rise on exercise (Groves et al. 1993) though the numbers studied were small. Neither do they develop the structural changes in their pulmonary arterial tree that are found in Andean highlanders (Gupta et al. 1992). The incidence of right ventricular hypertrophic signs in the electrocardiograph (ECG) was found to be only 17 per cent in Tibetans and 29 per cent in Han Chinese at the same altitude (Halperin et al. 1998).

Lifelong residents also have an increase in the number of branches to the main trunks of their coronary arteries (Arias-Stella and Topilsky 1971).

Another adaptation of high altitude residents is that, on exercise at altitude, their maximum heart rate does not seem to be limited, as is the case for acclimatized lowlanders. This is discussed more fully in Chapter 7 and in relation to the adrenergic system in Chapter 15. A recent study by Passino et al. (1996) looked at the spectral analysis of ECGs of high altitude residents compared with lowlanders at altitude. The high altitude residents did not show the reduced vagal tone seen in lowlanders, which may indicate the mechanism which allows this higher maximum heart rate in highlanders.

17.4.6 Adaptation to cold

Cold is a feature of life at high altitude (section 3.8.1). Further aspects of cold adaptation are considered in Chapter 24.

17.5 ADAPTATION TO HYPOXIA OVER GENERATIONS

Most of the adaptations to hypoxia that have been shown in humans appear to develop during a lifetime of exposure. Even the blunting of the hypoxic ventilatory response has been shown to develop in people of lowland stock over a period of decades (Weil *et al.* 1971). The lower hemoglobin concentration in Sherpa and Tibetan subjects has been suggested as an example of adaptation over many generations in Tibetan stock.

17.5.1 The hypoxic pulmonary pressor response

In animals, Harris (1986) has shown elegantly that in cattle the pulmonary pressor response, or lack of it, is genetically determined. The yak has little or no response, whereas the cow has a brisk response. The crossbred dzo has the blunted response of its yak parent, but the second cross of dzo and bull produces 50 per cent brisk and 50 per cent low response offspring. That is, the gene responsible for a low response is dominant and the characteristic is inherited in a Mendelian way. Presumably, a low response is an advantage at altitude, a brisk response being a risk factor for brisket disease (named after the brisket, the loose skin at the animal's throat). Thus, we have a true adaptation achieved presumably by environmental pressure selecting for the low response gene. Similar adaptation has been found in the llama.

There is evidence that in populations of Tibetan origin a similar adaptation may have taken place. Jackson (1968) found little ECG evidence of pulmonary hypertension in Bhutanese and Sherpa subjects at altitude, in that their mean frontal QRS axis differed by only 10° from healthy Edinburgh adults, in contrast to both lowlanders and Andean residents at altitude, who have marked right axis deviation due to pulmonary hypertension (Chapter 7). Groves *et al.*

(1993) found pulmonary artery pressures and resistance in five Tibetan subjects in Lhasa (3658 m) to be within normal sea level values at rest and exercise. If confirmed, this would mark out the Tibetan population as showing genuine altitude adaptation, presumably by natural selection over very many generations.

17.5.2 Arterial oxygen saturation

In 1994 Beall and her colleagues reported that the level of Sa_{O_2} was influenced by a single gene in a population of Tibetan women they had studied at 4850–5450 m (Beall *et al.* 1994). They later studied another Tibetan population in the Lhasa region (3800–4065m) and calculated that this gene accounted for 21 per cent of the variance in Sa_{O_2} (Beall *et al.* 1997b). More recently the same group compared Tibetan with South American Aymara women. They found that the Tibetans had Sa_{O_2} on average 2.6 per cent higher than the Aymara, and also that whereas much of the variance of Sa_{O_2} in the Tibetan women could be attributed to genetic factors, no significant proportion of the variance could be so attributed in the South American population (Beall *et al.* 1999). Therefore there is the potential for natural selection towards higher Sa_{O_2} in the Tibetan but not in the Aymara population.

17.6 DISEASES

It is clear from the biography of Yu-Thog the elder (786–911 CE), the physician-saint and founder of traditional Tibetan medicine, that a number of medical conditions were known at high altitude from the earliest times. These included lung disease, leprosy, venereal disease, a 'swelling of the throat' (possibly diphtheria) and rabies, as well as urinary retention and stones in the urinary tract (Rinpoche 1973, p. 72).

Travelers to Lhasa in the eighteenth and nineteenth centuries, such as Huc and Gabet (Pelliot 1928, vol. 2 p. 250), reported epidemics of smallpox and in 1925 it was estimated that 7000 people died in and around Lhasa from this cause. Because of the prevalence of smallpox in Tibet, in the eighteenth century the Chinese placed a tablet in Lhasa giving instructions on how to curb the disease, and it was also reported in south Tibet and Bhutan by Saunders (1789) and in the Pamir (Forsyth 1875). The Tibetan cure for smallpox was the skin of the ox and rhinoceros (Rinpoche 1973, p. 72), though a form of inoculation was used, apparently borrowed from China and India (Das 1902). A kind of snuff prepared from the dried pustules of smallpox patients was inhaled, which induced a mild form of the disease, protecting the snuff taker from the severe form as described by the Pandit A-K (Walker, 1885). These conditions (smallpox, rabies, leprosy, etc.) are not, of course, caused by altitude.

Gallstones, commonly perceived as a disease of the developed world, is also a common problem in high altitude populations. Commoner in women than men, increased alcohol consumption is associated with a lower risk (Moro *et al*. 1999).

17.6.1 Birth defects

Apart from congenital heart disease, considered in the next section, a high frequency of other birth defects has been noted by Castilla *et al*. (1999). In a collaborative study from three hospitals situated between 2600 and 3600 m in Bogota (Columbia) La Paz (Bolivia) and Quito (Ecuador) they found a high frequency of craniofacial defects, cleft lip, microtia, pre-auricular tag, brachial arch complex, constriction band complex and anal atresia; there was a low frequency of neural tube defects, anencephaly and spina bifida. The incidence of patent ductus arteriosus was not addressed.

17.6.2 Cardiovascular disease

CONGENITAL HEART DISEASE

Congenital cardiovascular malformations are common at altitude, with patent ductus arteriosus being 15 times commoner at Cerro de Pasco (4200 m) than at sea level in Lima (Peñaloza *et al*. 1964). Marticorena *et al*. (1959) reported an incidence of 0.72 per cent of patent ductus arteriosus in children born around 4300 m, compared with an incidence of 0.8 per cent for all congenital heart disease at sea level.

In Xizang (Tibet), among the resident Tibetan population the incidence of congenital heart disease has been shown to range from 0.51 per cent to 2.25 per cent, with patent ductus arteriosus being the most frequently encountered abnormality (Sun 1985). The greater the altitude the higher the prevalence; the highest documented incidence (2.5 per cent) occurred in Chinese emigrants (Zhang 1985). Presumably the cause of these high rates is the lack of a sudden increase in oxygen levels in the few hours after birth which normally triggers the reduction in pulmonary vascular resistance and the closure of the ductus.

ATHEROSCLEROSIS

Studies of populations in the Andes suggest that both coronary artery disease and myocardial infarction are uncommon amongst high altitude residents. No cases were found in one series of 300 necropsies carried out at 4300 m, and epidemiological studies in South America have shown that both angina of effort and ECG evidence of myocardial ischemia are less at altitude than at sea level (Ramos *et al*. 1967). In the Tibetan ethnic population of North Bhutan no autopsy studies were available but angina seemed uncommon, and, as judged by ECG recordings, evidence of coronary artery disease was minimal. Studies from the Tien Shan and Pamir also suggest that degenerative cardiovascular disease is rare in these regions (Mirrakhimov 1978).

In autopsy studies of 385 Tibetan adults living in the Lhasa area, arteriosclerosis of the aorta and its main branches occurred in 81.8 per cent and of the coronary artery in 65.5 per cent. In Qinghai, coronary artery disease was common and autopsies on Tibetans showed the same incidence as in lowlanders, but the incidence of coronary infarction was low (Sun 1985). Serum cholesterol levels were low in Andean natives and in the Bhutanese high altitude group studied; in the latter there was no progressive increase with age (Jackson *et al*. 1966, p. 96).

HYPERTENSION

Hypertension is uncommon in high altitude populations in South America. In a study of 300 high altitude natives in Peru no significant rise in either systolic or diastolic pressure occurred with age. Of individuals aged between 60 and 80 years in the same area, few had a systolic pressure above 165 mm Hg or a diastolic pressure above 95 mm Hg (Baker 1978). There was no significant hypertension in ethnic Tibetan populations of North Bhutan, and, of 70 individuals examined, levels of blood pressure above 165/90 mm Hg were found in 4 per cent. Hypertension was not found in a Sherpa population studied in Northeast Nepal nor in populations studied in the Tien Shan or Pamir. In an Ethiopian group, a slightly higher systolic pressure was found in males. By contrast, Sun reports (1985, 1986) a relatively high incidence of hypertension among indigenous Tibetans. He also found an age-associated increase in blood pressure. There was no tendency for hypertension to decline at higher altitudes and the blood pressure was higher in women than in men. The incidence was greater in the urban population around Lhasa than in rural populations. Similar observations have been made in Tibetans living in high altitude areas of western Szechuan. However, Han (Chinese) immigrants to Tibet showed a lower incidence of hypertension than did the Tibetans. In Qinghai province (which contains the northeastern part of the Tibetan plateau) the incidence of hypertension appears to be lower than in Xizang.

The incidence of hypertension and lack of rise in blood pressure with age in the South American and Himalayan populations studied may be the product of diet and behavior associated with a traditional lifestyle. The cause of hypertension among Tibetans is not clear. On the plateau, obesity is uncommon and traditionally few smoke (though this is changing). However, they do have a very high intake of salt, estimated at up to 1 kg per month, much of it taken in their tea. They also add yak butter, which is often slightly rancid. In the Bhutanese and Sherpa varieties of 'Tibetan' tea neither the salt nor the butter content appears, by taste, to be as high. In all houses and nomad dwellings there is a continuous supply of this tea, which is offered to every visitor. Even when they have migrated to low levels, Tibetans still drink large quantities of it and may become very obese. The high salt and butter intake may be a factor in the high incidence of hypertension in Tibetans.

However, a 15-year survey of Tibetan native highlanders living on the Tibetan plateau showed a low incidence of systemic hypertension. A total of 7797 men and 8029 women were studied. Just over 2 per cent of this group had hypertension compared with over 4 per cent of Chinese immigrants to Tibet. The intake of salt varied. Tibetans in Zadou county (4068 m) had the highest intake with an average of 14.6 g per day and an incidence of hypertension of 3.48 per cent. In Zhidou county (4179 m) the average

salt intake was 2.2 g per day and hypertension was found in 2.62 per cent (Wu 1994a). By contrast, in lowland Chinese the incidence of hypertension is 7.9 per cent (Liu 1986).

17.6.3 Infection

Direct exposure to increased solar radiation inhibits the growth of some bacteria because of the ultraviolet component of sunlight. *Staphylococcus aureus* is greatly inhibited, but *Escherichia coli* is more resistant (Nusshag 1954). The number of bacteria in ambient air decreases with altitude, and a study on the Jungfraujoch (3400 m) in Switzerland showed that, despite a large number of tourists, few bacteria were present in the air.

High altitudes do not influence human bacterial flora *per se*. However, a lower incidence of many common infections of bacterial, viral and protozoal origin was observed in soldiers at altitudes up to 5538 m (Singh *et al.* 1977). Examination of nasal swabs in a high altitude population in North Bhutan showed that there was only a 4 per cent carrier rate of coagulase positive staphylococci; normally the incidence is between 29 and 40 per cent in western communities. A high frequency of β-hemolytic streptococci, highly sensitive to penicillin, was found in throat cultures, whereas in western communities sensitivity to penicillin would be minimal (Selkon and Gould 1966).

In the highlanders of Peru, Colombia and Ecuador, oroya fever is found, which is caused by *Bacillus bacilliformis* becoming parasitic in the red blood cells. Various hemorrhagic fevers are described in the highlands of Bolivia. These are considered to be viral in origin, the virus belonging to the same group as that which causes lassa fever. Hemorrhagic disorders have also been described in north-eastern Nepal.

Mosquitoes, which transmit malaria and yellow fever, are absent at high altitude, but typhus appears to be commoner than at lower levels. This may be because bathing is not usual at higher altitudes, because of the cold, and so lice are common.

Pulmonary disease also appears common at altitude and this in part may be related to the exposure of highlanders to the smoke from open fires inside their houses or tents. In Xizang (Tibet) the incidence of chronic bronchitis was 3.7 per cent in a low altitude population and 22.9 per cent in a population at

4500 m. This was complicated by emphysema in 5–12 per cent of cases and by cor pulmonale in 0.98 per cent (Sun 1985). In Qinghai province, chronic obstructive airway disease is relatively common but smoking is prevalent, particularly amongst immigrants to high altitude. In the Pamir too, respiratory infections were noted by Forsyth (1875), though they seem less common now.

In Nepal and throughout the subcontinent, pulmonary tuberculosis was relatively common, whereas in Ethiopia it was rare. In Ethiopia the major communicable diseases were measles, malaria, dysentery, scabies and syphilis, and the total incidence of communicable disease was greater in the low altitude population (Harrison *et al.* 1969).

In northern Bhutan, respiratory infections appeared to be commoner in the younger age groups but were rare in adults; antibodies to a number of common viral infections were found. A high proportion of the population had been exposed to influenza, mumps, measles, herpes simplex and the common cold (Jackson *et al.* 1966, p. 96); in Lhasa, other parts of Tibet and the Pamir, measles epidemics with a high mortality have been reported in the past.

Leprosy occurs in Nepal and Bhutan (Ward and Jackson 1965) and was reported in Tibet in the nineteenth century (Das 1902) and in the western Himalayas (Moorcroft and Trebeck 1841, Vol. 1, p. 180). The incidence of venereal disease appears to have been high in Lhasa (Chapman 1938), south Tibet and Bhutan (Saunders 1789) and in the Pamir (Forsyth 1875). Where large flocks of sheep are found, as in Qinghai province, hydatid disease is common. European travelers in Central Asia (Deasy 1901, Grenard 1904, p. 249) have also mentioned plague.

Chronic eye infections are seen in the populations of the Pamir, Himalayas and Tibetan plateau; the smoke of yak dung fires exacerbates them. Instruments for the treatment of cataract were available to those who practiced traditional Tibetan medicine; in general, surgery was not commonly carried out.

In summary, where certain infections are common they are due to the low living standards of the people rather than to altitude *per se*.

17.6.4 Goiter

The frequency of goiter in mountainous areas has been recognized for centuries, but it is not confined to the mountains, and over 200 million people worldwide have goiter (Figure 17.1). Iodine deficiency is due to low iodine content of the soil and therefore the water. Soils poor in iodine are found where the land remained longest under quaternary glaciers. When the ice thawed, the iodine-rich soil was swept away and replaced by new soil derived from iodine-poor crystalline rocks. Seaweed, which is rich in iodine, and other folk remedies have been used since ancient times for prophylaxis and treatment (Hetzel 1989).

Scientific proof that goiter was due to iodine deficiency was not available until Marine and Kimball (1920) published a controlled trial in high school children in Akron, Ohio. They showed a reduction in the size of goiters and prevention of their development in children treated with iodine.

Iodine deficiency causes hyperplasia and retention of colloid in the thyroid, resulting in goiter and,

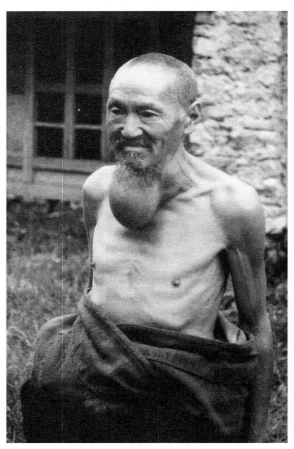

Figure 17.1 *Tibetan from north Bhutan with large pendulous goitre.*

eventually, hypothyroidism in adults. Children born to iodine-deficient mothers have a range of neurological and skeletal defects known collectively as cretinism, an association noted for centuries. This term covers a range of clinical conditions which seem to vary in frequency and importance from locality to locality and includes dwarfism, goiter, facial dysmorphism, deafness, deaf mutism and intellectual impairment.

In populations with goiter, the overall work capacity of the population may be impaired, as, in addition to cretinism, there is a marked morbidity, infant mortality is raised and mental subnormality common.

Iodine deficiency may result from insufficient intake, goitrogenic substances and deficiency in intrathyroidal enzymes; an excess of calcium or fluoride in the presence of iodine deficiency may increase the incidence of goiter.

McCarrison (1908, 1913) carried out a classical study of goiter and endemic cretinism in the Gilgit Agency of Kashmir (Karakoram), and more recently Chapman et al. (1972) worked in the identical area.

In 1906, McCarrison found a goiter incidence of 65 per cent; in Chapman's study it was 74 per cent. In the latter study, 10 of 589 individuals examined were cretins, and hypothyroidism, excluding cretinism, was found in 24 subjects. Although the population as a whole appeared to be iodine deficient, the majority had adapted well. No evidence was found that goiter was caused by an infectious agent, a theory put forward by McCarrison.

The incidence of goiter may vary widely within a few miles; some 100 miles (160 km) north of Gilgit where goiter was endemic, it was not observed in the semi-nomadic Kirghiz tribesmen who inhabit the Pamir plateau of southern Xinjiang. Direct questioning of the nomads revealed that they knew about goiter but they were adamant that there was no history of its occurrence amongst them (Ward 1983), though Marco Polo noted a large population of people with goiter in Yarkand (Shache) as did Forsyth (1875). However, hearsay evidence is notably unreliable. Anecdotal evidence of goiter in other regions of the Himalayas, the Shimshall region of the Karakoram, and west Bhutan, suggests also that the incidence may vary considerably within a few miles (Saunders 1789, Shipton 1938).

Moorcroft and Trebeck (1841, Vol. 2), while traveling in the western Himalayas and on the Tibetan border, comment on goiter that, 'scarcely a woman was free from it' (p. 25). Later they say, 'Goiter was here very common: the water was soft whilst at Gonh it was too hard to mix with soap: but so it was at Le where goiter does not prevail' (p. 30). Fraser (1820) alludes to surgical removal

> We understand it (goiter) was sometimes cured when early means were taken, and these are said to consist in extirpation of the part by the knife. We saw some persons who had scars on their throat resulting from this mode of cure which had in these instances been completely successful.

Waddell (1899), in a village where goiter was prevalent, writes, 'I was surprised to see that several of the goats and the domestic fowls, as well as some of the ponies, had the same large swellings'.

According to Dr Sun Sin-Fu (personal communication), in Lhasa, about 60 per cent of Tibetan indigenous inhabitants have goiter. Das (1902) commented too that Tibetan physicians recognized six varieties of goiter. Rockhill (1891, p. 265) also observed goiter, particularly in women in eastern Tibet, and other travelers noted the condition in northern Tibet (Bonvalot 1891, p. 116) and in the gorge country of south-east Tibet (Bailey 1957).

The incidence of goiter in Himalayan valleys is high, and in the Tibetan ethnic population of north Bhutan it was the commonest clinical condition. In subjects less than 20 years old it was less marked, and younger individuals had a diffuse enlargement, whereas with age a nodular goiter was more common. No cases of cancer or thyrotoxicosis were seen, and two cretins were found in 349 individuals examined. The incidence of goiter was 60 per cent in females and 19 per cent in males (Jackson et al. 1966, pp. 40–4).

Ibbertson et al. (1972), in a survey of Sherpas (also of Tibetan ethnic origin) in the Sola Khumbu region of north-eastern Nepal, found that 92 per cent had a palpable goiter, which was visibly enlarged in 63 per cent; 75 per cent had below normal protein-bound iodine levels in the blood and 30 per cent were clinically hypothyroid. Classical myxedema was present in 5.9 per cent of the population, deaf mutism in a further 4.7 per cent and isolated deafness in a further 3.1 per cent. Pitt (1970) describes Nepalese babies born with goiter. In many of these areas the incidence of goiter is much lower now after various projects for giving iodine by tablets or depot injections have been carried out. In a survey carried out in 1980–1 in Ethiopia, the gross goiter prevalence was found to be 30 per cent among schoolchildren and 19 per cent in household members (Wolde-Gebriel *et al.* 1993).

17.6.5   Sickle cell disease

Adzaku *et al.* (1993) reported on 136 patients resident at about 3000 m in Saudi Arabia and compared them with 185 patients living at sea level. Patients at both locations included those with homozygous disease (Hb SS), hemoglobin C (Hb SC) and sickle cell trait (Hb AS). The main finding was a marked increase in 2,3-diphosphoglycerate (2,3-DPG) in patients with sickle cell disease compared with normal controls at altitude and patients at sea level. Their hemoglobin concentration was not different from sea level patients; they were anemic, with values around 8.0–9.0 g dL^{-1}. Sickle cell patients resident at low altitude have a high risk of crises on going to altitude (section 27.4.3). Adzaku *et al.* (1993) attribute the relative well being of their patients at altitude to their high 2,3-DPG, which, at this relatively modest altitude, would help tissue oxygenation, in contrast to the situation at extreme altitude (Chapter 12).

17.6.6   Dental conditions

There is no evidence that altitude has any direct effect on the teeth but the economic conditions, dictated in part by altitude, may well affect diet and hence dental condition. Generally the diet of high altitude populations contains less refined sugars and more fiber, giving fewer caries than a more 'western' diet. Green (1992) reported a much higher incidence of caries amongst Sherpa children along the popular trekking routes in Nepal (76 per cent) than in villages off the routes (17 per cent). The latter had not had the 'benefit' of cadging sweets from generous but misguided tourists.

18

Acute mountain sickness

SUMMARY

Acute mountain sickness (AMS) commonly afflicts otherwise healthy men and woman who go rapidly to altitude. Symptoms, which come on a few hours after arrival, include headache, anorexia, nausea, vomiting, lack of energy, malaise and disturbed sleep. The symptoms are usually worst on days 2 and 3 at altitude and disappear by day 5. Symptoms may reappear on ascent to a higher altitude. This common self-limiting condition is termed simple or benign AMS. Two other forms of AMS are high altitude pulmonary edema (HAPE) and high altitude cerebral edema (HACE) which are the subjects of Chapters 19 and 20 respectively. These are potentially lethal and can be termed malignant AMS.

The incidence of AMS depends upon the rate of ascent and the height reached. It is uncommon below 2000 m but is almost universal among those flying directly to altitudes above 3800 m. It occurs in both sexes and at all ages. Fitness confers no protection and so far no physiological measurement gives reliable prediction of susceptibility for AMS. Strenuous exercise on arrival at altitude is possibly a risk factor, especially for HAPE. The mechanism underlying the symptoms is still debated but cerebral edema is considered the most likely immediate cause. The edema is probably due to vasogenic mechanisms in which cerebral blood flow and permeability play a part. There may be roles for fluid and sodium balance, also

for ventilation and its control in the mechanism of AMS. Subclinical pulmonary edema through its effect on blood gases may also be important.

Though there is debate about the mechanisms of AMS there is a consensus about its management. AMS can be prevented or ameliorated by a slow rate of ascent and by drugs, of which acetazolamide is the best studied and most widely used. Other drugs, including spironolactone, probably also help. Treatment is hardly needed in the majority of cases but ibuprofen and dexamethasone have been shown to be effective in the relief of headache; acetazolamide is also helpful as treatment and improves blood gases.

An agreed scoring system for AMS has been devised, the Lake Louise system, which is recommended for research into AMS. It is described at the end of the chapter.

18.1 INTRODUCTION

It has been known for many years that travelers to high mountains experience a variety of symptoms: an early description was given by de Acosta (Chapter 1.3). The first modern account of AMS was by Ravenhill (1913). He pointed out that fatigue, cold, lack of food, etc. complicated previous descriptions by explorers and mountain climbers. He was serving as a medical officer of a mining company whose mines at 4700 m in Chile were served by a railway, so that the patients he observed were suffering the uncomplicated effects of altitude alone. The local Bolivian name for AMS was *puna*; in Peru it was *soroche*. Tibetan names for AMS include *ladrak* (poison of the pass) *damgiri*, *duqri*, *yen chang* (from the Koko Nor region), *chang-chi* (from Szechuan), and *tuteck*. Ravenhill's description of simple AMS, which he calls puna of the 'normal' type, can hardly be bettered. He wrote:

> It is a curious fact that the symptoms of puna do not usually evince themselves at once. The majority of newcomers have expressed themselves as being quite well on first arrival. As a rule, towards the evening, the patient begins to feel rather slack and disinclined for exertion. He goes to bed but has a restless and troubled night and wakes up next morning with a severe frontal headache.

> There may be vomiting, frequently there is a sense of oppression in the chest but there is rarely any respiratory distress or alteration in the normal rate of breathing so long as the patient is at rest. The patient may feel slightly giddy on rising from bed and any attempt at exertion increases the headache, which is nearly always confined to the frontal region (Ravenhill 1913)

To this description should be added the symptoms of irritability and occasionally photophobia. Sleep is often disturbed, probably because of periodic breathing. The patient may wake with a feeling of suffocation during the apneic phase. It should be noted, however, that periodic breathing is not a symptom of AMS. At altitudes above about 5000 m it continues in many subjects long after any symptoms of AMS have resolved and there is no correlation between its severity and AMS scores (Eichenberger *et al.* 1996). It is not a cause of AMS though its presence, by causing more severe intermittent hypoxia, may make matters worse. Ravenhill then goes on to describe puna of the cardiac and nervous types, corresponding in our present nomenclature to

acute pulmonary edema and acute cerebral edema of high altitude (section 18.2).

After Ravenhill, although mountain sickness was well recognized, the distinction and importance of the two complicating forms seem to have been lost, at least in the English-speaking world, until rediscovered by Hultgren and Spickard (1960) and Houston (1960) in the case of HAPE and by Fitch (1964) for HACE. However, HAPE was well known to South American physicians with experience at altitude. Lizárraga (1955) gave the first detailed description of the condition after Ravenhill. A fuller account of the history of AMS is given in West (1998, pp. 132–63).

18.2   DEFINITIONS AND NOMENCLATURE

The nomenclature of mountain sickness is summarized in Table 18.1. The terms puna and soroche are used loosely in South America, not only for the symptoms of AMS but also for the dyspnea normal to exertion at high altitude (Ravenhill 1913). They are also used for chronic mountain sickness, a completely distinct clinical entity (Chapter 21). The term 'mountain sickness' needs to be qualified by the word 'acute' to distinguish it from this latter entity; the term 'acute mountain sickness' is now well accepted for this condition or group of conditions. Finally there is the recently described subacute mountain sickness affecting either infants or adults (Chapter 21).

Dickinson (1982) made the useful suggestion that the 'normal' or 'simple' AMS, which commonly affects most people going rapidly to high altitude and which is self-limiting, be termed 'benign', whereas the other two forms or complications of AMS be termed 'malignant', since they are life threatening. They are thus termed 'malignant pulmonary AMS' and 'malignant cerebral AMS'.

Table 18.1 *Nomenclature of mountain sickness*

Ravenhill (1913)	Puna of the normal type	Puna of the cardiac type	Puna of the nervous type	
Dickinson (1982)	Benign AMS	Malignant pulmonary AMS	Malignant cerebral AMS	
Others	Simple AMS	High altitude pulmonary edema (HAPE)	High altitude cerebral edema (HACE)	Chronic mountain sickness (CMS)

However, this terminology, emphasizing the crucial difference between the forms of AMS, has not been widely adopted. The terms more commonly used for the malignant forms are HAPE and HACE. Many cases of malignant AMS include features of both pulmonary and cerebral edema. There is a strong impression that HACE is an advanced form of simple AMS. The symptoms of both are due to cerebral edema. The difference is that in simple AMS the edema is self-limiting and reverses even at altitude, but in HACE it is progressive. HAPE has different mechanisms from simple AMS, involving pulmonary hypertension, and is more clearly a condition of individual susceptibility.

18.2.1   Definition, signs and symptoms

Benign AMS may be defined as a self-limiting condition affecting previously healthy individuals on going rapidly to high altitude. After arrival there may be an asymptomatic period of some 6–12 h. Symptoms, including headache, anorexia, nausea, vomiting, fatigue, light-headedness and sleep disturbance, then start gradually and usually peak on the second or third day. By day 4 or 5 symptoms are usually gone and do not recur at that altitude. The Lake Louise scoring system (section 18.8) requires mild headache and at least one of the above symptoms to make the diagnosis as well as a score of 3 or more. There must be a history of recent height gain and (if altitude is reached abruptly as by air or cable car) several hours must elapse before the symptoms start. The diagnosis is made on the history and there may be no signs. However, physical examination may reveal crackles in the chest and peripheral edema. This may show as periorbital edema after sleep or as ankle edema after being up and about (Figure 18.1). According to Hackett and Rennie (1979) the proportions of cases showing these signs were 23 per cent and 18 per cent respectively. Mild fever may be present. Maggiorini *et al.* (1997) found a rise in body temp of 0.5 °C in mild cases (AMS score = 3), 1.2 °C in more severe cases of AMS (score >3) and 1.7 °C in cases of HAPE. With the advent of small, portable pulse oximeters, Sa_{O_2} can be measured easily and this value is often low both in patients with AMS and in subjects who will subsequently develop AMS (section 18.4.8).

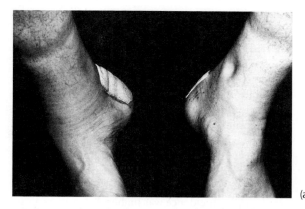
(a)

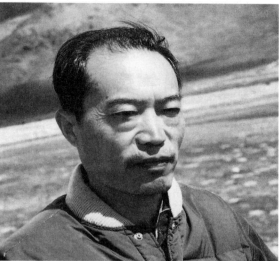
(b)

Figure 18.1 *(a) Pitting edema of ankle after hill walking at low altitude. (b) Periorbital edema at high altitude.*

Ascent to a higher altitude, even after acclimatization at a lower altitude, may precipitate a further attack. Descent and re-ascent after less than 7–10 days does not usually provoke symptoms but descent for more than about 10 days renders the subject susceptible to AMS on re-ascent. The period of risk for AMS therefore corresponds with the period before acclimatization has taken place. Acclimatization prevents AMS, though it is not clear how.

18.3   INCIDENCE OF BENIGN AMS

The incidence of AMS depends on the rate at which people ascend to altitude and the height reached as well as the exact definition of the condition. The lowest altitude at which some individuals can be affected is as low as 2000 m, the height of many ski resorts. Rapid ascent to 3100 m, for instance by the railway to the Gornergrat in Switzerland or by road to Leadville, Colorado, produces symptoms in a proportion of people by the next morning. Hackett and Rennie (1979) found an overall incidence of 43 per cent in trekkers reaching the aid post at Pheriche (4243 m), though some affected trekkers would have dropped out before reaching this altitude. Among those who flew into the airstrip at Lukla (2800 m), the incidence was higher than among those who walked all the way (49 per cent versus 31 per cent). Maggiorini et al. (1990) found incidences in climbers to European alpine huts of 9 per cent at 2850 m, 13 per cent at 3050 m and 34 per cent at 3650 m. A study of a general tourist population arriving at resorts in Colorado at altitudes of 1900–2940 m found an incidence of 25 per cent (Honigman et al. 1993). Among lowlanders who drive directly from Lima to Cerro de Pasco (4300 m) in Peru or who fly to La Paz in Bolivia (3700 m) there are very few who do not have at least mild symptoms on the morning after arrival. Murdoch (1995) reported an incidence of 85 per cent in tourists flying into the airstrip at Shayangboche (3800 m) in Nepal.

However, if the stay at altitude is only an hour or two the incidence of AMS is negligible. This is the case, for instance, for the great majority of tourists who drive or take the train to the summit of Pikes Peak, Colorado (4300 m).

18.4 ETIOLOGY

18.4.1 Individual susceptibility

The etiology of AMS is multifactorial. The most important factors are the rate of ascent and the height reached. Symptoms can be induced in almost all subjects if ascent is made rapidly to a sufficient height, but for any given altitude/time profile there is great variation in individual susceptibility.

18.4.2 AMS and fitness

There is no easy way to identify the susceptible individual, as Ravenhill (1913) says:

There is in my experience no type of man of whom one can say he will or will not suffer from puna. Most of the cases I have instanced were young men to all appearances perfectly sound. Young, strong and healthy men may be completely overcome. Stout, plethoric individuals of the chronic bronchitic type may not even have a headache. I have known several instances of this even when the persons have taken no care of themselves (Ravenhill 1913).

Certainly athletic fitness provides no immunity. A superbly fit French paratrooper on a family trek to Everest Base Camp had to be evacuated to lower altitude with severe symptoms of AMS while his mother and aunt were unaffected (Milledge, B.A. personal communication). One study found no correlation between fitness as measured by $V_{O_2 max}$ before an expedition to Mount Kenya and AMS symptom scores during the first days at altitude (Milledge et al. 1991a). Bircher et al. (1994), in a study of 41 mountaineers who went to 4559 m in the Alps in 20–22 h, found no correlation between a measure of fitness (PWC_{170}) and AMS scores, and Savourey et al. (1995) similarly found no correlation between $V_{O_2 max}$ and subsequent AMS on an Andean expedition.

18.4.3 Consistency in response to altitude

Individuals respond reasonably consistently, so that performance on one occasion is a guide to future performance. This clinical impression has been confirmed in a study by Forster (1984), who studied workers at Mauna Kea observatory in Hawaii, situated at 4200 m. These workers alternated 5 days at the observatory with 5 days at sea level so Forster was able to score the symptoms of AMS in 18 men on two altitude shifts. He showed that the rank order of scores correlated significantly on the two occasions. There is a tendency to acclimatize better on each subsequent trip to altitude.

However, there are numerous exceptions and case histories do show anomalies. For instance, someone who has had little trouble on the first two trips may develop AMS on a third. A respiratory or some other infection may be an added factor in such cases. The consistency in response is greater in the case of individuals who have had HAPE.

18.4.4 AMS, gender, age and body build

Both men and women are at risk. One study (Kayser 1991) of trekkers going over the Thorong pass in Nepal (5400 m) found women to have a higher rate of sickness than men (69 per cent versus 57 per cent), but perhaps women are more ready to admit to symptoms than men. The young are probably at greater risk than the old (Hackett et al. 1976, Roach et al. 1995) and the risk among boys, at least of HAPE, seems especially high in South America (Hultgren and Marticorena 1978). However, Yaron et al. (1998) found an incidence of benign AMS in young children similar to that in adults.

Subjects slimmer than average (body mass index < 22) may be less susceptible to AMS than those who are standard or obese, according to one study (Hirata et al. 1989); Kayser (1991) also found obesity to be a risk factor in men.

18.4.5 Smoking, diet and AMS

There has been an impression amongst mountaineers that smokers have less AMS than nonsmokers perhaps because, being habituated to a modest level of carboxyhemoglobin, they have, in effect, some pre-acclimatization. A recent chamber study (Yoneda and Watanabe 1997) seems to confirm that, at least for very acute, severe hypoxia, smokers had fewer symptoms, though their time of useful consciousness was not different from that of nonsmokers.

A high carbohydrate diet has some physiological benefit at altitude (section 14.8.1) and is preferred by many mountaineers, but does it reduce AMS? In a chamber study of 19 subjects given either a high (68 per cent) or normal (45 per cent) carbohydrate diet for 4 days before altitude exposure for 8 h, Swenson et al. (1997) found that there was no difference in the AMS scores between the two diets.

18.4.6 AMS and hypoxic ventilatory response (HVR)

There is some evidence that subjects with a low HVR (Chapter 5) measured at sea level are liable to develop AMS. The association has been shown by measurements of the response to acute hypoxia in the laboratory in studies of a few subjects (Lakshminarayan and Pierson 1975, Hu et al. 1982, Matsuzawa et al. 1989). In the last study, 2 of the 10 subjects had HVR within the normal range.

Richalet et al. (1988) studied a large group of climbers before they went on various expeditions to the great ranges. They found that low ventilatory and cardiac responses to hypoxia on exercise were risk factors for AMS. The same group recently reported a single case of high susceptibility in a subject who had had radiation to his neck as a child and had a very low HVR (presumably because of damage to his carotid bodies). He suffered severe AMS at only 3500 m (Rathat et al. 1993). However, a number of more recent studies in the field have failed to find a correlation. Two prospective studies found no correlation between HVR measured before going to altitude and symptom scores for AMS after arrival (Milledge et al. 1988, 1991b). Savourey et al. (1995) recently also reported no correlation with HVR measured before an Andean expedition and subsequent AMS. Interestingly, they did find that resting P_{O_2} at sea level or at simulated altitude was predictive for AMS. Selland et al. (1993) found that two of four subjects with a history of HAPE had HVR greater than their control subjects' mean value. Hackett et al. (1987b) in a study of 106 climbers on Mount McKinley found that, although a low Sa_{O_2} predicted the likely development of AMS, there was no good correlation between HVR and Sa_{O_2} on arrival at altitude. Hohenhaus et al. (1995) found that, compared with control fit subjects, HVR was significantly lower in subjects who developed HAPE but not in subjects with AMS. Highlanders, who generally have less AMS than low-landers, have a blunted HVR (section 5.5.2). Interestingly, Hackett et al. (1988b) found an abnormal (negative) HVR at altitude in patients with HAPE. They seemed to have hypoxic depression of ventilation, which was relieved by oxygen breathing.

In conclusion, it would seem that although susceptibility to HAPE is associated with a low HVR, susceptibility to AMS is not.

18.4.7 AMS, hypoxic pulmonary artery pressor and cerebral blood flow responses

A brisk increase in pulmonary artery pressure in response to hypoxia is possibly also a risk factor for AMS (Hultgren et al. 1971, Kawashima et al. 1989), although doubt is cast on this by the finding that nifedipine, which by lowering the pulmonary artery pressure is protective of HAPE, does not protect from AMS (Hohenhaus et al. 1994). The measurement of pulmonary artery pressure noninvasively with Doppler ultrasound in a short hypoxic test might be useful in identifying those subjects susceptible to HAPE since they have an abnormally brisk response (section 19.2.8).

A recent study looked at the cerebral blood flow response to a 15-min hypoxic and hyperoxic challenge in one group of subjects who had suffered HAPE, another who had been to altitude with no AMS and a third unselected control group. The test was found not to be predictive of altitude tolerance (Berre et al. 1999).

18.4.8   Oxygen saturation and AMS

Although hypoxia is not the immediate cause of the symptoms of AMS, the severity of hypoxia is important since the incidence increases with altitude. It is perhaps not surprising, therefore, that a number of studies have shown a correlation between Sa_{O_2} and AMS (Bircher et al. 1994, Roach et al. 1998). In the study by Bircher et al. subjects traveled to the Capanna Margherita (4559 m) in the Alps by helicopter and the saturations were measured on the second day when AMS symptoms were at their height. Some subjects had overt HAPE and no doubt others had subclinical edema. In the study by Roach and colleagues, 102 climbers on Mount Denali in Alaska were studied at Base Camp (4200 m) and then questioned about AMS symptoms on their return from their summit bids. The Sa_{O_2} measured before climbing from Base Camp correlated with subsequent AMS scores. Thus a low Sa_{O_2} on arrival at altitude is a good predictor for the later development of AMS. The authors comment that the reason for the low Sa_{O_2} in these subjects could be either hypoventilation or impaired gas exchange. However, Bircher et al. (1994) did not find a difference in Pa_{CO_2} between those with and without AMS and the collected results from over 90 subjects from a number of studies at this location by Bärtsch (personal communication) gave the same finding. However, other studies, mostly taking measurements earlier in altitude exposure, did find evidence of hypoventilation and higher P_{CO_2} in AMS subjects (section 18.5.2).

Another way of looking at the possible gas exchange abnormality was studied by Ge et al. (1997) who measured pulmonary diffusing capacity for carbon monoxide (D_{CO}) in a group of 32 subjects at 2260 m and after ascent to 4700 m. In non-AMS subjects there was an increase in D_{CO} at the higher altitude whereas in AMS patients the increase was insignificant. They also showed lower vital capacity (FVC), reduced expiratory flow in the middle of their FVC and greater $(A–a)O_2$ gradient. These differences were thought to be due to subclinical pulmonary edema. Pollard et al. (1997) also found reduced FVC and forced expiratory volume one second (FEV_1) at altitude and a correlation between these indices of lung function and arterial saturation. Probably a degree of subclinical pulmonary edema is common during the early days at altitude; and Anholm et al. (1999) found radiographic evidence of pulmonary edema in some well trained cyclists after an endurance ride at moderate altitude.

18.4.9   Exercise and AMS

AMS can and frequently does occur in the absence of any exercise, as in chamber experiments, or with only gentle walking short distances, as in helicopter transport to a mountain hut or a flight to La Paz, Bolivia. But until recently we could not answer the question of whether subjects climbing on foot to altitude would be more or less likely to have AMS than those who arrived there by air or motor transport given the same rate of ascent. Obviously, most people who fly to altitude have a more rapid height gain than those who walk and therefore more AMS. Again, the advice to people on arrival at altitude is to avoid exercise for some time but there are few hard data to support this. Bircher et al. (1994) did not find any difference in the incidence of AMS in relation to intensity of work (as assessed by heart rate) in groups of subjects who climbed to the Capanna Margherita. However, as the authors say, their study was not designed to look at this relationship and the differences in exercise rates were not great. Roach et al. (2000) carried out a crossover trial in which subjects were exposed to 4572 m altitude equivalent in a chamber for 10 h on one occasion with and on another without exercise. The AMS scores were significantly higher during the exposure with exercise. This one study lends some credence to the time-honored advice to avoid strenuous exercise in getting to and on arrival at altitude, in order to avoid AMS. The same advice is probably even more pertinent in relation to HAPE where exercise raises pulmonary artery pressure and increases the risk of HAPE.

18.5 MECHANISMS

18.5.1 Fluid balance and AMS

Clearly hypoxia is a crucial starting mechanism for AMS but it is not the direct cause of symptoms. Within a few minutes of exposure to high altitude P_{O_2} falls throughout the body, but symptoms of AMS are delayed for at least a few hours. This suggests that hypoxia initiates some process which requires a time course of 6–24 h before it, in turn, causes the symptoms.

Current thinking favors the hypothesis that hypoxia causes some alteration of fluid or electrolyte homeostasis with either water retention or shifts of water from intracellular to extracellular compartments (Hansen *et al.* 1970, Hackett *et al.* 1981).

In considering the possible role of disturbances in fluid balance in the mechanism of AMS we need to take into account two other variables apart from the rate of ascent:

- whether or not the subject exercises in getting to altitude or on arrival
- whether the subject has a physiological or a pathological response to altitude hypoxia; that is, whether or not he gets AMS.

Table 18.2 shows the effect on various fluid compartments of exercise (hill walking at low altitude)

and of going to altitude and responding physiologically or pathologically.

EXERCISE AT LOW ALTITUDE

The effect of day-long exercise (hill walking) continued for several days at low altitude was studied in the hills of north Wales. Full measurements of water and electrolyte balances were carried out before, during and after the exercise period. There was significant sodium retention, modest water retention, significant increases in plasma and interstitial fluid volumes at the expense of the intracellular compartment (Williams *et al.* 1979). In a later study this was shown to be due to activation of the renin–aldosterone system during exercise (Milledge *et al.* 1982; see section 15.3.3). The increased interstitial fluid volume can cause overt pitting edema in a few subjects (Figure 18.1) but all were in a state of subclinical edema.

ALTITUDE WITHOUT EXERCISE OR AMS

It is surprisingly difficult to obtain reliable data on the effect of altitude on fluid and electrolyte balance in the absence of exercise and AMS. Papers usually indicate if exercise has been excluded (though not always) but seldom make it clear which, if any, subjects were free of AMS. Few papers quote strict balance studies and those that do often give conflicting results. It is usually considered that the physiological response to hypoxia is a diuresis. This seems to be the case in animals and is effected by stimulus of the peripheral chemoreceptors (Honig 1989) but is less easy to demonstrate in humans. Studies in the field have given conflicting results, probably because of the difficulty in controlling factors such as temper-

Table 18.2 *Changes in sodium and water control with exercise at low altitude and in response to altitude in subjects with and without AMS*

	Exercise Low altitude	No AMS High altitude	With AMS High altitude
Urine volume	↓	↑	↓
Water balance	? Positive	? Negative	? Positive
Sodium excretion	↓	↑	↓
Plasma volume	↑	↓	?↑
Extracellular volume	↑	↓	?↑
Plasma aldosterone	↑	↓	↑

ature, sweating, sodium and water intake. However, Swenson *et al.* (1995), in a 6-h chamber study where these factors have all been controlled, have shown that there was an increase in urinary volume and sodium output with hypoxia. Further they found a good correlation between these two measurements and the individual's HVR. There were only minimal symptoms of AMS in the 6 h of the study. The diuresis and natriuresis did not correlate with changes in aldosterone, renin, atrial natriuretic peptide (ANP), vasopressin or digoxin-like immunoreactive substance.

There is a reduction of plasma, interstitial and intracellular volumes during the first few days at altitude (Frayser *et al.* 1975, Jain *et al.* 1980). Similar changes were found in a study by Singh *et al.* (1990) and are shown in Figure 18.2. Note that the changes, as a percentage of sea level values, are quite small, the greatest being a 6–7 per cent reduction in plasma and extracellular fluid (ECF) volumes at 2 days. The

changes in these compartments remained for up to 12 days whereas the reductions in total body water and intracellular fluid were restored by day 12 at altitude.

ALTITUDE WITH EXERCISE AND WITHOUT AMS

A study based on the Gornergrat (3100 m), Switzerland, involved baseline studies at rest at low altitude followed by exercise in climbing to the Gornergrat and daily while there (Milledge *et al.* 1983d). Full balance studies were continued throughout. The results were almost identical to those of exercise at low altitude. The plasma volume increased so that the hematocrit, instead of rising as is usual at altitude, actually fell as it did at sea level. Renin and aldosterone levels were high whereas subjects at rest at altitude have low aldosterone levels. The effect of exercise overrides the effect of altitude in this situation.

ALTITUDE WITH EXERCISE AND AMS

There are no balance studies that have addressed exactly this question, owing to the formidable problems of carrying out balance studies on sufficiently large numbers of subjects to cover both good and bad acclimatizers. Studies measuring just 24-h sodium excretion have shown an inverse correlation between sodium excretion and AMS symptom scores and a direct correlation with aldosterone concentration. That is, those who develop AMS have higher aldosterone levels and retain more sodium. All subjects have a reduced urine volume, with the AMS victims tending to have a greater antidiuresis but this did not reach statistical significance (Bärtsch *et al.* 1988, Milledge *et al.* 1989).

SODIUM AND WATER BALANCE IN AMS

Table 18.2 attempts to bring together these changes, showing that the subject with AMS is in a similar state of expanded plasma and ECF volume as a subject starting day-long exercise at low altitude. They are both in a state of subclinical edema.

These effects are shown in Figure 18.3, on the left. It is suggested that this increase in ECF in turn results in the dependent and periorbital edema often seen in patients with AMS (Hackett and Rennie 1979). It also causes mild cerebral edema, resulting in the

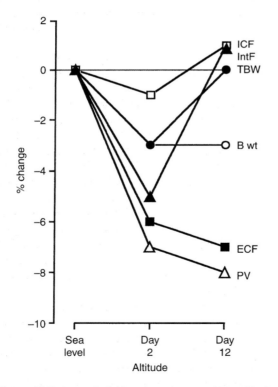

Figure 18.2 *Changes in fluid compartments on going to altitude in the absence of exercise or AMS. ICF, intracellular fluid volume; IntF, interstitial fluid volume; TBW, total body water; B wt, body weight; ECF, extracellular fluid volume; PV, plasma volume. (Data from Singh* et al. *1990.)*

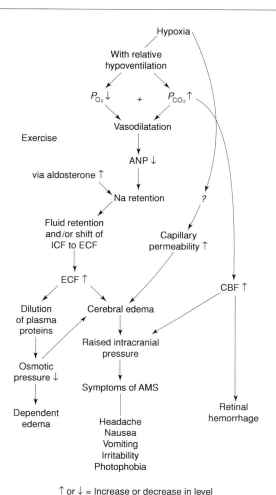

Figure 18.3 *Possible mechanisms underlying acute mountain sickness (AMS). ICF, intracellular fluid; ECF, extracellular fluid; CBF, cerebral blood flow; ANP, atrial natriuretic peptide.*

symptoms of AMS. More severe cerebral edema causes the full-blown malignant condition of HACE and pulmonary edema causes HAPE.

Some evidence of fluid retention is provided by the clinical observation of lower urine output in soldiers with AMS than in soldiers free of symptoms (Singh *et al.* 1969b) and by the finding that trekkers with the condition gained weight, whereas trekkers without AMS had lost weight by the time they reached 4243 m (Hackett *et al.* 1982). The 'normal' response to altitude seems to be a mild diuresis, whereas subjects destined to get AMS have an antidiuresis.

Because of this antidiuresis the antidiuretic hormone (vasopressin) might be thought to underlie this mechanism but that seems not to be the case; see section 15.2.3. The effect of altitude on the renin–aldosterone system is reviewed in section 15.3. Briefly, ascent to altitude alone has a variable effect on plasma renin activity but results in lower than normal aldosterone levels at rest. Exercise stimulates the release of renin which in turn, via angiotensin, stimulates aldosterone release and – if continued long enough – causes salt and hence water retention (Williams *et al.* 1979, Milledge *et al.* 1982). This may be important especially in HAPE, in which a history of exercise is often a prominent feature (Chapter 19). AMS symptom scores were found to correlate with aldosterone levels and with reduced 24-h urine sodium output on the first day at altitude in subjects who had ascended to 4300 m on foot on Mount Kenya (Milledge *et al.* 1989). A similar result was reported from a study in the European Alps (Bärtsch *et al.* 1988) although Hogan *et al.* (1973), in a chamber experiment, found that subjects with AMS had lower aldosterone concentrations than did asymptomatic subjects.

ANP, which increases urinary sodium excretion and hence fluid excretion, is elevated by hypoxia in rats (Winter *et al.* 1987a) and humans (Bärtsch *et al.* 1988, Cosby *et al.* 1988, Milledge *et al.* 1989). The relationship between ANP levels and AMS is variable. One study found a tendency to higher levels in subjects more resistant to AMS (Milledge *et al.* 1989) whereas two other studies found the opposite (Bärtsch *et al.* 1988, Cosby *et al.* 1988). It seems that despite its name ANP is not a very powerful natriuretic hormone. Subjects hill walking at low altitude have raised ANP levels while retaining sodium vigorously (Milledge *et al.* 1991b). ANP may have an effect by increasing capillary permeability but its significance in the etiology of AMS remains to be established (Bärtsch *et al.* 1988).

Although, as mentioned, the favored hypothesis is that fluid is retained and somehow causes AMS, it has proved very hard to obtain good evidence for this. Measurements of urine output have usually not shown a clear difference between those with and without AMS (Milledge *et al.* 1989), though this negative finding often goes unreported. Westerterp *et al.* (1996) applied the technique of labeled water and bromide to the problem. A group of 10 subjects was transported by helicopter to the Vallot observatory

(4350 m) on Mont Blanc and studied for 4 days. Fluid intake correlated closely with food intake and both were reduced in those with AMS. There was reduced evaporative water loss at altitude which resulted in increased urine output in the case of subjects without AMS but not in AMS sufferers. The change in total body water was small and not significantly different between those with and without AMS. However, those with AMS showed a fluid shift greater than 1 L between intracellular and extracellular compartments. The shift could be in either direction, making it difficult to understand the mechanism. However, only one AMS subject had a reduction in extracellular volume while three showed the expected increase.

18.5.2 Role of P_{CO_2} in AMS and cerebral blood flow

On going to high altitude the subject experiences not only hypoxia but also hypocapnia. The possibility that hypocapnia over a number of hours might be a factor in the genesis of AMS was tested by Maher *et al.* (1975c). They exposed two groups of subjects to simulated altitude in a hypobaric chamber. One group had carbon dioxide added to the atmosphere to maintain their P_{CO_2} at control levels; the other group breathed air and became hypocapnic. Hypoxia was similar in the two groups, though to achieve this the group with carbon dioxide added was taken to a lower barometric pressure. Far from alleviating symptoms of AMS, the added carbon dioxide increased their severity.

Sutton *et al.* (1976) found that in a group of subjects air lifted to a camp at 5360 m on Mount Logan in the Canadian Yukon, the severity of AMS correlated best with the P_{CO_2}. Forwand *et al.* (1968) found AMS symptom scores correlated well with P_{CO_2} but not with pH or P_{O_2}. In a study of 42 trekkers, Hackett *et al.* (1982) found that those who gained weight on ascent to 4300 m had the highest incidence of AMS and reduced their Pa_{CO_2} very little, whereas those who lost weight (presumably mainly fluid) had less frequent AMS and a low PA_{CO_2}. Two studies of men in decompression chambers also found a correlation between AMS and hypoventilation (King and Robinson 1972, Moore *et al.* 1986). Maher *et al.* (1975) suggested that the mechanism connecting P_{CO_2} and AMS was the well-known effect of carbon dioxide in increasing the cerebral blood flow.

Hypoxia also causes an increase in cerebral blood flow. In subjects with a brisk ventilatory response and low P_{CO_2} these two effects are, to a degree, counterbalanced, whereas in subjects with little increase in ventilation and P_{CO_2} close to sea level normal, cerebral vessels will be dilated and may contribute to cerebral edema and a rise in intracranial pressure. This is turn causes the symptoms of AMS and is shown in Figure 18.3 on the right of the diagram. Another possibility, referred to above, is that the higher P_{CO_2} and lower P_{O_2} would cause peripheral vasodilatation which, by lowering central venous pressure, would lower the level of ANP and result in an antidiuresis. Cerebral blood flow is increased on going to altitude and falls towards sea level values with acclimatization (Severinghaus *et al.* 1966b). One study, which confirmed this general pattern, found no difference in cerebral blood flow between subjects with and without AMS symptoms (Jensen *et al.* 1990). However, two more recent studies (Baumgartner *et al.* 1994, Jansen *et al.* 1999), using velocity in the middle cerebral artery measured by Doppler ultrasound, have shown greater increase on going to altitude in subjects with AMS than in nonsymptomatic controls. The Sa_{O_2} was lower in AMS subjects and accounted for much of the difference in flow. However, Jansen *et al.* (1999) showed that AMS subjects had greater response in flow to changes in P_{CO_2} (voluntary hyperventilation) than controls, suggesting brisker vasomotor response in these susceptible individuals.

18.5.3 Intracranial pressure and AMS

There is a striking similarity of symptoms between AMS and the effects of high intracranial pressure due to cerebral tumors, etc. The evidence for raised intracranial pressure in AMS is:

- The CSF pressure was found to be elevated by 60–210 mm H_2O during AMS compared with that after recovery (Singh *et al.* 1969b).
- In cases of malignant cerebral AMS, papilledema has been noted (Dickinson 1979).
- In those dying with cerebral AMS, cerebral edema with flattening of the cerebral convolutions has been found (Singh *et al.* 1969b, Dickinson *et al.* 1983).
- Computerized tomographic examination of the brain in patients with HACE showed diffuse low

density areas in the cerebrum representing edema (Fukushima *et al.* 1983).

- Direct measurement has been made in one unreported study (B. H. Cummings, personal communication). One of three subjects with pressure transducers implanted in their skulls before a Himalayan expedition was mountain sick on return from 5700 m to Base Camp at 4750 m. His intracranial pressure was normal at rest but elevated on the slightest exertion. Other subjects without AMS had normal pressures even on exercise.

- Using an indirect measure of intracranial pressure (tympanic membrane displacement) exposure to acute hypoxia at 3440 m was associated with a rise in pressure. However, on going to 4120 m and 5200 m the pressure returned to sea level values. There was no correlation between intracranial pressure and AMS scores (Wright *et al.*1995).

Despite the lack of good direct evidence, the consensus view seems to be that the symptoms of AMS are best explained as being due to cerebral edema and raised intracranial pressure (Hackett 1999). This is further considered in Chapter 20, where other factors that may be involved in the mechanism of cerebral edema are discussed.

18.5.4 Derangement of clotting mechanism

In reports on necropsy material, the presence of thromboses in lungs and brain figures prominently. No doubt parts of the pathological picture are secondary, such as the development of hyaline membrane in the alveoli and possibly some thrombi, but there is evidence of alterations in coagulation associated with altitude (Singh and Chohan 1972b). It has been suggested that thrombosis may form a basis for the development of both pulmonary hypertension and edema (Dickinson *et al.* 1983). However, Hyers *et al.* (1979) were unable to show differences in activated coagulation between those who are susceptible to pulmonary edema and more normal individuals at altitude.

Bärtsch *et al.* (1987) studied a range of clotting factors in 66 subjects presenting at the Capanna Margherita (4559 m) with varying degrees of AMS. They found that coagulation time, euglobulin lysis time and fibrin(ogen) fragment E were normal in all subject groups. Fibrinopeptide A (FPA), a molecular marker of *in vivo* fibrin formation, was elevated in patients with HAPE. However, FPA was not elevated in subjects with simple AMS even with widened $(A–a)O_2$, suggesting early HAPE. They conclude that the fibrin formation which takes place in HAPE is an epiphenomenon and not causative.

18.5.5 Microvascular permeability and AMS

Hypoxia may increase microvascular permeability directly or via mediators. Numerous animal studies have shown that hypoxia increases lymph flow with variable results on the lymph/plasma ratio for protein. The problem is to separate hemodynamic effects from permeability itself. Staub (1986) has reviewed the effect of hypoxia on microvascular permeability and concludes that, 'On best analysis . . . the change in permeability is slight, albeit statistically significant'.

However, there is no really good animal model and the failure to show an important change in an animal which does not get HAPE in no way excludes the importance of permeability changes in humans. Three findings have served to strengthen the evidence for some effect of hypoxia on microvascular permeability:

- Larsen *et al.* (1985) have shown in rabbits that neither hypoxia alone nor the infusion of cobra venom (which activates the complement system) alone caused pulmonary edema. However, the two insults together did cause permeability-type pulmonary edema. This suggests the possibility that hypoxia, with some other factor, may increase microvascular permeability.

- Schoene *et al.* (1986) and Hackett *et al.* (1986), by analysing bronchoalveolar lavage and pulmonary edema fluid respectively, have shown conclusively that in HAPE the edema is of the high protein permeability type rather than hemodynamic. They also found significant levels of leukotriene B4 and factors chemotactic for monocytes in the lavage fluid, suggesting that the release of these and other mediators of inflammation may be involved in the mechanism of HAPE.

- Richalet *et al.* (1991) found a rise in plasma levels of most of the six eicosanoids measured in subjects taken abruptly to the Vallot observatory on Mont Blanc (4350 m). All subjects had AMS. The levels of these vasoactive mediators affecting permeability had a time course parallel to that of AMS symptoms.

- Roach *et al.* (1996) measured urinary leukotriene E4 in subjects taken to 4300 m with a 4-day stopover at 1830 m. There was a significant increase in levels of urinary leukotriene though the correlation with AMS did not reach significance. The authors conclude that leukotrienes may be involved in the genesis of AMS.

Most of these studies have concentrated on the pulmonary microvascular permeability but the same mechanism could affect microvascular permeability generally, including cerebral microvessels and thus contribute to cerebral edema as shown in Figure 18.3 (center). Hypoxia has been shown to increase permeability of endothelial monolayers to a range of proteins *in vitro,* though quite severe hypoxia (12–19 mm Hg) and incubation for 48–72 h were needed to show the effect (Gerlach *et al.* 1992).

Proteinuria is also common during the first few days at altitude, especially in subjects with AMS (Chapter 15), and this may be due to increased microvascular permeability in the kidneys (Winterborn *et al.* 1986). If increased permeability has a role in AMS there is the question of whether it initiates or continues the process. Kleger *et al.* (1996) investigated this by measuring the escape rate of $[^{125}I]$-labeled albumin as well as various cytokines in the plasma of 24 subjects taken rapidly to 4559 m altitude. Ten subjects developed AMS and four HAPE. The authors found no significant increase in albumin escape in any group of subjects. The only significant increase in cytokine levels was in the HAPE patients and that was of IL-6 on days 2 and 3 at altitude when HAPE was established. Swenson *et al.* (1997) measured a number of cytokines in the plasma of 19 subjects exposed to 10 per cent oxygen for 8 h. They found no change in the concentration of the measured cytokines by the end of the exposure time. These findings suggest that if cytokines do play a role in AMS it is probably in the development of the illness towards HAPE or HACE. In Chapter 19 there is further consideration of mechanisms in relation to HAPE, some of which may also apply to benign AMS.

18.5.6 Anorexia, leptin and AMS

Leptin, a recently discovered hormone, produces the sensation of satiety and is thought to be important in body weight regulation. Tschop *et al.* (1998) measured its level in subjects in two field studies at the Capanna Margherita (4559 m). They found it to be elevated at altitude compared with sea level and to be higher in subjects with AMS than in those without. The neuropeptide cholecystokinin (CCK) also suppresses the appetite. Bailey *et al.* (2000) found it to be increased in plasma from subjects with AMS compared with subjects free of symptoms on the Kangchenjunga Medical Expedition 1998.

18.6 PROPHYLAXIS

AMS only occurs during the first few days at a given altitude. It seems, therefore, that acclimatization in some way confers protection from AMS. Allowing time for acclimatization is therefore the best way to prevent AMS. There is an impression that there are limits to acclimatization which vary for different individuals. At altitudes above this limit a person is therefore at risk of AMS, HAPE and HACE even after acclimatization to lower altitudes has been achieved.

18.6.1 Rate of ascent

A slow rate of ascent will prevent AMS but, because of the great variation in susceptibility to AMS, it is not possible to be dogmatic in advice on rate of ascent. A suggested rule of thumb is that, above 3000 m, each night should be spent not more than 300 m above the last, with a rest day (i.e. 2 nights at the same altitude) every 2–3 days. In addition, anyone who experiences symptoms of AMS should go no higher until they improve. It is not certain where the rule originated, possibly from the epidemiological study of trekkers on the route to Everest Base Camp (Hackett *et al.* 1976). Recently Murdoch (1999) has looked for evidence of its efficiency in preventing AMS in the same area. He surveyed 283 trekkers, asking about AMS symptoms and speed of ascent. There are two clear messages from this study:

- Firstly, that there is huge individual variation in susceptibility. Half the trekkers ascending at the very low mean rate of 100–200 m/day became sick whereas almost half the trekkers ascending at 500–600 m/day remained free of AMS. Obviously there was a process of self-selection, with those feeling fine going fast and those feeling less well going slowly.

- Secondly, that, overall, the incidence of AMS was higher the faster trekkers ascended.

Murdoch's conclusion is that, although the rule is slower than is really necessary for many, if not most, trekkers, it should continue to be the guideline, in the interest of a substantial minority. Basnyat et al. (1999) also found evidence from their questionnaire survey of the same trekking route that rate of ascent was an important risk factor. AMS risk decreased by 19 per cent for each additional day spent between the airstrip at Lukla (2804 m) and the place of survey, Pheriche (4243 m).

18.6.2   Fluid intake

Trek leaders often urge their clients to drink plenty as they gain altitude in order to avoid AMS. There seems no good scientific reason for this advice. Providing enough fluid is taken to avoid dehydration, further intake will only be excreted. However, there is a recent epidemiological study that appears to lend some support for this practice. Basnyat et al. (1999) gave questionnaires to Everest Base Camp trekkers at Pheriche (4243 m) and found that 30 per cent of them had AMS. They asked about daily fluid intake and found that the higher the intake (up to 5 L/day) the lower the incidence of AMS (odds ratio 1.54). But in the only controlled trial to address this issue, Aoki and Robinson (1971) found that there was no effect of hydration on AMS incidence. They achieved dehydration by treatment of one group with furosemide, and hyperhydration in another with vasopressin; a third group was given a placebo. All groups were decompressed at the same rate in a chamber. Clearly more work is needed to answer this question.

18.6.3   Drugs for prophylaxis

ACETAZOLAMIDE

Cain and Dunn (1965) were the first to show that acetazolamide (Diamox) increases ventilation and

Pa_{O_2}, and decreases Pa_{CO_2}. It has been shown to reduce the incidence and severity of AMS in a number of double-blind controlled trials in the field (Forwand et al. 1968, Birmingham Medical Research Group 1981, Larsen et al. 1982). All symptoms are improved, as well as general performance, as judged by peer review. Sleep was improved and the profound desaturation associated with periodic breathing (Chapter 13) was relieved (Sutton et al. 1979). Acetazolamide has been shown to prevent patients with asthma from developing AMS (Mirrakhimov et al. 1993). In these trials, the dose was 250 mg orally 8 hourly, started 1 day before ascent, except in the Birmingham trial where the dose was one 500 mg slow release tablet daily. This dose, or 250 mg normal release twice daily (which is cheaper), used to be the recommended regimen. More recently many are recommending half that dose morning and evening since it is believed that protection is adequate and side effects are fewer. However, although this may well be true, there are as yet no trials to support this recommendation. Treatment should be started 24–48 h before ascent to altitude.

The duration of treatment depends on the circumstance and situation. In many treks, the exposure to conditions when AMS may be a problem is limited to a few days and obviously treatment can be discontinued when the party has descended from altitude. In situations where subjects go to altitude and stay there, the risk of AMS is limited to the first 4–5 days so that treatment could reasonably be stopped after that.

However, a study by the Birmingham group (Bradwell et al. 1986) has shown that taking acetazolamide for 3 weeks at 4846 m conferred a benefit in that the group on treatment lost less weight, lost less muscle bulk and had superior exercise performance than those on placebo. Here the drug was being used not so much to prevent AMS as to reduce altitude deterioration.

The side effects of acetazolamide consist of a mild diuresis and paresthesiae in the hands and feet, which tend to diminish with continued use of the drug. A few people find this tingling very disturbing; some are troubled by gastric side effects. Also, fizzy drinks taste flat; this is due to the inhibition of carbonic anhydrase in the tongue so that the conversion of carbon dioxide to carbonic acid fails to take place in the time available as the drink passes over the tongue, and the acid-sensing buds are not stimulated. The safety of acetazolamide is assured by its widespread use in glaucoma where it is used for years at doses similar to that recommended for AMS prophylaxis.

The ethics of the use of acetazolamide (or that of any drug), especially if used throughout an expedition, need consideration but in the end it is for the individual or team to decide.

The mechanism of action of acetazolamide is thought to be due to its inhibition of carbonic anhydrase rather than its diuretic action. It is quite a mild diuretic and more powerful diuretics are said to be less effective though no direct comparisons have been made in controlled trials. Interference with carbon dioxide transport is thought to result in intracellular acidosis, including the cells of the medullary chemoreceptor. In this way it acts as a respiratory stimulant. It has been shown to shift the ventilatory carbon dioxide response curve to the left, as happens with acclimatization (section 5.12), although it does not affect the slope. The acute effect after a single dose results in a reduction in the hypoxic ventilatory response, though with a few hours administration this is restored (Swenson and Hughes 1993).

It probably also acts as a respiratory stimulant by promoting the excretion of bicarbonate by the kidneys, thus correcting the respiratory alkalosis due to hypoxic-induced hyperventilation. In effect the subject is given an artificial respiratory acclimatization. The importance of this renal effect is suggested by Swenson et al. (1991) in a study in which the drug benzolamide, a selective inhibitor of renal carbonic anhydrase, reduced high altitude periodic breathing, a feature of acetazolamide use. A recent trial of benzolamide as a prophylactic for AMS (Collier et al. 1997a) showed it to be beneficial compared with placebo, suggesting that inhibition of cerebral carbonic anhydrase may not be the important action of acetazolamide.

Another possible mechanism is via its effect on cerebral blood flow (Vorstrup et al. 1984). Acetazolamide increases cerebral blood flow, which would increase cerebral P_{O_2}. However, increased P_{CO_2}, which has the same effect on cerebral blood flow, seems to increase the symptoms of AMS at the same level of hypoxia (section 18.5.2). Additionally, the dosage used in this study (1 g i.v.) was very large compared with that used in AMS prophylaxis. Jensen et al. (1990) found that, although 1.5 g acetazolamide caused a 22 per cent increase in cerebral blood flow

after 2 h, there was no change in AMS symptoms. Also Hackett et al. (1988a) found no change in cerebral blood flow (as measured by transcranial Doppler ultrasound) in subjects with or without AMS after 0.25 g acetazolamide intravenously.

SPIRONOLACTONE

Jain et al. (1986) compared spironolactone with acetazolamide and placebo. They found both drugs to be effective in ameliorating AMS, with spironolactone being possibly superior. This confirms a previous uncontrolled report (Currie et al. 1976).

DEXAMETHASONE AND ASPIRIN

Dexamethasone (4 mg 6 hourly) has been tried on the grounds that it is effective in cerebral edema. In a double-blind crossover chamber study it was found to be an effective prophylactic (Johnson et al. 1984) and was found to be superior when compared with acetazolamide (Ellsworth et al. 1991). Rock et al. (1989) carried out a dose ranging chamber experiment and concluded that 4 mg 12 hourly was the minimum effective dose. The same group had previously found that, if dexamethasone was given for only 48 h after arrival at altitude, it was effective in reducing symptoms, but that after stopping the drug, symptoms of AMS began (Rock et al. 1989). The combination of acetazolamide and dexamethasone has been shown to be more effective than acetazolamide alone, especially in preventing the cerebral symptoms of AMS (Bernhard et al. 1998). Aspirin has been shown to be similarly effective as a prophylactic (Burtscher et al. 1998) but, like dexamethasone, does not affect oxygen saturation. A later study (Burtscher et al. 1999) found that aspirin alone was not very effective in preventing the headache of AMS in subjects skiing to a mountain hut, whereas aspirin in combination with dexamethasone was. There was no placebo arm in this trial.

NIFEDIPINE

Nifedipine has been shown to be beneficial for both treatment and prophylaxis of HAPE (sections 19.3.1, 19.3.2) so Hohenhaus et al. (1994) carried out a double-blind placebo-controlled trial of its use in benign AMS. They found that, even though pulmonary artery pressure was lower in the drug group, there was no effect on AMS scores.

OTHER DRUGS

Theophylline (300 mg) has been shown to be beneficial as a prophylactic in a placebo-controlled double-blind trial by Kuepper *et al.* (1999). This drug also reduces sleep disturbance and periodic breathing.

Herbal extracts have been advocated both as preventative and curative for AMS. As is usual in herbal medicine there are few good trials to guide us. However, some remedies have now been tested. An extract of *Ginko biloba* (EGb 761) was studied by Roncin *et al.* (1996) in a placebo-controlled trial and found to be very effective as a prophylactic. Coca, from the coca leaf, is very commonly taken in South America either infused as a tea or chewed. Many people are convinced of its efficacy in preventing AMS but there seem to be no trials to confirm this.

18.7 TREATMENT

Most cases of AMS will get better in 24–48 h with no treatment. If there is progression of symptoms to those of acute pulmonary edema, or serious cerebral edema, action is vital since these two disorders are frequently fatal in a matter of hours. Their treatment is discussed in Chapters 19 and 20 respectively.

18.7.1 Rest, acetazolamide

Rest alone often relieves the symptoms of AMS (Bärtsch *et al.* 1993), and this fact needs to be borne in mind in trials of therapy in AMS. Acetazolamide had been shown to be an effective treatment of AMS as well as a prophylactic (Bradwell *et al.* 1988, Grissom *et al.* 1992). The earlier study used a single large dose (1.5 g) whereas the later study used the more conventional 250 mg 8 hourly. Pa_{O_2} as well as symptoms were improved.

Dexamethasone was shown, in a double-blind trial, to be effective as an emergency treatment for acute AMS (Ferrazzini *et al.* 1987). The dosage used was 8 mg initially followed by 4 mg every 6 h. Levine *et al.* (1989) also found it to be effective in relieving AMS symptoms compared with placebo but it had no effect on fluid shifts, oxygenation, sleep apnea, urinary catecholamine levels, chest radiographs or perfusion scans. These findings emphasize the dictum that, in the event of HAPE or HACE, patients should be taken to lower altitude as soon as possible.

18.7.2 Aspirin, paracetamol, nonsteroidal anti-inflammatory agents, dexamethasone

For the headache of AMS, aspirin or paracetamol is often used but there are no controlled trials and they are often ineffective. A double-blind, placebo-controlled trial of ibuprofen (400 mg) showed it to be more effective than placebo in relieving headache (Broom *et al.* 1994). Keller *et al.* (1995) carried out a trial comparing dexamethasone with hyperbaria (in a Certec bag) for 1 h. Assessment 1 h after treatment found hyperbaria to be better but at 11 h dexamethasone was more effective.

18.7.3 Other drugs

SUMATRIPTAN

The possibility that the headache in AMS and in migraine might have a common mechanism stimulated a group from Heidelberg to carry out a placebo-controlled trial of sumatriptan, a 5HT antagonist effective in migraine. Although the pooled results failed to show significant benefit, analysis of male and female subjects separately showed significant benefit in men (Utiger *et al.* 1999).

18.7.4 Oxygen

Oxygen may help, but frequently does not, and its use, besides being impractical in most cases, would impede acclimatization. Voluntary hyperventilation often helps and probably does promote acclimatization. Inhalation of 3 per cent carbon dioxide in air has been claimed to alleviate symptoms in one study (Harvey *et al.* 1988) but not in another (Bärtsch *et al.* 1990). Both found a rise in Pa_{O_2}, due presumably to hyperventilation. In the latter study most subjects given air to breathe had a reduction in symptoms, indicating the importance of the placebo effect or perhaps the beneficial effect of rest.

The place of portable inflatable pressure chambers (the Gamow bag) is considered in Chapter 19.

Table 18.3 *Lake Louise consensus: scoring of AMS*

(a) AMS self-assessment. The sum of the responses is the AMS self-report score. Headache and at least one other symptom must be present for the diagnosis of AMS. A score of 3 or more is taken as AMS. It is suggested that this part of the scoring system be always used and reported separately. The question relating to sleep will not always be relevant, e.g. in short 1-day studies or in evening assessment when twice-daily scoring is used.

Symptom	Scoring
Headache	0 None at all
	1 Mild headache
	2 Moderate headache
	3 Severe headache, incapacitating
Gastrointestinal symptoms	0 Good appetite
	1 Poor appetite or nausea
	2 Moderate nausea or vomiting
	3 Severe, incapacitating nausea and vomiting
Fatigue and/or weakness	0 Not tired or weak
	1 Mild fatigue/weakness
	2 Moderate fatigue/weakness
	3 Severe fatigue/weakness
Dizziness/light-headedness	0 None
	1 Mild
	2 Moderate
	3 Severe, incapacitating
Difficulty sleeping	0 Slept as well as usual
	1 Did not sleep as well as usual
	2 Woke many times, poor night's sleep
	3 Could not sleep at all

(b) Clinical assessment. This portion of the scoring system contains information gained by examination. The clinical assessment score is the sum of scores in the following three questions.

Sign	Scoring
Change in mental status	0 No change
	1 Lethargy/lassitude
	2 Disorientated/confused
	3 Stupor/semiconscious
	4 Coma
Ataxia (heel/toe walking)	0 None
	1 Balancing maneuvers
	2 Steps off the line
	3 Falls down
	4 Unable to stand
Peripheral edema	0 None
	1 One location
	2 Two or more locations

(c) Functional score. The functional consequences of the AMS self-reported score should be further evaluated by one optional question asked after the AMS self-report questionnaire. Alternatively, this question may be asked by the examiner if clinical assessment is performed.

Overall, if you had any of these symptoms, how did they affect your activities?	0 Not at all
	1 Mild reduction
	2 Moderate reduction
	3 Severe reduction (e.g. bedrest)

Source: after Roach *et al.* (1993).

18.8 SCORING AMS SYMPTOMS

In studies on AMS there is obviously a need to score the symptoms in some way and it is preferable for all researchers to use the same system so that results of different studies can be compared. The most complicated scoring system is the Environmental Symptom Questionnaire (ESQ) (Sampson *et al.* 1983). This consists of 67 questions in its ESQ-III version, many of which are overlapping and of uncertain relevance to AMS. Most workers have used more simple formats, scoring only three to five symptoms often on a 0–3 scale, with 0 for no symptoms and 1, 2 and 3 for mild, moderate and severe symptoms. Either an observer can administer the questionnaire to all subjects or self-assessment by each subject can be used; the two methods give similar results. A document was produced at the Lake Louise Hypoxia Symposium in 1991, which, after defining AMS, suggested a simple method of scoring along these lines. This was modified at the next Hypoxia Symposium in 1993 and is shown in Table 18.3 (Roach *et al.* 1993). It is important to note that one of the modifications introduced was the caveat that headache must be present for the diagnosis, as well as at least one other of the symptoms listed. The importance of insisting that headache is present for the diagnosis is illustrated by a paper comparing a previous system (Hackett's) with the Lake Louise system (Röggla *et al.* 1996). It was found that the Lake Louise system gave a spuriously high incidence, 25 per cent, compared with 8 per cent using the Hackett system, at the moderate altitude of 2940 m. Unfortunately the authors used the earlier 1991 version. Only 9 per cent of their subjects had headache. Had they excluded from the diagnosis subjects without headache, the two systems would have given almost identical results.

There have been a number of studies comparing the ESQ with the Lake Louise system. Bärtsch *et al.* (1993) did just this and found the percentages of subjects diagnosed as having AMS in alpine huts at four altitudes were comparable whichever system was used. Maggiorini *et al.* (1998) applied questionnaires to 490 climbers in alpine huts up to 4559 m. Using a Lake Louise score of 4 or more as the cut-off, they found a sensitivity of 78 per cent and specificity of 93 per cent compared with the ESQ AMS-C. Ellsworth *et al.* (1991) found similar results in 400 climbers on Mount Rainier in Washington State, USA. The Lake Louise system, being much simpler, is therefore to be preferred.

There remains the question of the score at which AMS is said to be present. On the self-report section, five questions yield a possible top score of 15. The consensus report suggests a score of 3 or more (with headache) be deemed AMS, though from the study quoted above a score of 4 or more seemed to give better sensitivity and specificity. It is not clear what is to be done with the other two parts of the assessment, the clinical and functional scores, if they are used. Clearly if these scores are added to the self-reported scores a greater cut-off value would be appropriate. Bärtsch *et al.* (1993) suggested a figure of >5 for the total Lake Louise score. We would suggest that, until more data are available on the other parts of the assessment, reliance be placed mainly on the self-reported score, which has been well validated.

These systems have all addressed the situation in adults. The diagnosis of AMS in children presents especial problems. Children too young to express their symptoms verbally may be irritable, miserable or tearful and refuse food. This behavior is even more nonspecific than symptoms in adults. The only safe course is to assume that this behavior in a child who has gained altitude in the previous hours or days indicates AMS until proved otherwise. Yaron *et al.* (1998) have addressed the problem of scoring AMS in preverbal children, and devised a 'fussiness' scale derived from the Lake Louise system. For more details of this see Chapter 28.

19

High altitude pulmonary edema

SUMMARY

High altitude pulmonary edema (HAPE) is a potentially lethal form of acute mountain sickness (AMS) which, like AMS, affects previously healthy people who go rapidly to high altitude. A few hours after arrival the patient suffers the usual symptoms of AMS but then becomes more breathless than his companions. Over the next few hours the breathlessness increases, and a cough develops which is first dry but later productive of frothy white sputum. The sputum may become blood tinged. The signs of obvious pulmonary edema are found and cyanosis may be detected. As the patient literally drowns in his own secretions, he becomes comatose and dies if no action is taken. Investigations show raised pulse and respiratory rates, mild pyrexia and leukocytosis and a characteristic radiographic appearance. The pathology, in fatal cases, is of patchy hemorrhagic edema of the lungs.

The most important management is to get the patient down; if there is unavoidable delay, oxygen and calcium channel blocking drugs are helpful. Hyperbaric treatment in a Gamow (or Certec) bag gives temporary relief and may be useful in enabling a patient to walk down rather than having to be carried.

The mechanism of the edema formation is not left ventricular failure, as shown by normal wedge pressures on cardiac catheterization. However, there is severe pulmonary hypertension. There are a number of hypotheses about how this results in edema.

The most favored mechanism is that the hypoxic vasoconstriction is uneven, causing some areas to have less and some more blood flow. The hyperperfused areas have raised capillary pressure and suffer stress failure of these vessels allowing proteins and later blood cells to leak out into the interstitial space and then alveolar spaces. There is also evidence of inflammation; cytokines and arachidonic acid metabolites are found in the edema fluid, and these contribute to the vascular leakage. Exercise seems to be a risk factor, presumably by raising the pulmonary artery pressure.

Many patients who suffer HAPE show susceptibility to the condition on subsequent altitude exposure. These subjects are found to have a brisk hypoxic pressor response in their pulmonary circulation and it is thought that this susceptibility may have a genetic origin.

19.1 INTRODUCTION

There are a number of accounts of climbers dying of 'pneumonia' in early climbing literature. In retrospect it seems that many, if not most, of these fatalities were probably due to HAPE. One of the best known was the death of Dr Jacottet on Mont Blanc in 1891. He died in the Vallot hut (4300 m) after taking part in a rescue on the mountain. He spent 2 nights in the hut with obvious symptoms of AMS, refusing to go down. He died during the second night. The autopsy showed 'acute edema of the lung' (oedème considerable) (Mosso 1898, p. 179).

In 1913, Ravenhill described what he called 'puna' of the cardiac type as a lethal form or development of AMS. Though he was wrong in attributing the condition to cardiac failure, his description of three cases fits well with HAPE. However, his work was forgotten.

For the first half of the twentieth century the condition was uncommon in the European Alps because few unacclimatized people spent nights above 2500 m, or in the Himalayas because approach marches to the mountains were long enough for acclimatization to take place. But in South America, as Ravenhill's experience showed, railways had been built and later roads to altitudes up to 3000 or 4000 m, thus putting large numbers of people at risk. However, even in these countries the condition does not seem to have been recognized for many years after Ravenhill. West (1998, pp. 146–54) has unearthed a description of a case reported by Alberto Hurtado in 1937 in an obscure booklet. But the case is atypical in a number of ways and Hurtado says (in translation from the Spanish)

> this is undoubtedly a type of Soroche (mountain sickness) which is quite rare and infrequent and is characterized by of intense congestion and edema of the lung. Possibly in these cases there is a prior cardiac condition . . .

and this case did seem to have further long-term problems suggestive of a cardiac condition. Although this could be considered as the first case report of HAPE after Ravenhill, there was mention of some cases of soroche who had cough with frothy pink sputum and who made a rapid recovery on descent to low altitude. This was in an article by Harold Crane, the chief surgeon of the hospital at the mining town of Oroya (3750 m) in Peru. The article was published in the *Annals of the Faculty of Medicine*, Lima, in 1927. The first series of cases to be published was by Leoncio Lizárraga Morla in 1955 in the same journal. He mentioned that the condition was recognized by Carlos Monge M. as early as 1927. The seven cases described were typical of HAPE and included chest radiographs and electrocardiograms (ECGs) typical of HAPE. This paper was followed by others, including by Bardáles, from Peru in the later 1950s. The first reference in English to the condition we now call HAPE was in a letter to the *Journal of the American Medical Association* by Bardáles in 1956. In it he describes the condition briefly in high altitude residents returning to altitude, saying it is particularly common in young people. For a fuller description of these papers and the full references, see West (1998, pp. 146–54).

An interesting sidelight showing the situation in the English-speaking world in the mid 1950s is given by a letter to Dr Griffith Pugh which he published with a comment in *The Practitioner* (Pugh 1955a). Dr Pugh was the leading authority on altitude medicine and physiology in the UK at the time. The letter gave an excellent account of a fatal case of HAPE and asked whether acute pulmonary edema is a common symptom of high altitude sickness. Pugh, in his response, indicates that he knew of no such case from his experience or from the literature. The original letter and response together with a commentary are to be found in West (1999b).

Herbert Hultgren visited Peru in 1959 and saw cases of HAPE. He and his companion, Spickard, wrote up their experiences in the *Stanford Medical Bulletin* published in May 1960 under the title, 'Medical experiences in Peru'. In it they mention 41 cases of acute pulmonary edema in residents returning to altitude after a stay of 5–21 days at low altitude. They correctly suggested that the mechanism was not left ventricular failure but related to pulmonary hypertension. Not surprisingly this important observation was not recognized at the time and so the condition was brought to the notice of the English-speaking medical world by Houston (1960) who published his landmark paper on 'acute pulmonary edema of high altitude' later in the same year in the *New England Journal of Medicine*. Houston said 'this single case is presented in the hope of stimulating further reports' and 'pulmonary edema of high altitude deserves further study'. Both hope and declaration have been amply fulfilled in the succeeding years by the description of hundreds of cases from all the major mountainous areas and hundreds of studies aimed at elucidating the mechanism of the condition have been conducted, some of which will be reviewed in this chapter.

19.2 CLINICAL PRESENTATION

HAPE, like AMS, affects previously healthy individuals on ascent to altitude. There is a wide range of altitude of presentation of 2000–7000 m (Lobenhoffer *et al.* 1982). A typical history is that the subject ascends rapidly to altitude and is very active getting there or on arrival. The subject suffers the symptoms of AMS after arrival, though not necessarily very severely, and then becomes more short of breath and lethargic and may have chest pain. Physical signs are of tachycardia, tachypnea and crackles at the lung bases. A dry cough develops, which later progresses to one productive of frothy white sputum and eventually blood tinged sputum. Over a few hours the condition progresses with increasing respiratory distress, orthopnea, cyanosis, bubbling respirations, coma and death.

19.2.1 Case histories

CASE 1 (HOUSTON 1960)

A male patient left sea level on 18 June, reaching 16 700 ft (5090 m) by car and on foot 5 days later. He had no symptoms until 1 day later when he noted dyspnea progressing to severe orthopnea. Within a few hours his breathing became progressively more congested and labored. He sounded as though he was literally drowning in his own fluid with an almost continuous loud bubbling sound as if breathing through liquid. A white froth resembling cotton candy appeared to well up out of his mouth, which was open. This was even though he was sitting up with his head tilted back. The patient died within 8 h of the onset of symptoms.

CASE 2

A Sherpa on a large expedition had carried a load from 6400 m to 7000 m and returned. The following morning he complained of severe headache and malaise. He was anorexic and remained in his sleeping bag. On examination at mid-morning he was found to be breathless on the slightest exertion, cyanosed and had a dry cough. The pulse and respiratory rate were increased. Fine crackles were heard at the lung bases. At noon he started down for a lower camp at 5800 m accompanied by two expedition members. It was at once apparent that he could not carry even a light load. Every 100–200 yards (90–180 m) he had to stop, even though the route was over an easy downhill glacier. He began coughing frothy white sputum, which later became blood

tinged. At about 100 m above the camp he was given oxygen and was able to complete the journey without stopping. After breathing oxygen for about 3 h at the camp he declared himself well and refused any more oxygen. He descended unaided to a lower camp next day, carrying a load.

19.2.2 Incidence

It is difficult to obtain data on incidence of HAPE because of the problem of knowing the number of people at risk. As with AMS it will depend upon the rate of ascent and the height reached. Hackett and Rennie (1976) saw seven cases in 278 trekkers who passed through Pheriche (4243 m) on their way to Everest Base Camp, giving an incidence of 2.5 per cent. The incidence of AMS in the same group was 53 per cent. Menon (1965) found an incidence of 0.57 per cent in Indian troops flown to the modest altitude of Leh (3500 m). Hultgren and Marticorena (1978) gave an incidence of 0.6 per cent in adults going to La Oroya (3750 m) in Peru. In these series a diagnosis was only made in clear, overt cases. If the chests of all newcomers to altitude are auscultated, crackles will be heard in many who would not be otherwise diagnosed as having HAPE, and radiographic signs are also found on chest radiography in many subjects. Hence we now believe that a degree of subclinical edema is probably present commonly in subjects with simple AMS and contributes to the reduced Sa_{O_2} found at this time (section 18.4.8). However, in simple AMS the edema is self-limiting whereas in HAPE it is progressive.

The incidence will be affected by health education of people going to altitude. It is the impression of health workers at the aid post at Pheriche (4243 m) in Nepal that the incidence is less following some years of publicity about the dangers of HAPE amongst trekkers and the trekking agencies.

19.2.3 Symptoms of HAPE

Table 19.1 shows the symptoms from the largest series managed by a single physician, that of Menon (1965), who reported 101 cases. The frequency of chest pain, second only to breathlessness, is unusually high. Only 21 per cent of patients complained of

Table 19.1 *HAPE: symptoms in 101 cases*

Symptom	No. of cases
Breathlessness	84
Chest pain	66
Headache	63
Nocturnal dyspnea	59
Dry cough	51
Haemoptysis	39
Nausea	26
Insomnia	23
Dizziness	18

Source: after Menon (1965).

chest pain in a German series (Lobenhoffer *et al.* 1982). Hallucinations are not uncommon and, with confusion and irrational behavior, may make management difficult. Nocturnal dyspnea and the symptoms of AMS – headache, nausea and insomnia – are all common.

19.2.4   Signs

The signs depend upon the stage of the condition. Probably the earliest sign is of crackles at the lung bases. These may be heard in subjects with no other signs of HAPE and who do not progress to the full blown condition. The presence of early edema may be the cause of dry cough on exertion and of the shift to the left of the pressure/volume curve of the lung (Mansell *et al.* 1980, Gautier *et al.* 1982) and the reduction in forced vital capacity (Welsh *et al.* 1993). The pulse rate increases early and was over 120 in 70 of 101 patients in Menon's series (1965). The respiratory rate was over 30 in 69 cases; cyanosis was detected in 52 subjects. The pulmonary artery pressure is high in this condition (section 19.2.7) giving the signs of right ventricular heave and accentuated pulmonary second sound in about half the patients. Signs of right ventricular failure are not prominent but 15 of Menon's patients had raised jugular venous pressure and dependent edema is found in a number of cases. The temperature is normal in at least 25 per cent of cases but was found to be mildly elevated (37–39 °C) in 70 per cent of Menon's cases. In only two cases was it above 39 °C. Maggiorini *et al.* (1997) found temperature to be elevated by a mean of

0.8 °C compared with climbers without HAPE. The systemic blood pressure is either normal or mildly elevated (systolic 130–140 mm Hg) as is found in some subjects on ascent to altitude who do not have HAPE.

Some subjects (15 in Menon's series) have mental confusion and amnesia following recovery. This may be due to hypoxia or cerebral edema (Chapter 20).

19.2.5   Radiology

Figure 19.1 shows a chest radiograph of a patient with HAPE and a second radiograph 4 days later after treatment. The typical features are of cotton-wool blotches irregularly positioned in both lung fields. They are frequently asymmetrical, possibly being denser on the side which has been dependent. Very often, the right side is more densely shadowed (Menon 1965). Quite frequently, the lower zones, especially the costophrenic angles, are spared as well as the apices. The pulmonary vessels may be seen to be engorged (Marticorena *et al.* 1964). The radiographic appearance in early cases shows more pathology than would be expected from clinical examination (Menon 1965). In patients with a second attack of HAPE there is no consistent pattern in the areas of lung involved. This patchy distribution of edema is even more dramatically shown in computerized tomographic scanning of the chest.

In treated cases the radiographic lesions clear rapidly (see Figure 19.1), often within 2 days (Houston 1960), though usually lagging behind symptoms.

19.2.6   Investigations

ELECTROCARDIOGRAPHY

The ECG shows tachycardia. The P waves are often peaked (P pulmonale) and there is right axis deviation of the AQRS (mean +123 °). Some patients show elevation of the S–T segment (Marticorena *et al.* 1964). T-waves may be inverted in the precordial leads but this may be seen in asymptomatic subjects at altitude (Milledge 1963). The ECG appearances can be attributed to the very high pulmonary artery pressure and the consequent increase in right ventricular work.

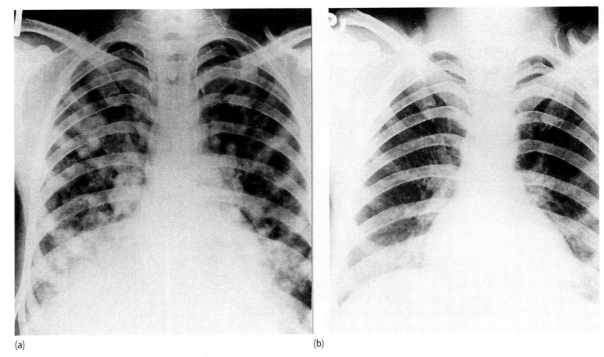

(a) (b)

Figure 19.1 *Radiograph of a patient with high altitude pulmonary edema: (a) on admission and (b) 4 days later. (Reproduced with permission of Dr T. Norboo of Leh, Jammu and Kashmir, India.)*

HEMATOLOGY

Menon (1965) found that hemoglobin concentration was 14.0–16.0 g dL^{-1} and the sedimentation rate was normal. The white cell count was raised in 75 of 95 cases. This elevation was due to an increase in neutrophil count.

BLOOD GASES

P_{O_2} and arterial oxygen saturation are low compared with normal values for that altitude. P_{CO_2} is very variable and is not significantly different from controls (Antezana *et al.* 1982, Schoene *et al.* 1985).

URINE

Proteinuria was present in 4 of 101 cases (Menon 1965), but using more sensitive tests there was an increase in urine protein in all subjects during the first few days at altitude, the degree of proteinuria correlating with the severity of AMS (Pines 1978; Chapter 15).

19.2.7 Cardiac catheter studies

There have been a number of catheter studies carried out on patients with HAPE before treatment (Peñaloza and Sime 1969, Antezana *et al.* 1982) or soon after starting treatment (Fred *et al.* 1962, Hultgren *et al.* 1964, Roy *et al.* 1969). In all these studies there was found to be a high pulmonary artery pressure compared with healthy subjects at the same altitude (Table 19.2). The wedge pressures were normal. The pulmonary artery pressure ranged up to 144 mm Hg systolic (Hultgren *et al.* 1964) and is usually 60–80 mm Hg (Table 19.2). The normal wedge pressure implies normal pulmonary venous and left atrial pressures; in one subject direct measurement of left atrial pressure was made via a patent foramen ovale and was normal (Fred *et al.* 1962). The cardiac output was within the normal range so the calculated pulmonary resistance was markedly raised. There was no evidence of left ventricular failure. Breathing 100 per cent oxygen resulted in a fall of pulmonary artery pressure to normal values within 3 min in two

Table 19.2 *Cardiac catheter studies in HAPE*

	n	Pulmonary artery pressure (mm Hg)		Wedge pressure (mm Hg)	Cardiac output (L min^{-1})
		Systolic	Diastolic		
HAPE	5	81	49	5	5.8
Controls	50	29	13	9	6.4

Source: data from Antezana *et al.* (1982).

of five subjects. However, in the other three, pressures fell but leveled out at 40–50 mm Hg pulmonary artery pressure, well above the upper limit of normal at that altitude (Antezana *et al.* 1982).

19.2.8 Etiology and susceptibility

The etiology of HAPE is similar to that of AMS (section 18.4), all ages and both sexes being susceptible. There is an impression that children and young adults are more prone to HAPE than older people. It seems that individual susceptibility is more clear cut than for AMS; that is, subjects who have suffered HAPE on one occasion are very likely to have problems on subsequent altitude trips.

Susceptible subjects are found to have a greater pulmonary pressor response to hypoxia than control subjects who have been to altitude previously without problems (Hultgren *et al.* 1971, Vachiery *et al.* 1995, Eldridge *et al.* 1996, Scherrer *et al.* 1996). Hohenhaus *et al.* (1995) studied both the pulmonary pressor and hypoxic ventilatory responses in HAPE-susceptible subjects and concluded that they had lower hypoxic ventilatory response (HVR) than controls but not significantly different from subjects who had simple AMS. The latter had a wide range of HVR. Some HAPE-susceptible subjects had very brisk pressor responses but not all subjects could be separated from controls by this test. One possibility is that HAPE-susceptible individuals have a restricted lung vasculature or just smaller lungs. A study by Steinacker *et al.* (1998) tested this idea by comparing eight such subjects with controls at rest and on exercise in normoxia and hypoxia. The HAPE-prone group had 35 per cent smaller functional residual capacity and 7–10 per cent smaller vital and total lung capacities, and did not increase their diffusing capacities as much on exercise under hypoxia. This lends support to the hypothesis

of smaller lungs in HAPE-susceptible individuals. A similar conclusion had been reached by Podolsky *et al.* (1996) who studied the pulmonary response to exercise in HAPE-susceptible subjects at sea level and 3810 m. They found greater vascular reactivity in HAPE subjects. The reactivity was not affected by altitude or oxygenation so was due to either flow-dependent pulmonary vasoconstriction or a reduced vascular cross-sectional area. Duplain *et al.* (1999a) measured sympathetic activity directly from postganglionic nerve discharge in HAPE-susceptible subjects in response to a short hypoxic test. They found at both high and low altitude that the test subjects had two to three times the response compared with controls, suggesting that sympathetic overactivation may be a part of susceptibility.

In HAPE subjects, Hanoka *et al.* (1998) found an association with certain HLA complexes (HLA-DR6 and HLA-DQ4). Morrell *et al.* (1999) reported that Khirghiz highlanders with pulmonary hypertension had a high incidence of the D allele of the ACE gene compared with subjects suspected but found not to have pulmonary hypertension. These studies support the idea that HAPE susceptibility has a genetic basis.

19.3 PREVENTION

19.3.1 Slow ascent

It is generally considered that HAPE is a progression or complication of benign AMS. Therefore, if precautions are taken to prevent AMS by making a sufficiently slow ascent (section 18.6.1), HAPE will also be prevented. However, people often have to ascend at a rate that puts them at risk of AMS and, of course, the great majority of patients who suffer from benign AMS do not progress to the malignant forms.

19.3.2 Exercise

Many case histories from Houston (1960) onwards emphasize the point that patients have been very energetic while getting to high altitude or on arrival there. Ravenhill (1913) was of the opinion that physical exertion rendered a man more susceptible to AMS in general. The Indian Army, with great experience of HAPE since the war with China in the Himalayas in 1962, advises all inductees to altitude to take no unnecessary exertion for the first 72 h. Exercise, by increasing cardiac output, raises the pulmonary artery pressure, especially in subjects susceptible to HAPE, and it is believed that the higher the pulmonary artery pressure, the greater the risk of HAPE. In healthy subjects at altitude, Eldridge et al. (1998) have shown that strenuous exercise results in the appearance of red cells, white cells and $\gamma\delta T$ cells in the lavage fluid. The latter cells indicate damage to the endothelium and play a role in inflammation. Anholm et al. (1999) found radiographic evidence of pulmonary edema in a group of cyclists at the end of a run at modest altitude. However, HAPE can occur in the absence of hard physical exertion; 66 of Menon's 101 cases had taken no exercise more strenuous than office work, traveling as a passenger in a truck or walking about on level ground (Menon 1965). Nevertheless, the anecdotal evidence is strong enough to advise people who have to make a rapid ascent to altitude to avoid hard physical exertion for 2–3 days.

19.3.3 Drugs

Acetazolamide (section 18.6.2), by preventing or at least reducing AMS, probably also reduces the risk of HAPE. Nifedipine has been shown in a controlled trial to reduce the risk of HAPE in susceptible subjects (Bärtsch et al. 1991b).

19.4 TREATMENT

19.4.1 Descent

The single most important maneuver in treating a case of HAPE is to get the patient down as fast and as far as possible. Even a descent of as little as 300 m may improve a patient's condition dramatically (report of case 2 in section 19.2). However,

there are often unavoidable delays while awaiting evacuation and there are a number of therapeutic possibilities.

19.4.2 Oxygen

Breathing air enriched with oxygen, if available, is an obvious treatment. It relieves hypoxia and reduces pulmonary artery pressure (section 19.2.6), but, although most patients benefit, in some the relief is only partial and in a few deterioration may continue, perhaps because of inefficiencies in the delivery system. The dosage of oxygen is usually dictated by its supply. If there is sufficient, a flow of 6–10 L min^{-1} is indicated for the first few hours, reducing to 2–4 L min^{-1} when there is improvement.

19.4.3 Diuretics

Since the patient has edema, diuretics have been used in the treatment of HAPE (Singh et al. 1965). However, physicians who see a lot of the condition now do not advocate their use.

19.4.4 Antibiotics

Antibiotics by themselves will not cure HAPE. However, many cases have mild fever and leukocytosis suggesting that infection may play a part. Therefore, it would seem prudent to add a broad spectrum antibiotic to the treatment regimen, although Menon (1965) discontinued their use in his last 44 cases with no apparent disadvantage.

19.4.5 Calcium channel blockers

Oelz et al. (1989) showed that nifedipine was of value in the treatment of HAPE. Six subjects with clinical physiological and radiographic evidence of HAPE were treated with 10 mg of nifedipine sublingually and 20 mg slow release orally 6 hourly thereafter. Despite continued exercise at 4559 m this treatment without oxygen resulted in clinical improvement, better oxygenation, reduced $(A–a)P_{O_2}$ gradient and pulmonary artery pressure, and clearing of alveolar edema. The sublingual preparation is very rapidly absorbed and occasionally results in systemic hypotension; most physicians now do not use it.

19.4.6 Nitric oxide

Nitric oxide produced by endothelial cells is a naturally occurring potent vasodilator. It was first used in the treatment of HAPE by Scherrer *et al.* (1996), who took 18 HAPE-susceptible subjects to 4559 m. Their pulmonary artery pressures were higher and Pa_{O_2} lower than control, nonsusceptible subjects. Nitric oxide lowered their pulmonary artery pressure and raised their Pa_{O_2} whereas in control subjects Pa_{O_2} fell. The latter was thought to be due to increasing ventilation/perfusion mismatching. In HAPE subjects, nitric oxide goes preferentially to ventilated, nonedematous areas dilating the vessels there. This shifts blood flow from edematous to nonedematous areas with improvement in V/Q matching. The beneficial effects of nitric oxide were confirmed by Anand *et al.* (1998) in 14 patients with established HAPE. They compared nitric oxide treatment with 50 per cent oxygen and nitric oxide plus 50 per cent oxygen. Both nitric oxide and oxygen were effective in reducing pulmonary artery pressure and improving Pa_{O_2} but the combination had an additive effect. These studies are of great interest in understanding the mechanisms of HAPE, but nitric oxide is not suitable for use in the field and if the patient reaches a hospital the descent, calcium channel blockers and oxygen are almost always effective in relieving the condition.

19.4.7 Other vasodilators

Hackett *et al.* (1992) have shown that several vasodilators are beneficial in HAPE as indicated by a reduction in pulmonary artery pressure, pulmonary vascular resistance and improved gas exchange (Figure 19.2). Nifedipine and hydralazine were of equal benefit but rather less effective than oxygen. Phentolamine, an alpha-blocker, was more effective than oxygen and, when combined with oxygen, was even more effective.

19.4.8 Other drugs

Digoxin has been used. Menon (1965) observed the effect of an intravenous dose of 0.5–1.5 mg in 66 patients and claimed that the response was uniformly good within a few hours, even in patients given only 1 L min^{-1} of added oxygen. However, there was no evidence of myocardial failure nor was there atrial fibrillation – the current indications for digoxin therapy – and its use is no longer advised.

Morphine (15–30 mg i.v.) has been used, again with the clinical impression that this resulted in a reduction in pulmonary edema. As it does in acute left ventricular failure, it also makes the patient more comfortable, possibly by causing peripheral vasodilatation and a shift of blood from central to peripheral circulations. However, its respiratory depressant effects should make for caution in its use.

Corticosteroids have been used in a few cases with no clear result but the beneficial effect of dexamethasone in simple AMS shown in a controlled trial by Ferrazzini *et al.* (1987) would justify its use in HAPE, especially in severe cases where there is often an element of HACE as well.

19.4.9 Expiratory positive airways pressure

Feldman and Herndon (1977) suggested that expiratory positive airways pressure might be beneficial in HAPE by analogy with its use in other forms of pulmonary edema. They proposed a simple device in which the subject exhaled through an underwater tube to achieve the desired positive pressure while inspiration was direct from atmosphere.

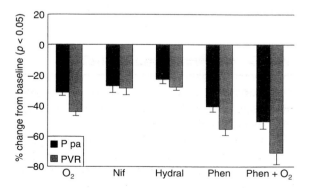

Figure 19.2 *Percentage change in mean pulmonary artery pressure (P pa) and pulmonary vascular resistance (PVR) with five different interventions in subjects with HAPE. Nif, nifedipine; Hydral, hydralazine; Phen, phentolamine. (Reproduced with permission from Hackett* et al. *1992.)*

Schoene *et al.* (1985) used a commercial expiratory positive pressure mask on four patients with HAPE on Mount McKinley in Alaska. They showed that, using the mask, arterial saturation was increased with increasing positive pressure (up to 10 cm H_2O). There was a concomitant rise in P_{CO_2} but not of heart rate. The intrathoracic pressure would be negative during inspiration so the cardiac output would probably not be reduced. A similar effect can be achieved by pursed lips expiration as used by patients with severe emphysema; mountain guides advise this, presumably because they have found it to be beneficial.

19.4.10   Portable hyperbaric chamber: the Gamow or Certec bags

A lightweight rubberized canvas bag has been developed into which a patient can be zipped and the bag pressurized using a foot pump. There is a pressure relief valve set to 2 psi (100 mm Hg). This pressure gives the equivalent altitude reduction of almost 2000 m from a typical base camp altitude of 4000–5000 m. There are currently two commercially available bags, the Gamow from the USA and Certec from France. There have been numerous accounts of their use in HAPE and HACE, with good results (Robertson and Shlim 1991). One report draws attention to the considerable placebo effect of the procedure. Roach and Hackett (1993) have reviewed the efficacy of hyperbaric treatment. They conclude that both oxygen and hyperbaria are effective. There may be a rebound effect some hours after treatment (typically 1–2 h duration). A recent controlled trial in benign AMS has shown that 1 h in the bag at pressure (193 mbar, equivalent to 147 mm Hg) was significantly more effective in reducing symptoms than control (1 h at the trivial pressure of 20 mbar, equivalent to 15 mm Hg) (Bärtsch *et al.* 1993). The effort of maintaining the necessary pumping for even 1 h is considerable, especially at altitude and if the number of rescuers is limited. Duff (1999), reporting a case, makes the useful point that some patients with severe HAPE or HACE may be orthopneic when made to lie flat in a compression bag and in their confused state may become belligerent. Their condition may be confused with claustrophobia. The solution is to position the bag at a 30° head-up angle.

19.4.11   Summary of treatment

The treatment of HAPE is:

- Get the patient down in altitude as fast and as low as possible.
- While awaiting evacuation, or if evacuation is not possible, give oxygen or hyperbaria. Nifedipine 20 mg slow release (or possibly phentolamine) should be given and a broad spectrum antibiotic should be considered. If there is any suspicion of cerebral edema as well give dexamethasone 4 mg (Chapter 20).
- The use of expiratory positive airways pressure, with a respiratory valve device or, failing that, by pursed lips breathing, will give some temporary improvement.

19.5   OUTCOME

In fully established cases, where evacuation to lower altitude is impossible, death within a few hours is usual. If cases are recognized early and taken down, patients usually recover completely in 1–2 days but occasionally they continue to deteriorate and die even after being brought down to lower altitude, especially if there are symptoms of cerebral edema (Dickinson *et al.* 1983). Only one case has been reported as progressing to adult respiratory distress syndrome (Zimmerman and Crapo 1980). Usually the pulmonary hypertension reduces rapidly on going to low altitude and the inverted T-waves on the ECG return to normal (Singh *et al.* 1965, Figure 3). But Menon (1965) mentions two soldiers (out of 101 cases) who having recovered from HAPE had to be evacuated later because of breathlessness, precordial pain and inverted T-waves in their EGC, and Fiorenzano *et al.* (1997) recently reported one case with prolonged T-wave inversion in the precordial leads suggesting prolonged pulmonary hypertension. Even patients who have apparently fully recovered have been shown to have significant hypoxemia and widened $(A–a)P_{O_2}$ gradients for up to 12 weeks (Guleria *et al.* 1969). However, after recovery at lower altitudes, many climbers have returned to climb their peaks without further trouble.

19.6 PATHOLOGY

19.6.1 Postmortem examination

There have been a number of postmortem studies which have shown a similar pathology in the heart and lungs (Hultgren *et al.* 1962, Arias-Stella and Kruger 1963, Marticorena *et al.* 1964, Nayak *et al.* 1964, Singh *et al.* 1965, Dickinson *et al.* 1983). The lungs are heavy and feel solid. The cut surface weeps edema fluid, usually blood stained, but a striking feature is the nonuniform nature of the edema. Areas of hemorrhagic edema alternate with clear edema and with areas which are virtually normal (or overinflated). Pulmonary arterial thrombi are commonly found.

On microscopy, alveoli are filled with fluid containing red blood cells, polymorphs and macrophages, though not in great numbers. Hyaline membranes are found in the alveoli, identical with those seen in respiratory distress syndrome of the newborn. The pulmonary capillaries are congested with small arteries and veins containing thrombi and fibrin clot. Perivascular edema and hemorrhage are found. In postmortem studies of high altitude natives from South America the pulmonary arteries are very muscular and the right ventricle is hypertrophied. In lowlanders the pulmonary vessels have normal musculature (Dickinson *et al.* 1983).

19.6.2 The edema fluid

The hyaline membranes are probably formed by coalescence of proteins, suggesting a high protein edema. It has been shown in life that the edema fluid is rich in protein. Hackett *et al.* (1986) sampled pure edema fluid by bronchoscopy in one case and showed it to have a plasma/fluid ratio of 0. 8:1.1 for total protein. Schoene *et al.* (1986) took bronchoalveolar lavage (BAL) fluid from three cases of HAPE and compared it with lavage fluid from three controls at the same altitude (4400 m). The fluid from patients was rich in high molecular weight protein, red cells and macrophages. These findings suggest a 'large pore' leak type of edema. In further studies the same group (Schoene *et al.* 1988) also found that the fluid was rich in alveolar macrophages. There was evidence of activation of complement (C5a) and release of thromboxane B_2 and leukotriene B_4. Tsukimoto *et al.* (1994) also showed, under tightly controlled laboratory con-

ditions in the rat, that elevation of the capillary pressure alone resulted in the appearance of leukotriene B_4 in the BAL fluid. Recently a Japanese group (Kubo *et al.* 1998) has carried out BAL in seven patients with early HAPE and found increased cell counts of macrophages, lymphocytes and neutrophils plus markedly elevated concentrations of proteins, lactate dehydrogenase, IL-1β, IL-6, IL-8 and TNF-α. IL-6 and TNF-α were shown to correlate with the Pa_{O_2} and pulmonary artery driving pressure ($P_{PA} - P_{wedge}$).

19.7 MECHANISMS

HAPE develops from AMS and the mechanisms that cause the symptoms of AMS (section 18.5) are already operating in these patients. Indeed, there is evidence suggesting that a degree of subclinical pulmonary edema is common during the second and third days at altitude. That is, there is a reduction in vital capacity, a shift of the pressure/volume curve of the lung (Mansell *et al.* 1980, Gautier *et al.* 1982) and an increase in alveolar arterial oxygen difference (Sutton *et al.* 1976). This might simply be part of a generalized increase in extracellular fluid (ECF) volume which shows itself as subcutaneous edema in the face on rising and in the ankles later in the day. In the skull, the same edema raises the intracellular pressure and gives rise to the symptoms of AMS, but the progression from this mild edema to clinical pulmonary edema requires a further mechanism or mechanisms.

19.7.1 Facts to be explained

Any hypothesis that seeks to explain the mechanism of HAPE must take into account the following facts:

- The edema is of the high protein type.
- The patchy distribution of the edema seen on postmortem and radiology (Figure 19.1).
- The very high pulmonary artery pressure and normal wedge (and left atrial) pressures (Table 19.2); the improvement which follows treatment with different drugs which reduce the pulmonary artery pressure indicates the importance of this factor in the mechanism of HAPE.
- The presence of vascular thrombi and fibrin clots in pulmonary vessels (section 19.4.1).

- The individual susceptibility which is associated with an increased hypoxic pulmonary pressor response (Hultgren *et al.* 1971) and response to exercise (Kawashima *et al.* 1989).
- The increased risk of HAPE with exercise on arrival at altitude.

19.7.2   Left ventricular failure

Although HAPE resembles left ventricular failure (LVF) clinically, which is why Ravenhill (1913) called it puna of the cardiac type, it is not now thought to be due to heart failure. Catheter studies have shown normal wedge pressures and the edema fluid is of the high protein permeability type. Also the chest radiograph and pathology are not typical of LVF.

19.7.3   Pulmonary hypertension

The extraordinarily high pulmonary artery pressure found in HAPE must play a role in the mechanism of the condition. High pulmonary artery pressure by itself does not cause edema, as for instance in primary pulmonary hypertension, or in a group of men studied by Sartori and colleagues (1999). These individuals had suffered an episode of hypoxia in the neonatal period and as a result had exaggerated pulmonary hypoxic pressor responses. When taken up to high altitude they had high pulmonary artery pressures but did not get HAPE. This is perhaps not surprising since the resistance vessels, the arterioles, are upstream of capillaries and therefore capillary pressure should be normal. One must therefore postulate some further mechanism as well as, but related to, the pulmonary hypertension. The following have been proposed.

19.7.4   Uneven pulmonary vasoconstriction and perfusion

Hultgren (1969) suggested that the edema is caused by a very powerful, but uneven, vasoconstriction so that there is reduced blood flow in some parts of the lung and torrential blood flow in others. He showed (Hultgren *et al.* 1966) that if one progressively ties off more and more of the pulmonary arterial tree in a dog, thus forcing the total cardiac output through only a portion of the lung, pulmonary edema results in the part of the lung that remains perfused.

A case report by Dombret *et al.* (1987) provides confirmation in humans of Hultgren's experimental findings. The reported patient had a massive pulmonary embolus resulting in perfusion being reduced to only the left upper and middle lobes. She developed symptoms and signs of pulmonary edema, which on radiograph were shown to be confined to those same perfused lobes.

Evidence in favor of this mechanism as being the cause of HAPE is provided by Viswanathan *et al.* (1979) who, at sea level, studied 12 subjects who had recovered from HAPE. They showed that, on being given 10 per cent oxygen to breathe, they had a greater pulmonary pressor response than controls and on lung scanning their perfusion was more uneven.

This hypothesis accounts well for the patchy distribution of the condition. High flow through less severely constricted areas might well produce edema by capillary stress failure (section 19.7.5). Added support for this hypothesis came from a paper by Hackett *et al.* (1980a), who collected four cases of HAPE occurring at very modest altitudes (2000–3000 m) in subjects who had a congenital absence of the right pulmonary artery. The edema developed in the left lung, which received the total cardiac output. That four cases of HAPE developed in such an uncommon condition (only 50 cases have been described in the world literature) strongly suggests a causative rather than a coincidental association.

19.7.5   Stress failure of pulmonary capillaries

It has been proposed that HAPE is caused by damage to the walls of pulmonary capillaries as a result of very high wall stresses associated with increased capillary transmural pressure (West *et al.* 1991, West and Mathieu-Costello 1992a). These high capillary pressures are the result of uneven hypoxic pulmonary vasoconstriction as originally proposed by Hultgren (1969). Extensive laboratory studies have now shown that raising capillary transmural pressure causes ultrastructural damage to the capillary walls, including disruption of the capillary endothelial layer, alveolar epithelial layer, and sometimes, all layers of the wall (West *et al.* 1991, Tsukimoto *et al.* 1991, Costello *et al.* 1992, Elliott *et al.* 1992, Fu *et al.* 1992). The result is a high permeability form of pulmonary edema (Tsukimoto *et al.* 1994). Figure 19.3

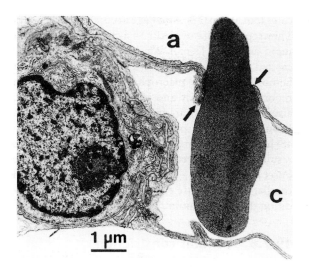

Figure 19.3 *Electron micrograph of a pulmonary capillary in a rat exposed to a barometric pressure of 294 mm Hg for 4 h. Note rupture of the capillary wall with a red cell moving out of the capillary lumen (c) into an alveolus (a). (From West* et al. *1995.)*

is an electron micrograph showing rupture of a pulmonary capillary wall in a rat exposed to a barometric pressure of 294 mm Hg for 4 h. Note the red cell in the process of moving from the capillary lumen to the alveolar space (West *et al.* 1995).

The work on stress failure began because of two key observations about HAPE. The first is that, as described above, there is a very strong relationship between the occurrence of HAPE and the height of the pulmonary arterial pressure. This suggests that HAPE is caused in some way by high vascular pressures in the pulmonary circulation. The second observation was that samples of alveolar fluid obtained by bronchoalveolar lavage in patients with HAPE show that the fluid is of the high permeability type with a large concentration of high molecular weight proteins and many cells. This observation strongly suggests that HAPE is associated with damage to the walls of the pulmonary capillaries by some mechanism. The problem therefore was to reconcile a hydrostatic pressure basis for the disease with the development of abnormalities in the capillary walls. As a result, extensive studies of the effects of raising pulmonary capillary pressure on the ultrastructure of pulmonary capillaries were carried out. These showed that stress failure is common in rabbit lung when the capillary transmural pressure rises to 40 mm Hg and that when it occurs it causes a high permeability type of pulmonary edema.

It is not at all surprising that pulmonary capillaries break under these conditions because the calculated wall stress of the capillary is extremely high (West *et al.* 1991, West and Matthieu-Costello 1992b). The surprising thing is not that the capillaries fail, but that they do not fail more often. Stress failure is now believed to play a role in a number of lung diseases (West and Mathieu-Costello 1992c) and is also the

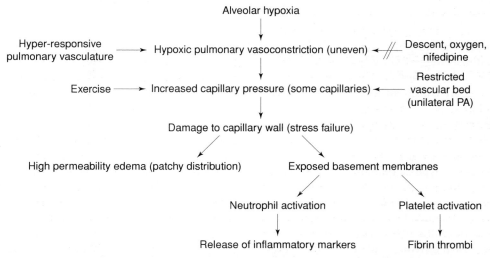

Figure 19.4 *Diagram summarizing the pathogenesis of HAPE based on stress failure of pulmonary capillaries. PA, pulmonary artery. (From West and Mathieu-Costello 1992a.)*

cause of bleeding into the lungs of racehorses, which is extremely common (West *et al.* 1993).

Bronchoalveolar lavage studies in patients with HAPE show the presence of inflammatory markers including leukotriene B4, other lipoxygenase products of arachidonic acid metabolism, and C5a complement in the lavage fluid (Schoene *et al.* 1988). At first sight these findings might seem to argue against stress failure of pulmonary capillaries as a mechanism. However, an important feature of the ultrastructural changes in stress failure is that the basement membranes of capillary endothelial cells are frequently exposed (Tsukimoto *et al.* 1991). The exposed basement membrane is electrically charged and highly reactive, and can be expected to activate leucocytes and platelets. In bronchoalveolar studies of the rabbit preparation, leukotriene B4 is seen in the lavage fluid (Tsukimoto *et al.* 1994). Platelet activation will result in the formation of fibrin thrombi, which are a feature of the pathology of HAPE (Arias-Stella and Kruger 1963). Figure 19.4 summarizes the mechanism of HAPE.

A striking feature of stress failure of pulmonary capillaries is that some of the breaks are rapidly reversible when the pressure is reduced. In one study carried out in rabbit lung, it was found that about 70 per cent of both the epithelial and endothelial breaks closed within a few minutes of the pressure being reduced (Elliott *et al.* 1992). This rapid reversibility of most of the disruptions may explain why patients with HAPE often quickly improve when they descend to a lower altitude.

Stress failure of pulmonary capillaries had not previously been suggested as the mechanism of HAPE. However, Mooi and co-workers (1978) studied the ultrastructural changes that occurred in rat lungs when the animals were exposed to acute decompression in a hyperbaric chamber. The appearances that they described are consistent with the findings seen in stress failure.

The mechanism of stress failure has clear implications for therapy. The main objective should be to reduce the pulmonary artery pressure. The pressure is high because of hypoxic pulmonary vasoconstriction, and the best way to reduce it is by rapid descent to a lower altitude, which reduces the alveolar P_{O_2}. In addition, oxygen should be given if this is available. Calcium channel blockers such as nifedipine are also effective because they reduce pulmonary artery pressure (Oelz *et al.* 1989).

A recent case report by Grissom *et al.* (2000) indi-

cates that alveolar hemorrhage occurs early in HAPE. They report a case of HAPE in a climber who made a rapid ascent of Denali, Alaska, and on whom they carried out BAL. The fluid yielded an abundance of hemosiderin-laden macrophages. These have been reported at necropsy and indicate bleeding into the alveoli. They appear from 48 h after bleeding. Bronchoscope was performed in this case less than 48 h after symptoms started so the timing of this result indicates bleeding occurred well before the onset of symptoms. This finding is consistent with capillary stress failure early in the course of the condition due to high pulmonary artery pressure.

19.7.6 Venular constriction

Since patients with HAPE have such a powerful arteriolar constriction in response to hypoxia, perhaps they have some degree of venular constriction as well. There is some pathological evidence for this from Wagenvoort and Wagenvoort (1976). This would not give high wedge pressures because when the catheter is wedged the blood in that segment runs off even through constricted venules and the wedge pressure reflects only the large vein and left atrial pressures, not the pressure in capillaries when the blood is flowing. To explain the patchy nature of the condition one must further postulate that the venular constriction is uneven.

19.7.7 Arterial leakage

Severinghaus (1977), impressed with the extraordinarily high pulmonary artery pressure in these patients, suggested that perhaps the fluid leak was upstream of the resistance vessels (i.e. in the arteries). He pointed out that when there was generalized arterial vasoconstriction, Laplace's law would mean reduction in diameter of small vessels but distension of large vessels (even though their wall tension was as great or greater). Radiography frequently shows distended hilar vessels (Marticorena *et al.* 1964). These larger vessels, not designed for such high pressure, suffer minor ruptures or fenestrations, which then leak high protein fluid and eventually red cells. The leakage is into the perivascular spaces which, when full, 'back up' to eventually cause alveolar flooding. This sequence occurs wherever the initial leak takes place since the perivascular space is the low pressure region of the lung.

Some evidence for such a mechanism was provided by two studies in animals (Milledge *et al.* 1968, Whayne and Severinghaus 1968) and in excised dog lungs (Iliff 1971). This evidence was reviewed by Severinghaus (1977) who quoted Hultgren's report on two horses that died suddenly after running at altitude. Both were found to have a ruptured pulmonary artery. Both this and the preceding hypothesis would account for exercise being a risk factor since it increases both flow and pressure in the pulmonary artery.

19.7.8 Multiple pulmonary emboli

Multiple scattered pulmonary emboli, even of inert substances, such as glass beads, cause a rapid profuse pulmonary edema in animals (Saldeen 1976) and this has been shown to be of the protein-rich, increased permeability type (Ohkuda *et al.* 1978). The finding in postmortem studies of frequent vascular thrombi and fibrin clots has led to the microembolization hypothesis for HAPE on the premise that there is a derangement of the clotting system. The effect of hypoxia on coagulation has been studied by a number of workers (section 18.5.4). It seems that most clotting factors are unaffected by hypoxia; they are not disturbed in AMS. Some evidence of *in vivo* fibrin formation was found by Bärtsch *et al.* (1987) in patients with HAPE but this was considered to be an epiphenomenon and not causative. If it does occur it will cause further deterioration in the patient. It is possible that changes in the red cells with hypoxia might alter their rheological properties and be a factor in AMS and HAPE. However, Reinhart *et al.* (1991) found no difference between subjects with and without AMS with respect to a number of rheological parameters.

It has even been suggested that rapid ascent may cause bubble formation by decompression and thus air microembolization (Gray 1983). If this were the case, HAPE should be much more common in chamber studies than in the mountains, but this is not so.

19.7.9 Hypoxia, vascular permeability and inflammation

Hypoxia may increase vascular permeability, either directly or, more likely, via the release of chemical mediators. Against this suggestion is evidence that, in

dogs, hypoxia does not alter the threshold for edema formation at a given microvascular pressure (Homik *et al.* 1988). However, it may require some other agent acting with hypoxia to produce the effect, as suggested by the work of Larsen *et al.* (1985). They showed in rabbits that neither hypoxia alone nor activation of the complement system (by infusion of cobra venom) alone caused pulmonary edema, but the two insults together did. Such a mechanism may well produce secondary intravascular coagulation, which would result in further pulmonary edema. On the other hand Duplain *et al.* (1999b) found in a group of HAPE-susceptible individuals, some of whom developed HAPE at altitude, that there was no tendency for the exhaled nitric oxide to increase with HAPE. Exhaled nitric oxide is a marker for inflammation, so this is evidence against inflammation being a factor in the genesis of HAPE.

Recently Swenson *et al.* (2000) found, in a group of HAPE-susceptible subjects taken to 4559 m, that their BAL fluid did not show an increase in inflammatory markers or neutrophils on the day after arrival at altitude, whereas increased red cells and protein (compared with control subjects) were found. Most of the subjects progressed to overt HAPE. This finding also suggests that inflammation, if it plays a part in HAPE, does so late in the course of the condition and that capillary stress failure is likely to be the initiating mechanism.

19.7.10 Hypoventilation

Grover (1980) has pointed out that hypoventilation has two disadvantages for a subject in relation to HAPE. It will mean that the subject is more hypoxic at a given altitude than a subject with the normal altitude hyperventilation and also has a higher P_{CO_2}. The higher P_{CO_2} means that there is no peripheral vasoconstriction and reduction in plasma volume on going to altitude; hence the plasma osmotic pressure is not raised. The subject is, therefore, more susceptible to pulmonary edema. A number of studies have found subjects with a history of HAPE to have low HVR (Hackett *et al.* 1988b, Matsuzawa *et al.* 1989). This might lead to relative hypoventilation at altitude, although Hackett *et al.* concluded that the low HVR played a permissive rather than a causative role in the pathogenesis of HAPE, allowing hypoxia to cause depression of ventilation. They found oxygen breathing increased ventilation in some of their subjects at altitude.

19.7.11   Neurogenic pulmonary edema

In some cases of head injury, a form of acute pulmonary edema is found which can be mimicked in experimental animals by creating lesions in the fourth ventricle. High levels of catecholamines are found, and the edema can be prevented by pretreatment with α-adrenergic blocking drugs. It is assumed therefore that the edema is caused by a surge of sympathetic activity. During the first few days at altitude there is increased sympathetic activity and possibly a similar mechanism is at work. The effectiveness of the α-blocker phentolamine in HAPE (Hackett *et al.* 1992) suggests that this may be the case.

19.7.12   Infection

Before 1960 many cases of HAPE were attributed to pneumonia. Although in many cases infection plays no part in HAPE, in some it may be a factor, especially in those individuals who are not normally susceptible to AMS but on one occasion succumb.

Carpenter *et al.* (1998) showed that rats given a mild respiratory infection and allowed to recover had greater lung edema and higher cell counts and protein concentration in BAL fluid when exposed to 10 per cent oxygen a week later than control rats. This gives support to the clinical impression that a concomitant or even previous respiratory infection is an important risk factor for HAPE.

19.7.13   Defective transepithelial sodium transport

Recent studies by Scherrer and colleagues have reinforced the proposition that pulmonary hypertension by itself does not cause pulmonary edema (section 19.7.3; Sartori *et al.* 1999). However, in transgenic mice with disruption of the gene for the α subunit of the amiloride-sensitive epithelial sodium channel, hypoxia did induce pulmonary edema. The same group has found a similar defect in epithelial ion transport in HAPE-susceptible human subjects (Lepori *et al.* 1999).

19.7.14   Mechanisms: conclusions

The various mechanisms discussed are not mutually exclusive and it is probable that the genesis of HAPE is multifactorial. The importance of various factors may be different in individual cases. For example, infection may play a role in some subjects, though certainly not in the majority. Some mechanisms may be important in the initiation of the condition, others in its progression. At present it is not possible to be dogmatic about which mechanism is most important in the initiation and development of HAPE. However, the mechanism of abnormally powerful pulmonary hypoxic vasoconstriction, which is uneven and leads on to capillary stress failure, seems to have the most evidence in its favor.

High altitude cerebral edema

SUMMARY

High altitude cerebral edema (HACE) is a severe form of acute mountain sickness (AMS) characterized by the same symptoms, headache, malaise, fatigue, etc., but progressing to ataxia, hallucinations, coma and death. Signs include papilledema, extensor plantar responses and other neurological signs. There may be mild fever, cyanosis, increased pulse and respiratory rates. Computerized tomography and postmortem appearance indicate cerebral edema and magnetic resonance imaging (MRI) scans show lesions in the splenium and corpus callosum. In untreated cases remaining at altitude, death occurs in a few hours or days.

The incidence of HACE is rather less than for high altitude pulmonary edema (HAPE). Many patients have a mixed picture with signs and symptoms of both conditions.

Prevention of HACE is the same as for AMS, that is, to make a slow ascent to altitude and to descend if symptoms do not improve. The diagnosis is made on the history and clinical examination. In a patient with symptoms of AMS, if any neurological signs appear or if there is any clouding of consciousness or hallucinations then HACE is the likely diagnosis. Often the earliest sign is ataxia, which is easily missed in a patient lying in a tent with a headache, especially as the patient may be irritable and insist that he is all right.

The most important action in treatment, as in HAPE, is to get the patient down. If this is impossible, or while awaiting evacuation, oxygen will help if available. Dexamethasone 4–8 mg has been shown to relieve the neurological symptoms and signs and treatment in a portable compression bag (Gamow or Certec) is also beneficial, at least for a few hours. Recovery is often rapid on descent but a number of cases have been described in which recovery was delayed by days or weeks.

The mechanism of development of cerebral edema is not understood. It is probably the same as in benign AMS to start with but instead of being self-limiting it progresses to an advanced stage giving rise to the signs and symptoms described and eventually to death. The consensus at present is that the edema is vasogenic in origin with an increase in the permeability of the blood–brain barrier. Various hypotheses have been advanced to account for this and are discussed.

20.1 INTRODUCTION

The symptoms of benign AMS are probably due to mild cerebral edema, which, though unpleasant, is not serious. In a small minority of cases the condition progresses to more severe symptoms. Unmistakable signs of cerebral edema and increased intracranial pressure become manifest and progress to coma. Death can be expected if the patient is not treated. This malignant form of AMS is called high altitude cerebral edema (HACE).

Ravenhill (1913) called the condition 'puna of a nervous type'. He describes three cases who recovered on being sent down to low altitude. As with acute pulmonary edema of high altitude, his work was forgotten and it was only during the 1960s that this serious form of acute cerebral edema of high altitude was again described (e.g. Fitch, 1964; Singh *et al.* 1969b).

20.2   CLINICAL ASPECTS

20.2.1   Symptoms and signs

Patients usually have the symptoms of benign AMS (Chapter 18). They may have headache, loss of appetite, nausea, vomiting and photophobia. Their climbing performance falls off, they may be irritable and wish only to be left alone. It can be difficult to decide the point at which these benign symptoms have progressed to malignant AMS, but the appearance of ataxia, irrationality, hallucinations or clouding of consciousness should alert one to the likelihood that the patient now has HACE. The patient may report blurring of vision which may be due to retinal hemorrhage (section 22.9) or to papilledema, which may be evident on examination of the retina. The reflexes may be brisk and later the plantars may become extensor.

There may be ocular muscle paralysis with diplopia. The pulse is often rapid and cyanosis usual.

Often there is also an element of pulmonary edema with signs and symptoms of that condition as well (sections 19.2.3, 19.2.4). As the condition progresses all symptoms and signs become more evident. The headache becomes worse, the ataxia intensifies so that the patient can no longer sit up (truncal ataxia). As coma comes on, the breathing becomes irregular. Death may occur in a few hours or in a day or two in untreated cases.

20.2.2   Case histories

CASE 1 (HOUSTON AND DICKINSON 1975)

A 39-year-old Japanese woman flew from 1500 m to 2750 m and during the next 2 days climbed to 3500 m, where she developed a severe headache. On day 4 at 3800 m she began to vomit. On day 5 at 3960 m she became breathless and weak, was vomiting and needed assistance to walk. On day 6 she lost consciousness and was carried down to 3350 m where she was found to be deeply unconscious and cyanosed, with a temperature of 40.6 °C and a pulse of 140 beats/min⁻¹. Crackles filled the chest. Reflexes were brisk and plantars flexor. Slight papilledema was present. She was treated with oxygen, frusemide and penicillin. On day 8 she was flown to hospital at 1500 m where she was found to be in the same condition but with extensor plantar reflexes. Lumbar puncture showed a pressure of 270 mm H_2O and the cerebrospinal fluid (CSF) was normal. She slowly improved over 2 weeks and eventually recovered completely.

Comment

The symptoms of HACE are dominant in this case but the patient also had signs of HAPE.

CASE 2 (DICKINSON ET AL. 1983)

A 46-year-old man trekked from 1500 m to 3650 m in 2 days. On the way he began to feel unwell, was tired, anorexic and later began to vomit. At 3650 m he became unconscious and was evacuated to hospital at 1500 m. On examination he was deeply unconscious, responding only to pain. He was cyanosed and hyperventilating. There were crackles and wheezes in the lungs; papilledema and retinal hemorrhage were present. Respirations were 40 min⁻¹, the pulse was 120 min⁻¹, and the temperature 40 °C. He remained unconscious and died after 4 days in hospital.

Comment

This is a typical case of HACE, which seemed to have reached an irreversible stage before descent.

CASE 3 (HOUSTON AND DICKINSON 1975)

A 42-year-old fit man reached 3600 m from sea level in a few days. He spent 2 days at this altitude and on day 3 climbed to 4940 m, returning to sleep at 3960 m. On day 4, after carrying about 25 kg to 4940 m, he complained of severe headache, and went to sleep on arrival at the camp. Next morning he was confused and unable to talk coherently. He could not coordinate hand and foot movements and was disorientated in time and space. He was carried down to 3600 m where he became coherent and was able to walk without assistance. He was given an intramuscular steroid and by late afternoon seemed normal. The next day he was taken down to 2130 m where he was completely normal.

Comment

A typical case of HACE, where prompt action in bringing the patient down saved his life.

CASE 4 (ABRIDGED FROM HOWARTH 1999)

A 42-year-old member of a scientific expedition had trekked to Kangchenjunga Base Camp (5100 m) in Nepal and spent a week at this altitude including climbing twice to about 5400 m on day outings. He had had no sickness during all this time. With three companions he set out to climb a 6200 m peak on the return trek. On the first day from Base Camp their porters took the wrong route to their intended camp at 5500 m, necessitating some climbing over very rough ground. During the early part of the day the patient had been going strongly but in the later part he was slow and reached camp at 2.45 p.m., cold and exhausted. He complained of a bad headache but took some hot soup and painkillers. AMS was diagnosed and it was hoped he would improve with rest. However, over the next 2 h he deteriorated and became ataxic. He was given acetazolamide and dexamethasone but vomited most of the tablets. Evacuation was started but it required a man on each side to support him and over the boulder-strewn ground going was very slow. He continued to deteriorate and they had to stop for rest every 20 yards or so. The party was benighted but fortunately was able to radio other members of the expedition for help. The rescue party met them with oxygen and injectable dexamethasone after which the patient improved though descent, over now steepening scree, was still very slow. A temporary camp at about 4900 m was reached at 11.30 p.m. By next morning the patient was much better and during the day was able to walk slowly back to Base Camp.

Comment

This case illustrates the unpredictability of AMS in that typical HACE developed in a climber who would seem to have acclimatized well. In some subjects who have no problems up to a certain point there seems to be a critical altitude above which they quite abruptly start having symptoms. It also emphasizes the importance of making an early diagnosis and getting the patient down as soon as possible – easier with hindsight of course.

20.2.3 Investigations

Blood counts and blood biochemistry are usually normal. Chest radiograph may show evidence of concomitant pulmonary edema, whilst lumbar puncture (which is not normally indicated) usually shows raised pressure but normal CSF. Computerized tomographic scanning of the brain in 12 patients with HAPE and HACE (Koyama et al. 1984) showed evidence of cerebral edema with diffuse low density of the entire cerebrum and compression of the ventricles. Recovery to normal computerized tomography findings occurred within a week in three cases but persisted for 1–2 weeks in two cases; one case took over a month to clear. MRI findings are detailed in section 20.3.1.

20.2.4 Treatment

The treatment for HACE is very similar to that for HAPE; that is, get the patient down to lower altitude as soon as possible. Oxygen therapy is obviously advised while awaiting evacuation, but often is only of marginal benefit. Dexamethasone has been shown to be of benefit in a double-blind, randomized, placebo-controlled trial in AMS (Ferrazzini et al. 1987). It is particularly the cerebral symptoms which seem to be helped by this drug, so it should certainly be used in this situation. The dose used in the trial was 8 mg initially, followed by 4 mg 6 hourly. Probably dexamethasone is to be preferred to diuretics, although they can be tried if response to the former is not adequate,. Enthusiasm for dexamethasone should be tempered by the finding that, although symptoms are relieved, the physiological abnormalities (fluid shifts, oxygenation, sleep apnea, urinary catecholamine levels, chest radiograph, perfusion scans and the results of psychomotor tests) were not improved (Levine et al. 1989). The drug is no substitute for descent. Portable hyperbaric bags (Gamow bags) are now available and their use in HAPE is discussed in Chapter 19. In HACE their use is less well documented but, if available, they can certainly be tried. Their use may make it possible for a patient to then descend unaided instead of having to be carried. Recovery after descent may not be as rapid as is usually the case with HAPE (Dickinson 1979; and see Cases 1 and 2).

20.2.5   Postmortem appearance

There have been a few reports of postmortems in HACE (Singh *et al.* 1969b, Houston and Dickinson 1975, Dickinson *et al.* 1983). The usual findings in the brain are of cerebral edema with swollen, flattened gyri, and compression of the sulci. There may be herniation of the cerebella tonsils and unci. Spongiosis, especially in the white matter, may be marked. In many cases there are widespread petechial hemorrhages; in some there are ante-mortem thrombi in the venous sinuses or there may be subarachnoid hemorrhages, but there seems to be considerable variation in the findings. It must always be remembered that the few cases that reach autopsy are highly selected and may well be unrepresentative of the condition as seen clinically in the field.

20.2.6   Incidence and etiology

The incidence – like that of HAPE – is difficult to determine and depends upon the rate of ascent and therefore on terrain, logistics and the pattern of movements of people from sea level to altitude. It also depends upon definition, where the distinction between severe cases of benign AMS and mild HACE is impossible. Many cases show a mixed picture of HAPE and HACE. However, Hackett *et al.* (1976) had five cases out of 278 trekkers arriving at Pheriche (4243 m) in Nepal giving an incidence of 1.8 per cent, rather less than that for HAPE.

The age and sex distributions, like those for AMS, show no group to be immune. Possibly the younger male is rather more at risk, perhaps because he is more likely to push on to higher altitude with symptoms, a feature of many histories in fatal cases. People native to high altitude can become victims of HACE. The impression is that the incidence in them is lower but there are no good published data.

20.3   MECHANISMS

The mechanism for the development of cerebral edema at altitude is reviewed in Chapter 18. Hypoxia seems to induce an increase in extracellular fluid (ECF). It may also cause increased microvascular permeability. Hypoxia certainly increases cerebral blood flow (Severinghaus *et al.* 1966b), particularly

when there is no marked reduction in P_{CO_2}. However, a study by Jensen *et al.* (1990) found no correlation between increase in cerebral blood flow and AMS. These same factors may become more pronounced to cause the symptoms of HACE, but there may be others. The question of why certain individuals are susceptible whereas others are not is as puzzling in HACE as in other forms of AMS, although one possible factor might be the relative sizes of the brain and cranial cavity. In a recent review of etiology, Hackett (1999) discusses this 'tight fit' hypothesis: those with a tight fit brain in the box of their cranial cavity will have a greater rise in pressure for a given increase in fluid volume in the brain. Those with looser brains are less susceptible. As we get older our brains shrink and this may be a why older people are less susceptible to AMS and HACE.

20.3.1   Cytogenic or vasogenic cerebral edema

There is no doubt that the symptoms of HACE (and probably those of AMS) are due to cerebral edema and increased intracranial pressure. A recent point of debate has been whether the edema is cytogenic, edema of the brain cells, or vasogenic, movement of fluid and protein out of the vascular compartment. Hackett *et al.* (1998) reported MRI scans in nine patients with HACE compared with three with HAPE and three who had been to altitude with no illness. They found intense T_2 signals in white matter, especially in the splenium and corpus callosum. There were no lesions in the gray matter. These findings suggest that the edema was vasogenic and that the problem may lie with the blood–brain barrier.

20.3.2   Venous thrombosis

Venous thrombosis has been found on computerized tomographic scan in one patient (Asaji *et al.* 1984) and in some postmortem studies of HACE. It may develop late in the condition as a consequence of intracranial hypertension. It will certainly exacerbate the condition.

20.3.3   Cellular edema

In profound hypoxia, the ATP-dependent sodium pump eventually begins to fail; sodium concentration rises in the cell and water follows to maintain osmotic equilibrium (Fishman 1975). This may be the cause of further cerebral edema in established cases, especially in those with pulmonary edema causing further hypoxia. However, it cannot be the cause of problems at the start of HACE because the hypoxia is not sufficiently profound.

20.3.4   Vascular endothelial growth factor

Severinghaus (1995) suggested that the same factors, operating in situations of angiogenesis, may be involved in HACE. Hypoxia stimulates the release of transforming growth factor (TGF) which attracts macrophages. These in turn release vascular endothelial growth factor (VEGF) and other factors which eventually give rise to growth of new capillaries. The more immediate effect is to increase capillary permeability as capillary basement membranes are broken down. Severinghaus suggests that, even earlier than these events, hypoxia may cause osmotic brain swelling. Dexamethasone is very effective in preventing angiogenesis and it may be this action which explains its effectiveness in HACE. This theory received support from the finding of VEGF mRNA in rat brains after only 3 h of hypoxia. The level reached a peak of three times control at 12–24 h (Xu and Severinghaus 1998). This could explain the increased permeability of the blood–brain barrier and the vasogenic edema.

20.3.5   Nitric oxide and cerebral edema

Clark et al. (1999) suggested that the mechanism of cerebral edema in HACE may be via the induction of inducible nitric oxide synthase (iNOS) in the brain by hypoxia. This gives rise to increased levels of nitric oxide which causes edema by increasing vascular permeability. In most cases this is quite mild and self-limiting, giving rise to the symptoms of benign AMS. However, if there are even low levels of cytokines as well, due to a mild infection for instance, there will be a synergistic effect on iNOS induction and permeability. This results in HACE.

21

Subacute and chronic mountain sickness

SUMMARY

Subacute mountain sickness is a condition affecting either infants born or brought up to altitude within their first year, or adults remaining at extreme altitude for weeks or months. In Tibet, the infants are usually the children of lowlanders, Han Chinese; the highland Tibetan infants are relatively immune. As the condition develops the infants become breathless, irritable and edematous. The pathology is of pulmonary hypertension and right heart failure. In adults, it has been reported in Indian soldiers stationed at about 6000 m for long periods. Again the signs of right heart failure are prominent. Descent results in reversal of signs and symptoms.

Chronic mountain sickness (CMS) was first recognized by Carlos Monge M. in Peru and is also known as Monge's disease. It is found in all populations who remain at altitude for a number of years. The incidence is increased with altitude and with age; it is higher in males than in with females. In Tibet at least, it is more common in immigrant Han Chinese than in native Tibetans.

In cases without overt lung disease various factors which cause relative hypoventilation, such as a reduced hypoxic ventilatory drive or disturbed breathing patterns during sleep, may be involved in the mechanism. The commonest underlying condition is chronic obstructive lung disease (chronic bronchitis, emphysema) often associated with smoking; tuberculosis, kyphoscoliosis and other lung diseases are also found as contributory causes. These conditions make the patient more hypoxic and increase the stimulus to erythrocytosis.

The symptoms that result from this excessive erythrocytosis are rather vague and include headache, dizziness, physical and mental fatigue, anorexia and breathlessness. Signs are few and include cyanosis and a florid complexion.

Prevention, apart from remaining at low altitude, can only be directed at secondary risk factors such as smoking and occupational dust air pollution. Relocation to low altitude cures the condition but many patients are not able to take this option. The removal of a unit of blood is beneficial but needs to be repeated as the hemoglobin concentration rises again. Respiratory stimulants have been used with reported success.

21.1   SUBACUTE MOUNTAIN SICKNESS

21.1.1   Introduction

Two forms of subacute mountain sickness have been described, one in infants born at low altitude and taken to high altitude (Sui *et al.* 1988) and the other in adults who have spent some months or more at extreme altitude (Anand *et al.* 1990).

21.1.2 Infantile subacute mountain sickness

The Spaniards who first colonized the Andes became well aware that their infants did not thrive if born at high altitude. They made it their practice to arrange delivery at low altitude and not to bring their babies to high altitude before 1 year of age. The lowland Han Chinese colonists of Tibet face the same environmental problem. Wu and Liu (1995) described a Chinese infant of 11 months born in Lhasa (3658 m) who presented with dyspnea, cyanosis and congestive heart failure. At postmortem, marked right ventricular hypertrophy and muscular thickening of the peripheral pulmonary artery tree was found. There was no other pathology such as congenital heart disease and the authors called the condition high altitude heart disease. Sui et al. (1988) reported the postmortem findings on 15 infants who died in Lhasa of a syndrome they called infantile subacute mountain sickness. The presenting symptoms were commonly dyspnea and cough, with often sleeplessness, irritability and signs of cyanosis, edema of the face, oliguria, tachycardia, liver enlargement, rales in the lungs and fever. The majority of infants had been born at low altitude but two were born at high altitude, one of Han and one of Tibetan parents. The condition was usually fatal in a matter of weeks or months. The postmortem findings were of extreme medial hypertrophy of muscular pulmonary arteries and muscularization of pulmonary arterioles. There was massive hypertrophy and dilatation of the right ventricle and of the pulmonary trunk.

21.1.3 Adult subacute mountain sickness

Anand et al. (1990) described the adult form in 21 soldiers who, after a full acclimatization period, had been posted to between 5800 m and 6700 m for several months (mean 1.8 years). They presented with dyspnea, cough and effort angina. The signs were of dependent edema. They were treated at high altitude with diuretics with improvement. When they were evacuated to low altitude by aircraft they were found to have cardiomegaly with right ventricular enlargement and, in most cases, pericardial effusion. The pulmonary artery pressure was elevated (26 mm Hg) and rose significantly on mild

exercise to 40 mm Hg. Recovery was rapid after descent from high altitude. The mechanism includes a generalized increase in the volume of the fluid compartments of the body and total body sodium, even in subjects without overt disease at these altitudes for this length of time (Anand et al. 1993). The increase in central blood volume is the probable cause of the decrease in forced vital capacity, and the radiographically engorged pulmonary vessels found in the subjects of Operation Everest II (Welsh et al. 1993). It would seem that this subacute mountain sickness is the human form of a similar condition affecting cattle taken to high altitude, and known as brisket disease (Hecht et al. 1959). The brisket is the loose skin area of the cow's neck, which is dependent and becomes swollen with edema fluid in this condition.

21.2 CHRONIC MOUNTAIN SICKNESS

21.2.1 Historical

In 1925 Carlos Monge M. reported a case of polycythemia in a patient from Cerro de Pasco (4300 m) in Peru to the Peruvian Academy of Medicine (Monge 1925). In 1928 he reported a series of such patients with red cell counts significantly higher than normally found at altitude (Monge C. and Whittembury 1976). (Note: Carlos Monge M. is the father and Carlos Monge C. the son: the M and C are the initial letters of the mothers' names, as is Spanish custom.) This condition of CMS has come to be known also as Monge's disease. The 1935 international expedition, led by Bruce Dill, reported one case of CMS in the English literature (Talbott and Dill 1936). In 1942 Hurtado published detailed observations of eight cases, outlining the symptomatology and hematological changes at altitude and the effect of descent to sea level and return to altitude (Hurtado 1942).

Outside South America, CMS was observed in Leadville (3100 m), a mining town in Colorado, USA, by Monge M. in the late 1940s (Winslow and Monge 1987, p. 15) and from the 1960s the condition has been studied there by Weil and colleagues (1971) from Denver (section 21.3.3). Reports of CMS from the Himalayas indicate the condition to be prevalent in immigrant Han Chinese in Lhasa (3658 m) but rare in the indigenous Tibetan population (Pei *et al.* 1989).

21.2.2 Clinical aspects of CMS

SYMPTOMS

Patients typically have rather vague neuropsychological complaints including headache, dizziness, somnolence, fatigue, difficulty in concentration and loss of mental acuity. There may also be irritability, depression and even hallucinations. Dyspnea on exertion is not commonly complained of, but poor exercise tolerance is common and patients may gain weight. The characteristic feature of the disease is that the symptoms disappear on going down to sea level, only to reappear on return to altitude.

SIGNS

Although normal people are mildly cyanotic at an altitude of 4000 m, patients with CMS stand out since, with a high hemoglobin concentration and lower oxygen saturation, they have a far higher concentration of reduced hemoglobin. In Andean Indians, the population with the greatest number of patients, the signs may be florid:

> The combination of virtually black lips and wine red mucosal surfaces against the olive green pigmentation of the Indian skin gives the patient with Monge's disease a striking appearance (Heath and Williams 1995, pp. 193).

The conjunctivae are congested and the fingers may be clubbed. In Caucasians and at lower altitudes such as Leadville (3100 m), the appearances are rather less striking, resembling patients with polycythemia secondary to hypoxic lung disease at sea level. Some patients show very little in the way of signs.

INVESTIGATIONS

The red cell count, hemoglobin concentration and packed cell volume are raised; values as high as 28.0 g dL^{-1} hemoglobin and a packed cell volume of up to 83 per cent have been recorded (Hurtado 1942). Like secondary polycythemia at sea level and unlike polycythemia rubra vera there is no increase in white cell numbers. Blood gases, compared with healthy controls at the same altitude, show a higher Pa_{CO_2} and lower Pa_{O_2} and oxygen saturation

(Peñaloza and Sime 1971, Kryger *et al.* 1978a). The lower Pa_{O_2} is partly due to hypoventilation as shown by the increased Pa_{CO_2} and partly (in many cases) by an increased alveolar–arterial oxygen tension $((A-a)O_2)$ gradient. Manier *et al.* (1988) found a mean of 10.5 mm Hg in CMS patients at La Paz (3600 m) compared with the normal $(A-a)O_2$ of 2.9 mm Hg at this altitude. Using the multiple inert gas technique, they attributed most of this to increased blood flow to poorly ventilated areas of lung rather than to true shunting. Tewari *et al.* (1991) found a reduced diffusing capacity in lowland soldiers with excessive polycythemia, which improved after descent and return to a normal hematocrit. In some cases standard pulmonary function tests show abnormalities indicating obstructive and/or restrictive defects, suggesting that patients have coexisting chronic lung disease.

HEMODYNAMICS AND PATHOLOGY

The very high hematocrit increases the viscosity of the blood enormously. The systemic blood pressure may be moderately elevated and the pulmonary artery pressure is significantly higher than healthy high altitude residents. Peñaloza *et al.* (1971) found a mean pulmonary artery pressure of 64/33 mm Hg in 10 cases of CMS compared with 34/23 mm Hg in controls. Cardiac output was not significantly different, so that calculated resistance was just over twice that of controls.

As might be expected these hemodynamic changes lead to increased right ventricular hypertrophy and associated electrocardiogram (ECG) changes. A recent study found that 90 per cent of cases of CMS had ECG evidence of right ventricular hypertrophy (Halperin et al. 1998). There is also thickening of the pulmonary arteries to a greater degree than in normal residents at high altitude (Arias-Stella *et al.* 1973).

PREVENTION

Descent to low altitude without return is a sure preventative but not an option for many altitude residents whose livelihood depends upon their work at altitude. Attention to any secondary risk factors such as smoking is obvious. Since many patients are miners, efforts can also be made to avoid occupational health risks such as dust and air pollution, but these are frequently difficult to eliminate.

TREATMENT

As already mentioned, symptoms and signs classically clear up on going down to sea level. However, many patients want to remain at altitude for family or economic reasons. In these cases, venesection is beneficial. Venesection not only lowers the raised hematocrit but also improves many of the neuro-psychological symptoms. It also improves pulmonary gas exchange (Cruz *et al.* 1979) and exercise perform-ance in some subjects (Winslow and Monge 1987, p. 212). In Leadville, Colorado, with about 60 patients being regularly bled for therapeutic purposes, the blood bank has no need of any other donors (Kryger *et al.* 1978a)!

An alternative to venesection for residents at high altitude is the long-term use of respiratory stimu-lants. Kryger *et al.* (1978b) have reported success with medroxyprogesterone acetate. They showed a fall in hemoglobin concentration after 10 weeks' treatment in 17 patients. The drug increased venti-lation and P_{O_2} and reduced P_{CO_2} by a modest amount. Although the changes in blood gases were small, they suggest that the main benefit may have been in oxygenation at night since hypoxemia may be much greater then. The only side effect reported was of loss of libido in four patients. In all but one, this could be overcome by lowering the dose to a level that still kept the hemoglobin concentration down. In one patient the dose had to be reduced to a point which did not hold down the hemoglobin concentration.

There do not seem to have been any reported trials of other stimulants such as acetazolamide, which has been shown to be effective in preventing AMS (Chapter 18).

21.2.3 Epidemiology of CMS

ANDES

CMS is found most commonly in the Andes, where it was first described mainly affecting the local Amerindians, especially the Quechuan population living on the altiplano at altitudes about 3300–4500 m. Men are affected far more commonly than women. The average age is 40 years with a range from 22 to 51 years in one reported series (Peñaloza *et al.* 1971). Occasional cases are seen in expatriate mining company staff. It used to be thought that CMS was virtually confined to the Andes but this is not the case, as is discussed below.

HIMALAYAS AND TIBET

Until recently there have been few reported cases of CMS in the Himalayas. Winslow noted one Sherpa on the American Medical Research Expedition to Everest to have a hematocrit of 72 per cent (Winslow and Monge 1987, p. 17). Pei *et al.* (1989) describe their experience of CMS in Lhasa (3658 m). The condition is not uncommon among male cigarette-smoking Han Chinese. These subjects had immigrated some years before becoming poly-cythemic and then displayed the usual signs and symptoms of CMS. In a 12-month period there were 24 patients admitted to their hospital with CMS. All were male, 23 were Han and only 1 Tibetan. Six were nonsmokers, the rest, including the one Tibetan, were smokers. The mean duration of altitude expo-sure in the lowlanders was 26 years (range 9–43 years). However, though the incidence in Tibetans may be less than in Han immigrants, CMS is now being reported in this population. Wu *et al.* (1992) reported a series of 26 cases in native-born Tibetans living at between 3680 m and 4179 m with typical symptoms of CMS and hemoglobin concen-tration of 22.2 g dL^{-1} mean compared with 16.6 g dL^{-1} in healthy controls at the same altitude.

In Himalayan residents, hemoglobin concentra-tion tends to be lower than the values from the Peruvian Andes, although much of this difference disappears if results from mining towns are excluded (Frisancho 1988). It is speculated that this may be because the geography allows residents to move to lower altitudes more easily than from the altiplano of the Andes, and the way of life of the Sherpas, with seasonal migration, contributes to this movement in altitude. Like the inhabitants of the Andes, Tibetans live on a high altitude plain and cannot easily move up and down.

Although more evidence is needed it would seem that people of Tibetan stock are less at risk of CMS than Andean highlanders, and certainly than lowland Han subjects long resident at altitude. This may be due to genuine genetic adaptation to altitude over very many generations.

A recent review comparing incidence of CMS in the Andes with that in Tibet seems to bear out this earlier speculation (Moore *et al.* 1998b). This review also presents more evidence on incidence at various altitudes, men versus women, and Tibetan versus Han Chinese.

NORTH AMERICA

The condition is well recognized in Leadville, Colorado (3100 m). Kryger *et al.* (1978a) described 20 cases, all male, and mentioned that, of about 60 cases known to physicians there, only 2 were female. One case of apparently classical CMS in a 67-year-old woman has been reported from as low as 2000 m in California (Gronbeck 1984).

21.2.4   Terminology

POLYCYTHEMIA OF ALTITUDE

Opinions differ about the hemoglobin value required for diagnosis of CMS. A value of 23 g dL^{-1} has been used, but it would seem wiser to take into account the normal value and range for that particular altitude (Chapter 8), and even then, any given value is rather arbitrary. Indeed, it has been argued that CMS does not represent a distinct entity at all and that the hemoglobin values represent merely the 'tail' of a normal distribution curve (Monge C. and Whittembury 1976). For practical purposes, a value of two standard deviations above the mean for that altitude can be considered the cut-off for 'normal'. The 'tail' population may then be considered abnormal and polycythemic for that altitude. Since at this value symptoms occur, treatment is indicated and therefore this definition has practical implications.

This concept is in line with the conclusions of a monograph on CMS by Winslow and Monge, C. (1987, p. 204), who define it in terms of a hematocrit 'above the statistical maximum for the altitude in question'. However, they also draw attention to the work of Cosio who found important differences in hemoglobin concentration between two populations living in two towns at the same altitude (4600 m) (Winslow and Monge, C. 1987, p. 37). This illustrates the difficulty of assigning a 'normal' value for a given altitude.

LUNG DISEASE AND POLYCYTHEMIA

It is well known that hypoxic lung disease causes polycythemia in patients even at sea level. Many patients in the mining towns of the Andean altiplano smoke and work in dusty occupations. Is their polycythemia simply secondary to lung disease which has greater effect because of the altitude? Arias-Stella (1971) initiated discussion at the Ciba Symposium on high altitude physiology with a paper describing a postmortem on a woman with CMS and kyphoscoliosis. He suggested the use of the term 'Monge's syndrome' for cases like this, where there was lung or chest wall disease as a primary cause, and 'Monge's disease' proper for cases with no lung disease. The challenge was thrown out for some pathologist to report a case of polycythemia in which lung disease had been excluded by rigorous modern pathological methods. This challenge has yet to be taken up. The usage of 'Monge's syndrome' has not been generally adopted and most workers simply refer to patients as having CMS, Monge's disease or polycythemia of high altitude, with or without overt lung disease.

CONSENSUS GROUP ON CMS

In 1998 at the World Congress on Mountain Medicine at Masumoto a group was established to try to define the terminology of CMS. They had great difficulty in reaching a consensus on the definitions to be used. Among other problems discussed were how to define the level of hemoglobin concentration, what to do about obvious lung disease and if signs of pulmonary hypertension should be included in the definition. However, the following was agreed as a working definition:

> CMS is a syndrome, which occurs in persons long resident at high altitude and which is characterized by excessive erythrocytosis and hypoxemia and by reversibility on descent. It may be classified as primary (without identified cause) or secondary (due to underlying condition) (Leon-Velarde 1998).

At the same meeting a scoring system was proposed by Leon-Velarde but it has yet to be adopted widely.

21.2.5   Mechanisms of CMS

CMS WITH LUNG DISEASE

In cases of CMS with definite lung disease, it is easy to understand that the combination of altitude with fairly mild lung disease precipitates polycythemia and cor pulmonale (Fig. 21.1). Removal of altitude

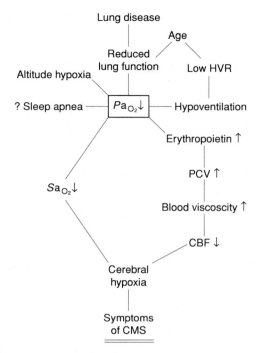

Figure 21.1 *Possible mechanisms in the development of chronic mountain sickness (CMS). HVR, hypoxic ventilatory response; CBF, cerebral blood flow; PCV, packed cell volume.*

hypoxia by descent to sea level is sufficient to reverse the process. At altitude, these patients are more hypoxic than normal people because of their lung disease, hence their stimulus to erythrocytosis via erythropoietin secretion is greater and they become abnormally polycythemic. The importance of lower respiratory tract disease is emphasized in a study by Leon-Velarde *et al.* (1994) which shows that subjects with chronic lower respiratory disease had higher hemoglobin concentration, lower Sa_{O_2} and higher CMS symptom scores than healthy controls or subjects with chronic upper respiratory disease.

CMS WITH NORMAL LUNGS

The mechanism in cases with apparently normal lungs is less clear.

HYPOXIC VENTILATORY RESPONSE (HVR)

Severinghaus *et al.* (1966a) found that such patients have an extremely blunted HVR compared with healthy resident controls of the same age. Maybe people at the low end of the spectrum for HVR in the

population are destined to get CMS if they remain for years at altitude. The HVR decreases with age (Kronenberg and Drage 1973) and with duration of stay at altitude (Wiel *et al.* 1971); perhaps patients with CMS are those in whom the process is faster than average (Fig. 21.1).

Kryger *et al.* (1978a), however, found no difference in HVR between patients and age-matched controls in Leadville, Colorado. They did find that their patients had a greater dead-space/tidal volume ratio and that their ventilation increased on breathing 100 per cent oxygen; they therefore appeared to have hypoxic ventilatory depression. They concluded that blunted chemical drive to breathing is not the cause of CMS.

SLEEP

During sleep, even in normal subjects, the ventilation is depressed. If there are frequent periods of apnea, either central or obstructive, Sa_{O_2} will be further reduced and could contribute to the etiology. A recent study by Sun *et al.* (1996) found that CMS patients had more disordered breathing and lower mean Sa_{O_2} values when asleep than a group free of CMS.

GENDER

Women (at least before the menopause) seem to be protected from CMS as from the hypoventilation syndrome (the Pickwickian syndrome) at sea level, possibly by the stimulating effect of female sex hormones on ventilation. Leon-Velarde *et al.* (1997) compared premenopausal and postmenopausal women at Cerro de Pasco (4300 m) in Peru and found significantly higher hematocrit and Sa_{O_2}, and lower peak expiratory flows in the postmenopausal group, supporting the protective role of female sex hormones.

AGE

Age has effects on lung function as well as its effect on HVR. The Pa_{O_2} declines with age and, although this has little effect on oxygen saturation at sea level, it has much more effect at altitude because subjects are already on the steep part of the oxygen dissociation curve. A study by Leon-Velarde *et al.* (1993) at 4300 m in Peru found an increasing incidence of CMS with age. Taking a hemoglobin concentration of above

21.3 g dL^{-1} (the mean plus 2 SD of the total population aged 20–29 years) as 'excessive erythrocytosis', the incidence at 20–29 years was 6.8 per cent which increased to 33.7 per cent at age 60–69 years. This study also found a decreasing vital capacity with age at altitude, in both those with and without CMS, but the reduction was significantly more marked in the CMS group. Sea level subjects showed no reduction in vital capacity between 20–29 years and 60–69 years.

SUMMARY

Polycythemia results in reduced cerebral blood flow (Thomas *et al.* 1977) due to increased viscosity. There do not seem to have been studies of cerebral blood flow in CMS but there is no reason to doubt the assumption that it is reduced. Figure 21.1 shows the interaction of factors involved in CMS. Altitude hypoxia and hypoventilation will result in a low Pa_{O_2}.

This hypoventilatory response may be due to a low HVR, to hypoxic depression of ventilation or some unknown cause. If lung function is also reduced by lung or chest wall disease, this will reduce Pa_{O_2} still further. Aging results in both reduced lung function and reduced HVR, especially in a life spent at high altitude, thus further lowering the Pa_{O_2}. The low Pa_{O_2} results in a low Sa_{O_2}. It also stimulates secretion of erythropoietin and hence an increase in packed cell volume. However, it should be noted that a study of erythropoietin levels in subjects at Cerro de Pasco (4300 m), although showing the expected higher mean values at altitude than at sea level, did not demonstrate any difference between subjects with and without CMS (Leon-Velarde *et al.* 1991). The rise in packed cell volume causes a rise in blood viscosity and a fall in cerebral blood flow, which, with a low Sa_{O_2}, results in chronic severe cerebral hypoxia and symptoms of CMS.

22

Other altitude related conditions: neurovascular disorders, eye conditions, altitude cough, anesthesia at altitude

SUMMARY

A cluster of neurovascular signs and symptoms has been reported in mountaineers for many years. These vary from transient ischemic attacks (TIA), often with symptoms of dysphasia or transient visual disturbance or even blindness, to longer lasting strokes with hemiplegia, etc. The problems usually occur after some time at altitude and so are not considered part of acute mountain sickness (AMS). The condition usually resolves rapidly and recurrence is unusual. However, few patients expose themselves to altitude risk again. Also reviewed in this chapter is the effect of altitude on factors involved in clotting, which in general seem little disturbed at altitude. Risk factors for thrombosis and mechanisms are discussed.

Eye problems at altitude include retinal hemorrhage, transient visual disturbance or blindness, which may be neurovascular or migrainous in origin, and problems following corneal surgery. Retinal hemorrhage is normally a symptomless, benign condition diagnosed only if the retina is inspected. Small hemorrhages are seen which clear in a few days. The incidence is variable, often being over 50 per cent when looked for. It is usually seen early in altitude exposure. Only in rare cases, when the hemorrhage affects the macula, is vision disturbed. Problems after corneal surgery are confined to patients who have had radial keratotomy for myopia. In these patients the hypoxia of altitude results in a change in the refractive properties of the operated eye, making for long-sightedness. At extreme altitude this can render the patient almost blind. The problem resolves after descent.

Altitude cough, though known for many years, has only recently been scientifically investigated. It afflicts most climbers who remain at altitude for more than a few days and in severe cases can cause sleep disturbance, fatigue and even fracture of ribs. Although hyperventilation of the cold dry air at altitude may be a factor, it seems that hypoxia itself is important. The cough threshold for citric acid is lowered by stay at altitude and this can be prevented by therapy with antiasthma inhalers. Altitude also affects mucociliary function in the nose and this can be prevented by regular moistening of the nasal mucosa with saline.

General anesthesia at altitude is dangerous because of the respiratory depressant effects of anesthetics. They abolish the hypoxic ventilatory response (HVR) so that ventilation is reduced and with the low inspired P_{O_2} the risk of severe hypoxia is considerable. This risk of hypoxia extends into the postoperative period because even small concentrations of anesthetic gases depress the HVR. It is therefore advised that general anesthetic be avoided at altitude. Either local anesthetic should be used or the patient brought down to low altitude. If general anesthetic must be given at altitude, oxygen should be added at high concentrations.

22.1 INTRODUCTION

Apart from AMS in its various forms and cold injury, altitude can result in a variety of disorders. Transient ischemic attacks, attacks of dysphasia or strokes are encountered indicating an effect of altitude on the blood supply of the central nervous system (CNS). The eyes can be affected by retinal hemorrhage and various disturbances of vision, altitude cough may be a problem for climbers especially at extreme altitude, and it may be necessary to give anesthesia at altitude. These conditions are discussed in this chapter.

22.2 NEUROVASCULAR DISORDERS

22.2.1 Historical background

Increasingly, cases with neurological signs, some transient and others permanent, are being reported from expeditions at altitude in both lowlanders and highlanders. These are not associated with AMS, or high altitude cerebral or pulmonary edema (HACE, HAPE). It is likely that some have a vascular origin, such as spasm, thrombosis, embolus or hemorrhage. Others may be focal neurological disorders or are of unknown etiology.

Sporadic cases of vascular disorders have been described in the mountain and geographical literature over the last century (Table 22.1).

In 1895, while exploring the Amne Machin range in eastern Tibet, Roborovsky, a Russian traveler, suffered a 'stroke' in crossing the Mangur Pass (4270 m). He described 'a stroke of paralysis which attacked the right part of my body from head to the toes of my right foot; my tongue hardly obeyed my will. I lay in a disgusting and unbearable state for eight days.' Over the next few weeks he gradually recovered and continued his journey (Roborovsky 1896).

Cases of hemiplegia also occurred on Everest expeditions in 1924 and 1936. One, a Gurkha soldier, died, and the other, a Sherpa porter, recovered (Norton 1925, p. 68, Tilman 1948). Evans (1956, p. 169) on Kangchenjunga recorded a further fatal case of hemiplegia in a Sherpa. Each of these three cases was in a fit young man who had spent a considerable period above 6000 m.

In 1954, a young American mountaineer, stormbound in a tent at 7465 m on K2, developed thrombophlebitis in the calf and, after a further 2 days, had a hemoptysis. A provisional diagnosis of pulmonary embolus was made and he was evacuated; however, during the descent he was swept away in an avalanche (Houston and Bates 1979).

Shipton (1943), after climbing to 8865 m on Everest, described an episode of transient aphasia with severe headache. This was possibly due to a migraine attack. Apart from severe headache he had no other symptoms and was fully recovered by the next morning

Coronary and cerebral thrombosis and cases of phlebitis of the limbs have been reported (Fujimaki et al. 1986), as have TIA and transient blindness (Hackett et al. 1987c, Wohns 1987). Cases of lateral rectus palsy and diplopia have been described at altitude (Murdoch 1994). At sea level the development of lateral rectus muscle palsy is usually due to lesions in the sixth cranial nerve or its nucleus. It is found in cases of diabetes mellitus, neoplasm and raised intracranial pressure. At altitude, although raised intracranial pressure may be present in AMS and especially HACE, rectus palsy may occur in their absence.

Migraine with ophthalmoplegia has been reported at altitude. Its pathogenesis remains uncertain, although vascular mechanisms are considered important. Psychological factors may also be important (Jenzer and Bärtsch 1993). Unsuspected cases of

Table 22.1 *Cerebrovascular accidents at altitude. All subjects were male adults. The two patients who died were Sherpas; the remainder were climbers from low altitude*

Date	Altitude (m)	Time at altitude	Signs	Outcome	Source
1895	4300	?	Right hemiparesis	Recovered	Roborovsky (1896)
1924	6000	?	Hemiparesis	Died	Norton (1925)
1938	6400	?	Right hemiparesis	Recovered	Tilman (1948)
1943	6400	6 weeks	Dysphasia	Recovered	Shipton (1943)
1954	6000+	?	Hemiparesis	Died	Evans (1956)
1961	6400	7–8 weeks	Right hemiparesis	Recovered	Ward (1968)
1978	6400	?	Hemiparesis	?	Messner (1979, p. 137)
1982	8200	7 weeks	Left hemiparesis	Recovered	Clarke (1983)
1983	6100	?	Semi-conscious	Recovered	Asaji *et al.* (1984)
1986	4900	Several days	Headache, visual disturbance Numb right hand, ?migraine	Recovered	Jenzer and Bärtsch (1993)
1990	4800	9 days	Right hemiparesis	Recovered	Sharma *et al.* (1990)
1990	5300	Several days	Headache, weak right hand and right leg, ?migraine	Recovered	Jenzer and Bärtsch (1993)
1994	3867	4 days	Right lat. rectus palsy	Recovered	Murdoch (1994)
1994	4242	12 days	Right lat. rectus palsy	Recovered	Murdoch (1994)
1995	3660	100 mile race	Diplopia	Recovered	Murdoch (1994)
1997	7600	Several days	Right hemiparesis, CT scan edema, left parietal lobe	Recovered	Basnyat (1997)

brain tumor have become symptomatic at altitude (Shlim and Meijer 1991).

The term high altitude global amnesia (HAGA) has been used by Litch and Bishop (1999, 2000) to describe a variety of neurological features associated with transient loss of memory and confusion but not associated with obvious HAPE. As the cerebral cortex is vulnerable to hypoxia, local hypoxia of the limbic cortex may be implicated. Cases of HAGA, rectus palsy and TIA may be commoner than realized. There are many anecdotal accounts, but few cases are recorded in detail (Murdoch 1996). In Operation Everest III (Comex), a 40-day chamber study of eight subjects, there were three cases of TIA towards the end of the study at an altitude equivalent of above 8000 m. They all recovered rapidly (Richalet *et al.* 1999).

22.2.2 Cortical blindness and transient visual defects

Transient blindness has been reported in otherwise healthy individuals at altitude. Six cases at an altitude

of 4300 m were reported by Hackett *et al.* (1987c), four on Denali in Alaska and two at Pheriche near Everest. These individuals were not suffering from pulmonary edema or severe AMS. They did not have retinal hemorrhage. The blindness lasted from 20 min to 24 h, with intermittent periods of normal vision. Oxygen breathing relieved it and recovery was complete. It was thought to be due to hypoxia or ischemia of the visual cortex. Houston (1987) also reported various visual disturbances on acute exposure to altitude in chambers. There is some suggestion that subjects with a history of migraine are more susceptible and that aspirin may help prevent attacks, which may be related to platelet aggregation and microemboli.

22.3 PLATELETS AND CLOTTING

There has been considerable interest in factors in the blood associated with clotting, and the effect of hypoxia, with and without symptoms of AMS, on these systems. This is because of the frequent finding of thrombi in various organs at postmortem in cases of AMS and its complications (Dickinson *et al.* 1983), and the frequency of cases of cerebrovascular accidents at altitude.

22.3.1   Platelet counts

In mice, there is a profound fall in platelet count on exposure to hypoxia. Counts are down to 36 per cent of control by day 12 (Birks *et al.* 1975). In humans, no such fall has been found. It has been reported that in the first few days there is either no change (Maher *et al.* 1976, Sharma 1982), or a small fall of 3 per cent in subjects with AMS and a rise of 3 per cent in asymptomatic subjects (Sharma 1980). Chatterji *et al.* (1982) found a 12–26 per cent reduction in platelet count on day 2 or 3 at altitude in two studies at 3200 m and 3700 m. Counts increased towards control values over the next 10 days. These small changes may simply reflect hemoconcentration or dilution. With more prolonged exposure Sharma (1981) found a 14 per cent increase by 21–31 days followed by a fall to sea level values at 180 days. At 4300 m, a rise of between 50 per cent and 100 per cent has been found, both on arrival and 2 weeks later, after climbs to higher altitude (Simon-Schnass and Korniszzewski 1990).

22.3.2   Platelet adhesiveness

Under a variety of conditions platelets become more sticky, and this property may be important in initiating platelet thrombi. Sharma (1982) has also studied the effect of altitude on platelet adhesiveness. On acute exposure to altitude he reported an increase in platelet adhesiveness in subjects with AMS, compared with their sea level results. However, this was only on days 2 and 10 of altitude exposure and not on days 1 and 4. Also, the sea level values for symptomatic subjects were markedly less than for the asymptomatic group. Actual values at altitude were the same for both groups. He also reported (with others) that high altitude residents had significantly higher platelet adhesiveness than lowlanders at sea level (Sharma *et al.* 1980).

22.3.3   Coagulation

Singh and Chohan (1972a) found an increase in fibrinogen level and fibrinolytic activity in 38 sub-

jects at altitudes between 3670 m and 5470 m, but, in six subjects thought to have pulmonary hypertension on clinical grounds, the fibrinogen levels were lower, suggesting consumption coagulopathy. In these patients, factors V and VIII were increased, as was platelet factor III. Maher *et al.* (1976) also found a fall in fibrinogen level in eight subjects in a simulated altitude of 4400 m but no change in thrombin or prothrombin times; platelet factor III was normal. Partial thromboplastin time was shortened and factor VIII activity was reduced. Hyers *et al.* (1979) found accelerated fibrinolytic activity in subjects with and without susceptibility to AMS but no change in fibrinogen, partial prothrombin time, platelet lysis time or fibrinopeptide A. In patients with HAPE, fibrinogen levels and venous clot lysis time have been reported to be increased (Singh *et al.* 1969a, Singh and Chohan 1972a).

Bärtsch *et al.* (1982) showed, in 20 subjects taken rapidly to 3700 m, that there were no changes in coagulation tests 1 h after arrival. After strenuous exercise there was shortening of clotting time, euglobulin lysis time, and increase in factor VIII activity – changes that are all found on exercise at sea level. There was no change in fibrinopeptide A and no rise in fibrin degradation products or fibrin fragment E (i.e. no evidence of intravascular clotting). In a later project the contact phase of blood coagulation was studied in subjects who had ascended to 4559 m in 3 days. There was no evidence of activation of this system even in subjects who developed acute HAPE (Bärtsch *et al.* 1989).

An extensive study of the clotting cascade during a 40-day chamber experiment, Operation Everest II, when subjects were taken in stages up to the simulated equivalent altitude of Mount Everest, showed no significant changes in clotting factors, though thrombosis round the sites of Swan–Ganz catheters was common (Andrew *et al.* 1987).

In summary, it seems that the physiological response to hypoxia has not been shown to involve any important changes in platelet count or adhesiveness or in other clotting factors. However, there may be changes associated with AMS and especially HAPE (Singh and Chohan 1972b). These may include changes suggesting disseminated intravascular coagulation but this is still not proved. The changes so far demonstrated seem to appear rather too late in the course of altitude exposure to be considered causative, so, even if present, they may represent an effect or a complication of AMS rather than being essential in its genesis.

22.4 SPLINTER HEMORRHAGES

Splinter hemorrhages may occur under the finger-nails of high altitude natives, and are more pro-nounced in those with CMS and in climbers at extreme altitude (English 1987). In South American high altitude dwellers, the incidence appears to increase with altitude, rising from 34.9 per cent at 150 m to 57.9 per cent at 4200 m (Heath and Williams 1995, pp. 311–13). In over 1000 healthy Chinese children born at altitude, examination of the nails showed an increase in number of capillary loops and abnormal loops (Han *et al.* 1985). The cause of these hemorrhages may be associated with increased capillary fragility or it may be embolic or traumatic in origin.

22.5 RISK FACTORS FOR THROMBOSIS

The risk factors for thrombosis include decreased physical activity, dehydration, increased hematocrit and cold.

Physical activity may be greatly decreased at alti-tude. Individuals may spend several days recumbent in a sleeping bag in bad weather and, even in good weather, activity can be restricted by fatigue to a shorter working period each day than at lower levels.

Dehydration is common, with increased respira-tory water loss owing to cold and a high respiratory rate. A diminished sensation of thirst, together with the practical difficulties of melting snow to produce water, results in an inadequate fluid intake.

A hematocrit of 45–60 per cent is normal for sea level visitors to altitude and some high altitude resi-dents. When the hematocrit exceeds 50 per cent the apparent viscosity increases steeply. Vasoconstrict-ion further increases viscosity and thus cold will con-tribute (Whittaker and Winton 1933, Pappenheimer and Maes 1942). Cold can also damage vessel walls and by causing coronary vasoconstriction may be implicated in 'heart attacks'. Cerebral venous throm-bosis has been reported (Fujimaki *et al.* 1986, Song *et al.* 1986).

22.6 MECHANISMS OF VASCULAR ACCIDENTS

The mechanism of vascular accidents is debatable. Short-lived attacks may be due to spasm, or possibly a manifestation of migraine. Thrombosis is another possibility, due to a high hematocrit and dehydration (Ward 1975, pp. 289–92), and disturbances of coag-ulation and platelet function may also occur. In some cases hemorrhage cannot be ruled out. As with 'stroke' at lower altitudes, there may be different causes. However, the risk of a cardiovascular acci-dent in an otherwise fit person at altitude, though small, would appear to be greater than would be expected from such a population at sea level.

22.7 CASE HISTORIES

22.7.1 Patient A

A white man, aged 32, while climbing at 8400 m, sud-denly experienced a severe pain in the right side of his chest and collapsed. He was unable to move for 30 min and then started to cough up dark red blood. After a night at 8200 m he crawled down to a lower camp at 7800 m, continuing to complain of severe pain and coughing up blood.

Three days later, that is, 5 days after the initial inci-dent, he reached camp at 7800 m. He was barely con-scious and his feet and hands were gray-white in color and had the consistency of wood. He was evac-uated to a camp at 6400 m where his general condi-tion was poor and he was still coughing up blood. On examination, air entry at the base of the right lung was found to be greatly diminished, and there was deep frostbite to both legs below the knees, but both popliteal and femoral arteries were palpable. Deep frostbite was also present in the distal parts of all fin-gers and both thumbs.

In the next 2 days he was evacuated to 4600 m and then flown to hospital at 1100 m. Here a chest radio-graph showed shadowing in the right lower zone, presumably an infarct. Later he developed a lung abscess in this part of the lung and then an empyema with bronchopleural fistula. After a rib resection and drainage this resolved (Figures 22.1–22.3).

Eventually, bilateral below-knee amputation was carried out and all fingertips on both hands were

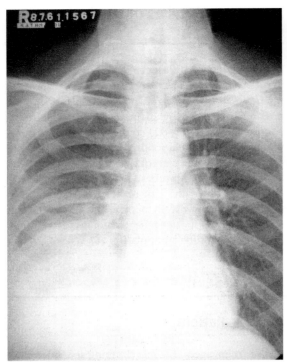

Figure 22.1 *Patient A: thrombosis of the right lower lobe, which occurred at 8350 m.*

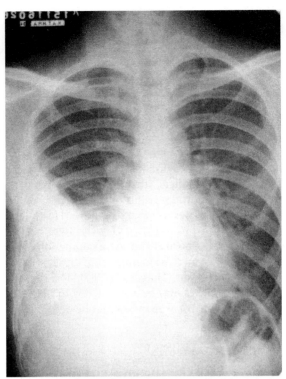

Figure 22.2 *Patient A: after the development of a right pleural effusion.*

removed after mummification. There remained some scarring of the right hand with restriction of finger and thumb movement (Ward 1968).

22.7.2 Patient B

A white man climbed from 7850 m to 8750 m in 13 h using supplementary oxygen and then spent 35 min on the summit. He bivouacked for the night a few hundred meters lower. The night temperature was estimated at −30 °C with winds gusting to 80–95 km h^{-1} (50–60 mph). During the night his supply of oxygen ran out and he shivered continuously. Later he estimated that he had had nothing to drink for 30 h while above 7900 m.

Next day he descended and developed a persistent cough. A day later he complained of pain in the left side of his chest and, when examined, was told that he had pneumonia and pleurisy. He continued to have chest pain and then 4–5 days later began coughing up blood. Eleven days after he had reached the summit, chest radiograph showed a left pleural effusion. Three days later he was admitted to hospital in the USA. Six weeks after the initial incident, at operation, a fibrous

tissue mass occupying 50 per cent of the lower half of the left thorax was excised. He made an uneventful recovery and postoperatively reached an altitude of 5800 m. His stamina has in no way been impaired (Wickwire 1982).

22.7.3 Patient C

A white man, aged 40, complained of severe headache at 6400 m. This continued for 3 days and was relieved by codeine tablets. By the evening of the third day he noticed that he could not speak properly. On examination he had nominal aphasia but could understand the spoken word. There was some evidence of right facial weakness with involuntary movements confined to the right side of the face. Both carotid arteries were palpable. There was loss of power in the right arm, but no loss of sensation. The lower limbs could not be examined as the patient was in a sleeping bag.

After sedation and continuous oxygen by mask for 8 h, he was able to descend to 5000 m, with some difficulty due to weakness of the arms and legs. For a

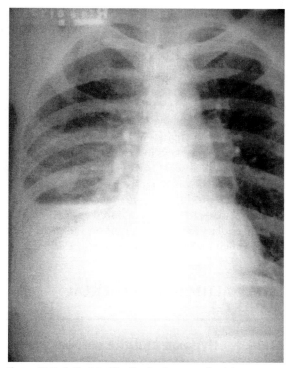

Figure 22.3 *Patient A: After the development of a right pyopneumothorax and bronchopleural fistula.*

further 3 days speech remained slurred, he was often at a loss for a word and individuals' names were mixed. After 15 days there were no residual signs; a note written at this time contained lucid statements and logical arguments and his writing was normal. There appeared to be no permanent after-effects (Ward 1968).

22.8 MANAGEMENT

22.8.1 Prevention

Adequate hydration is extremely important and, as the majority of mountaineers at extreme altitudes appear to be dehydrated, the danger of thrombosis occurring probably increases with length of stay.

Posture too may be significant, particularly while bivouacking, when a fetal position is assumed to prevent too much heat loss. As the knees, hips and arms are kept flexed there is an increased risk of thrombosis, so arm and leg stretching should be carried out regularly. Lying in a sleeping bag, particularly if the calves are constricted, may lead to the formation of 'silent' calf thrombosis. Regular movement is therefore important. In subjects with an abnormally high hematocrit (e.g. over 0.65), after adequate hydration, venesection should be considered if the subject plans to remain at altitude. Hemodilution has been used for treating polycythemia in mountaineers; it is considered to be a potentially hazardous maneuver (Sarnquist *et al.* 1986).

22.8.2 Treatment

Treatment will depend upon the diagnosis but all patients will benefit from descent and hydration. Oxygen may improve those who are severely shocked. Anticoagulants are potentially dangerous and adequate laboratory facilities should be available before they are used. However, in exceptional circumstances in cases of thrombosis and if the physician is experienced, small doses of a short-acting anticoagulant may be given. Return to altitude after a vascular episode should be considered with caution, but some have returned with future expeditions to climb at high altitude without recurrence of symptoms.

22.9 RETINAL HEMORRHAGE

22.9.1 Clinical features

In 1970 Frayser *et al.* reported retinal hemorrhages in 35 per cent of subjects flown to 5330 m. Since then retinal hemorrhages have been found in a proportion of climbers on a number of expeditions (Rennie and Morrissey 1975, Clarke and Duff 1976). The condition is almost always symptomless and self-limiting. The hemorrhages are usually multiple, often flame shaped and adjacent to a vessel. If near the disc there may be some blurring of vision.

Besides hemorrhages, 'cottonwool' spots have been reported in one case (Hackett and Rennie 1982) and some mild papilledema may be present as well. There is usually engorgement of both arteries and veins (Figure 22.4).

The hemorrhages are usually found during the first few days after ascent to altitude (the 'at risk' time for AMS) and subjects are often suffering from AMS, though the correlation with severity of AMS is not

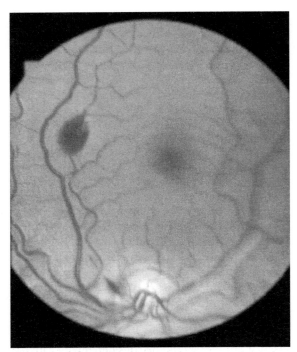

Figure 22.4 *Retinal hemorrhage at altitude.*

strong (Rennie and Morrissey 1975). A recent study by Wiedman and Tabin (1999) found a significant correlation between retinopathy and HACE ($p = 0.02$).

22.9.2   Incidence of retinal hemorrhage

The incidence varies from zero on one 10-member expedition to Mount Kongur (7719 m) in Xinjiang, to 15 of 16 members on an expedition to Peak Communism (7495 m) in Russia (Nakashima 1983). It seems that people going to altitude for the first time are especially liable to show this phenomenon (Clarke and Duff 1976) whereas experienced high altitude climbers and Sherpa residents are relatively immune. Wiedman and Tabin (1999) found retinopathy in 19 of 21 climbers who went to over 7500 m and in 14 of 19 who ascended to between 5000 and 7500 m.

22.9.3   Mechanism of retinal hemorrhage

At the time when retinal hemorrhage appears, the cerebral blood flow is increased (Severinghaus *et al.* 1966a). The blood flow through the retinal vessels is

increased by 105 per cent (Frayser *et al.* 1970). Rennie and Morrissey (1975) found arterial diameter to be increased by 24 per cent and venous diameter by 19 per cent. They suggest that, in the presence of these dilated vessels, the sudden rise in vascular pressure associated with coughing and straining may cause a microvessel to rupture; cough is common and severe at altitude (see section 22.11). However, Sakaguchi and Yurugi (1983) have produced retinal hemorrhage in monkeys in a chamber when presumably cough was absent. In 16 exposures 5 monkeys showed retinal hemorrhage, whereas no retinal hemorrhage was produced in 46 rabbits. The authors point out that rabbits, unlike monkeys or humans, have arteriolar–venular anastomotic vessels in their retina, which may protect them.

22.10   ALTITUDE AND CORNEAL SURGERY

22.10.1   Hypoxia and the cornea

The cornea relies on the direct diffusion of oxygen from the air for its oxygen supply. At altitude it therefore suffers from hypoxia but, unlike other tissues in the body, there can be no compensatory mechanisms of acclimatization such as increased ventilation and hemoglobin concentration. The effect of hypoxia on the cornea is to increase its hydration, causing it to swell. Shutting the eyes as in sleep results in lowering the P_{O_2} further so that any swelling will be worse after a night's sleep. Normally this swelling is not noticed and causes no change in the refraction of the eye in either normal eyes or myopia (short sight).

22.10.2   Surgery for myopia

A number of operations have been devised to change the refraction of the cornea in myopia, one of the most successful and frequently performed being radial keratotomy (RK). Millions of young people have now benefited from this operation. In this operation four to eight radial incisions are made in the cornea from the edge of the central area to the periphery. The effect of this maneuver is to cause a flattening of the cornea as the incisions heal and contract, reducing the power of the cornea/lens system and thus correcting much or all of the refractive error of the eye. Originally the incisions were made by a diamond scalpel but now a laser is usually used. Another operation is photorefractive keratectomy (PRK). Here a laser is used to ablate and remodel the anterior surface of the cornea, reducing its curvature.

22.10.3 Hypoxia and the postsurgical myopic patient

Mader and White (1995) and Mader *et al.* (1996) have studied the effect of hypoxia on subjects following surgery. In the first study four normal corneas were compared with four which had undergone RK at 12 000 ft (3658 m) and 17 000 ft (5182 m) for 24 h. They found that from sea level to 12 000 ft there was a change in refraction of the operated eyes of −0.59 diopters and at 17 000 ft of −1.75 diopters after 24 h. There was no change in the normal eyes. In the second study at 14 100 ft (5182 m), six subjects with RK, six with PRK and nine with myopia were studied daily for 3 days. There was no change in refraction in the subjects with myopia or PRK, whereas the RK subjects had significantly changed refraction. The mechanism of this change is probably due to the swelling of the cornea because of hypoxia causing further flattening of the RK cornea. The effect is to make the subject farsighted. These changes are all reversible after return to sea level. However, although the changes at moderate altitude are probably only of nuisance value, at extreme altitude they can result in near blindness which in turn can lead to catastrophe as in the case of an American climber on Everest in 1996 (Krakauer 1997). If subjects who have had RK wish to climb high they should be advised to take a selection of cheap positive lens glasses to correct the change in refraction that can be expected. It is not possible to predict this change accurately.

22.11 HIGH ALTITUDE COUGH

22.11.1 Background

It has been common knowledge amongst mountaineers that cough is a problem at high altitude, especially after some time spent at extreme altitude. Tasker writes in his account of the winter expedition on Everest's west ridge:

Alan (Rouse) . . . was still racked by frequent coughs and periodically, as if by auto-suggestion I found that I too was succumbing to a bout. Once started, there was no escape. The cold dry air compounded the irritation in the throat and the victim's body would be shaken by the hacking cough until randomly flung free of its spell. The nights at Base Camp as well as on the mountain were often punctuated by staccato bursts of noise disturbing the sleep of the sufferer and all those around (Tasker 1981).

Apart from disturbing the sleep of climbers, cough is quite debilitating and can even cause rib fracture (Steele 1971).

Although well known to climbers, altitude cough attracted no scientific study until Barry and colleagues carried out their work on the British Mount Everest Medical Expedition (BMEME) in 1994. They first documented the reality of increasing cough frequency with altitude and length of stay. They did this by using voice-activated tape recorders and showed that the number of coughs at night increased from zero at sea level to a mean of 60 per night at 7000 m (Barry *et al.* 1997a).

22.11.2 Mechanism

It has been generally assumed that the cause of altitude cough is the cooling and drying of the upper airway due to hyperventilating cold, dry air at altitude. However, anecdotal reports of cough in long-term chamber studies such as Operation Everest II, where the temperature and humidity were controlled at comfortable levels, gave pause for thought as to whether this was the whole story. In Operation Everest III (COMEX '97) cough frequency was monitored, again with voice-activated tape recorders, and shown to increase with altitude (Mason *et al.* 1999). In 1994 Barry and his team also measured the cough threshold to citric acid. In this test the subject is given a nebulizer of increasing concentrations of citric acid and the concentration which first provokes cough is noted. This threshold was reduced at altitude (Barry *et al.* 1997a). In the Operation Everest III study the cough threshold for citric acid also was shown to decrease at 8000 m even though the temperature was kept at 18–24 °C and relative humidity at 30–60 per cent

Barry *et al.* (1997b) also documented a decrease

in mucociliary clearance by the saccharin time test and also found that the sensation of nasal blockage was increased at Everest Base Camp. In a double-blind, placebo-controlled trail on Kangchenjunga in Nepal in 1998, the same team showed that salmeterol or nedocromil could prevent the reduction in cough threshold, though the effect on cough frequency was not significant (Bakewell *et al.* 1999). Also it was shown, in a controlled trial, that moistening the nasal mucosa by saline spray four times a day prevented the increase in saccharin times seen in the control group.

It is probably too early to make a coherent hypothesis taking into account the results of all these studies. It is apparent that altitude cough is not simply an effect of cold dry air and hyperventilation, though these may be factors. Results from chamber studies suggest that hypoxia *per se* is at least a factor. The importance of the changes in the nasal mucosa is also not clear. Finally, combining results of two separate studies from BMEME '94 showed that those individuals who had the greatest change in cough threshold also had the greatest increase in dynamic carbon dioxide ventilatory response (see section 5.16)(Barry *et al.* 1997c). This is in line with an earlier finding by Banner (1988) of a correlation between cough induced with hypotonic aerosol and the ventilatory response to carbon dioxide. This raises the possibility that central mechanisms may be involved.

22.12   ANESTHESIA

22.12.1   Summary

A considerable number of major medical centers are at altitudes of 1500–2000 m. General anesthetics are administered there safely, and with only minor modifications of techniques. Above 2000 m, increasing attention must be paid to the effects of decreased barometric pressure. Anesthetics are not normally administered above 4000 m, and the response to general anesthesia in this situation has not been systematically studied. Anesthesia above this altitude might, however, be required in an emergency and is potentially very dangerous This is because anesthesia abolishes the peripheral chemoreceptor response to hypoxia. This, together with the low PI_{O_2}, means that the patient is at serious risk of severe hypoxia. The

use of intravenous ketamine with oxygen enrichment may be the technique of choice but local anesthetic is considered safer at altitude (Stoneham 1995). Patients requiring general anesthetic should, wherever possible, be evacuated to lower altitude.

22.12.2   Avoidance of hypoxia

During anesthesia with spontaneous ventilation, breathing is almost always depressed and alveolar ventilation may be reduced to half the value appropriate to the metabolic rate. Whether breathing is spontaneous or artificial, there is usually an increase in the alveolar/arterial P_{O_2} gradient, equivalent to a shunt of about 10 per cent of pulmonary arterial blood flow. For these reasons maintenance of a normal arterial P_{O_2} requires, at sea level, an increase in the inspired oxygen concentration to 35–40 per cent. The inspired P_{O_2} is thus about 300 mm Hg and this should be maintained regardless of barometric pressure. The concentration of oxygen breathed by the anesthetized patient should therefore be increased in accordance with altitude, as shown in Table 22.2.

Nitrous oxide is an effective anesthetic at an alveolar partial pressure of about 750 mm Hg (70 per cent nitrous oxide at sea level is only a partial anesthetic). It will be clear from Table 22.2 that it cannot make a very effective contribution to anesthesia above 2000 m, at which altitude only 46 per cent of the inspired gas is available for nitrous oxide. It is contraindicated at any higher level and general anesthesia must then be based on potent volatile anesthetic agents vaporized in oxygen enriched mixtures. Intravenous anesthetics should only be used with oxygen enrichment of the inspired gas according to Table 22.2.

Table 22.2 *Minimal concentrations of oxygen in the inspired gas required to maintain a normal arterial* P_{O_2} *in the anesthetized patient*

Altitude (m)	P_B (mm Hg)	Oxygen concentration (%)	PI_{O_2} (mm Hg)
Sea level	760	40	285
2000	596	54	296
4000	462	72	298
6000	354	100	307

P_B, atmospheric pressure; PI_{O_2}, partial pressure of inspired oxygen.

22.12.3 Hypoxic ventilatory drive

Survival at altitudes much in excess of 5000 m depends upon hyperventilation in response to hypoxic drive, although this is counteracted by negative feedback, resulting from reduction of the P_{CO_2}. It is now established that anesthesia (and even subanesthetic concentrations of anesthetics) will totally abolish the peripheral chemoreceptor response to hypoxia (Knill and Celb 1978). It is therefore possible to envisage a situation in which a patient at 6000 m, who would normally have an arterial P_{O_2} of 45 mm Hg and a P_{CO_2} of 23 mm Hg, might perhaps be anesthetized with halothane and air. There would be rapid inactivation of peripheral chemoreceptors with decrease of P_{O_2} to about 23 mm Hg, which would threaten life. An increased oxygen concentration is therefore essential, not only during anesthesia, but in the postoperative period, because the peripheral chemoreceptors are severely depressed by as little as one-tenth of the anesthetic concentration of volatile anesthetic agents.

22.12.4 Performance of vaporizers

Calibrated vaporizers depend upon known dilution of saturation concentrations of volatile anesthetics. The saturation concentration equals the vapor pressure divided by the barometric pressure. Vapor pressure depends only on temperature. Thus, if the barometric pressure is halved, the saturation concentration is doubled. If the dilution ratio of the vaporizer is unaffected by the reduction in barometric pressure (a reasonable assumption), it may be expected that the vaporizer will then deliver twice the concentration shown on the dial. However, the pharmacological effect depends on partial pressure. Twice the concentration at half the barometric pressure gives the same partial pressure as at sea level. Therefore, as a first approximation, probably adequate for clinical purposes, a temperature controlled calibrated vaporizer may be expected to produce the same effect for the same dial setting at altitude as at sea level.

These concepts have never been tested at altitude. However, one of the authors (MPW), Nunn and Woolmer anesthetized one another in a chamber at a pressure of 375 mm Hg in 1961, in preparation for the Himalayan Scientific and Mountaineering Expedition (Silver Hut) 1960–1. The apparatus was based on equipment designed for use in Antarctica (Nunn 1961). With a carrier gas of 60 per cent oxygen in nitrogen, obtained with oxygen flow through an injector, and a standard halothane vaporizer (Fluotec Mark 2), uneventful anesthesia was easily obtained in all three subjects and recovery was rapid and uneventful. In view of the subsequent discovery of the effect of anesthetics on the peripheral chemoreceptors, we would now favour 100 per cent oxygen at this simulated altitude of nearly 6000 m.

22.12.5 Practical considerations

The greater the altitude the lower is the possibility of a trained anesthetist and appropriate equipment being available. Dangers are multiplied by anesthesia being attempted in this very hostile environment by someone who is untrained. The first rule must be to avoid anesthesia above 4000 m if at all possible and to evacuate rather than attempt surgical intervention on the spot.

If anesthesia is essential, then oxygen enrichment of the inspired gas is essential for both patient and anesthetist throughout the perioperative period. The safest technique is probably a nonirritant volatile anesthetic (halothane, enflurane or isoflurane) vaporized in oxygen-enriched air according to Table 22.2. It was demonstrated that this technique could be accomplished at sea level by medical officers without special training in anesthesia who were destined for the Antarctic (Nunn 1961). Transport of sufficient oxygen, the vaporizer and the gas delivery system would clearly present logistic difficulties. Use of the open mask is not recommended because of the difficulty in controlling the inspired oxygen concentration. Ruttledge (1934) described a near disaster when chloroform was administered on an open mask at 4300 m on the Tibetan plateau during the march in on the 1933 Everest expedition. This would be expected on present understanding.

Intravenous anesthesia should not be attempted at altitude by those without experience because of the dangers of respiratory obstruction and depression. However, ketamine (2–4 mg kg^{-1}) might well be satisfactory because the patient's airway and respiratory drive are well maintained with this drug. This is logistically very attractive for major disasters, mass casualties and warfare. There is good analgesia, and duration is sufficient for any procedure likely to be considered. Hallucinations may occur but would be the least of the patient's problems. Ketamine should only be administered with oxygen enrichment. A study of the use of ketamine anesthesia at 1850 m without supplementary oxygen found that saturation values fell below 90 per cent in significant numbers of patients, particularly in adults. However, the authors conclude that ketamine was acceptable provided that supplementary oxygen and staff experienced in airway management were readily available (Pederson and Benumof 1993). A recent report from Khunde Hospital (3900 m) in Nepal describes the successful use of ketamine in 11 cases. A low dose (2.0 mg kg^{-1}) was used and premedication with midazolam prevented the nightmares commonly encountered with ketamine. Oxygen saturation was maintained either with supplemental oxygen or by encouraging the patient to breathe faster and deeper (Bishop *et al.* 2000).

Reliance on injectable solutions must be tempered by the hazard of freezing and breakage of ampoules. Local anesthetic techniques are obviously safer and should be used if at all possible in preference to general anesthesia at altitude.

22.12.6   Postanesthetic period

In the postanesthetic period, after a general anesthetic, the hazard of hypoxia due to respiratory depression discussed above is still very real. Indeed, in the hours after the operation, the danger may be greater since the patient may not be so closely watched as during anesthesia.

It should be remembered that, even at sea level, patients are normally mildly hypoxic during this stage. Hypoxia may cause restlessness, irritability and confusion, which may be misinterpreted as being due to pain. Additional analgesics may then be administered which further depress respiration and the patient may die from hypoxic cardiac arrest. This was probably the sequence of events in a Sherpa operated upon for debridement of frostbitten fingers at an altitude of 3900 m. Clearly, supplementary oxygen must be given during the postanesthetic period if available. The patient must be closely watched and stimulated to breathe either by verbal encouragement or, possibly, by the use of a respiratory stimulant such as doxapram.

Thermal balance and its regulation

SUMMARY

To maintain cell function, the core temperature must be kept between 36°C and 38°C and this enables humans to be almost independent of the environmental temperature. The price paid is a relatively high metabolic rate. The regulation of core temperature depends on physiological and cultural mechanisms, whereas thermal exchange relies on convection, conduction, radiation and evaporation. At high altitude the balance between heat production and loss is tilted, because of hypoxia, towards poor heat production and increased loss. Indeed, hypothermia and frostbite can occur despite subjects being fully clothed and mobile. Solar radiation may be critical in preventing hypothermia. Clothing insulation is of great importance, but malnutrition, fatigue, food and fluid intake also all influence temperature regulation.

23.1   GENERAL PRINCIPLES

For the past 70 million years mammals (homeotherms) have developed a system of temperature regulation which keeps the core temperature between 36°C and 38°C to maintain cell function.

This enables them to be almost independent of the temperature of the environment, which may vary from +40°C to –40°C, and is therefore of considerable evolutionary advantage. The price that is paid is a relatively high metabolic rate compared with poikilotherms, or cold-blooded animals, whose core temperature is more closely allied to that of the environment.

To maintain cell function, the core temperature of humans has to remain within a narrow band, though small variations occur during the menstrual cycle, the circadian rhythm and fever. A core temperature higher than 41°C (hyperthermia) or lower than 35°C (hypothermia) may cause death.

The relationship between heat production by the body and heat loss to the environment obeys two physical laws.

- **Fournier's law** states that the rate of heat transfer between an object (or animal) and the environment is proportional to its surface area and the difference in temperature between the body and the environment. As all living organisms produce heat by metabolism and since heat flows from a hot to a cold object, all living animals that usually have a higher body temperature than the environmental temperature will therefore lose heat to the environment.

When heat production is exactly balanced by heat loss a steady-state temperature will have been achieved. As poikilotherms have no control mechanisms to alter the relationship between heat loss and heat production, their metabolic rate, body temperature and activity will be dependent on the environmental temperature.

- **Arrhenius's law,** put simply, states that, as temperature increases, so does the metabolic rate and therefore the rate of heat production.

23.2 REGULATION OF CORE TEMPERATURE

Two main mechanisms regulate core temperature and keep it at 37 °C. There are physiological or reflex mechanisms, which are involuntary, and behavioral mechanisms, which are voluntary.

23.2.1 Physiological mechanisms

PHYSICAL

Physical mechanisms include vasomotor control, which can alter blood flow to the skin by a factor of more than 100, and sweat production. In the cold, to reduce heat loss from the periphery, blood is shunted from the surface to the deeper vessels. Conversely, as the ambient temperature rises, so more blood flows through the surface vessels to dissipate heat.

When the ambient temperature is higher than the temperature of the body surface, and heat loss by radiation, conduction and convection is not possible, then active sweat production starts and heat is lost by evaporation.

Thus by physical means alone humans can tolerate a wide range of environmental temperatures and still maintain a constant core temperature.

CHEMICAL

Chemical mechanisms enable adjustments of metabolism to be made by hormonal and neural methods. These come into play when physical methods have been overtaxed, for example when maximal vasoconstriction has taken place but heat loss remains larger than heat production.

First, muscle tone is increased, then muscle tremors occur and finally shivering starts. Intense shivering can raise the metabolic rate by three to four times the basal level. Heat is produced very efficiently as no external work is done and virtually all the energy from contraction is produced as heat within the muscle. In addition, nonshivering thermogenesis can increase basal metabolism by 30–40 per cent.

In humans, therefore, physiological mechanisms alone are capable of maintaining a constant core temperature at widely varying environmental temperatures.

23.2.2 Behavioral mechanisms

Behavioral mechanisms include all voluntary actions that make the individual thermally comfortable. In hot conditions, taking cold drinks, seeking the shade, and air conditioning are common; in cold climates extra clothing is worn, exercise is increased, and the individual stays indoors and lights a fire.

These mechanisms give us the greatest independence from the environment and, through our ingenuity and the application of modern technology, we can survive in the hottest, coldest, deepest and highest places on Earth and even in space.

23.3 THERMAL BALANCE

A useful but oversimplified concept is to imagine the body as consisting of a central core at a fairly uniform temperature of 37 °C, with some organs such as the liver at 1–2 °C higher, and an insulating shell some degrees lower. The body is therefore continually losing heat and in a cold environment has to maintain a balance between heat production and heat loss (Burton and Edholm 1955). In reality there is no physical or anatomical boundary separating the central core from the insulating shell and the difference can be thought of in terms of the temperature of the tissues.

- In hot weather, or during periods of increased exercise, some heat loss is necessary to maintain thermal balance, and the core is enlarged, extending into the root of the extremities. During exercise most heat production occurs in the proximal muscles of the limbs and the skin vessels are dilated to bring warm blood to the skin surface to lose heat; as a result the insulating shell is thin.

- In a cold climate, or when heat production falls and it is important to conserve heat, skin vessels contract and venous return is confined to the deeper vessels. The core decreases in size and is restricted to the head, neck, thorax and abdomen, and the thickness of the insulating shell increases. As blood flow to the skin can be increased to 100 times that of normal by vasomotor activity, and as much of the transfer of heat in the body is by convection via the blood flow, this is a very important method of heat conservation.

As well as vertical temperature gradients between skin and vessels there are also longitudinal gradients down the length of the limbs where countercurrent heat exchange takes place between the arteries and veins.

23.4   COLD-INDUCED VASODILATATION

The object of thermal regulation is to maintain the central core temperature at 37 °C and, if the environmental temperature falls, the body will 'sacrifice' the extremities to maintain the core, but it does put up a considerable fight to maintain the temperature of the extremities. To this end, under certain conditions and in some individuals only, the extremities exhibit the phenomenon of cold-induced vasodilatation. When this occurs the normal response to cold, which is peripheral vasoconstriction to reduce blood flow and heat loss, is reversed, and vasodilatation occurs. Warm blood flows to the periphery and the temperature is raised. This surge is transient only and vasoconstriction then sets in. The mechanism is not certain but, although it could be central in origin, the neural mechanism for vasoconstriction may be inhibited by local cooling causing the vessels to relax.

The magnitude of the heat input to the extremity caused by cold-induced vasodilatation is small and cannot prevent frostbite at below-zero temperatures, or nonfreezing cold injury, but it may result in less finger pain when working in cold conditions (Hoffman and Wittmers 1990).

23.5   THERMAL EXCHANGE

The body is continually losing heat to the environment and heat exchange occurs by convection, radiation, conduction and evaporation.

23.5.1   Convection

Convection is a molecule-to-molecule transfer of energy. The medium accepting heat is either a gas in motion or a fluid. Although the thermal conductivity and heat capacity of a gas may be low, its movement ensures a high thermal gradient between the body and the environment. The wind chill factor describes the increased heat loss by convection due to air movement, either by wind or body movement. Convection is also an important avenue of heat exchange during immersion in water; even in still water it is 26 times that of air. Heat transfer within the body is by convection, that is, by the flow of blood, which is a factor of great physiological importance.

In a cold environment warm air currents are generated adjacent to the skin and slowly rise to be replaced by cold air, which in turn is heated at the expense of body temperature. The rate of convective heat exchange depends on the amount of exposed skin surface area (which is almost always less than the total body surface) and the extraneous air movement, which will accelerate the movement of warm air currents; this is so-called 'forced convection'.

Posture is important and the surface area may be reduced by curling up in the fetal position, which is a behavioral response. The heat required to maintain a constant internal temperature is heavily dependent on the body mass/surface area ratio. The heat loss from a squat individual is significantly less than from a tall, thin person of the same weight. Children have a particularly unfavorable ratio and easily become hypothermic.

WIND AND WIND CHILL

An important influence on the rate of heat exchange by convection is the wind. Forced convection, either by wind or by relative air movement (e.g. downhill skiing or riding in open vehicles), is a major cause of heat loss in a cold environment; this is known as wind chill.

Wind chill correlates the effects of wind and temperature and provides an index which corresponds to the degree of discomfort that is experienced in the field (Siple and Passel 1945). This effect can be quantified by quoting the equivalent still air temperature produced by any given wind speed. This is shown in Table 23.1. For instance, at a temperature of −1°C the effect of a 10 mph (16 km h⁻¹) wind on the skin is equivalent to a still air temperature of −9 °C.

Under field conditions, however, the tolerance of humans to cold and wind is determined by those parts that are unprotected, often the face and hands. Exposing the face when walking into the wind is less tolerable than walking at an angle and with some protection.

The chilling power of the wind can produce extreme cooling of the skin and, without protection, frostbite of the nose, chin and cheeks is common at ambient temperatures of 0 °C or above. At high altitude, because of decreased air density, the wind chill factor for a given temperature and wind velocity is less than at sea level, but the wind velocity is frequently very high.

As the skin temperature falls from −4.8 °C to −7.8 °C the risk of frostbite increases from 5 per cent to 95 per cent. The risk of frostbite above an air temperature of −10 °C irrespective of wind speed is low, but below −25 °C there is a pronounced risk even at low wind speed (Danielsson 1996).

CONVECTION CURRENTS

Warm air rises and, if cooled, falls, setting up convection currents. Around the neck this produces a feeling of a draught as warm air from the skin rises around the collar to be replaced by cold air. A close-fitting collar reduces heat loss by this means.

AIR MOVEMENT

Air in the clothes is displaced by body movement, which has a balloon effect on the trunk and a pendulum effect in moving limbs. This effect is reduced by close-fitting garments. However, in so-called windproof clothing, some wind penetration and increased heat loss always occur. With increased relative air movement as the outer layers of clothing are cooled there is an increase in the thermal gradient across the layers beneath.

23.5.2 Radiation

The transfer of heat by electromagnetic energy (i.e. movement of photons from a warm surface to a cooler one), can be a most important source of heat loss and would still take place even if a vacuum replaced the air. It is independent of air movement.

All objects warmer than absolute zero emit radiation and therefore lose heat but they also gain heat from objects around them by the same process.

Table 23.1 *Wind speed and equivalent chill temperature*

Wind speed (mph)	Equivalent chill temperature (°C)									
0	4	−1	−7	−12	−18	−23	−29	−34	−40	−46
5	2	−4	−9	−15	−21	−26	−32	−37	−43	−48
10	−1	−9	−15	−23	−29	−37	−34	−51	−57	−62
15	−4	−12	−21	−29	−34	−43	−51	−57	−65	−73
20	−7	−15	−23	−32	−37	−46	−54	−62	−71	−79
25	−9	−18	−26	−34	−43	−51	−59	−68	−76	−84
30	−12	−18	−29	−34	−46	−54	−62	−71	−79	−87
35	−12	−21	−29	−37	−46	−54	−62	−73	−82	−90
40	−12	−21	−29	−37	−48	−57	−65	−73	−82	−90

Little danger   Increasing danger — Flesh may freeze within 1 min   Great danger — Flesh may freeze within 30 s

Source: data redrawn from Mills (1973a).
10 mph = 16.1 km h⁻¹.

Heat loss by radiation can be considerable in a cold environment if the body is not covered and insulated. Exposed face and hands lose heat to the clear cold night sky by radiation, and gain heat from the bright sun even in cold conditions. The greatest source of heat gain by radiation is from the sun and, in the clear polar or mountain regions where snow forms a reflection, this effect is enhanced. An overcast sky diminishes radiation, and at night the Earth loses heat by radiation to the black sky, with clear nights being cooler than those when cloud acts as a blanket and heat is retained.

The heat received by the body in full sunshine may be two or three times greater than that generated by normal metabolic processes. The amount adsorbed on the surface of clothing will depend on posture, the reflecting power of clothing surface, the absorption of radiation by dust and moisture, and reflection from the ground.

The amount of heat gained from solar radiation will vary with the degree of cloud cover and type of clothing. Black clothing adsorbs about 88 per cent of solar radiation, khaki 57 per cent and white clothing 30 per cent.

In Antarctica, because of the clean air, solar radiation reaches levels which at lower latitudes are found only at high altitude. Heat gain from snow reflection – the albedo – is an important factor at high altitude and polar regions and may vary from 75–90 per cent in snow to 25 per cent if it is absent. Heat gain also varies with the sun's 'altitude' in the sky; it is low at dawn and increased at midday (Chrenko and Pugh 1961).

In polar regions in summer, solar heat gain may be two to four times greater than in desert, and at high altitude the gain will be comparable. At extreme altitude this may be crucial to survival, as diminished oxygen uptake reduces heat output from exercise with the result that body temperature may fall, and heat from solar radiation keeps the climber in thermal balance.

23.5.3 Conduction

Conduction involves a molecule-to-molecule transfer of energy between two solids in physical contact. Under most conditions heat exchange by this method is small because the contact surface area between individuals and the environment is small. However, it may be of great importance during the rescue or transporting of casualties; extra insulation must be provided under the body when lying or sitting on a cold surface. Localized frostbite may occur should the body surface come into contact with materials of a high thermal conductivity below zero temperature. Touching the cold metal of an ice axe with bare hands or spilling liquids onto the body can result in frostbite or hypothermia. When clothing becomes soaked it can lose up to 90 per cent of its insulating value.

Different tissues conduct heat at different rates. Fat is a good insulator and skin over areas of fatty tissue will cool more rapidly and to lower temperatures than areas where fat deposits are scanty. For most tissues thermal conductivity is a function of fluid content and tissue blood flow in a cold climate. Prolonged vasoconstriction leads to fluid shifts and increases central blood volume, which in turn leads to a diuresis. A decrease in tissue conductivity results but this is marginal considering the total insulation required under cold conditions.

23.5.4 Evaporation

Unlike conduction, convection and radiation, where heat may be both gained and lost, with evaporation heat can only be lost.

During heavy exercise and in hot climates evaporation of sweat is essential, and in a very hot climate, where environmental temperatures exceed skin temperature, the body may be actually gaining heat by radiation, conduction and convection. Evaporation therefore is the only method of heat loss and means of preventing hyperthermia.

About 25 per cent of the total heat loss in humans is by evaporation from the skin and respiratory tract. Significant heat loss will occur by evaporation in the process of drying clothes by body heat, particularly in a wind or at altitude where the air is dry.

SKIN

As the epidermis is only slightly permeable to water, the rate of loss by passive diffusion is small. Insensible water loss and sweating account for 66 per cent of the evaporative heat loss under normal conditions. Sweating occurs as a result of exercise and emotion, particularly fear. During exercise thermal balance is maintained by the heat of increased metabolism being balanced by the heat loss from the evaporation of sweat. However, if exercise is stopped abruptly, heat continues to be lost from evaporation of sweat on the skin and in clothing but as the metabolic rate falls the individual cools.

Large amounts of fluid, over 1 L h^{-1}, may be lost by sweating, particularly with severe exercise or in a hot environment. If the air is dry and there is a wind, heat loss by evaporation is limited only by the rate of sweat secretion. If the air is moist and still, loss is limited by the rate of water evaporated from the skin. In very cold conditions considerable loss may result from the sweat generated through exercise first evaporating, but then condensing and freezing inside the outer layers of clothing. Increased sweating therefore results in both heat and water loss.

RESPIRATORY TRACT

The temperature of expired air is below body temperature and is probably not fully saturated with water even at this lower temperature (Ferrus *et al.* 1984, Milledge 1992). Even so, with normal ventilation, heat loss amounts to about one-third of the total loss from evaporation. At high altitude, with higher ventilation rates, this will increase particularly as the air is drier. In the cold, even at sea level, the volume of body water lost through respiration is large enough to cause dehydration and weight loss, and may damage the upper respiratory tract.

23.6 REGULATION OF BODY TEMPERATURE

In a cold environment normal maintenance of body temperature is by balancing heat loss against heat production, the main control being a central 'thermostatic' mechanism in the hypothalamus. This regulates the body temperature within narrow limits but it is not a simple on–off device. There is a complex system of neurones linking input and output with many cross-links, which produces a graduated response.

Sensory input comes from central receptors along the internal carotid artery, reticular part of the mid-brain, the pre-optic region and the posterior hypothalamus. Peripheral receptors are situated in the skin and stomach, and there is also clinical evidence of receptors inside peripheral veins (Lloyd 1979).

23.6.1 Variation of body temperature

CIRCADIAN RHYTHM

Adult rhythm develops after the age of 2 years. Body temperature shows cyclic changes throughout the day, with an early morning low (oral temperature 36.6 °C) and a late afternoon high (37.4 °C). This may be upset when prolonged daylight, as in polar summer or darkness as in polar winter (Colquohoun 1984), disturbs the normal day/night ratio. Sleep and mental depression lower the temperature settings (Crawford 1979).

INDIVIDUAL VARIATION

Normally there is little temperature difference between individuals but there are occasional exceptions. A persistent core temperature of 35.5–36.0 °C has been recorded.

LEVEL OF ACTIVITY

Activity leads to an increase in body temperature. Heavy exercise will result in a high body temperature; sleep or quiet resting causes a fall in temperature.

AGE

Shivering is not present in infants but develops as the nervous system matures. Sweating occurs in children and obesity retards heat loss. Over the age of 60 years thermoregulatory capacity declines, less sweating occurs and the vasoconstrictor response is reduced.

GENDER

The thermoregulatory response in women is similar to that in men. However, the normal increase in subcutaneous fat in women may make them less at risk of cold injury under similar climatic conditions. During a winter climb on Mont Blanc in France Raymond Lambert, a well known Swiss climber who reached 8530 m on Everest in 1952, suffered severe frostbite with amputation of fingers and toes, but his female companion Lulu Boulaz escaped unhurt.

During the menstrual cycle the core temperature is 0.5 °C lower in the follicular than in the luteal phase, probably due to increased progesterone levels.

During pregnancy the thermoregulatory system is more sensitive to heat produced by exercise.

With the menopause both thermoregulation and cardiovascular irregularities have been observed and exercise at high environmental temperatures may be particularly stressful.

23.7 HEAT PRODUCTION

Between 27 °C and 29 °C, the critical air temperature, an unclothed person at rest can maintain the body temperature, as basal metabolic heat is balanced by heat loss.

Eating increases basal heat whereas malnutrition decreases it and may result in hypothermia; exercise increases heat production considerably.

23.7.1 Shivering thermogenesis

Exposure to cold increases muscle tone and metabolism and leads to shivering, which may increase oxygen uptake up to fivefold. The onset of shivering is controlled by central and peripheral stimuli working independently (Lim 1960) and may be triggered by external stimulus. It is progressive, starting from the neck muscles, proceeding to the pectoral and abdominal musculature and then the extremities. Shivering metabolism is proportional to lowered mean skin temperature when the core temperature is constant and to the core temperature when the skin temperature is constant (Hong and Nadel 1979).

Although shivering is useful for increasing metabolism in an emergency it makes coordinated motor tasks difficult and energy resources are depleted, hastening the onset of fatigue and hypothermia. If cold exposure continues, considerable stored glycogen is burnt and the associated water loss may be as high as 1.5 L. However, under normal conditions this should be replenished in the next 48–72 h.

23.7.2 Nonshivering thermogenesis

Nonshivering thermogenesis (NST), or lipolytic thermogenesis, is the production of heat from adipose tissue, especially brown fat. There is controversy over the occurrence of NST in adult humans (Hervey and Tobin 1983, Rothwell and Stock 1983). Although in humans, brown fat persists into the sixth decade in the neck, mediastinum, kidneys and suprarenal glands and around the aorta (Heaton 1972), it constitutes only a very small fraction of the total body fat.

The infant relies, for the most part, on NST to maintain thermal balance, brown fat accounting for 25–35 per cent of its fat stores.

It is debatable how much norepinephrine can increase heat production in tissues other than brown fat. The breakdown and resynthesis of neutral fat are a possibility, and protein catabolism is increased on acute cold exposure (Goodenough et al. 1982).

The insulation of subcutaneous fat enables obese people to withstand cold better than the lean, but a lowered NST response has been found in post-obese individuals (Jequier et al. 1974).

23.7.3 Activity

Maximal physical exercise ($V_{O_2 max}$) increases heat production by 20 times the basal rate; about five times the normal basal heat production can be maintained for several hours (Maugham 1984). In cold conditions, additional heat may be produced through shivering and, as this can occur during exercise, oxygen consumption will be increased.

Limitation will be imposed by altitude where oxygen uptake falls and shivering may be inhibited. In very cold conditions too, oxygen uptake may be insufficient to meet the demand imposed by both exercise and cold. Exhausted individuals and those with malnutrition cannot increase metabolism because of lack of substrate (Wang 1978) and will be at increased risk from hypothermia.

23.8 HEAT LOSS

Overheating may, at times, be a problem in the mountains, particularly on glaciers in still, sunny weather. When body temperature rises due to increased exercise or too much insulation, body heat must be lost and vasodilatation occurs which raises the skin temperature. Vasodilatation also increases the transfer of heat from the core to the shell and the amount of fluid available to the sweat glands.

Sweating is an important method of heat loss which may be impaired by dehydration and drugs;

there are also individual differences in regional sweating patterns (Hertzman 1957).

23.9 HEAT CONSERVATION

Heat conservation occurs by physiological methods and by insulation of clothing and shelter.

23.9.1 Vasoconstriction

Below the critical ambient temperature of 27–29 °C cold receptors in the skin initiate subcutaneous vasoconstriction which limits blood flow to the peripheral shell and this results in a decrease in skin temperature and reduced heat loss. The thermal insulation of skin varies from 0.15 CLO on vaso-dilatation to 0.9 CLO on vasoconstriction (Burton and Edholm 1955). (The definition of the CLO is given in section 23.9.3.)

In the scalp there is minimal vasoconstriction and this makes the scalp less liable to cold injury by comparison with the limbs. At rest at –4 °C, heat loss from the head may be half the resting heat production in a clothed subject (Froese and Burton 1957). However, the nose, face and ears do vaso-constrict and hence are liable to frostbite.

23.9.2 Countercurrent heat exchange

SUBCUTANEOUS GRADIENT

Subcutaneous temperature varies with the depth and location of arteriolar and venous plexuses, being highest at about 0. 8 mm from the skin. A drop in temperature superficial to this is due to returning venous blood being cooler than arterial blood and heat from the arterioles being lost to the veins.

Fluctuations in temperature are controlled by arteriolar–venous anastomoses; their opening results in warm blood passing to the veins and the dissipation of heat.

LONGITUDINAL GRADIENT

Arterial blood loses heat in the surface capillaries and returns to cool the body. Heat lost in this manner is reduced as arteries and their accompanying veins exchange heat through their walls along the length of the limb. Thus the blood reaching the skin capillaries is precooled and the temperature gradient between capillaries and the skin surface is reduced; venous blood is warmed and heat conserved.

The temperature gradient down the length of a limb may be more important in the control of insulation than the gradient from the deep tissues to the skin (Bazett and McGlone 1927).

23.9.3 Insulation

The CLO, which was introduced in 1941, is a practical unit of thermal insulation for describing heat exchange in humans. One CLO will maintain a resting, sitting subject, whose metabolic rate is 50 kcal m^{-2} h^{-1} (209 kJ m^{-2} h^{-1}), comfortable indefinitely in an environment of 22 °C with a relative humidity less than 50 per cent and air movement 6 m min^{-1}.

The CLO is not a rigorously scientific unit of heat resistance but nevertheless is a useful working unit for the comparison of insulation. It is equivalent to the insulation afforded by ordinary business clothing and underwear for a sedentary worker in comfort-able indoor surroundings (Burton and Edholm 1955). The value for insulation of tissues is 0.15–0.9 CLO, for air 0.2–0.8 CLO and clothing 0–6.0 CLO. The importance of the insulating values of clothes is obvious. Under certain extreme conditions, tissue insulation may be important.

23.9.4 Tissue insulation

Heat transfer in the body occurs by mass flow along the blood vessels, but, as the capillaries do not extend to the superficial parts of the epidermis, heat is transferred from the capillaries to the skin surface by conduction. This rate of heat transfer is determined by the number of capillaries and their caliber. The thermal insulation of tissues varies from 0.15 CLO on vasodilatation to 0.9 CLO on vasoconstriction; countercurrent heat exchange prevents excessive heat loss. Subcutaneous fat is the most important form of natural insulation and, as fat has few blood vessels, thermal conductivity is less than in muscle. The greater the fat layer, the lower the skin temperature and the smaller the gradient between skin surface and environment (Keatinge et al. 1986).

Individuals with a good layer of subcutaneous fat will still shiver, as the temperature receptors are in the skin and thus superficial to the insulating layer. However, the heat produced by shivering will be retained by the subcutaneous fat and result in a smaller fall in rectal (central) core temperature and less increase in heat production. Obesity is, however, rare in indigenous people in cold climates or at altitude.

Sites where subcutaneous fat is thin or absent are more liable to local cold injury. These include the tips of the fingers, nose and ears.

23.9.5 Air insulation and wind chill

In the cold, air density increases and loss of heat by radiation decreases, but this is almost completely compensated for by an increase in heat loss by convection. Heat loss varies with wind velocity and the loss increases up to about 16 km h^{-1}. At higher speeds there is little further increase in heat loss.

23.9.6 Clothing

Insulation and protection from the wind are the most important functions of clothing in dry conditions. In wet conditions waterproofing is an important factor in maintaining insulation. Insulation depends on trapped, still air and is proportional to the volume of this air. To maintain insulation, the trapped, still air must remain immobile to prevent air currents and loss of heat by convection. A windproof outer layer should prevent a large proportion of wind penetration. Materials should maintain their thickness after compression or when wet, and the actual bulk of the material must be low to prevent heat loss by condensation. To maintain thermal balance it is as necessary to facilitate heat loss as it is to maintain heat production and preserve insulation (Adam and Goldsmith 1965, Keighley and Steele 1981).

A variety of clothing is necessary in order to change the amount of insulation to meet the demands of heat production and ambient temperature. If only one material, such as fur, is used, this causes difficulties; to vary insulation, clothing must be available in layers which can be put on and taken off as required to avoid overheating. Adequate and easily adjustable ventilation improves clothing

adaptability and clothing should fit correctly without pressure on underlying tissues.

As wetting may decrease insulation by up to 90 per cent, this should be prevented, but at the same time allowing sweat to evaporate. If a completely windproof and waterproof garment is used in freezing conditions, evaporated sweat will condense and freeze on the inner surface and clothing will become soaked, thereby reducing insulation. The outer layer should therefore be permeable to water vapor, water resistant to retard water entry and windproof to prevent excessive air movement and diminish insulation (Jackson 1975).

Clothing assemblies may now be so effective that after many months in cold conditions there is a possibility that an individual may become heat adapted (Wilkins 1973).

The choice of materials varies, and wool and cotton are popular. The crimped fibers of natural wool retain 40 per cent of their insulating value when wet, compared with 10 per cent for cotton. Natural down provides excellent insulation when dry but not when wet. Synthetic fibers are becoming increasingly important. Some are hydrophobic (Stephens 1982) and do not retain moisture. When used as a padded jacket or trousers, these may not have such good insulation when dry but insulate well when wet. Clothing assemblies are very much an individual matter, but recently several equipment innovations have helped climbers at extreme altitude. Plastic boots with insulating liners have reduced weight and increased warmth and, when knee-length gaiters are added, foot protection is excellent.

Underwear that absorbs sweat as well as giving some warmth under a fiber pile garment seems a thermally efficient combination, especially with an outer layer of 'breathable' fabrics like Goretex. Over the past few years a number of synthetic fibers have been developed for insulation in jackets, trousers and sleeping bags. Their qualities rival down and they have the merit of not losing as much insulation when wet.

TRUNK

Insulation of the trunk is relatively easy as little movement takes place and bulky garments are more acceptable than on the arms and legs. A nonirritant garment should be worn next to the skin; this will absorb sweat and skin debris. Whether this has sleeves is an individual choice. Shirts or sweaters usually form the next layer. A polo neck is often used in continuously cold conditions as it diminishes loss of heat around the neck by convection currents. If more than one layer is worn, the size must be graduated. Drawstrings around the waist or wrists may prevent heat loss due to the bellows effect.

Padded jackets of natural down or artificial fibers, with or without sleeves, are common and they should extend over the buttocks to overlap the trousers by a wide margin. Often these have a wind-proof outer layer. They should open down the front and be easy to take off and put on.

LOWER TRUNK AND LEGS

The amount of movement at the hip and knee and the close proximity of the skin of the inner thigh, which can cause severe chafing if garments are badly fitted, influence insulation. Long close-fitting under-pants of soft weave wool or synthetic fiber are commonly worn. They should fit well around the ankles to prevent heat loss.

Padded trousers should not be so thick as to prevent easy leg movements. Breeches or trousers should be of hard-wearing material and the fly opening should be easily operated. Gaiters are often used, and prevent snow from entering the top of the boot. Some boots have gaiters attached to the sole. One-piece padded suits may be used in extremely cold conditions; these should have convenient zips for ventilation and excretion. Salopettes, which extend up to the upper chest, are increasingly worn; they provide a large overlap with the upper jacket and are very warm.

FEET

Feet remain covered all day and are not inspected as easily or as regularly as hands and, as a result, frostbite and nonfreezing injury may remain hidden for a long period. The design of footwear for dry or cold conditions has improved markedly with the development of a boot containing a molded plastic outer shell, including the sole, and an inner detachable boot of artificial fiber. As these are separate, the outer shell is removed when in a sleeping bag. The inner boot may be changed if it gets damp. Friction occurs between the inner and outer compartments when walking rather than between the skin of the foot and boot. Because of

this blisters are less common, despite the rigidity of the outer shell.

Leather boots are seldom used now in severe dry/cold conditions but in World War II, the Russian army issued leather boots several sizes too large which could be stuffed with straw or paper, whereas the German army had well fitting boots but suffered more from cold injury of the feet.

The ideal boot has yet to be designed for wet/cold conditions and most rely on the leather boot with or without an insole, and regular changes of socks. Both Thinsulate and Goretex have been incorporated in boot design. Once the foot gets wet its temperature falls quickly owing to small heat stores. Overboots or gaiters improve insulation and should extend to the knee. Crampon straps constrict the circulation of the foot in leather boots, but clip-on crampons and plastic boots avoid this problem.

Socks must fit well and be kept dry; spare pairs must be available in the rucksack. Feet should be inspected regularly so that incipient cold injury, blisters and infections are dealt with quickly. Meticulous care of the feet by the British Army in World War II resulted in a lower incidence of non-freezing cold injury than in any other army in the same theater of war.

HANDS

The multilayer principle is best, and a mitten with four fingers in one compartment and a thumb is warmer than a glove. Individual insulation of a finger is less effective because the heat loss from the curved surface of a small cylinder is greater than from a large cylinder. As the diameter decreases to 6.5 mm, any increase in the thickness of insulation makes little or no difference to the total insulation.

Mittens or gloves should be windproof, water resistant, permeable to water vapor and robust. Dachstein mittens made of uncured wool are very effective. As metals are good conductors, contact of cold metal with a dry finger will cause a 'cold burn', whereas a wet finger freezes to the metal and tissue may be left attached. If it is necessary to use fingers for fine work, contact gloves should be worn.

It is worth noting that few indigenous mountain inhabitants wear gloves; this is partly due to local cold acclimatization, but native garments do have long fold-back sleeves that can extend beyond the fingers.

THE HEAD

The head is an important avenue of heat loss. The most likely areas to freeze are the tip of the nose, and ears and cheeks. The ears are easy to protect with muffs or a hat, and a painful ear is a warning of incipient cold injury. The nose and cheeks are less easy to protect and face masks, though increasingly used, tend not to be comfortable and therefore are not popular.

A well designed anorak hood is essential for protecting the face from the wind, driving ice and snow particles. It must project well forward from the face and have a stiff but malleable wire in its leading edge. This enables the hood to be arranged so that it protects the face from whichever angle the wind comes; if necessary, only a minute hole need be left through which the individual can see.

The use of a visor of tinted glass provides more protection than individual goggles or dark glasses. An oxygen mask may be incorporated into the visor.

METABOLIC COST OF CLOTHING

Working with multilayered Arctic clothing increases the metabolic rate by 16 per cent by comparison with carrying the weight of the clothing. This increase can be attributed to the frictional resistance of one layer sliding over the other layer during movement, and the hobbling effect which interferes with movement.

WIND, MOVEMENT AND WETTING

If wind penetrates clothing, movement of the trapped, still air can result in a 30 per cent fall in insulation. The magnitude of this effect depends on the degree of wind resistance of the clothes and the effectiveness of the sealing at the neck, wrist and ankle. Movement also can lower insulation to half its resting value. Exercise in the cold may cause overheating and sweating; rain may also wet clothing and as much as 50 per cent of insulation may be lost by this means alone.

The combination of movement, wind and wetting may cause a 90 per cent loss of insulation, as a result of which the individual is essentially unprotected from the environment.

23.9.7 Insulation and oxygen consumption

From Table 23.2 it will be apparent that at 0 °C ambient temperature, to maintain a core temperature of 37 °C with a total thermal insulation of 3.0 CLO it is only necessary to work at a rate equivalent to an oxygen consumption of 0.5 L min^{-1}. At sea level this is not difficult but, at 7000 m and above, a steady rate of 0.5 L min^{-1} may represent 50 per cent of $V_{O_2 max}$. To remain in thermal balance at an ambient temperature lower than 0 °C necessitates either working harder or wearing more clothes. If neither is possible, the individual will become gradually hypothermic.

If insulation falls to 1 CLO, work rate has to increase threefold to 1.5 L min^{-1} to maintain thermal balance. If insulation falls even lower due to wetting, a work rate in excess of 3.0 L min^{-1} is necessary. This will not be possible for an exhausted or unfit individual who will become hypothermic.

Table 23.2 *Calculated final body temperature (°C) at an ambient temperature of 0 °C for a 75-kg man dependent upon the total thermal insulation (clothes plus tissue) and activity, measured as oxygen consumption*

Total thermal insulation (CLO units)	Oxygen consumption (L min^{-1})					
	0.5	1.0	1.5	2.0	2.5	3.0
0.2	2	4	6	8	10	12
0.4	4	9	14	18	23	28
1.0	12	24	36	48	60	72
1.4	23	34	50	66	–	–
2.0	24	48	72	–		
2.5	32	58	–			
3.0	38	–				
4.0	52					

Source: from data of Pugh (1966).

23.9.8 Shelter

The main value of a tent is to provide protection from the wind, though some modern double skinned tents also have quite good insulating properties.

Igloos and snow caves provide good insulation by virtue of the air trapped in the snow. This is illustrated by an incident in 1902 on one of Scott's early Antarctic expeditions. One member went missing and a blizzard developed which lasted 48 h. He took shelter and was covered by snow, falling asleep for 36 h, after which he awoke and returned unscathed (Brent 1974, p. 61.). Adequate ventilation is important to prevent the accumulation of carbon monoxide given off by stoves (Pugh 1959).

23.10 THERMAL BALANCE AT HIGH ALTITUDE

Many factors common at high altitude contribute to a negative thermal balance. Chronic fatigue, the result of great exertion, loss of sleep and decreased food intake are associated with loss of tissue insulation and result in reduced metabolic heat production (Young et al. 1998). Previous severe physical exertion may result in increased heat loss (from sweating) and decline in core temperature (Castellani et al. 1999b).

Severe dehydration could impair maintenance of body temperature (O'Brien et al. 1998) and if shivering is inhibited for any reason the core temperature is likely to fall (Giesbrecht et al. 1997).

An altitude of 5800–6000 m seems to represent the limit of permanent habitation (West 1986a); although at this height exhaustion is not uncommon after physical exertion, recovery with improvement in work capacity does occur, though it takes longer than at lower altitude.

Over 7000 m deterioration, both physical and mental, is more marked, $V_{O_2 max}$ falls, climbing rate falls and frequent stops are necessary. In 1978 Messner (1979, pp. 178–92), in the first account of climbing Everest without supplementary oxygen, comments, 'We can no longer keep on our feet while we rest . . . every 10–15 steps we collapse into the snow and then crawl on again.' As a result negative thermal balance is more common without supplementary oxygen because heat production is reduced

while heat loss, including respiratory loss from excessive hyperventilation, is considerable. As the $V_{O_2 max}$ near the summit of Everest is down to about 1.0 L min^{-1} (West et al. 1983c) the sustained oxygen uptake cannot be more than about 0.6–0.7 L min^{-1} and heat production is diminished.

Heat gain from solar radiation, both direct and indirect, plays an important part in maintaining thermal balance. In sunshine the gain from this source at 5800 m in snow is estimated at 1.463 MJ m^{-2} h^{-1} (350 kcal m^{-2} h^{-1}), compared with 0.522 MJ m^{-2} h^{-1} (125 kcal m^{-2} h^{-1}) in desert conditions at sea level (Pugh 1962b). Heat gain from solar radiation at altitude is estimated to be equivalent to a rise of about 20 °C in ambient temperature. The difference between day and night temperature at 6000 m may be 60–70 °C, a considerable cold stress.

At extreme altitude, although clothing may be adequate when moving, it may not be adequate to maintain thermal balance at rest.

The climber without supplementary oxygen at extreme altitude, despite being fully clothed, is never far from hypothermia and frostbite (Ward 1987). The use of supplementary oxygen at extreme altitude combats cold and hypoxia. It restores warmth to cold extremities and increases the chances of survival and success by increasing the endurance and climbing rate. Sudden failure of an open circuit oxygen set causes shortness of breath, limb paresthesia and incontinence of urine: in the closed circuit set, collapse and partial unconsciousness have been recorded.

23.11 FACTORS ALTERING TEMPERATURE REGULATION

23.11.1 Introduction

Trauma, hemorrhage and nausea increase heat loss, whereas exhaustion reduces heat production. Sleep, anesthesia and alcohol also affect regulation of temperature, and the extremes of age are associated with increased risk of hypothermia. Abnormal thermoregulatory patterns are found in some ethnic groups living in cold environments. The core temperature of sleeping aborigines drops further than that of Europeans before causing discomfort, and natives of Tierra del Fuego maintain a high metabolic rate (Hammel 1964). Meditation by Tibetan lamas may result in cutaneous vasodilatation and possible increased metabolic rate (Benson *et al.* 1982).

Certain medical disorders and drugs predispose to hypothermia.

23.11.2 Malnutrition

Malnutrition, by depleting the body stores, renders the subject more liable to hypothermia. The metabolic demands of cold are similar to, though less marked than, those of exercise, and the combination of cold, fasting, exercise and altitude will impose a considerable strain on the body. As a result, mild degrees of hypothermia are probably commoner than realized at altitude (Guezennec and Pesquies 1985).

23.11.3 Sleep

The central thermostat is set at a lower level when the individual goes to sleep, and the basal metabolic rate is reduced (Shapiro *et al.* 1984). Heat production when asleep is 9 per cent lower than when at rest and awake. During rapid eye movement (REM) sleep the skin temperature rises if the rectal temperature is high and falls if the rectal temperature is low (Buguet *et al.* 1979).

In non-REM sleep, oxygen consumption and metabolic rate are at their lowest. During the night there is a gradual reduction in heat production, which rises just before wakening. The skin temperature drops during sleep, which may wake the individual because of a feeling of cold. Theoretically, there is no danger from falling asleep in extreme cold since each bout of shivering would wake the person; however, an exhausted individual may not shiver and thus will fall into a dangerous cooling sleep.

Mountaineers bivouacking in extreme conditions will try to keep each other awake; there seems to be sound physiological reasons for this as the lower body temperature set point will allow body heat content to fall before discomfort due to cold is appreciated.

23.11.4 Alcohol

It is now recognized that alcohol may be an important contributory cause of death in cold environments. Its role is complex, but even quantities which result in levels below those of legal drunkenness are dangerous before working in the cold.

The inhibitory action of alcohol on cerebral function can cause bravado and lessen the ability to assess risk. Before exercise in the cold alcohol is associated with a decrease in blood glucose (Haight and Keatinge 1973) which will increase the risk of exhaustion leading to hypothermia and further impairment of gluconeogenesis (Drinking and drowning 1979). Cooling also decreases the elimination of alcohol (Krarup and Larsen 1972); as it is also a sedative, there will be an increased tendency to sleep with resulting failure to maintain body heat. Freund *et al.* (1994) suggest that alcohol reduces central core temperature during exposure to cold and that the degree of reduction is related to the blood alcohol concentration; also hypoglycemia increases the reduction in body temperature caused by the ingestion of alcohol.

23.11.5 Regular exposure to cold

Normal responses to cold may be modified by regular exposure. Divers regularly exposed to cold may be susceptible to progressive and symptomless hypothermia resulting in poor judgment and death (Hayward and Keatinge 1979). During experimental cooling it is possible, by slightly raising the skin temperature at the start of shivering, to abolish both shivering and the sensation of cold without arresting the continued cooling (Keatinge *et al.* 1980).

Reaction to thermal extremes: cold and heat

SUMMARY

Cold is as important a factor as hypoxia in the stress of high altitude. Humans react to cold more efficiently by behavioral means than by physiology and the majority of the body's systems are involved. As a result Inuits can live at environmental temperatures of −70 °C and similar temperatures are recorded by mountaineers at great altitude.

Local cold tolerance but not general acclimatization occurs. Children, because of their greater surface area to weight ratio, are at greater risk of cold injury than adults.

Because of the high solar load found on enclosed glaciers and snowfields, minor forms of heat injury can be a problem at high altitude. In addition snow blindness and sunburn are common and may be severe if adequate protection is not taken. Because of temperature extremes at high altitude, it is possible to suffer from frostbite and minor heat injury at the same time.

24.1   COLD

24.1.1   Introduction

Humans reacts to cold more effectively by behavioral rather than by physiological means. Clothing and shelter enable Inuits to live in an environmental temperature of −70 °C. The opportunity to become cold tolerant is limited in Europeans as, even at polar bases, people may be out of doors for only 10–15 per cent of the time. Mountaineers, because they live in unheated tents or snow caves, may spend longer periods exposed to cold.

However, protective clothing is now so efficient that the microclimate (environment beneath the clothing) may be as warm as a temperate zone and some degree of heat acclimatization occurs. Only exposed parts, such as the hands, become cold adapted and those used to working out of doors are less liable than newcomers to frostbite. Local acclimatization has an essentially vascular basis with an increase in blood flow; improved tactile discrimination and less appreciation of pain occur in the cold adapted (Hoffman and Wittmers 1990).

Most people respond to cold stress by cardiovascular and metabolic changes, but not all respond equally. Some tend to raise their heat production by shivering; others adjust more by peripheral vasoconstriction.

In subjects of different body size and composition there is a wide variation in the amount of heat production resulting from shivering thermogenesis; thin men shiver more intensely than fat ones. In small to medium sized individuals, vasoconstriction with light shivering precedes heavy shivering, whereas in large men, because of their body size and subcutaneous fat, metabolic heat production is less (Strong *et al.* 1985). Children, because of their greater surface area to weight ratio, are at greater risk of cooling than adults.

Acclimatization is a term that has been used in relation to cold by many workers and certainly changes, both short and long term, have been shown after repeated exposure (Shephard 1985). However, the term has been used in so many different ways that it tends to confuse rather than clarify.

24.1.2 Metabolic response to cold

Hammel (1964) distinguishes three distinct patterns of human response to moderate exposure of the whole body:

- those who increase their metabolic rate as body temperature falls (urban dwellers)
- those whose metabolic rate falls gradually as rectal and skin temperatures fall below those of urban controls (Australian aborigines)
- those who start with a high metabolic rate which declines slightly and is accompanied by a fall in rectal temperature to a level no lower than that of a white control (Alaculuf Indians).

Repeated exposure to cold results in a greater sympathetic response and improved cutaneous insulation (Young *et al.* 1986). It appears that the type of physiological response varies according to the degree, length and frequency of exposure.

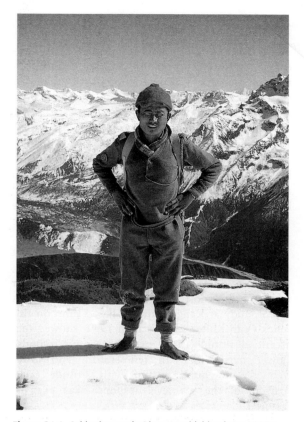

Figure 24.1 *Cold tolerance in Bhutanese highlander at 4800m.*

24.1.3 Cold tolerance

Those who are used to working out of doors in the cold can work longer than newcomers, are less liable to frostbite and are less likely to need additional clothing when the temperature drops (Butson 1949). Brown and Page (1952) noted that both the skin temperature and blood flow in the hands of Inuits were higher in cold temperature than in controls and when immersed in water the blood flow did not decline so abruptly. It has been noted too that when Tibetan highlanders are exposed to cold they complain of less pain and shiver less than lowlanders. A similar phenomenon is seen in Australian aboriginal bushmen who may sleep virtually naked in the cold desert without shivering (Hammel 1964).

Pugh (1963) describes a remarkable degree of cold tolerance in a Nepalese pilgrim who normally lived at 1800 m. During the Silver Hut Expedition 1960–1 in the Everest region he spent 4 days at 4550–5300 m in midwinter, wearing only cotton clothing and no shoes, socks or gloves. The temperature fell to –13 °C at night and he slept in the open with only a coat for covering but no protection from the ground at a temperature of 0 °C to –5 °C. He maintained a relatively high metabolic rate without shivering but with further cooling exhibited only light continuous shivering which did not interrupt sleep, rather than the usual violent intermittent shivering. The surface temperature of his hands never fell below 10–12 °C and his toes 8 °C. He complained of neither pain nor numbness and as his skin temperature did not drop below freezing he did not suffer from frostbite. He did, however, develop fissures in the skin of his feet, which failed to heal, and became infected. It was for this reason that he returned to lower levels. A similar ability to withstand cold has been observed in Tibetan practitioners of g tum-mo yoga, who are able to increase the temperature of their fingers and toes by as much as 8.3 °C (Benson *et al.* 1982).

24.1.4 Skin and peripheral vessels

The initial response to cold on the skin is the contraction of the erector pili muscles with the development of 'gooseflesh'. Constriction of the cutaneous vessels occurs and there is increased blood viscosity with decreased blood flow.

On immersion of a finger in iced water, skin temperature falls to nearly 0 °C and then rises. With continued immersion, the finger temperature fluctuates, known as the 'hunting' phenomenon. This is due to reflex (cold-induced) vasodilatation and increased blood flow through arteriovenous anastomoses. The temperature rise is greater in the distal than in the proximal phalanges.

The explanation of 'hunting' appears to be that cold paralyses the vasoconstrictor muscle fibers, the vessels dilate, blood flow increases, the finger warms, heat is lost and the cycle repeats itself. A recent study at Kangchenjunga Base Camp on this reflex (Van Ruiten and Daanan 1999) showed that ascent to altitude (5100 m) blunted this response (lower maximum skin temperature and lower frequency of hunting) but with altitude acclimatization, the sea level response was partially restored.

Pain is related to blood flow, being severe on vasoconstriction and improving on vasodilatation. With increasing cold, tissue metabolism ceases, the skin blanches and becomes waxy and pale due to continuous vasoconstriction. The bloodless region cools to the environmental temperature and frostbite may occur.

The general thermal state affects the peripheral circulation, and local vasodilatation is greatly increased when the individual is warm and reduced when cold. The extent of peripheral vasodilatation depends too on the area heated. Heating the face is far more effective than the chest or leg in varying skin temperature and blood flow to the hand.

Cooling of one part of the body surface results in diminished blood flow to other regions also. When the whole body surface is cooled there is a general cutaneous vasoconstriction with diminished blood flow to peripheral tissues (Burton and Edholm 1955, pp. 140-1).

Both cold phlebitis and cold arteritis may occur on prolonged exposure. Those with varicose veins should consider treatment prior to long periods in the cold.

24.1.5 Nerves

Exposure of the hands to cold, even above freezing, impairs nerve function after a period of about 15 min, and this is not immediately reversed by warming and may occasionally persist for more than 4-5 days (Marshall and Goldman 1976). There is diminished skin sensation followed by a lessening of manual dexterity. The critical air temperature for tactile sensitivity is 8 °C and for manual dexterity it is 12 °C (Fox 1967). Above these temperatures performance is little affected, though the hands may feel cold, but at lower temperatures performance falls markedly. Not all tasks are equally affected and impairment may persist after the hands have been rewarmed to normal temperatures. Many climbers returning from high altitude have some loss of sensation in their fingertips, which may last several weeks.

24.1.6 Muscle

Cold also decreases the power and direction of muscle contraction and seems to have a direct effect on the muscle fiber, as blood flow is not decreased (Guttman and Gross 1956). Handgrip diminishes considerably when the forearm is immersed in water at 10 °C (Coppin et al. 1978).

Increasing failure of muscle function may be due to a combination of failure of nerve conduction, neuromuscular function and the direct action of cold on muscle fibers. Cold muscles are notoriously liable to rupture and the more explosive the activity the greater the risk, hence the need for a warm-up before taking exercise. Muscle is more vulnerable to cold than skin or bone (Kayser et al. 1993).

24.1.7 Joints

The temperature of the joints falls faster than that of muscles, and cold joints are stiff joints (Hunter et al. 1952). Cold increases the viscosity of synovial fluid and, by reducing its lubricating qualities, it increases the resistance of joints to movements, increasing the risk of tearing tendons and muscles.

24.1.8 Cardiovascular system

A number of thermoregulatory systems designed to reduce heat loss are brought into play immediately on exposure to cold; these affect the cardiovascular system with an increase in cardiac output, blood pressure and pulse rate (Hayward *et al.* 1984). Initially, catecholamine excretion increases but, as core temperature falls from 31 °C to 29 °C, this decreases (Chernow *et al.* 1983).

BLOOD PRESSURE

In normal people and untreated hypertensives, the blood pressure is higher in the winter. This rise in systemic blood pressure increases with age and in thin people (Brennan *et al.* 1982). Exercise in the cold usually decreases diastolic pressure but this may be countered by the inhalation of cold air (Horvath 1981) and may precipitate angina because, with the associated increase in ventricular pressure, the oxygen needs of the myocardium increase (Gorlin 1966).

On cold exposure, constriction of the peripheral vessels shunts a large volume of blood into the capacitance vessels causing an increase in cardiac load. With the same volume of blood restricted to a smaller vascular bed a rise in blood pressure results and angina or cardiac failure may be precipitated as a result. A rise in systemic blood pressure is associated with a risk of cerebral hemorrhage; the incidence of stroke is increased in the UK in winter (Haberman *et al.* 1981).

INTRAVASCULAR CHANGES

Subjects exposed to cold for 6 h show an increase in packed cell volume, circulating platelets and blood viscosity. These increase the risk of thrombosis and also the incidence of myocardial infarction, which often occurs within 24 h of the onset of a cold spell, as a house takes approximately this time to cool (Keatinge *et al.* 1984). Mortality from ischemic heart disease increases in direct proportion to a fall in environmental temperature and the rate rises after a few cold days, especially in the elderly (Blows from the winter wind 1980).

The factors of both cold stress and hypoxia should therefore be taken into account in cases of vascular disorders in young men at altitude (Ward 1975, pp. 289–92) (Chapter 22).

24.1.9 Pulmonary artery

Acute exposure to cold is known to cause pulmonary hypertension in sheep and cattle and this involves peripheral sensory stimulation and the efferent innervation of the pulmonary vessels (Bligh and Chauca 1978, 1982, Will *et al.* 1978). At altitude this may be added to the rise in pressure produced by hypoxia, which is a local effect on these vessels. However, Yanagidaira *et al.* (1994) found that rats exposed to cold over a long period had no right ventricular hypertrophy.

In the Arctic many middle-aged and elderly Inuit develop chronic obstructive lung disease which leads to pulmonary hypertension and right heart failure, or 'Eskimo lung'. These Inuit had been hunters and trappers when young, which involved hard physical work in very cold conditions. Similar respiratory problems have been noted in white trappers and in native and immigrant Russian workers exposed to extreme conditions in Siberia. Inuit women and men who did little or no winter hunting were relatively free of pulmonary hypertension due to cold (Schaefer *et al.* 1980).

24.1.10 Fluid balance

Exposure to cold causes peripheral vasoconstriction with shunting of blood into the deep capacitance vessels. This results in an increased circulating volume in a diminished vascular bed and an increased arterial pressure. The body responds to this excess volume of fluid by a diuresis (Hervey 1973), initially caused by the release of atrial natriuretic peptide (Atrial natriuretic peptide 1986, Chapter 15.4). With further body cooling, diuresis results from the failure of tubular reabsorption of sodium and/or water and occurs despite diminished renal blood flow and glomerular filtration (Tansey 1973). The often severe weight loss experienced by people exposed to cold over a long period is due to fluid loss (Rogers 1971).

Complicating factors are numerous. Respiratory fluid loss occurs during exercise in the cold and at altitude (Hamlet 1983). Vigorous exercise in the cold can also produce marked fluid loss due to sweating, which the individual may not notice because the air is dry and evaporation rapid. This loss may amount to 1–2 L per day or between 0.74 per cent and 3.4 per cent of total body mass in 24 h (Budd 1984). Cold also has a tendency to depress the sensation of thirst, as does hypoxia and, as water may not be easily available to mountaineers at altitude, dehydration is common.

The severity of fluid shifts is directly related to the time exposed to cold. Another complicating feature is that the type of exercise associated with hill walking results in appreciable sodium retention and expansion of the extracellular fluid at the expense of the intracellular fluid. This may result in overt clinical edema of the face and ankles due to activation of the renin–aldosterone system (Williams *et al.* 1979, Milledge *et al.* 1982).

During rewarming the circulating blood volume may increase to up to 130 per cent of its value prior to cooling. This is probably due to a reversal of fluid shifts, and the volume of fluid available for return will depend on the duration of cooling. If rewarming is too rapid, therefore, fluid overload may cause either cerebral or pulmonary edema (Lloyd 1973).

24.1.11 Respiratory tract

It is generally believed that the mechanisms available in the upper respiratory tract for warming cold inspired air remove the possibility of cold injury to the lungs. Certainly there has been no evidence of damage to the lungs in those working at the South Pole, in winter joggers or cross-country skiers (Buskirk 1977). The inhalation of cold dry air can, however, damage the epithelium of the upper respiratory tract in humans and dogs (Houk 1959) and at 7500 m on Everest Somervell, a surgeon, nearly suffocated from the sloughing of the mucosa of his nasopharynx. He gives a graphic account:

> When darkness was gathering I had one of my fits of coughing and dislodged something in my throat which stuck so that I could breathe neither in nor out. I could not of course make a sign to Norton or stop him for the rope was off now; so I sat in the snow to die whilst he walked on . . . I made one or two attempts to breathe but nothing happened. Finally, I pressed my chest with both hands gave one last almighty push – and the obstruction came up (Somervell 1936).

Because the environmental air is never fully saturated there is a net loss of heat and water when air is exhaled and as much as 50-60 per cent of the heat transferred to inhaled air may be lost on expiration.

If the individual is breathing quietly and at rest the inspired air is equilibrated with body temperature and has achieved full saturation by the time it has reached the tracheal bifurcation. As the tracheal temperature falls during hyperventilation, the mucosa shrinks and becomes pale in the same way as skin does; this will prevent the temperature of the upper airways from rising and provide a thermal gradient for the recovery of heat and moisture during expiration.

Exercise may induce bronchospasm in patients with asthma. Its severity is directly related to the rate of respiratory heat loss and can be prevented by inhaling warm humid air (Strauss *et al.* 1978). However, asthmatic subjects seem to do well in general on high altitude expeditions, possibly because the beneficial effects of removal from their usual allergens more than outweigh any detrimental effects of inhaling cold air.

Exercise in a cold environment can cause bronchoconstriction. During severe exercise in extremely cold conditions horses may develop frosting of the lungs and sled dogs show evidence of pulmonary edema (Schaefer *et al.* 1980). There are also anecdotal reports of Arctic hunters having 'freezing of the lung'.

24.1.12 Alimentary tract

Cold stress can significantly delay gastric emptying and acid secretion. The initial reduction in both gastric secretion and pancreatic trypsin output is followed in the post-stress period by an increase. This appears to be a nonspecific response, as normal postprandial function of the upper gastrointestinal tract can be disturbed by other stressful stimuli (Thompson *et al.* 1983).

24.1.13 Hormonal responses

ADRENOCORTICAL FUNCTION

In those with no prior exposure to cold, a rise in 17-OHCS levels has been found. This may reflect the nature and severity of the stress. There is disturbance of sleep and shivering together with the painful sensation of cold. Cold-adapted individuals showed no increase in 17-OHCS activity (Radomski and Boutelier 1982).

ADRENOMEDULLARY FUNCTION

Norepinephrine secretion increases in the nonadapted and remains raised (Weeke and Gundersen 1983), whereas the well adapted showed no such increase.

Epinephrine secretion increased in both the non-adapted and adapted individuals (Radomski and Boutelier 1982).

THYROID FUNCTION AND GROWTH HORMONE

In rats and some other animals T_3 secretion increases in response to cold exposure but there is also evidence that the main stimulus to nonshivering thermogenesis is a hypothalamic activity via the sympathetic system (Galton 1978).

In humans, the possibility of an increased metabolic rate due to thyroid activity has been considered but there is little evidence that it takes place in response to cold exposure. Korean women divers have a higher basal metabolic rate (BMR) in winter, greater utilization of thyroxine (T_4), increased thermal insulation and changes in peripheral blood flow (Hong 1973). However, most studies designed to show increased thyroid activity in response to cold have failed to show any change that could not be accounted for by increased physical activity (Galton 1978).

On acute exposure to cold there is inhibition of growth hormone secretion (Weeke and Gundersen 1983).

24.1.14   Immune response

Hypothermia may compromise the immune response with severe infection and little inflammatory response (Lewin *et al.* 1981). However, an acute fall in the core temperature does not necessarily affect the immune system (Brenner *et al.* 1999). McCormack *et al.* (1998) consider that immuno-suppression occurs in cold exposure with reverse T_3 (rT_3) being raised above normal values. The uptake of rT_3 on lymphocyte nuclear receptors increases and this rise suggests a response to general physiological stress.

Clinically, superficial wounds seem to heal more rapidly when the patient is removed from the cold and hypoxic environment of high altitude.

24.1.15   Fatigue and cold

Chronic fatigue combined with sleep loss, reduced fluid intake and poor tissue insulation may result in blunted metabolic heat production, and this can lead to a fall in body temperature (Young *et al.* 1998). Previous severe exercise may also lead to greater heat loss and decrease in body temperature (Castellani *et al.* 1999b). However, a short period of rest, sleep and adequate food restores the normal response to cold but thermal balance may be compromised until tissue insulation is back to normal, which can take several weeks (Westerterp-Plantagna *et al.* 1999).

24.1.16   Mental function

The decrease in cerebral blood flow associated with hypothermia results from a drop in metabolism (Hernandez 1983). There is an ideal level of temperature and humidity at which mental tasks may be carried out, and an increase in cold stress decreases the standard of performance, as well as decreasing the rate of work (Enander 1984). Cold causes apathy and distracts individuals from their tasks. Performance in the cold depends on familiarity; well motivated subjects can complete given tasks even if the central core temperature has dropped (Baddeley *et al.* 1975).

Individuals exposed to both fatigue and cold stress adjust their performance so that they maintain as steady a core temperature as possible and limit their heart rate to about 120 beats min^{-1}. To maintain maximum 'comfort' between various stresses, a physiological compromise is reached, and, rather than increase work output so that anaerobic exercise is performed, a lowered core temperature is accepted (Cabanac and LeBlanc 1983).

Accidents show an increase with low environmental temperature, possibly owing to loss of manual dexterity (Goldsmith and Minard 1976). Workers in cold stores have a reduction in the ability to concentrate, and personal irritability increases (Andrew 1963). Silly errors (verbal, mechanical and clerical) may occur as a result of the inability to concentrate. Subjects may not be aware of the drop in performance and consider that they had done particularly well when, in fact, they had the greatest impairment in function. The individual developing hypothermia is not aware of any mental impairment, and may totally lack insight (Hamilton 1980).

Exposure to cold produces mental stress and changes in personality. Hallucinations are a sign of incipient or actual hypothermia (Ogilvie 1977).

There are many accounts in the mountain literature of people seeing and talking to a nonexistent presence, feeling abnormal fear or pleasure and hearing footsteps or sounds when none exist. In the majority of cases cold, hypoxia, fatigue, starvation or a combination have been present.

Hallucinations are said to occur when the core temperature drops below 32 °C, but they often occur above this level (Hirvonen 1982). Although mountaineers at great altitude report hallucinations, similar findings have been recorded at sea level. Acute hypoxia is not usually associated with hallucinations (Hatcher 1965), which seem to occur when cerebral hypoxia has been present for some time, suggesting that this may be the result of the biochemical changes resulting from hypoxia rather than the hypoxia *per se*. Some individuals respond to hallucinations, for example by paradoxical undressing, going berserk or attempting to kill their companions (Wedin *et al.* 1979). Even on reaching safety, a hypothermic hypoxic patient may be unable to identify exactly where he has been.

24.2   HEAT

24.2.1   Heat injury

Heat injury occurs when heat production is greater than heat loss and the combination of high temperature and high humidity blocks the mechanisms for heat loss and predisposes to heat injury.

Basal metabolism alone can produce heat at 271–355 kJ h^{-1} (65–85 kcal h^{-1}), enough to raise core temperatures by 1°C h^{-1}, were it not for the various mechanisms for heat removal. Moderate work done can increase this fivefold, to 1254–2508 kJ h^{-1} (300–600 kcal h^{-1}) and solar radiation may increase heat gain by 627 kJ h^{-1} (150 kcal h^{-1}). Raised body temperature, of itself, increases cell metabolism and therefore heat production (Arrhenius's law).

As long as the air temperature is lower than body temperature, 65 per cent of cooling occurs by radiation or the transfer of heat from the body to the environment.

Above an environmental temperature of about 37 °C, evaporation is the only method of heat loss and, if humidity exceeds 75 per cent, heat loss by this method falls and sweating exacerbates dehydration without cooling.

Overheating can be a problem at altitude because very high solar temperatures are common on enclosed glaciers and snowfields such as the Western Cwm of Everest. Climbing at night or before dawn should be considered under these circumstances.

Temperatures inside a tent may be as high as 30 °C and a sun temperature of 59 °C measured with a black bulb radiation thermometer has been recorded on Everest (Pugh 1955b).

PREDISPOSITION TO HEAT INJURY

Elderly people are less able to maintain cardiac output and dissipate heat and may be dehydrated. A previous myocardial infarct may also limit the ability for vasodilatation. Obese individuals have more insulation and less relative surface area from which to lose heat, hyperthyroidism increases heat production, and large areas of skin affected by disease may interfere with heat loss by sweating. Various drugs may predispose to heat illness, such as beta-blockers inhibiting a compensatory increased cardiac output.

ACCLIMATIZATION TO HEAT

In contrast to cold, some general acclimatization to heat does occur. It takes about 10 days to reach its maximum benefit and requires up to 2 h a day of daily exercise.

The mechanisms, though poorly understood, are associated with increased aldosterone production and sodium conservation. Sweating occurs at a lower core temperature and may be more than double the normal amount. An increased cardiac output results in the increased delivery of heated blood from core to periphery and, in addition, there is increased density of mitochondria per unit of muscle which allows for increased oxygen usage (Weiss 1991).

CLINICAL FEATURES OF HEAT INJURY

There are two main clinical stages: heat exhaustion, of which 'glacier lassitude' is a part, and heat stroke.

- Glacier lassitude has been well recorded since the start of mountaineering over 150 years ago. It is associated with extreme lethargy and dehydration, and loss of salt. It occurs when heat uptake from solar radiation is considerable, and is described particularly when climbing in a 'bowl of snow'.

- Heat exhaustion is a further stage, but the core temperature remains normal. There may be 'flu-like symptoms with faintness, anorexia, nausea, vomiting and muscle cramps. Sweating is usually present but diminished. The central nervous system is usually normal.
- Heat stroke is a true medical emergency. It is not common among mountaineers but its possibility should be recognized during an approach to the mountain across hot desert. Sweating stops and characteristically the core temperature is above normal. Onset is rapid with the victim becoming confused and uncoordinated; hypotension, tachycardia and tachypnea are common. All untreated cases die with brain damage. The degree of residual cerebral damage in treated cases is directly related to the time that has elapsed before treatment. A core temperature of 41 °C or above has a poor prognosis.

TREATMENT

For heat exhaustion, the patient must be taken out of the sun and given fluids and salt.

For heat stroke, treatment must start immediately. The body must be cooled as rapidly as possible. Cooling must be promoted by any means, and fluid (even urine) does not have to be cold to provide heat loss by evaporation. Packs of snow or ice should be placed on the body where the large blood vessels come to the surface: at the neck, axilla or groin. The limbs should be gently massaged to prevent peripheral stagnation and accelerate cooling. This technique avoids generalized vasoconstriction and shivering. Cooling rates of 0.1 °C min^{-1} have been recorded. No fluids should be given by mouth and patients should be taken to hospital as soon as possible and cooled rapidly.

In hospital the optimum treatment is controversial and includes peritoneal lavage, water spray and fans, ice water baths and gastric lavage. One or more methods may be used. Evaporation techniques to keep the skin at about 20 °C, together with ice packs to the axilla and groin, are practical in that monitoring is easy to manage. Most patients can be cooled to a core temperature of 38 °C in less than 40 min by this method. Cooling should be stopped at 37 °C to prevent overcompensation and hypothermia. Intravenous fluids should be started if necessary.

Rapid and prompt evacuation of heat stroke casualties to a hospital emergency department is mandatory. Rapid reduction in body temperature, control of fits and adequate rehydration result in a 90 per cent survival rate (Hubbard *et al.* 1995).

COMPLICATIONS OF HEAT STROKE

- Decreased renal perfusion can lead to tubular necrosis and renal failure.
- Muscle damage and rhabdomyolysis can produce myoglobulinuria and exacerbate renal failure.
- Hypoglycemia and hypocalcemia may occur.
- Total body potassium usually decreases.
- Liver enzymes may be raised.
- Thermal damage to vessel endothelial cells can occur with disorders of blood coagulation (Weiss 1991).

24.2.2   Injury from solar radiation

Light from the sun includes radiation of wavelengths of 290–1850 nm; the proportion reaching the Earth's surface varies with the season and atmospheric conditions. Much solar radiation is filtered out by smoke or fog, but less by cloud. At high altitude these screens are less effective and reflection from the Earth's surface, especially where there is snow, increases exposure.

SNOW BLINDNESS (PHOTOPHTHALMIA)

Snow blindness is an inflammation of the cornea and conjunctiva due to ultraviolet light of wavelength 200–400 nm. At altitude this makes up 5–6 per cent of solar radiation, compared with 1–2 per cent at sea level. Snow reflects 85 per cent of light waves and the eyes are particularly vulnerable.

Acute

Within a few hours the epithelial cells of the cornea die. There is loss of surface adhesion and the cells are brushed off the cornea by the mechanical act of blinking. The corneal nerve endings are then exposed. Within about 4 h, symptoms are felt that range from a feeling of 'grit in the eye' to excruciating pain and sensitivity to light. The slightest eye movement causes spasm of the eyelids, pupillary vasoconstriction, eye pain and headache. There is conjunctival inflammation, the eyelids are swollen and the secretion of tears profuse. The condition lasts 6-8 h and disappears in 48 h.

Treatment includes cold compresses, hydrocortisone eye ointment, an eye patch to exclude light, and the avoidance of light. The pupils should be dilated with atropine and an ocular antibiotic used in case corneal ulceration occurs. Analgesics may be necessary.

Chronic

Chronic snow blindness occurs in those inhabitants of mountainous and snowy regions over a long period. Visual disturbances, with sensitivity to light and chronic conjunctival inflammation, are reported.

Prevention

Inhabitants of mountainous regions have used primitive prevention methods for centuries. These include yak wool and hair pulled forward over the eyes, slits in wood, or cardboard strapped to the head (see Figure 3.3, which shows yak hair gogles).

Glasses or goggles with lenses that cut out radiation of wavelength 250–400 nm are normally used for protection. The quality of the lens is important, and it can be made of plastic or glass. The main advantage of plastic is that it is lightweight and unbreakable, but it does not filter out all the ultraviolet light; glass is heavier, but filters out most of the ultraviolet light. Ideally, the external surface is mirror finished to reflect light, and the internal surface should not reflect light onto the cornea. The upper and lower parts of the lens should be darker than the central part, through which the wearer is able to see clearly. Frames should have side and nasal shields for protection against sun, and a safety cord must always be firmly attached. A spare pair of glasses or goggles should always be carried. Goggles should have adequate ventilation to stop them steaming up (Lomax et al. 1991, Petetin 1991).

SUNBURN

Overexposure to ultraviolet radiation of wavelengths 200–400 nm can damage the skin. Ultraviolet B (UVB) (290–320 nm) is primarily responsible for burning, tanning and the formation of skin cancer. Ultraviolet A (UVA) (320–400 nm) contributes to skin aging. Melanin is the ideal sunscreen, and burning, aging and skin cancer are decreased in blacks, whereas blondes and redheads are particularly susceptible.

Seasonal variation is striking. The intensity of UVA doubles in the summer, whilst that of UVB increases tenfold in the same period.

Certain drugs make the skin sensitive to the effects of solar radiation. These include sulfonamides, phenothiazines, dimethylchlortetracycline and thiazide diuretics. Visual reactions to sunlight can occur in those suffering from lupus erythematosus, porphyria and albinism. In patients with abnormal sensitivity, prolonged use of antimalarial drugs such as chloroquine may suppress or reduce this sensitivity. Cold sores may be exacerbated by prolonged exposure to stray sunlight (Lomax et al. 1991).

Acute

Clinical features of acute sunburn, which vary from slight erythema to considerable blistering, appear within a few hours. The severity of the patient's condition varies with the surface area involved. Treatment should include removal from the sun, cold compresses, and corticosteroid cream. Secondary infection should be treated with antibiotics. Following exposure to ultraviolet radiation the rate of melanin formation increases and protects the skin from further damage.

Chronic

Recurrent exposure over many years causes atrophy of the skin and loss of elastic tissue with scattered pigmented areas (liver spots). Most of the skin characteristics attributed to aging are due to exposure to the sun, as skin on protected sites such as the buttocks appears 'young' even in the elderly.

24.2.3   Skin cancer

Ultraviolet radiation causes skin cancer in mice, and the epidemiological evidence for sunlight causing skin cancer in humans is overwhelming. It is one of the common cancers in the USA. The possible depletion of the ozone layer may cause a further increase in skin cancer.

PREVENTION

Sunburn is preventable and exposure should be graded so that skin can become pigmented. Clothes protect better than sunscreens; dark, dry fabrics are more effective than white, wet garments. The under-surface of the nose and the chin, also the lips and ears, are susceptible to reflected ultraviolet light. Sunscreens containing molecules that absorb ultraviolet radiation are now commonly used. Dibenzoylmethanes absorb UVA and, in combination with screening agents against UVB, provide effective sun protection over a broad range of wave lengths.

It is important that children and young people get into the habit of using sun screens as this will decrease the incidence of sunburn, photo-aging and skin cancer (Kaplan 1992).

25

Hypothermia

SUMMARY

Hypothermia or general cold injury occurs when the core temperature falls to below 35°C.

Trekkers and mountaineers suffer from subacute or exhaustion hypothermia which can happen in both wet cold and dry cold conditions. In wet cold when the environmental temperature is above zero, the dangerous combination of wind and wetting can decrease the effectiveness of insulating clothing to such an extent that the core body temperature may fall despite shivering and exercise. In dry cold when the environmental temperature is lower, a similar sequence of events can occur, particularly if an impermeable outer shell is worn and insulating clothing becomes soaked with sweat. Wind not only lowers the temperature of exposed skin by direct wind chill but also reduces the insulating properties of clothing by blowing away entrapped warm air near the skin.

Disorientation is an early feature of hypothermia and may occur at a core temperature above 35 °C. At high altitude supplementary oxygen, adequate food and fluid combat hypothermia, though many climbers suffer from both hypoxia and incipient general cold injury. Those who are not fit may be at risk, whether in wet or dry cold conditions, as they cannot maintain thermal balance by sufficient exercise.

Management in the field depends on preventing exhaustion and maintaining body heat. In hospital, treatment by either surface or airway rewarming can be successful. Severe cases should be treated in a cardiothoracic unit by central rewarming.

Death should never be assumed while the core temperature is below normal, even though the patient may appear dead. A number of cases have recovered from very low core temperatures.

25.1 INTRODUCTION

Worldwide populations of 100 million or more may be at risk due to cold injury, yet in civilian life the condition is less common than in wartime. In all campaigns carried out at an environmental temperature around freezing point cold injury is common and environmental hazard is now a major factor with armies in the field.

Early descriptions of cold injury do not distinguish between hypothermia, freezing cold injury (frostbite) and nonfreezing cold injury (immersion injury). However, a Tibetan medical text thought to date back to 889 BCE mentions frostbite (Parfionovitch *et al.* 1992).

Hippocrates wrote on the climate of different lands and the influence of the climate on their inhabitants, making many pertinent observations on cold injury, including the occurrence of blisters, blackening of the skin and tingling in the hands.

The number suffering from cold injury in badly equipped armies was considerable. During the winter of 400 BCE Xenophon led his Greek army of 10 000 through the deep snow in the mountains of Armenia where they suffered greatly from cold. In 218 BCE Hannibal crossed the European Alps and lost approximately 20 000 men in 14 days, mainly from cold. In 1812 Napoleon invaded Russia with 250 000 men and returned 6 months later, his army decimated by 'General Winter' and Russian resistance, his dreams of an eastern empire shattered. In the Crimean War French troops had 5000 cases of cold injury in an army of 300 000, and in World War I the numbers of casualties due to cold in the British, French and Italian forces were respectively 115 000, 80 000 and 30 000.

In World War II the Germans suffered 100 000 cold injuries requiring 15 000 amputations in November–December 1942 alone (Vaughn 1942). Of the 9000 US casualties in Korea 10 per cent were due to cold (Orr and Fainer 1951) and in the Falklands Campaign in 1982, 13.6 per cent of casualties were due to nonfreezing cold injury (Marsh 1983).

It has been suggested that the high survival rate among exsanguinated casualties in the Falklands War was partially due to the cold climate which facilitates clot formation and lowered metabolic rate. William Harvey knew about this, for at the Battle of Sedgehill, 1642, when there was a frost, he remarked that it 'staunched the bleeding'. He was familiar with a good method of treating hypothermia: 'A pretty young wench which he made use of for warmth's sake' (Harbinson 1999).

In peacetime, cold injury occurs particularly after natural disasters such as earthquakes during the winter months. Polar travelers, mountaineers and skiers are also at risk, despite improvements in clothing, technique and equipment. Cavers, divers, fishermen and swimmers are also exposed to cold injury (Washburn 1962). Elderly and very young people can be particularly liable, especially if their nutrition is poor or if they are ill.

Accidental hypothermia is not confined to high latitudes or altitude. In the Sahara where there are peaks up to 3010 m the temperature may fall to freezing at night (Pierre and Aulard 1985). Even in Kampala, Uganda, where the temperature never falls below 16°C cases have been recorded (Sadikali and Owor 1974, Barber 1978). In the mild English climate it is estimated that over 200 000 cases of hypothermia occur each year. In Yekaterinburg, 1368 km east and north of Moscow, where the mean winter temperature is −6.8°C, lower than anywhere else in Europe, mortality increases when the mean daily temperature falls below 0°C (Donaldson *et al.* 1998a,b).

25.2 DEFINITION

Hypothermia is defined as a lowering of central core body temperature below 35°C. This is rather an artificial definition as it takes no account of total body heat and some people drop their normal diurnal temperature as low as 35.5–36°C (RCP 1966).

Exposure is a nonmedical term used in relation to cold to describe a serious chilling of the body surface and is usually associated with exhaustion leading to a progressive fall in body temperature with the risk of death from hypothermia.

Cold stress is the term used to describe the stimulus which starts the physiological thermoregulatory response to cold.

25.3 CLASSIFICATION

Hypothermia may be classified according to the central core temperature:

- mild: core temperature 35–32°C
- severe: core temperature below 32°C.

It may also be classified according to length of exposure:

- acute: the cold stress is severe and overwhelms normal heat production in minutes or hours
- subacute: exhaustion is a critical factor together with depletion of the body's food stores
- chronic: a mild cold stress operates over perhaps days or weeks.

25.3.1 Acute hypothermia

Acute hypothermia is seen in victims of cold water immersion. The cold stress of ice-cold water is such that hypothermia supervenes rapidly despite normal or increased heat production by shivering or exercise at a time when food stores are still almost replete. There is no exhaustion in these cases. Injured climbers in cold environments may fall into this category. There is little time for fluid shifts to occur, and a victim who is rescued from cold water and dried is likely to warm spontaneously.

25.3.2 Subacute hypothermia

Subacute hypothermia is the type usually seen in mountaineers. The victim will have been out in severe weather conditions for hours, perhaps inadequately clothed and fed, suffering from exhaustion, with low food stores. The cold stress is not excessive and is combated by vasoconstriction and increased heat production by exercise and shivering. This maintains the body temperature until exhaustion supervenes and core temperature falls. Spontaneous rewarming is unlikely or slow and every route by which heat is lost must be blocked and additional heat added (see section 25.6). Fluid shifts between body compartments are likely.

25.3.3 Chronic hypothermia

Chronic hypothermia is associated with elderly people living in inadequately heated houses, especially if there is even a mild degree of hypothyroidism. There is mild, prolonged cold stress and although the thermoregulatory response is not overwhelmed it is insufficient to counteract the cold. The temperature falls over days or weeks. There are considerable fluid shifts between compartments leading to cerebral and pulmonary edema and occasionally death.

25.4 PATHOPHYSIOLOGY

Basal heat production generated by the body rises and falls with body temperature. During exercise or shivering when oxygen consumption may quadruple, heat production can increase up to 15 times normal and catecholamine secretion is increased to augment heat production. Shivering muscles use free fatty acids, and some are converted by the liver into low density lipoprotein, which is important as a source of heat production (Hartung et al. 1984). The main sources of energy in endurance activities are free fatty acids and lipoproteins and fitness depends on the ability to use these.

Fat utilization appears to be increased by exercising in the cold (Timmons et al. 1985), and a high body fat may retard cooling of the core during exercise (Weller et al. 1997). At high altitude enhanced fat metabolism spares muscle glycogen (Costil et al. 1977, Sutton 1987).

The lower the level of fitness the lower the level at which catecholamines are required to maintain adequate heat production.

Heat production is linked to muscular work and maximal oxygen uptake so that at altitude heat production is inevitably diminished.

Increasing fitness increases $V_{O_2 max}$, efficiency of oxygen uptake and cardiac output and combats cold and altitude. In cold conditions oxygen uptake and cardiac output need to be higher to maintain exercise rates and this explains the occurrence of angina in cold conditions (Lloyd 1996).

At sea level, even in very fit individuals, vigorous exercise in severe cold may not provide adequate heat and hypothermia can occur; in the unfit exhaustion and hypothermia occur sooner and more rapidly.

Wind can also increase oxygen uptake by as much as 60 per cent. In a gale, speed of walking is diminished and skin cooling, which is almost entirely dependent on the environmental temperature, is increased. Obviously clothing insulation will modify cooling but if protective clothing is soaked externally by rain, or internally by sweat, loss of insulation occurs.

In wet cold, the combination of wind, movement and wetting can reduce clothing insulation to a negligible figure and is the reason why hypothermia occurs at temperatures above zero.

Older men too have a faster drop in core temperature when exercising in cold conditions (Falk et al. 1994). There are no data on older women.

At high altitude, $V_{O_2 max}$ falls and with associated dehydration and malnutrition heat production is further diminished and hypothermia becomes more likely. Climbers at great altitude on pre-World War II expeditions often felt cold despite 'adequate' clothing. However, this clothing was inadequate by modern standards and, with their poor general physical condition, incipient hypothermia and frostbite were common.

Alcohol decreases awareness of cold, increases bravado and impairs both mental and physical ability and thus increases the likelihood of hypothermia.

During cooling, vasoconstriction occurs which reduces the volume of the active vascular bed; when cold stress is removed the vascular bed is increased and surface warming further increases this. With peripheral vasoconstriction, fluid is transferred to the deep capacitance vessels and this overload is countered by a diuresis due to a decrease in the antidiuretic hormone.

Depending on the diuresis of cold exposure, fluid may shift from the intracellular to the extracellular compartment and this will reverse on warming.

25.4.1 Exhaustion

A high work rate can maintain heat production and body temperature in cold conditions. However, if the work rate is too low, a fall in core temperature occurs with increased shivering and sympathetic activity, which is more marked in leaner subjects, and would impair performance still further (Weller et al. 1997).

With poor insulation, prolonged exercise in wet cold conditions can lead to exhaustion, fall in core temperature, diminution in shivering and resultant hypothermia. In one case the individual cooled so rapidly that he was unable to continue walking (Thompson and Hayward 1996).

Dehydration for short periods may reduce the vasoconstrictor response to cold but it does not cause a decline in core temperature. Severe dehydration may, however, impair fluid balance and therefore maintenance of body temperature (O'Brien et al. 1998).

If shivering is inhibited for any reason, the fall in core temperature is likely to be increased and rewarming inhibited (Giesbrecht et al. 1997) but neither shivering nor vasoconstrictor response to cold is affected by the time of day (Castellani et al. 1999a).

Previous severe physical exercise may predispose to greater heat loss and a greater decline in core temperature when subsequently exposed to cold conditions. Indeed, it has been suggested that further exercise could in the short term increase the risk of hypothermia (Castellani et al. 1999b).

Chronic fatigue, the result of exertion combined with loss of sleep, decreased food intake and reduced tissue insulation are the types of conditions that occur frequently on the battlefield and in the mountains especially at high altitude. They result in blunted metabolic heat production which compromises the maintenance of body temperature (Young et al. 1998). However, a short period of rest, sleep and adequate food restores the thermogenic response to cold; but thermal balance in cold conditions may remain compromised until tissue insulation is restored, which may take several weeks. (Westerterp-Plantagna et al. 1999).

In some cases of death due to hypothermia, unfit individuals have become exhausted and their shivering inadequate to maintain core temperature (Tikusis et al. 1999). Pugh (1967) has shown that the oxygen uptake of a subject exercising at a given work rate in wet cold conditions is 50 per cent higher than it is in a dry cold environment. Continuing exercise may, therefore, result in complete collapse, increased heat loss and hypothermia, and shelter must be found immediately.

A feature of hypothermia is amnesia, but a case of amnesia has been recorded at a core temperature of 35.6°C, that is, above the level set as the criterion for hypothermia (35°C). This has implications for both mountaineers and hill walkers (Castellani et al. 1998).

Exhaustion may lead to a reduced cardiac stroke volume, a falling peripheral resistance and shift in the distribution of blood to the capacitance vessels (Ekelund 1967). The failure of vasomotor regulation with pooling of peripheral venous blood will cause maximum heat loss in cold conditions. A low blood pressure state has also been observed after ascent to extreme altitude (Pugh and Ward 1956). The fall in skin blood flow during exhaustion might render the fingers and toes more susceptible to frostbite (Wiles et al. 1986).

During a demanding and strenuous climb, energy intake may not equal work output (Guezennec and Pesquies 1985), and depleting the body's glycogen stores increases the likelihood of fatigue. If blood sugar is kept above fasting level, deterioration in performance is prevented but an exhausted person cannot increase heat production in response to cold, and heat loss is inevitable with possible hypothermia and death.

25.4.2 Death

Fluid overload occurs when the circulating fluid volume exceeds the active vascular capacity, and death may result from pulmonary and cerebral edema and cardiac failure.

Continuous cooling may also cause death due to ventricular fibrillation with the risk increasing as the central core temperature falls. The commonest trigger is mechanical irritation.

Hypoxia too may contribute to some deaths as shivering can quadruple oxygen demand. Supplementary oxygen should therefore be considered for all hypothermic patients.

Temperature is a poor guide to death, as recovery has occurred from a core temperature of 9 °C (Niazi and Lewis 1958). Absence of cardiorespiratory activity or a flat electrocardiogram is not an indication as the heart may still be working, but undetectably and 'as hard as stone'. However, cardiac arrest due to cold does occur.

25.5 CLINICAL FEATURES

25.5.1 Mild hypothermia

Individuals suffering from mild hypothermia complain of feeling cold and lose interest in any activity except getting warmer. They also develop a negative attitude towards the aims of the party and, as cooling continues, become uncoordinated, unable to keep up and then start to stumble. There may be attacks of violent shivering.

25.5.2 Severe hypothermia

At core temperatures below 32 °C there is altered mental function and the patient becomes careless about self-protection from the cold.

Thinking becomes slow, decision making difficult and often wrong, and memory deteriorates. There

may be a strong desire for sleep and eventually the will to survive collapses with the individual becoming progressively unresponsive and lapsing into coma. Slurred speech and ataxia may be confused with a stroke. Gastrointestinal mobility may slow or cease, and gastric dilatation and ileus are common (Paton 1983).

Individuals show a great range of response to cold and loss of consciousness may occur with a core temperature as high as 33 °C or as low as 27 °C, depending on the rate of cooling. Consciousness is usually lost at around 30 °C but patients have been reported to be conscious though confused at lower temperatures than this (Lloyd 1972, Paton 1983).

Though shivering usually stops as the temperature drops below 30 °C, it has been observed at a core temperature of 24 °C (Alexander 1945). Some cases have been reported to cool without shivering (Marcus 1979) (Chapter 23).

When the temperature drops to below 30 °C, ventricular fibrillation may supervene.

Survival depends on sufficient cardiac function to maintain output adequate for brain and heart perfusion. Cardiac function is more relevant to survival than brain temperature.

The patient with profound hypothermia may be indistinguishable from one who is dead. The skin is ice cold to touch and the muscles and joints are stiff and simulate rigor mortis. Respiration may be difficult or impossible to register, the peripheral pulses may be absent and blood pressure unmeasurable. In profound hypothermia pupils do not react to light and other reflexes are absent.

The electrocardiogram (ECG) shows a slow rhythm with multifocal extrasystoles, broad complexes and atrial flutter (Jessen and Hagelstein 1978). There may also be J waves present (Osborne 1953).

Both hemoglobin and white cell count will be raised because of a shift of fluid from plasma to the interstitial space. Thrombocytopenia has been reported (Vella et al. 1988).

Even when there is evidence of a total stoppage of cardiorespiratory function, survival is possible (Siebhke et al. 1975). A flat electroencephalogram (EEG) is not a certain indicator of death in hypothermia. The only certain diagnostic factor is failure to recover on rewarming (Golden 1973, Lilja 1983). Before brain death can be diagnosed the core temperature must be normal (NHS 1974); however, brain death may be a cause of hypothermia (Table 25.1).

Table 25.1 *Clinical features of hypothermia*

Temperature (°C)	Clinical features
37.6	Normal rectal temperature
37	Normal oral temperature
35	Maximal shivering/delayed cerebration
34	Lowest temperature compatible with continuous exercise
33–31	Retrograde amnesia, clouded consciousness
	Blood pressure difficult to measure
30–28	Progressive loss of consciousness
	Muscular rigidity
	Slow respiration and pulse
	Ventricular fibrillation may develop if heart irritated
27	Appears dead
	Voluntary movement lost
	Deep tendon reflex and pupil reflex absent
25	Ventricular fibrillation may develop spontaneously
24–21	Pulmonary edema develops
20	Heart stops
14	Lowest temperature in accidental hypothermia patient with recovery (MacIntyre 1994)
9	Lowest temperature in cooled hypothermic patient with recovery
1–7	Rats and hamsters revived successfully

Source: adapted from Lloyd (1986a).

25.6 MANAGEMENT

The principles of management are to prevent further heat loss, to restore body temperature to normal and to maintain life while doing so.

Choice of technique will depend upon circumstances, facilities available and the experience and skill of the doctor. In mildly hypothermic patients a slow rewarming technique is acceptable, but for severe hypothermia rapid, active rewarming should be carried out. If there is no circulation the patient should be transferred to a unit where rewarming by heat exchange is possible. A summary of the technique is given in Table 25.2.

25.6.1 In the field

The management of hypothermia in the field is 'the art of the possible'. Hamilton and Paton (1996) carried out a survey and concluded that most rescue groups attempting to measure temperature did so by the oral method. A low-reading thermometer was carried by a majority of teams. For reheating, commercial heating pads were used by most groups. The incidence of hypothermia was, surprisingly, the same for summer and winter. Cardiorespiratory resuscitation in the field was started in 76 per cent of cases and the criteria for starting were the absence of a pulse, cardiac arrest and the likelihood of rapid evacuation.

MILD HYPOTHERMIA

Individuals should be stopped from walking and placed in shelter out of the wind, rain or snow. They should be protected from further cooling and warmed by any method available.

Ideally, wet clothing should be replaced by dry, but if dry clothing is not available wet clothing should be wrung out and put back on. If wet clothing, which has some insulating value, is left on, it should be covered with an impermeable material to prevent further heat loss. As large amounts of heat may be lost from the head, it should be covered. Warm fluids should be given, but never alcohol.

A patient with mild hypothermia can recover with these simple procedures, but recovery will be hastened if external heat is added (e.g. getting into a sleeping bag with another person). Central rewarming methods have been described (Lloyd 1973, Foray and Salon 1985) using warmed inhaled air which can be applied in the field with suitable apparatus.

Table 25.2 *Summary of rewarming technique*

Mild hypothermia 35–32 °C	Surface rewarming Warm intravenous fluids Warm inspired oxygen
Severe hypothermia 32 °C and below	Warm intravenous fluids Airway warming via endotracheal tube Warm bath immersion Peritoneal dialysis Gastric lavage
If circulatory arrest occurs	Cardiopulmonary resuscitation Airway rewarming Peritoneal dialysis Gastric lavage Central rewarming via heat exchanger

SEVERE HYPOTHERMIA

The management of severe hypothermia in the field will depend upon the local situation, possibilities for evacuation and access to specialist medical facilities. Where these are good, as in the mountains of Europe and North America, patients should be evacuated as soon as possible with the minimum of treatment in the field. However, active treatment in the field has been successful (Fischer *et al.* 1991). Aluminium foil 'blankets' and suits provide good thermal protection in rescue situations (Ennemoser *et al.* 1988). When bad weather delays evacuation the patient should be rewarmed slowly and treated as gently as possible to avoid ventricular fibrillation.

If cardiac arrest occurs in a hypothermic patient this produces a dilemma for rescuers because it may be due to some other cause because the heart may be beating even if clinically undetectable. Mechanical irritation of chest compression may trigger ventricular fibrillation with total loss of cardiac function. However, a consensus seems to be:

- If breathing is absent, becomes obstructed or stops, then standard airway management should be started including mouth-to-mouth resuscitation.
- Chest compression should be started if no carotid pulse is detected for 60 s, if the pulse disappears, or if cardiac arrest occurred within the last 2 h.
- Resuscitation should be started only if there is a reasonable expectation that it can be continued effectively with only brief interruption until the

patient can be brought to a hospital where full advanced life support is available (Lloyd 1996). Cardiac resuscitation has been continued for 6.5 h with ultimate success (Lexow 1991).
- Misguided attempts at cardiac massage may precipitate ventricular fibrillation (Mills 1983a). The mortality rate from hypothermia in the field is of the order of 50 per cent but with increasing expertise in management this figure should improve.
- The diagnosis of death in hypothermia should be made with caution because profound hypothermia can simulate death. Strictly, the diagnosis of death can only be made when the patient fails to revive after the core temperature has been brought to normal.

25.6.2 In hospital (Bohn 1987, Danzl *et al.* 1995, Lloyd 1996)

Those patients with mild hypothermia (32–35 °C) can be allowed to rewarm slowly on a general ward and warm humidified oxygen can be given by mask. Those with severe hypothermia (32 °C and below) should be admitted to an intensive care unit.

Intubation and ventilation should be carried out by a skilled anesthetist with adequate preoxygenation to prevent cardiac arrhythmia, if there is:

- absence of vital signs
- coma
- apnea
- hypoxemia not corrected by oxygen by mask

- cardiac arrhythmia
- aspiration pneumonia
- hypercarbia.

If there is no pulse or respiration then full cardio-respiratory resuscitation should be carried out, regardless of ECG activity. Between 30 °C and 28 °C the heart may fibrillate spontaneously but the presence of sinus rhythm does not mean that there is a useful cardiac output, so immediate external cardiac massage should be started.

Below 28 °C the fibrillating heart will not convert to sinus rhythm, so there is little point in using shock therapy until the core temperature is above this value. Cardiac pacing and atropine seem of little benefit; dopamine can improve cardiac output. An increase in filling pressure can be achieved by using pneumatic trousers to decrease peripheral volume.

25.7 METHODS OF REWARMING

Even in hospital, with perfect insulation, the rate of warming varies greatly at between 0.14 °C to 0.5 °C h^{-1}, and failure to rewarm may occur. Too rapid rewarming may result in fluid shifts with pulmonary and cerebral edema. Young people, particularly those in whom acute hypothermia was precipitated by drug overdose, have a high survival rate when allowed to warm spontaneously (Tolman and Cohen 1970). In the elderly with chronic hypothermia, there is a high mortality rate (Treating accidental hypothermia 1978) unless treatment is carried out in an intensive care unit (Ledingham and Mone 1980).

In severe hypothermia, when the patient no longer shivers, some method of active rewarming is necessary, as metabolic heat production is so low.

25.7.1 Peripheral (surface) rewarming

Peripheral rewarming may be carried out either rapidly or at a slow to moderate rate; it is only advisable for conscious patients suffering from acute accidental hypothermia.

RAPID REWARMING

The conscious patient should be placed in a bath which is then heated to 40–42 °C, hand hot, as rapidly as possible. The advantages are that it is the fastest way of transferring heat, needs unsophisticated equipment, suppresses shivering and speeds the feeling of well being. The main benefits occur within the first 20 min of rewarming and the method should only be used in the patient who is conscious, shivering and uninjured and able to get into and out of the bath with only minimal assistance (Handley et al. 1993).

The disadvantages are that, by dilating the peripheral circulation before the body temperature has been fully restored, there is a danger of 'rewarming shock' (Golden 1983). Also, because of the problem of maintaining the airway, this method of treatment is not advocated in an unconscious patient because cardiorespiratory resuscitation cannot be used.

SLOW TO MODERATE REWARMING

This includes the use of hot water bottles, blankets, hot water packs, temperature controlled cabinets and cradles and hot water sarongs (Paton 1983). This method requires an effective peripheral circulation and most, but not all, patients do rewarm (Ledingham and Mone 1980).

Superficial burns are an important hazard associated with all forms of surface heating, and may occur even when the temperature is quite low (e.g. hand-warm hot water bottles) (De Pay 1982). Another disadvantage is that, with peripheral vaso-dilatation, heat is further dissipated and cold blood returns to the heart causing irregularities of rhythm (Anderson et al. 1970).

Surface hot water warming abolishes shivering and oxygen demand is reduced. However, not all methods of surface rewarming provide enough heat and abolition of shivering may put the patient at further risk.

25.7.2 Central rewarming

With central rewarming the heat is applied to the central core of the body and warming proceeds outwards from within. The organs of the core, 8 per cent of the body weight, contribute 56 per cent of the heat production at rest in normothermic patients and a higher proportion in hypothermia, as the muscles and superficial tissues have cooled more than the core. By concentrating the heat gain to the core, thermal benefit will be significantly greater.

AIRWAY REWARMING

The main thermal input comes from the body's own metabolism and the main benefit is to stop heat and moisture loss through breathing, rather than by the additional heat supplied (Lloyd 1973). It is therefore of value only when the rest of the body is adequately insulated. This method is widely recommended in hypothermia as it accelerates rewarming with beneficial effects on cerebral and cardiorespiratory function (Lloyd and Mitchell 1974). It accelerates return to consciousness, restores respiratory drive, stabilizes cardiac rhythm and improves output and blood pressure. It abolishes shivering thus reducing oxygen demand and reduces mortality in hypothermia secondary to exhaustion.

The aim is to produce warm moist air for the patient to breathe without burning the face or larynx.

Various types of equipment are available:

- condenser–humidifier, which traps heat and moisture during expiration, returning both on the next inspiration
- electrically powered humidifier
- closed circuit consisting of a soda-lime canister and oxygen cylinder. The reaction between soda-lime and expired carbon dioxide produces heat and moisture (Lloyd 1986, pp. 199–203).

Portable equipment of this type has been used satisfactorily at 6000 m.

For first aid one can use a heat and moisture exchanger with mask and tubing covered by clothing and breathe the prewarmed boundary air close to the skin. It weighs only a few grams and is easy to carry.

Airway warming has the advantage that it can be used in the field and continued into the hospital. It is noninvasive and can be combined with other treatments.

VIA A HEAT EXCHANGER

In open heart surgery total body cooling and rewarming is routine. From experience gained by this method it was natural to suggest that similar methods be used in severe hypothermia. This may be considered the ideal method of rewarming since the vital organs of the core are warmed first with oxygenated warm blood and circulation is artificially supported, though it is invasive. Blood is removed from the femoral vein, warmed in a heat exchanger and returned by the femoral artery. Heat may be supplied very rapidly by this method and the body temperature raised by 10 °C in 1 h.

The heart is perfused directly with warm blood and cardiac irritability is reduced. If hypovolemic shock due to peripheral vasodilatation occurs, then a warm heart can compensate better than a cold or irritable one. A definite indication for extracorporeal rewarming is ventricular fibrillation associated with hypothermia (Braun 1985), and patients who are 'frozen solid and dead' with a core temperature as low as 17.5 °C have been resuscitated by this means. The method is safe in experienced hands and is becoming more popular in centers where open heart surgery is routine or where cases of severe hypothermia are seen frequently.

25.7.3   Irrigation of body cavities

MEDIASTINAL

Thoracotomy and mediastinal irrigation have been successful, but this is an open, invasive method requiring a sophisticated team. It causes more trauma to the patient, there is a risk of infection, and it is doubtful if it is more effective than central warming by heat exchange (Paton 1983).

PERITONEAL

Peritoneal lavage is an efficient method of heat transfer. The temperature gradients throughout the body are more normal than with surface rewarming. The inferior vena cava is warmed directly and thus venous blood returning to the heart is selectively warmed. Additional heat to the heart and lungs is transferred via the diaphragm, and cardiac, liver and renal functions are improved. It is a simple method not requiring highly trained personnel and sophisticated equipment (Patton and Doolittle 1972, Pickering et al. 1977).

Problems include peritonitis, which is related to perforation of the bowel, and respiratory insufficiency due to the pressure of fluid in the peritoneal cavity. Recent abdominal surgery is a contraindication because of the possibility of adhesions.

25.7.4   Other methods

Intragastric balloons have been used, in which a double lumen tube transports the warm fluid to and from the balloon. A double lumen esophageal tube with a thermostat controlled pump has also been tried (Kristensen *et al.* 1986). These offer some promise as a method of warming the central core without the sterile precautions needed for peritoneal lavage. A technique using a modified Sengstaken tube through which Ringer's lactate solution is circulated at 41°C has been described (Ledingham 1983). Enemas and gastric lavage have been described but require larger amounts of fluid. Intracolonic balloons may also be used.

Diathermy requires sophisticated and expensive equipment, but it has considerable potential for delivering significant amounts of heat by transmitting energy through the superficial tissues to the deeper ones where it is converted to heat. Three main types are considered by Harnett *et al.* (1983): ultrasonic, short-wave and microwave. There is a considerable number of hazards and disadvantages (Lehmann 1971).

25.8   ASSOCIATED THERAPY

25.8.1   Drugs

There is controversy over the use of corticosteroids in hypothermia. Some recommend their use from clinical experience and steroids have been given as a last resort to apparently moribund mountaineers with some success (MacInnes 1971).

25.8.2   Electrolyte abnormalities

Electrolyte abnormalities may be found in hypothermic patients, but the pattern is completely inconsistent. Hypokalemia should be treated by giving potassium; calcium will protect against the effects of hypokalemia on the myocardium.

25.8.3   Glucose

Hypoglycemia was an important factor in one series of hypothermic patients (Fitzgerald and Jessop 1982), but a high blood sugar may be found in cases of hypothermia (nondiabetic) probably due to non-utilization of glucose by cold muscles; on rewarming, the glucose level will fall. Hypoglycemia may precipi-

tate hypothermia and the center controlling heat production may be impaired. In cases of exhaustion hypothermia, glucose may be given to provide metabolic substrate for rewarming (MacInnes 1979).

25.8.4   Intravenous fluids

All intravenous fluids should be warmed to 35°C during resuscitation in treating hypothermia. In hospital a dedicated warmer is used, but in the field heat packs or body heat can be used.

25.8.5   Oxygen

Hypothermia will have the effect of shifting the oxygen dissociation curve to the left (i.e. increasing the hemoglobin affinity for oxygen) (Chapter 9). This means that there may be difficulty in giving up oxygen in the tissues, which may then be hypoxic. Therefore, there is a theoretical advantage in the use of oxygen (which should be warmed) in cases of hypothermia, though this has not been demonstrated. Bohn (1987) considers that all hypothermic patients should be considered hypoxemic until proved otherwise.

25.9   OUTCOME

All methods of rewarming have been used successfully but each has disadvantages and problems. Some require equipment and expertise found only in hospitals and, except for the simplest methods, medical supervision is necessary. The majority of methods are safe provided the patient is monitored in intensive care. The method of choice depends on the environment, availability of equipment and experience of those who have to treat the patient. A high serum potassium following prolonged cardiac arrest may suggest an inability to recover (Bender *et al.* 1995). Hypothermia compromises the host defense mechanism with the possibility of bacterial infection but with minimal inflammatory response (Lewin *et al.* 1981). However, contrary to popular belief that cold exposure can precipitate a virus infection, the immune system is not affected by short periods of cold exposure. The fall in core temperature resulting from cold leads to a consistent, significant mobilization of circulating immune cells, and increase in natural killer cell activity and elevation in interleukin-6 plasma levels (Brenner *et al.* 1999).

25.10 AFTER DROP

The core temperature continues to fall before rising after the individual has been removed from cold water; this has been termed the 'after drop'. As many deaths have occurred after removal from cold water and because this collapse coincided with the time that the rectal temperature was at its lowest (Golden 1983), it was assumed that death and the after drop were connected and that ventricular fibrillation had been precipitated by the continued cooling of the heart.

However, Golden and Hervey (1981) have now challenged the belief that the after drop is caused by cold blood returning to the core from the cooled peripheral circulation. In fact, if the rate of heat production from core to periphery is high enough to balance heat flow there is no after drop (Golden and Hervey 1981). The way that heat flows through the body tissues can explain the rectal temperature fall (Webb 1986). Savard *et al.* (1985) have shown that the after drop in core temperature *precedes* peripheral vasodilatation in human volunteers exposed to hypothermia. Moreover, at the time of maximum peripheral vasodilatation, core temperatures had already started to rise. Slow passive rewarming may therefore be used in mild hypothermia and rapid active rewarming is only indicated for severe hypothermia. Inhibition of shivering may increase the after drop and attenuate rewarming in hypothermic patients (Hayward 1997).

25.11 VENTRICULAR FIBRILLATION

The exact mechanism involved in the production of ventricular fibrillation due to cold has so far not been defined. Changes in electrolyte concentration occur but there is no general agreement on their interpretation. Hypoxia of the myocardium might be a cause but, in hypothermia, oxygen carried in the blood is adequate for the reduced myocardial work, though

sudden hypoxia may precipitate ventricular fibrillation in hypothermia.

Cardiac temperature may be very low without ventricular fibrillation (Laufmann 1951) and the direct effect of cold is often asystole. However, it seems probable that the effect of cold blood on the Purkinje fibers selectively cools them relative to the cardiac muscle. This could result in ventricular fibrillation following cardiac irritation (Lloyd and Mitchell 1974).

Defibrillation below 28 °C is unlikely to be successful, although there are some exceptions. Ideally one should manage such patients in a cardiac surgical unit. The circulation should be maintained artificially until cardiac temperatures exceed 28 °C before attempting defibrillation, as too many attempts are likely to burn the pericardium. However, with direct core rewarming, a heart in asystole has started spontaneously at 24 °C, and defibrillation has been successful at 22.5 °C. Bretylium tosylate is a most effective antifibrillatory drug at low temperature and can be used prophylactically (Paton 1991).

25.12 INTRAVASCULAR FLUID VOLUME

The intravascular fluid volume is depleted in all hypothermic patients, especially when hypothermia is associated with septicemia and trauma. Incidents of cardiovascular collapse and cardiac arrest during rewarming may be due to vasodilatation in a volume-depleted patient and not to after drop, the toxic effects of metabolites or the effect of cold blood on the heart.

Death may therefore be due to hypovolemia. During cooling, there is a shift in body fluids from the intravascular to the interstitial compartment, causing overt edema, which is increased on rewarming. The severity of the shifts is directly related to the duration of cold exposure.

During rewarming, reversal of fluid shifts occurs most rapidly in the peripheral vascular bed, causing a rise in central venous pressure.

Survival from hypothermia depends, therefore, on a balance between the size of the vascular bed, controlled by vasomotor tone, and the circulating blood volume, dependent on the extent of dehydration. It is also dependent on the extent and rate of reversal of the fluid shifts that occur during cooling. If vaso-

Table 25.3 *Complications of profound hypothermia*

Pneumonia and pulmonary edema
Gastric erosion or ulcer
Acute pancreatitis
Acute renal failure and hematuria
Temporary adrenal insufficiency
Hemolysis and disseminated intravascular coagulation
Myoglobinuria

Source: adapted from Wilkerson *et al.* (1986).

motor tone is poor, death from hypovolemia may occur, and fluid overload may cause heart failure; dehydration may affect either.

The only sure method of distinguishing these is by central venous pressure monitoring; this should be done routinely in hospital. If the blood pressure falls, a rapid infusion of 500 mL of warmed fluid will, if hypovolemia is present, raise the blood pressure temporarily (Lloyd 1986, p. 74).

25.13 COMPLICATIONS

For the previously healthy hypothermic patient the risk of serious complications is low. Many of those listed in Table 25.3 result from pre-existing conditions, chronic disease, malnutrition and alcoholism (Wilkerson *et al.* 1986).

Frostbite and nonfreezing cold injury

SUMMARY

Frostbite and nonfreezing cold injury are both forms of local cold injury and may be associated with hypothermia. Frostbite occurs when the tissues freeze but its clinical features are related to both freezing and thawing. Blisters may lead to superficial or deep gangrene and prevention is by the use of adequate protective clothing and avoidance of wind-chill. Management is conservative with rapid rewarming being most effective; infection must be avoided and surgical intervention delayed. The sequence of freeze–thaw–freeze, which is especially detrimental, must be avoided. The sequelae of frost-bite may last for many years.

Immersion or nonfreezing cold injury occurs at tissue temperatures between 0 °C and 15 °C. It is commoner than is generally realized and nerve involvement is usual. It may progress to frostbite. Treatment is by rewarming but sequelae are common. It is often found associated with accidents and bivouacs when maintaining body temperature is difficult.

Local cold stress may be associated with chilblains, Raynaud's disease, Raynaud's phenomenon and coronary artery spasm and other conditions.

injury (immersion injury, trench foot) and freezing cold injury (frostbite) may be present in the same limb and both may be associated with hypothermia.

Nonfreezing cold injury normally occurs at 0–15 °C, though the upper limits are not precisely known and feet exposed for some time in water at 26 °C may become swollen, hyperemic and painful. Freezing cold injury (frostbite) occurs at temperatures below 0 °C in dry cold conditions, especially if there is a wind or the tissues are wet. Frostbite may occur in fully clothed individuals at extreme altitude at subzero temperatures if oxygen uptake is insufficient for adequate heat production when the tissues cool to the environmental temperature. Local cold injury is not common in civilian situations, though 1500 cases were reported on 300 expeditions to the Karakoram Mountains of central Asia (Hashmi *et al.* 1998).

In World War I about 115 000 British soldiers suffered from immersion injury and frostbite. In 2 months in World War II, 100 000 cases of local cold injury occurred in the German army with about 15 000 amputations (Vaughn 1942).

26.1 INTRODUCTION

Many are cold, yet few are frozen – and frostbite is not common. However, both nonfreezing

26.2 FROSTBITE

Many clinical factors may precipitate local cold injury. These are shown in Table 26. 1.

Table 26.1 *Factors which may precipitate frostbite*

Excessive reaction to cold, e.g. Raynaud's syndrome
Diabetes
Endarteritis – local (result of previous cold injury)
Endarteritis obliterans
Vascular damage due to trauma or infection
Arteriosclerosis
Thyroid hypofunction
Hyperhidrosis (congenital or acquired)
Hypovolemia (loss of blood or through shock)
Dehydration due to gastrointestinal disease or exercise
Nicotine
Metal spectacle frames or seats

26.2.1 Clinical features

DISTRIBUTION OF FROSTBITE

Any area may be affected but some are more prone to cold injury because of pressure, position, lack of insulating fat or liability to wetting. These include:

- face: bridge of nose (due to spectacles), tip of nose, chin (double chin especially), ear lobes, cheeks, lips, tongue (due to drinking or sucking snow or ice)
- upper limb: fingers (particularly the index finger in rifle shooting), head of radius, lower end of ulna, olecranon, medial and lateral epicondyle of humerus
- lower limb: patella, head of fibula, subcutaneous border of tibia, medial condyle of tibia, lower end of fibula, lateral edge of foot, plantar aspect of toes, dorsal surface of foot joints, soles of feet, heels
- male genitalia: penis and testicles (difficulty in fastening zip; wetting due to overflow incontinence); jogging in conditions of severe wind chill (Hershkowitz 1977)
- buttocks and perineum (sitting on metallic seats).

Cultural patterns may influence the site of frostbite. With long hair frostbite of the ears is unusual, whereas short hair is associated with frozen ears. Some activity at low temperatures associated with inadequate foot gear (e.g. running shoes) may also predispose to the development of cold injury; a similar type of shoe is used for cross-country skiing.

Drug abuse may also contribute to cold injury, as nasal 'snorting' of cocaine causes vasoconstriction, and this makes the nose more prone to cooling in a cold environment.

26.2.2 Epidemiology

In the Finnish army, 1.8 per 1000 recruits suffer from frostbite (Lehmuskallio *et al.* 1995). A retrospective study of a 10-year period (1986–95) of personnel in the British Antarctic Survey (BAS) showed that of 61 new consultations for cold injury in 43 individuals, 95 per cent were for superficial frostbite, 3 per cent for hypothermia and 2 per cent for trench foot. The incidence was 65.5 per 1000 individuals per year, higher than that reported for soldiers stationed in Alaska.

The prevalence of cold injury increases with a fall in temperature in the BAS survey. It was not possible to find any correlation between smoking and frostbite; however, prior cold injury was a significant risk factor (Sumner *et al.* 1974, Cattermole 1999).

At the district hospital in Chamonix in the French Alps, about 80 cases of frostbite are seen each year. About 75 per cent are superficial; 57 per cent affect the feet, 46 per cent the hands and 17 per cent the face (Marsigny 1998).

26.2.3 Classification

- First degree: superficial frostbite with redness and swelling.
- Second degree: blebs or vesicles occur in addition.
- Third degree: deep frostbite; the tissue becomes gray, dark blue or black.

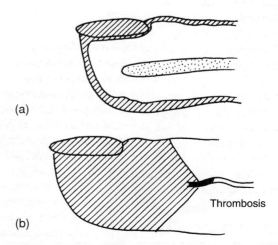

Figure 26.1 *(a) Superficial frostbite: gangrene (shaded area) is limited to the superficial 2–3 mm of tissue. (b) Arterial thrombosis: gangrene extends through all tissues.*

26.2.4 Clinical features

SUPERFICIAL FROSTBITE

In frostnip, the exposed skin (often of the tip of the nose, cheeks or ears, which have been painful), blanches and loses sensation, but remains pliable. On rewarming, the part tingles, becomes hyperemic and may have some skin desquamation several days later.

In superficial frostbite (Figure 26.1a), skin and subcutaneous tissues are affected; the skin becomes white and frozen, with the deep underlying tissues remaining fairly pliable. On rewarming the skin becomes mottled and blue or purple and will swell. Paresthesiae are common.

Within 24–48 h, blebs, initially filled with colorless serum, appear. They are usually found where the skin is lax, such as the backs of the hands or dorsum of the feet (Figure 26.2). Later they may be filled with serosanguineous fluid, which is absorbed, and a black carapace forms (Figure 26.3). Often white frostbitten tissue may become black without the formation of blisters.

The gangrene is superficial, not more than a few millimeters thick (Figure 26.1a), in contrast to that seen commonly in hospital due to arterial thrombosis (Figure 26.1b), where the gangrene involves all tissue layers. This means that the surgical approach must be more conservative in the case of frostbite (section 26.2.9).

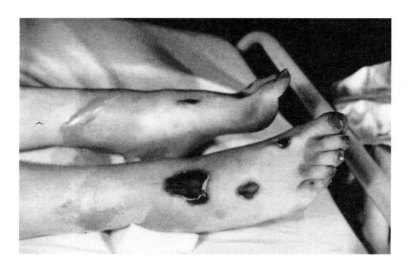

Figure 26.2 *Blister formation, swelling and gangrene on feet and ankles several days after freezing cold injury.*

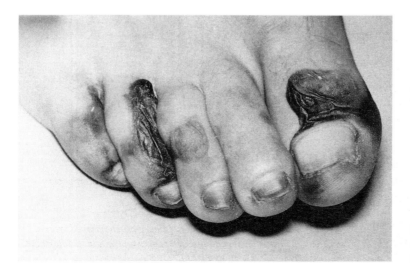

Figure 26.3 *Superficial frostbite showing black carapace developing after collapse of blisters on the toes.*

The carapace is insensitive and fits like a lead glove over the underlying tissue. If the contour of the blackened tissue corresponds to the original part, tissue loss is unlikely, but if contour is lost, tissue loss is almost certain. After some weeks, the blackened carapace begins to separate at the line of demarcation, and a black, mummified cast of tissue peels off like a glove or sock (Figures 26.4, 26.5). Hidden pockets of infection or pus may lead to tissue loss in both superficial and deep frostbite (Figure 26.6).

The underlying tissue is pink, unduly sensitive 'baby-skin' and there may be abnormal sweating. In 2–3 months it will take on a normal appearance.

DEEP FROSTBITE

Deep frostbite involves the deeper structures (muscle, bone and tendons), as well as the skin and subcutaneous tissues (Figure 26.7). The part is insensitive, wooden and gray-purple or white marble in color. Because tendons are less sensitive to cold and the associated muscle groups are distant from the injury, the part can be moved (Figure 26.8). Blisters filled with dark-purple fluid may appear after some weeks. Eventually dry gangrene and mummification occur and a cast of the affected tissue separates.

Permanent loss of tissue is almost inevitable with

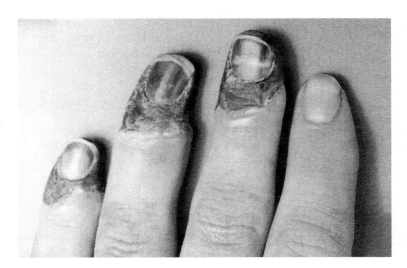

Figure 26.4 *Frostbitten fingertips showing blackened carapace and line of demarcation.*

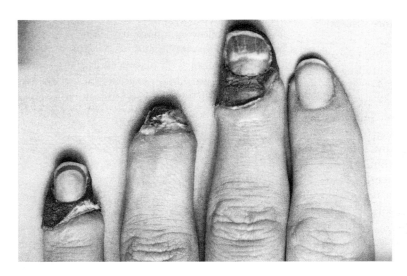

Figure 26.5 *Same fingers as in Figure 26.4, now showing separation of carapace from the ring finger leaving a conical stump.*

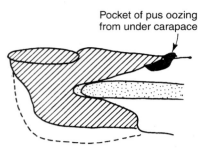

Figure 26.6 *Deep frostbite showing loss of contour and mummification with development of a pocket of pus.*

deep frostbite. However, the limbs may return to normal over a period of months, and amputation should never be carried out precipitately. A deep boring pain may be present throughout much of the period.

26.2.5 Pathophysiology

Classically there are four stages of frostbite:

- The pre-freezing stage occurs secondary to chilling and before ice crystal formation and is the result of vasoconstriction. The tissue temperature is 3–10 °C and cutaneous sensation is usually abolished at 10 °C.
- The freeze–thaw stage is caused by extracellular ice crystal formation, with the tissue temperature below 0 °C. The environmental temperature is usually between –6 °C and –15 °C. Because of underlying heat radiation from deeper tissues, skin must be supercooled before it freezes. Susceptibility to freezing varies. Endothelium, bone marrow and nerve tissue are more susceptible than muscle, bone and cartilage.
- In the vascular stage, changes in the blood vessel, plasma leakage, coagulation and shunting of blood occur.
- In the late ischemic stage, thrombosis, ischemia, gangrene and autonomic dysfunction supervene (McCauley *et al.* 1995). On thawing, capillary patency is restored but blood flow declines 3–4 min later. Three almost simultaneous phenomena occur on thawing: momentary vasoconstriction of arterioles and venules; restoration of capillary blood flow; and showers of microemboli. On freezing, the cells remain in a 'metabolic icebox' while frozen, but on rewarming, perfusion restarts and a number of biochemical reactions

come into play. The part swells and ischemia may increase as a result of sludging, emboli and thrombosis. Frostbite should therefore be considered as an injury both of freezing and of rewarming (Paton 1987).

SKIN

Skin freezes at –0.53 °C but, provided the period is short, this causes no lasting injury. After 11 min at –1.9 °C it becomes red and tender for days, and repeated exposures for 20 min or more at this level cause blistering (Keatinge and Cannon 1960). To freeze properly skin must be supercooled to –4 °C, to counter underlying radiant heat.

Cold injury is associated with hyperkeratosis of the skin and atrophy of elastic fibers. The sebaceous glands and hair follicles also show change; there is atrophy of the root sheaths of hair and the nails become brittle, thick and cracked.

BLOOD VESSELS

Considerable evidence points to the primary alteration in cold injury being changes in the vascular endothelium. Seventy-two hours after freeze–thaw injury there is loss of vascular endothelium in the capillary walls accompanied by fibrin deposition – the endothelium may be totally destroyed (Zacarian 1985)

Venules appear to be more sensitive to cold than other vascular structures because of their low flow rates. Arterioles with a flow rate twice that of venules are less damaged by freezing; capillaries show the fewest direct effects of cooling.

Normally, following intense vasoconstriction, the skin temperature equilibrates with environmental temperature, the stagnant plasma cools and viscosity increases. On rewarming, vasodilatation occurs and there is immediate recovery of microvascular

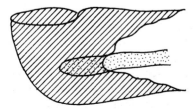

Figure 26.7 *Deep frostbite showing profile of tissue loss (cf. Figure 26.1b).*

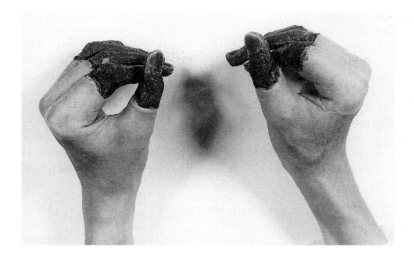

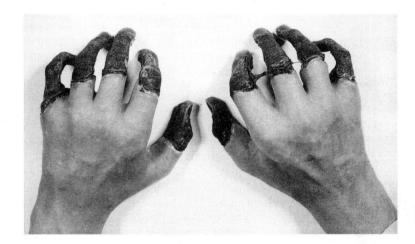

Figure 26.8 *Deep frostbite of fingers with mummification showing that movement is possible because muscles are unaffected and tendons are still intact.*

perfusion, provided no thrombosis is present. If pathological vasodilatation occurs with release of histamine or other tissue metabolites, this results in blood with a high hematocrit reaching the capillaries and the velocity of the blood flow is decreased, red cell aggregates appear and an increase in viscosity occurs. This may trigger further retardation of blood flow and further aggregation leading to complete occlusion of microvessels with complete stasis and gangrene.

Damage to blood vessels depends on the duration of freezing with resulting plasma leakage and blister formation. The blisters contain tissue breakdown products associated with vasoconstriction, increased leukocyte sticking and platelet aggregation. Analysis of the blister fluid shows prostaglandins and high levels of thromboxane to be present (Heggers *et al.* 1990). Due to the action of precapillary sphincters, arteriovenous shunts open and close in cycles and blood bypasses the frozen area. Complete closure of the arteriovenous shunts renders the part avascular and protects the body core from cooled blood and the patient from hypothermia (Greene 1943, Washburn 1962, Schmid-Schonbein and Neumann 1985). Both phlebitis and arteritis may occur as a result of frostbite.

ICE CRYSTAL FORMATION

If freezing is slow, interstitial ice crystals form which enlarge at the expense of intracellular water, osmotic pressure rises, and enzyme mechanisms are disturbed with resulting cell death. If freezing is rapid, ice crystals form everywhere and rupture of cell membranes is the result.

NERVES

Increasing cold and nerve malfunction are matched by severe morphological changes to peripheral nerves.

The main findings are an immediate increase in the mean diameter of myelinated and nonmyelinated fibers, marked edema, axon degeneration, and infrequent, segmented and paranodal demyelination. There is selective vulnerability to cold, based on nerve fiber diameter, with myelinated fibers being more susceptible than nonmyelinated. Degeneration of nerve fibers is probably due to increased permeability of endoneural vessels which leads to diffuse edema, toxin production, changes in osomolarity and increase in endoneural pressure. Although there is clear evidence of ischemia in freezing cold injury this is less clear in nonfreezing injury, though some changes in vascular endothelium occur.

Once the temperature falls below freezing for more than a few seconds degeneration occurs affecting all nerve fibers equally. There is complete necrosis of all structures within the perineurium, except the endothelial lining of the blood vessels (Peyronnard *et al.* 1977, Nukada *et al.* 1981).

MUSCLE

In freezing cold injury to muscle, the degree of injury depends on the amount of exposure. The superficial, coldest layer shows coagulation necrosis, slow necrosis occurs in the intermediate zone and muscle atrophy alone in the deepest layer; repair is by fibrous tissue (Lewis and Moen 1952). Biopsy and ultrastructural analysis have shown vascular damage and damage to membrane structure, contractile elements and mitochondria (Kayser *et al.* 1993).

EDEMA

- Primary edema: normally cold is associated with tissue dehydration. However, the longer the limbs take to cool the more likely edema is to occur, possibly as the result of changes in tissue pH.
- Secondary edema is the result of rewarming and vasodilatation and forms within 12–25 h. Plasma passes through the cold damaged capillaries into the interstitial tissue. Associated exercise may cause swelling of the feet, so-called exercise edema (Williams *et al.* 1979).

BONES AND JOINTS

Bone cells are more sensitive to cold than overlying skin. A clear line of demarcation occurs, but the damage extends proximal to this. Epiphyseal cartilage is more sensitive than bone, and periosteal new bone formation can occur. The direct action of cold, or microvascular changes with end artery thrombosis, or both, may be the cause of the damage (Hunter *et al.* 1952, McKendry 1981).

EYE DISORDERS

The eye and optic nerve are protected from cold by the paranasal sinuses. Impairment of vision occurs only in hypothermia and not with local cooling. Conjunctivitis due to cold has been observed, along with cold injury to the cornea, in downhill skiers and ice skaters unprotected by goggles.

26.2.6 Factors concerned with frostbite

ENVIRONMENTAL FACTORS

The presence or absence of wind (wind chill) and degree of temperature are important. As the skin temperature falls from $-4.8\,°C$ to $-7.8\,°C$ the risk of frostbite increases markedly. This risk is minor above an air temperature of $-10\,°C$ irrespective of wind speed, but below $-25\,°C$ the risk of frostbite is pronounced even at low air speeds (Danielsson 1996). The type of task, shelter available, duration of cold exposure and whether the part is wet are also factors (Molnar *et al.* 1973).

PERSONAL FACTORS

The type of clothing is important, as are intercurrent disease, low morale fatigue, previous cold injury and smoking. Previous vascular disease and use of vibrating tools will predispose to frostbite (Virokannas and Anttonen 1993).

26.2.7 Frostbite and altitude

Though few statistics are available, frostbite at great altitudes appears to be commoner for comparable environmental temperatures than at lower altitudes. Both cold and altitude raise the packed cell volume and viscosity and slow the peripheral blood flow, whilst cold injury to capillary walls leads to plasma leakage and intravascular sludging. This local hemoconcentration will be increased at altitude and impaired tissue nutrition and necrosis may occur more rapidly. Dehydration, from whatever cause, will also increase viscosity of the blood, and thrombosis may be encouraged due to relative inactivity.

Maximal oxygen uptake is progressively lowered and, with it, the ability to increase heat production through exercise and probably the ability to shiver are decreased (Gautier et al. 1987). Hypoxia also blunts mental function and precautions taken against cold injury may be inadequate. Poor appetite will lower calorie intake and loss of insulating subcutaneous fat will occur (Ward 1974).

The effect of altitude hypoxia on the tone of the peripheral microvasculature is important in determining the risk of frostbite at altitude. However, studies of this effect have given conflicting results (Durand and Martineaud 1971, Durand and Raynaud 1987).

26.2.8 Prevention

Different parts of the body may be subjected to widely varying temperatures at any one time. For example, the foot may be at below freezing in deep powder snow with the environmental temperature many degrees above freezing. Temperature variation throughout the day is considerable and both feet and hands should be kept as dry as possible. Footwear has to perform many functions other than the prevention of cold injury, and there is no footwear available at present that will prevent local cold injury under all circumstances.

The most useful preventative measures are to limit the period exposed to the possibility of cold injury, keep warm, maintain hydration, and keep the part dry and free from abrasion. In many situations, particularly wartime, these measures are not always practicable.

The 'buddy' system is valuable for preventing frostbite, especially in large groups. The party is paired off and each member of a pair is responsible for keeping a close rather than a casual watch on the other. This is done at regular intervals to note early signs and is the most effective form of early detection.

26.2.9 Treatment

Both superficial and deep frostbite may be associated with hypothermia, which has priority in treatment. In any event few patients present with simple frostbite and the temperature gradient down the affected limbs ensures that, if frostbite is present in the extremities, some degree of nonfreezing cold injury will be present proximally. In addition, many patients will have been exposed to a freeze–thaw–freeze sequence with potentially disastrous results whatever the treatment; if there is skin loss the tissues will have frozen solid. Associated fractures may interfere with blood supply. At high altitude, dehydration, raised hematocrit, and exhaustion with poor heat output will enhance cold injury.

The ten principles of management are:

- 'buddy' system (see above)
- avoid further trauma
- avoid freeze–thaw–freeze
- avoid infection
- keep clean
- rewarm
- maintain morale
- delay surgery
- treat associated conditions
- avoid subsequent frostbite.

IN THE FIELD

Frostnip
The part should be warmed out of the wind by the gloved hand or by placing the affected part in the arm pit or under clothing. It should not be rubbed. Within a few minutes sensation is restored and normal working can be resumed.

Frostbite
Under no circumstance should the part be beaten, rubbed or overheated. Excessive heat from wood

fires, heat from exhaust pipes of cars or from stoves can give disastrous results and the part will become burnt or baked because of cold anesthesia (Flora 1985). Rubbing with ice or snow does not rewarm and causes tissue damage. Thawing in the field is contraindicated, as this will immediately be followed by freezing and the catastrophic freeze–thaw–freeze sequence precipitated.

Before thawing, the frozen part should be protected to avoid trauma, but during mountain rescue this may not be possible. Once thawing has started it must continue and refreezing must be avoided. It is better to walk on frozen feet to a low camp from which evacuation is possible than to start warming and have to be carried, or walk on partially rethawed feet (Mills and Rau 1983).

IN HOSPITAL

Patients should be kept in pleasant surroundings and given a high energy, high protein diet and antitetanus serum. Broad spectrum antibiotics should be given if there is any likelihood of infection; because of devitalized tissue this may take hold very rapidly, causing considerable tissue loss. The affected part should be inspected daily. Morale must be maintained.

INVESTIGATIONS .

Tissue viability should be assessed by clinical examination and Doppler ultrasound. Tissue and bone scintillography allows perfusion to be assessed more accurately than with Doppler ultrasound (Salimi 1985, Ikawa et al. 1986, Shih et al. 1988). Other research methods include: thermal clearance and measures of skin blood flow (Roussel et al. 1982), xenon-133 muscle blood flow (Sumner et al. 1971, Nugent and Rogers 1980), muscle biopsy (Kayser et al. 1993) and thermography. The temperature of the deeper tissues can be measured by means of a special probe, thus distinguishing between superficial and deep frostbite (Hamlet et al. 1977). Phosphorus-31 nuclear magnetic resonance (NMR) scans can be used daily to follow the state of the tissue with time (Kayser et al. 1993).

THAWING

Various methods of thawing have been used but, at present, rapid rewarming is the most favored, as greatest tissue preservation seems to occur and the results in deep frostbite are reasonably good (Mills and Whaley 1960, 1961, Mills 1983b, Foray and Salon 1985). Gradual rewarming gives satisfactory results with superficial frostbite but variable results with deep frostbite. Rapid rewarming should be carried out in warm water, containing an antiseptic (e.g. Phisohex) in a whirlpool bath or tub at 40–42 °C for 15–30 min until thawing is complete. The temperature should be continuously monitored. Analgesics are usually required and antitetanus prophylaxis and antibiotics should be given.

Blisters should be left or fluid aspirated. After thawing, the extremities should be elevated, and enclosed in a 'burns' bag which has the advantage of protecting from infection. Protection by cradles avoids further trauma or pressure. Treatment in whirlpool baths containing an antiseptic is continued twice daily; in this way necrotic and infected tissue is gently removed.

On discharge patients should be warned that they will be more susceptible to frostbite.

MINOR SURGERY

Blebs are left intact if the contents are sterile or, if infected, they are drained but the tissue left as a cover. However, as the fluid contains tissue breakdown products which can cause continued vasospasm, some advise repeated aspiration.

A thickened eschar, which may limit joint movement or even constrict normal tissue, can be split or removed (Mills 1983b). Debridement or amputation should be delayed for up to 90 days so that mummification is complete. Fasciotomy to release pressure due to edema in tissue compartments has been advocated (Franz et al. 1978). Fractures should be treated conservatively by closed rather than open methods. Dislocations should be reduced immediately to prevent tissue pressure.

DEHYDRATION

The majority of patients are dehydrated, so rehydration with warmed fluids is important. Decreasing blood viscosity with a plasma expander after blood has been removed from the patient may be effective. Dextran (or newer colloids) can also be given.

PAIN RELIEF

Pain in the lower limbs may be controlled with epidural bupivacaine.

Sympathectomy reduces pain and decreases edema. After this, the line of tissue demarcation is said to appear more rapidly, and become more proximal. However, increased tissue preservation does not necessarily occur and possibly the nonsympathectomized limb does better. Medical sympathectomy by means of intra-arterial reserpine and intravenous blockade by the Bier technique has been used with some success. Evidence in this area is still anecdotal and there is need for good clinical trials.

NEW DRUGS

Iloprost, a stable metabolite of prostocyclin I_2, together with warming has also been used with some success (Groechenig 1994).

Oxygen free radicals have also been postulated as being important in the mechanism of frostbite tissue damage. Pegorgotein is a product of conjugating a long-acting version of the endogenous scavenger enzyme superoxide dismutase with polyethylene glycol. It has been shown to make no difference to tissue survival in rabbit frostbite injury (Muelleman *et al.* 1997). Aloe vera cream and oral ibuprofen have been used for their local inhibitory effect on thromboxane synthetase (Marsigny 1998).

PROTECTIVE FACE CREAMS

Cold-protective ointments on the face have traditionally been used by many in Finland during the winter. Recently doubts have been cast on the effectiveness of these creams and a higher incidence of frostbite has been associated with their use. An experimental study using a skin model has confirmed that the thermal insulation was at best negligible and at worst reduced by creams (Lehmuskallio 1999, Lehmuskallio and Anttonen 1999).

OTHER THERAPIES

Hyperbaric oxygen appears to have been discarded though it may be of value in the post-thaw period.

Unless infection is present, there is no indication for antibiotics, but infection can take hold very rapidly in devitalized tissue, causing considerable tissue loss. The affected part should be inspected daily for signs of infection and, if there is any doubt, a broad spectrum antibiotic should be started.

Thrombolytic enzymes have been evaluated (Flora 1985), but there is a risk, especially if intracranial injuries are present.

Both anticoagulants and vasodilators have been used but there is disagreement about their effectiveness. Tobacco should be prohibited. Biofeedback training has been tried (Kappes and Mills 1984).

AMPUTATION

Premature surgery is a most potent cause of morbidity and surgical intervention should be minimal. When amputation is necessary (Figure 26.9) closure should, if possible, be by skin flaps rather than grafts, and sufficient deep tissue should be removed to achieve this. However, skin grafts have been successful. If infection is present a modified guillotine procedure is recommended with secondary closure. Irrigation of the infected stump is often successful. Necrosis of the stump is a hazard because of cold endarteritis and trophic changes may also occur. Active movements of the fingers after amputation must be encouraged to avoid stiffness and the development of a claw hand. Isolated ulcers of the stump may develop owing to deep-seated bone necrosis, or osteomyelitis. Marsigny (2000) reports a case in which amputation of both hands and both feet had to be carried out to save the patient's life. Deaths from frostbite have also been reported (Ward 1975, p. 340).

Patients should be mentally prepared for treatment that can last months and involve many amputations and reconstructive surgery. They may need much psychological support.

TRAUMA

The risk of frostbite in exposed subdermal tissue is considerable. Devitalized flesh freezes in 1 min at $0\,°C$ if wind speeds rise above 2 m s^{-1}. As exposed wet tissues rapidly become frozen, tissue necrosis, wound sepsis and delayed healing are common. Immediate thermal protection by suture or a wound dressing is necessary. The patient should then be evacuated. Routine wound debridement should be carried out and secondary suture performed as circumstances dictate (Butson 1975).

If hypotension or hemorrhagic hypovolemia is present the normal signs of hypothermia may be masked. The risk of hypothermia is also increased when partially perfused exposed tissue is at subzero temperatures. When warmed, these hypothermic

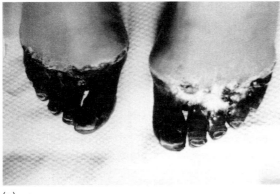

(a)

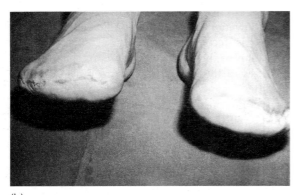

(b)

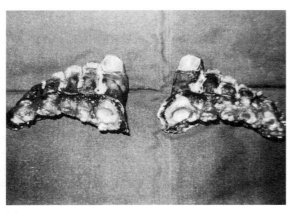

(c)

Figure 26.9 *Deep frostbite of forefeet (a) before and (b) after disarticulation at the metatarsophalangeal joints; (c) the disarticulated forefeet. (Reproduced with permission of C.J.C. Renton.)*

patients may start to bleed profusely from injured tissues. The analgesic protection afforded by cold will also be lost on rewarming (Pearn 1982).

26.2.10 After effects

Both short-term and long-term sequelae of local cold injury have been reported. Even at normal temperatures skin may crack, causing painful fissures and ulceration. Fungating and ulcerating squamous cell carcinomas of the heel have been reported 40 years after frostbite. These were well differentiated, of low malignancy and with no evidence of spread. Treatment was by local excision and skin grafting. Unstable scar tissue, chronic irritation and pressure were factors in etiology (Rossis *et al.* 1982).

Fibrosis follows cold injury to muscle. There may be persistent vasomotor paralysis, analgesia, and paresthesia; both early anhidrosis and late hyperhidrosis have been reported. Axon regeneration in both myelinated and nonmyelinated fibers, with full return of nerve function, may take 9 months or longer. A burning sensation in the feet has been noted in 61 per cent after full recovery and intractable pain may be present for up to 35 years (Suri *et al.* 1978, Kumar 1982).

There may be persistent and marked vasospasm to cold stimuli which continues long after the initial stimulus has been removed. Re-exposure to cold is likely to cause a relapse since a high incidence of nonfreezing cold injury occurs in those with a history of local cold injury.

Problems with rigidity of the feet, fallen arches and osteoporosis are reported. New bone formation usually restores the normal radiographic appearance (Francis and Golden 1985). Changes in the epiphyses of children with frostbite can lead to cartilage and bone abnormalities due either to the direct action of cold on chondrocytes or to microvascular changes with end-artery thrombosis, or both (McKendry 1981).

POLAR HANDS

This is the name given to superficial and often very painful fissures extending from the dorsal nail folds distally. It affects those who work in cold conditions, in the polar regions, in mountains or in those who have had frostbite. It may recur even after healing when the hands again get cold. Treatment is by closing the fissures with a human tissue adhesive,

N-butyl-2-cyanoacrylate, a form of superglue (Ayton 1993).

RENAL FAILURE

Following severe frostbite of both lower limbs and in nonfreezing cold injury of the feet in children, rhabdomyolysis with incipient renal failure has been recorded. Severe, long continued exercise may also be a factor in muscle breakdown (Raifman *et al.* 1978, Ross and Attwood 1984).

PAIN AND NUMBNESS

Ten of 14 patients with pain and numbness in the feet had a good response to continuous epidural blockade with recurrence after blockade had ended. Those with a limited response did well after lumbar sympathectomy (Taylor 1999).

26.3 NONFREEZING COLD INJURY

Prolonged exposure of tissue to temperatures below 15 °C, or to marginally higher temperatures in water, will result in nonfreezing cold injury, often with lasting damage to muscles and nerves.

'Trench foot' is the commonest form of this condition and is a significant cause of injury in military operations when, for combat reasons, long periods have to be spent with feet in water or in deep snow. Water both increases and accelerates the risk of injury, as does any factor that impedes circulation to the extremities, such as a cramped position, immobility, tight clothing, tight boots and tight socks. Mountaineers are at risk when powder snow gets into their boots by the ankle or is melted by foot warmth; damp socks will increase cooling.

Exactly the same sequence occurs with the hands in mittens or gloves made sodden by water or snow. However, because the hands are easier to inspect and keep dry and warm, 'trench hand' is uncommon.

Nonfreezing cold injury, though initially reversible, becomes irreversible if cooling is prolonged. It often occurs in tissues immediately proximal to frostbite.

26.3.1 Clinical features

It is convenient to classify the features into mild, moderate and severe (Table 26.2).

Table 26.2 *Clinical classification of nonfreezing cold injury*

Mild	Moderate	Severe
Erythema	Edema	'Blood' blisters
Edema	Hyperemia	Gangrene
Temporary sensory change	Blisters	Permanent disability
	Persistent sensory change	

When first seen, the affected part will be pale and sensation and movement poor. The pulse may be absent, but freezing has not occurred. If these features do not improve on warming, nonfreezing cold injury is present.

After a few hours the part becomes swollen, numb, blotchy pink-purple and heavy. After 24–36 h a vigorous hyperemia develops with a bounding pulse and burning pain proximally but not distally. Edema with 'blood blisters' appears and, if the skin is poorly perfused, it will become gangrenous and slough. At night a pain like an electric shock makes sleep difficult.

In severe cases there is a progressive reduction in sensation. The joints become stiff and muscles cease to function. To maintain balance the legs are kept apart and the sensation of movement has been likened to walking on cotton wool (Ungley *et al.* 1945). Repeated minor trauma, such as running, associated with the neuropathy encountered in nonfreezing cold injury, may result in severe blister formation with partial thickness skin loss (Reichl 1987).

Hyperemia appears to be due to vasomotor paralysis with paleness on elevation and redness when the part is dependent. This phase may last from days to weeks, as may changes in sensation. Persistent anesthesia suggests neurone degeneration with the prospect of long-term symptoms (Burr 1993).

A late feature is hyperhidrosis; this may lead to blistering, maceration of the skin and infection. After some months sensation and blood flow return to normal but gangrene may also occur. Severe changes occur more commonly and are more extensive in dependent, immobile tissues, whilst poor nutrition, fatigue, stress, injury and associated illness exacerbate the condition. Individuals who have had trench foot have a significant risk of subsequent cold injury in wet cold conditions (Ahle *et al.* 1990).

26.3.2 Pathophysiology

Because water is such a good conductor of heat, stored heat is lost rapidly and the deeper tissues, nerves, muscles, blood vessels and bones may be affected before there is any recognizable skin change. Changes in nerve conduction and sensation are common, as are changes in vessel permeability, which result in edema, blistering, and compression of peripheral vessels (Francis and Golden 1985).

There is clear clinical and pathological evidence of ischemia in frostbite, but this is less so in nonfreezing cold injury, though some evidence suggests that a cyclical reperfusion type of injury may occur (Irwin *et al.* 1994, 1997).

Initially, there is vasoconstriction followed by vasodilatation. Limb arteries exposed to nonfreezing cold injury are not normally thrombosed, but this may occur in injured limbs. Muscle damage may occur due to direct cooling, as may fat necrosis and atrophy (Friedman 1945). Infected wet gangrene may result, but dry gangrene and mummification can also occur.

After weeks or months, blood flow returns to normal but limbs may remain very sensitive to temperature changes, with cooling causing intense vasoconstriction and warming intense vasodilatation. Profuse sweating, sensory loss and loss of muscle power may persist. Amputation may have to be carried out.

26.3.3 Prevention

Some degree of nonfreezing cold injury is much commoner than normally recognized and the majority of those who spend long periods in cold conditions or at high altitude have some minor symptoms, usually paresthesiae, that persist over a few months and then disappear.

If the risk of nonfreezing cold injury is recognized then commonsense measures are normally adequate to prevent its occurrence. The feet are particularly at risk, as they remain covered throughout the day.

In World War I the British Army reduced the incidence of trench foot from 29 172 cases in 1915 to 443 cases in 1916–18 by rigorous and simple measures. In 1988 the incidence in one USA marine unit of 355 soldiers was 11 per cent. Tobacco smoking (but not

race) was associated with a higher incidence of trench foot (Tek and Mackey 1993).

Preventive measures include:

- Heavy socks should be worn in well fitting boots.
- Clothes should be loose fitting, and the trunk kept warm.
- Boots and socks should be removed twice a day. Feet should be washed, dried, massaged and warmed.
- Those at risk should sleep with dry feet. Wet socks and boots should be removed and dried.
- Keep feet out of water, snow and mud when bivouacking; elevate them if possible and keep toes and feet moving.
- Numbness and tingling are signs of trench foot; warm the feet immediately.
- Always carry a spare pair of socks (dry). They can double as gloves.

Modern mountaineering boots with a plastic outer shell and inner detachable boot of artificial fiber are better for high altitudes than leather boots.

26.3.4 Treatment

The patient should be removed from the cold; whole body warming should be started (Lahti 1982) and dehydration corrected. Rapid warming of the part has been advocated but not universally adopted. Because of pain, analgesics should be given, the patient rested and the part raised. Blisters that develop should be left unless infected, when drainage should be carried out. Sympathectomy does not appear to be very effective as hyperemia occurs naturally.

Gangrene may occur later, and this may be more widespread and affect deeper tissues more extensively than freezing cold injury. Conservative management should be adopted and surgical procedures kept to the minimum. In the long term, nonfreezing cold injury may be more serious than freezing cold injury because of the unrecognized cooling effect on deeper and more proximal structures.

26.4 AVALANCHES, CREVASSES AND BIVOUACS

Frostbite and hypothermia many occur in victims of avalanches, in those who fall into crevasses and those who bivouac.

26.4.1 Avalanches

About 80 per cent of avalanche victims survive if they remain on the surface. In those buried to a mean depth of 1.06 m, 30–40 per cent are alive after 1 h, but only 10 per cent after 4 h. The victims should therefore be located as quickly as possible (Dubas *et al.* 1991a). The main injuries caused by an avalanche are asphyxia, hypothermia, frostbite and blast injury.

The main cause of death is asphyxia. This may be due to inhalation of snow, rupture of the lungs, compression of the thorax, airway obstruction in an unconscious patient, brain damage resulting in depression of ventilation, or the air around the victim's face being used up. Gray (1987) records a woman who survived after 20 min in a wet snow avalanche where she was unable to breathe. He suggested that the 'diving reflex', which causes bradycardia, was triggered by the direct contact of the snow with the face, and this, together with the relatively rapid onset of hypothermia, was an important factor in survival.

Because there is variable permeability of air and carbon dioxide according to the type of snow, a victim completely covered by snow must not be assumed to have asphyxiated. It is because of this permeability that dogs are able to scent buried victims. People have been known to survive for several days if an air pocket is created.

The development of hypothermia is not inevitable after being buried, because of the low heat conductivity of snow and because the individual is protected from the wind. If clothing insulation is good and it remains dry the individual is likely to remain normothermic (Dubas 1980). Removal from the protection of avalanche snow will increase heat loss in a wind and the rate of cooling may be as much as 9 °C h^{-1}. If the victim is unconscious, mouth to mouth respiration or intubation and ventilation should be tried.

26.4.2 Crevasses

A fall into a crevasse can be fatal but, if not, the weight of the victim's body can leave him wedged with compression of the thorax. This is often associated with multiple injuries. The victim's body heat will melt the ice and the climber will sink deeper and deeper. The body will cool rapidly and many instances are recorded where the victim has been found dead from hypothermia.

The only way to unwedge the individual is to remove the ice with a drill or ice axe, although a thawing liquid can be very effective. A tripod leaning over the crevasse is the best method of extraction. A method of airway warming which can be carried out while the victim is still trapped has been developed (Foray and Cahen 1981, Dubas *et al.* 1991b).

26.4.3 Bivouacs and tents

Crevasses, snow caves and snow slots make good bivouacs because of the low thermal conductivity of snow. They should be out of the line of stone fall or avalanche, and provide protection from wind, fatiguing wind noise and heat loss. In both Himalayan and Alpine crevasses temperatures of 0 °C at 3 m from the surface have been recorded when the outside air temperature was well below this. A constant day and night temperature of –7 °C was noted in a snow cave at 5800 m when the outside temperature dropped to –20 °C at night; it was used for sleeping throughout the Silver Hut Expedition in the Everest region in the winter of 1960–1.

The temperature inside a tent is more liable to considerable variation. At 6000 m in the Western Cwm on the 1953 Everest Expedition, the temperature inside a tent dropped from 30 °C to 0 °C in 4 min as the tent went into the shade at dusk and rose from –5 °C to 30 °C in 2 h as the sun struck the tent at dawn (Pugh 1955b).

When bivouacking on snow, individuals must always protect themselves from the snow with which their bodies are in contact. They should huddle together and be enclosed as much as possible so that exhaled warm air heats the body. The fetal position exposes only 60 per cent of the body surface to cooling and therefore should be adopted. Occasional movement will diminish the possibility of thrombosis. Crampons should always be removed, as metal conducts heat away from the foot. If boots and socks are tight they must also be removed; a rise of up to 8 °C in skin temperature has been observed on removing a tight sock (Pugh 1950).

Attempts should be made to stay awake and not slip into sleep with subsequent body cooling and hypothermia. At extreme altitude, oxygen even at low flow rates will counter exhaustion and cold injury.

26.5   CONDITIONS ASSOCIATED WITH COLD STRESS

26.5.1   Cold allergy

The clinical features of cold allergy, described by Horton and Brown (1929) and Wanderer (1979), are malaise, shivering, aching joints and generalized urticaria. Susceptibility is transmitted as a genetic dominant (Eady *et al.* 1978). Sensitized mast cells are found in the skin; exposure to cold causes degranulation with release of mediators causing hypersensitivity both generally and locally. Wheals occur at the sites of local cooling, and even inside the mouth on taking cold drinks. Swimming may produce familial cold urticaria. It has been suggested that cases of sudden death within a few minutes of entering the water are due to undiagnosed cold urticaria (Cold hypersensitivity 1975, Ting 1984).

26.5.2   Chilblains

Chilblains are local inflammatory conditions developing as a result of exposure to cold and are more frequent in humid conditions than in a cold dry climate, probably because humidity increases local thermal conductivity. Women are more affected than men, and inadequate clothing with subsequent cooling is an important predisposing factor. Central heating reduces the incidence of chilblains (Cold hypersensitivity 1975, Lahti 1982).

26.5.3   Raynaud's disease

Raynaud's disease is a condition found most commonly in young women. On exposure to cold, intense vasospasm occurs in the small arteries and arterioles causing skin color to change from white (ischemia) to blue (cyanosis) and then to red (hyperemia), usually with pain or paresthesia. This is believed to be an exaggeration of the normal vasomotor response to cold. No organic lesion has been found.

26.5.4   Raynaud's phenomenon

In Raynaud's phenomenon arteriolar narrowing occurs secondary to a systemic disease such as sclerodema or lupus erythematosus and patients may suffer long-term sequelae including chronic nail and skin changes and muscle atrophy. In some this condition may be due to cold agglutinin disease characterized by clotting and hemolysis in tissues exposed to cold.

26.5.5   Asthma

Asthma may be exacerbated by breathing cold dry air during winter activities such as skiing, trekking or climbing, though in practice asthmatics generally do well at high altitude (see section 27.3.1).

26.5.6   Coronary and cerebral thrombosis

About 50 per cent of cold-related deaths are due to coronary and cerebral thrombosis. Most deaths from thrombosis appear to be due to a short outdoor exposure rather than long exposure in poorly heated rooms. Normal physiological responses to cold, an increase in erythrocyte count, platelet count, blood viscosity, plasma cholesterol and fibrinogen, platelet aggregation and sympathetic tone, all contribute to an increased risk of thrombosis. For a discussion of the risk of altitude for coronary disease patients see section 27.2.1.

Patients with underlying arterial disease are thought to be prone to arterial spasm in response to cold and therefore are at increased risk of death if they exercise in the cold (Caplan 1999).

A case of acute myocardial infarct at 5900 m has been recorded in a 29-year-old man. Within 6 h he was helicoptered to Kathmandu where he recovered. Eight months later he had a normal electrocardiogram. This may have been a case of coronary spasm associated with a raised hematocrit (Hutchinson and Litch 1997).

26.5.7   Acrocyanosis

Acrocyanosis occurs almost exclusively in women and is characterized by cold and blue extremities. It is worse in cold weather but is also present in warm weather. All peripheral pulses are present and the symptoms are symmetrical and constant.

26.5.8 Livedo reticularis

Livedo reticularis is characterized by persistent patchy red-blue mottling of the legs, and occasionally the arms, and is worse in cold weather. Chronic ulceration may occur. It is due to intermittent and random spasm of cutaneous arterioles with secondary dilatation of capillaries and vessels.

26.5.9 Cold hypersensitivity following trauma and cold exposure

A number of conditions with a vasospastic component follow frostbite and trauma. Pain is a prominent feature, and the limb is pale and cold and may show evidence of disuse atrophy.

27

Medical conditions at altitude

SUMMARY

As increasing numbers of people go to high altitude and at a greater age, medical advice on the advisability of these trips in those with existing medical conditions is more often being sought.

Clearly some illnesses make a trip to high altitude foolhardy, but with many conditions which are well under control it is possible to enjoy an adventure holiday of at least modest proportions. However, patients must understand their limitations and be realistic in their expectations. It is also necessary to plan ahead for eventualities, take any drugs that may be required and understand their use and actions. It is also important to be open and frank with the leader of the trek or expedition and with one's companions since any medical problem affects not only the patient but also the whole party.

27.1 INTRODUCTION

With more and more people going to altitude for adventure holidays, expeditions and skiing, doctors are more frequently being asked to counsel patients on the advisability of their trip. People are also continuing these pursuits into later life (including the authors of this book) and thus are increasingly likely to be suffering from chronic diseases which may prompt questions about their fitness for altitude. There are not many hard data on which to base one's advice to such people but such as there is will be reviewed in this chapter.

The effect of any condition that interferes with oxygen transport will be increased by altitude, so cardiac and respiratory conditions are particularly likely to interfere with performance at altitude.

Apart from the effect of altitude itself, the mountain environment poses other hazards. The great ranges are situated mostly in developing countries and in wilderness areas where gastrointestinal problems are common and medical help uncertain. Altitude holidays usually involve quite strenuous exercise and put a strain on the joints, especially knees, hips and backs. Finally, the different culture and lifestyle of such a holiday impose psychological stresses which may be too much for some people unused to the difficulties and privations of such a trip.

There is also the consideration that on an expedition or trek the aphorism 'No man is an island' applies with greater force than in normal urban life. One member's illness affects the whole team and may even imperil the safety of other members. Therefore it is ethically imperative that if people know of some pre-existing condition that might affect their performance, they should make it known, at least to the leader or medical officer if there is one.

As a general rule individuals should be as fit as possible before they leave for a holiday at altitude, though fitness is not protective for acute mountain sickness (AMS).

Those who have problems with their health should find out as much as possible about their condition before setting out. The action of specific medicines they use must be understood and an adequate supply taken, particularly when regular doses are necessary as with diabetes mellitus or asthma (Rennie and Wilson 1982).

27.2 CARDIOVASCULAR DISORDERS

27.2.1 Coronary artery disease

Coronary artery disease is one of the major causes of death in men and women aged 40 or over. If angina of effort is present at sea level it is likely that ascent to altitude will increase symptoms, especially in the first few days before acclimatization has occurred. If exercise is limited by pain and the exercise capacity reduced, it is likely that symptoms will occur at altitude and the risk of cardiac irregularities and infarction may be increased. Clearly such patients should not consider an active holiday at high altitude and even nonstrenuous trips for business or pleasure should be avoided. Visits to moderate altitude by asymptomatic patients with coronary artery disease are probably safe. Roach et al. (1995) surveyed 97 older people visiting Vail, Colorado (2500 m); 20 per cent had coronary artery disease. They reported no adverse signs or symptoms. Erdmann et al. (1998) studied a group of cardiac patients with impaired left ventricular function but no residual ischemia up to an altitude of 2500 m. They were compared with a group of controls. In both groups exercise capacity was reduced by altitude but there were no complications or sign of ischemia. Elderly subjects, even those with coronary artery disease, acclimatize well at altitude (Levine et al. 1997), so elderly people should not be debarred from going to altitude by their age but it would be prudent for patients with such disease to limit their activities during the first few days at altitude to allow time for acclimatization.

CARDIAC INFARCTION

A recent cardiac infarction is a contraindication to ascent, but after a mild infarct – providing the patient has been symptom free for several months – there is probably little risk in going to altitude (Halhuber et al. 1985). The exercise of hill walking at low altitude (470–1220 m) has been shown to be well tolerated in patients with a history of myocardial infarction and stable disease (Huonker et al. 1997). There was no evidence of coronary insufficiency on continuous electrocardiography (ECG) and echocardiography. A patient (known to the author) with auricular fibrillation and good left ventricular function has been to moderate altitudes (4000 m) with no problem.

Patients with poorly controlled heart failure due to coronary artery disease should obviously be advised not to go to high altitude. Those with well controlled disease who can manage a high level of exercise such as hill walking at low altitude may well be able to cope with the added strain of altitude.

It must be remembered that cold tends to make the platelets stickier and theoretically could increase the possibility of infarction. Cold is also thought to predispose to coronary artery spasm.

CORONARY BYPASS SURGERY AND ANGIOPLASTY

Patients who have had successful coronary bypass surgery before any myocardial infarction and have a good exercise tolerance can certainly enjoy an altitude holiday. One such patient was the subject of correspondence in the *Journal of the American Medical Association* and a subsequent editorial (Berner et al. 1988, Rennie 1989). He enjoyed a trek to 5760 m with no adverse effect. Another was a 67-year-old climber who enjoyed two Himalayan expeditions after his operation, although on the second expedition his altitude ceiling was limited to 4700 m. Ambulatory monitoring of his ECG when climbing and asleep at 4700 m did not show any evidence of ischemia. Patients can be warned that their condition may limit their performance and accept that. However, their fear, and that of their companions, centers on the risk of sudden death due to cardiac causes. Clearly there is a risk that the graft may block at any time but there is no evidence that altitude may precipitate this event. The same considerations apply to patients who have had coronary angioplasty.

RISK IN CARDIAC PATIENTS

In the wider context of cardiac disease Halhuber et al. (1985) found a negligible morbidity in 1273 'cardiac patients' who ascended to 1500–3000 m. These patients included 434 with coronary artery disease of whom 141 had had myocardial infarction. Only one of these had a new infarct at altitude.

A larger question is that of occult coronary artery disease, especially in those with known risk factors such as a family or smoking history, obesity, a sedentary lifestyle, etc. Risk factors that can be modified obviously should be, although there will be little benefit in the short term.

MEDICAL CHECK UP

Should doctors carry out 'check ups' and tests to identify any patients at risk? Is altitude a significant risk factor for sudden cardiac death? Shlim and Houston (1989) reviewed deaths amongst trekkers in Nepal. By obtaining the number of trekking permits issued, they were able to give a number for the denominator as well. Out of 148 000 trekkers in 3.5 years there were eight deaths, none of which was known to be cardiac in origin although two were of unknown cause. There were six helicopter rescues for cardiac reasons out of a total of 111 evacuations. Two were men in their late fifties with severe known cardiac disease; one was a young man with persistent ectopic beats and three had chest pain thought eventually to be noncardiac. Thus the incidence of sudden death from heart attack is low and if altitude is a risk factor for sudden cardiac death the figures suggest it is a minor one.

So should a symptomless subject be advised to have an exercise ECG test before undertaking an altitude trip? In view of the apparent low risk and the known poor sensitivity of the test (50 per cent) the answer should be no. Rennie (1989) argues that the predictive value of such a test might be 0. 001 per cent, i. e. it would identify only one patient with silent disease who would have a fatal event during a trip, for every 100 000 tests carried out! Further, the specificity of the test being only 90 per cent, the great majority of positive tests will be false positives.

So what should the general practitioner do when asked for advice from someone proposing to go on an adventure holiday to altitude?

- Take a history including coronary disease risk factors, advise on these and encourage the patient to get fit.
- Check the weight and blood pressure; in the absence of any evidence of disease, no further tests are indicated.

- Point out that 'getting away from it all' also involves getting away from easy access to medical treatment and that people going on such holidays must take a greater responsibility for their own health than they would on a standard package holiday.

27.2.2 Systemic hypertension

Acute hypoxia has a variable effect on blood pressure in hypertensive subjects but there is a tendency to elevation both at rest and at exercise at 3460 m (Savonitto et al. 1992). However, Halhuber et al. (1985) found that mild hypertensives who ascended and lived at up to 3000 m had few symptoms and both systolic and diastolic pressures fell. No cases of cerebrovascular accident or cardiac failure were noted in 935 patients. This improvement was continued for 4–8 months after returning to lower levels. Those with well controlled hypertension may go to altitude. In two treated hypertensives, a 6-week stay at altitudes of 3500–5000 m produced little change in either systolic or diastolic pressure. Subjects with borderline hypertension may well have higher pressures on going to altitude but at present there is no evidence that this means greater risk of vascular incidents (though no evidence of risk does not mean evidence of no risk).

27.2.3 Other cardiac conditions

Patients who have had valve replacements should, in general, not take hard physical exercise. Poor lung function is more often associated with mitral than aortic valve replacement. The risks of going to moderate altitude, provided anticoagulants are taken and hard exercise avoided, are probably acceptable.

After repair of a ventricular septal defect, residual pulmonary hypertension is not uncommon and patients who have had a correction of Fallot's tetralogy may often have some residual strain on the right ventricle due to obstruction of the pulmonary outflow tract. Ascent to altitude in both will increase pulmonary artery pressure and may put the individual at risk of high altitude pulmonary edema (HAPE).

Following operation for coarctation of the aorta some residual cerebral hypertension may be present and in theory cerebral edema may be more common.

Providing cardiac pressures are normal, the ascent to altitude following repair of patent ductus arteriosus and atrial septal defect is probably acceptable.

27.3 LUNG DISEASE

27.3.1 Asthma

Asthma is very common and sufferers are often young and active so the question of the advisability of an asthmatic individual undertaking an altitude trip is a common one. An attack of asthma may be provoked by cold air and exercise but in fact many asthmatic patients have less trouble at altitude than at home, possibly because the freedom from inhaled allergens is of greater importance than the effect of hyperventilation in cold air. This impression is born out by a recent study by an Italian team working at the Pyramid laboratory at Lobuje (5050 m) in Nepal. They found that bronchial responsiveness in a group of asthmatics was reduced at altitude compared with sea level (Allegra *et al.* 1995). Also the increased sympathetic and adrenocortical activity will counter the bronchoconstriction of asthma in the first few days at altitude. The importance of taking a sufficient supply of medication and using it regularly must be stressed. There is no evidence that asthmatics are at greater risk of AMS than nonasthmatics, though it must be presumed that poorly controlled patients must be at some risk. Acetazolamide helps prevent AMS in asthmatic patients (Mirrakhimov *et al.* 1993).

27.3.2 Chronic obstructive lung disease

Chronic obstructive lung disease includes chronic bronchitis and emphysema. Ventilatory capacity is reduced and oxygen uptake impaired. If patients are short of breath on exercise at sea level they will certainly be worse at altitude. Even mild cases will find their performance markedly diminished at altitude. The reserve capacity of the lung may be further diminished by infection, and antibiotics should be started at the first sign of an infective exacerbation. Such patients should probably be advised to select holidays which avoid high altitude. However, at modest altitude patients with mild disease may have no trouble. Roach *et al.* (1995) found that there were no adverse signs or symptoms in their group of older subjects, 9 per cent of whom had pulmonary disease.

27.3.3 Interstitial lung disease

Interstitial lung disease includes pulmonary fibrosis from whatever cause, sarcoidosis, etc. In these conditions there is both restriction of the lung and interference with gas exchange. Altitude has a marked effect on this aspect of lung function and patients will find themselves much more short of breath. Cystic fibrosis patients with bronchiectasis have problems of both airways obstruction and gas exchange. One paper describes two cases where an altitude holiday appeared to tip the patients into cor pulmonale (Speechley-Dick *et al.* 1992). In all but the mildest cases they should be advised against going to altitude.

Cystic fibrosis patients with stable disease who are proposing to go to altitude or indeed to fly in commercial aircraft can be tested in the laboratory by breathing a hypoxic gas mixture (15 per cent oxygen in nitrogen) for 10 min. The arterial oxygen saturation measured by a pulse oximeter gives a good indication of how they will fare at altitude (Oades *et al.* 1994). Other patients with stable lung disease might also benefit from the test.

27.3.4 High altitude pulmonary edema (HAPE)

A previous attack of HAPE indicates susceptibility and the need for caution on future ascents. However, many individuals have made subsequent ascents without trouble, possibly because their one attack was partly due to a respiratory infection. The prophylactic use of acetazolamide should be discussed and nifedipine should be included in the first aid kit.

27.4 BLOOD DISORDERS

27.4.1 Anemia

Anemia, when oxygen carrying capacity is reduced, should be treated prior to ascent. Premenopausal women may have inadequate iron stores (Richalet *et al.* 1994) and might benefit from iron therapy before or during an excursion to altitude.

27.4.2 Patients on anticoagulants

Patients with recurrent clotting or bleeding problems may be taking unnecessary risks, but for those on anticoagulants, if well controlled, there is no increased risk from altitude *per se* but their being remote from medical help will be a risk.

27.4.3 Sickle cell trait

Individuals with sickle cell trait may not be aware of the problem. Reports in the literature indicate that there is a 20–30 per cent risk that altitude travel over 2000 m may precipitate a crisis in patients with either homozygous sickle cell disease (Hb SS), sickle cell/hemoglobin C disease (Hb SC) or sickle cell trait (Hb AS) (Adzaku *et al.* 1993). These crises are either vaso-occlusive (mainly in Hb SS patients) or abdominal, splenic infarcts (mainly in Hb SC patients).

Two cases of white men with splenic crisis caused by sickle cell trait have been reported at 2750 m. Both were treated conservatively with satisfactory results (Tierman 1999).

27.5 DIABETES MELLITUS

Glucose tolerance is normal at altitude when energy expenditure and food intake balance one another. Exercise at altitude may improve sugar uptake and for well controlled diabetics there appears to be no contraindication to mountaineering.

Those taking insulin should appreciate not only the considerable energy output that may be demanded over a few days, up to 25 MJ (6000 kcal) or more per day, but also the variation from day to day and within the day. During severe exercise they may need less insulin than on rest days because of increased glucose uptake by muscle metabolism. During rest days at altitude, insulin requirement will be similar to that at sea level. Because of these great variations diabetics should be encouraged to use quick acting insulin, use three to four injections each day and monitor the blood sugar closely.

Ready access to glucose in the form of sugar or chocolate is necessary and for emergencies intravenous glucose should be available, as hypoglycemia can be produced very rapidly by severe activity.

Insulin freezes at 0 °C, so it should be kept warm close to the body. Frozen insulin may be thawed out without loss of potency, but care should be taken to prevent breakage and spare ampoules carried. Accidents to diabetics may be complicated by diabetic coma.

The companions of diabetic trekkers or mountaineers should be made aware of the problems that diabetics face, should be able to recognize hypoglycemia and diabetic coma and know what to do in emergencies. Hypothermia can produce hypoglycemia and exhausted diabetic mountaineers are at considerable risk. Extra easily assimilated carbohydrates must be taken for bivouacs. Clearly insulin dependent diabetes does present patients, their companions and trip leaders with problems. Many will consider the risks of serious mountaineering at altitude to be unjustifiable. However, many diabetics on well controlled insulin treatment have made successful, rather more modest trips to altitude. It is essential to discuss the situation with the expedition or trek leader and doctor (if there is one) at an early stage in planning.

27.6 GASTROINTESTINAL DISORDERS

Intestinal colic and diarrhea are frequently encountered in mountainous areas but altitude *per se* is not a factor. Simple traveler's diarrhea can be treated by loperamide unless there is evidence of parasitic infection when specific medicine should be given.

The incidence of peptic ulcer appears to be less at altitude (Singh *et al.* 1977). However, Wu (2000), reviewing experience in over 5000 road workers in Tibet, reported that gastrointestinal bleeding 10–70 days after arrival at altitude was not uncommon, with an incidence of 1–2 per cent.

Clearly, patients with known peptic ulcer should be well controlled prior to the expedition as complications in the field can be fatal. Drugs such as nonsteroidal anti-inflammatory agents taken because of joint problems or aspirin for headache may cause gastric hemorrhage, which should be considered as a cause of unexpected weakness. These drugs should not be taken on an empty stomach.

Those with inflammatory disorders of the bowel, such as Crohn's disease or ulcerative colitis in an active phase, should not go on expeditions. An expedition, which lasts weeks or months, should be considered very carefully for an individual in the quiescent phase and medication and diet planned to ensure that the condition gets no worse. Adequate treatment for an acute exacerbation must be available and evacuation of the patient should be easy.

Hemorrhoids, perianal hematoma and fissure-in-ano are often considered trivial conditions except by sufferers. They are not, and pre-expedition treatment must be undertaken. On an expedition a prolapsed pile should be replaced as soon as possible; perianal hematoma is classically a self-limiting condition lasting 5 days before resolution, but the clot may be evacuated under local anaesthetic. Acute fissure-in-ano may be exquisitely painful. Anesthetic ointment should always be available and, if necessary, a fissurotomy may be carried out under local anesthetic. Any recurrent perineal or ischiorectal abscess must be dealt with prior to an expedition, as must fistulae and pruritus ani. Abscesses can be drained in the field, but even when an adequate anesthetic is available this is painful postoperatively.

Patients with hernias must have these repaired prior to an expedition. Any hernias occurring in the field should be reduced and kept reduced by a home-made truss. Irreducible and strangulated hernias can be and have been operated on under local anesthetic, and the simplest operation consistent with the operator's skill and the patient's condition should be carried out.

Patients with recurrent appendicitis should consider an appendectomy prior to an expedition. In the past prophylactic appendectomy has been advised before very long periods away from good medical cover, but this is not necessary. If appendicitis occurs during an expedition it should be treated conservatively with antibiotics, intravenous fluids and nothing by mouth. Often it resolves; if an abscess or appendix mass forms this may either resolve or it will point on the abdominal wall or rectum and can be drained. Ruptured appendix and peritonitis should be drained under local anesthetic.

27.7 ORTHOPEDIC CONDITIONS

Those with arthritis, particularly of the joints of the lower limb, should carefully consider the degree and

amount of exercise that has to be taken on a mountain trek. Nonsteroidal anti-inflammatory drugs can be very beneficial and should be started early rather than being heroic about the pain. Treatment of painful joints, particularly of the hip, whether by replacement prosthesis, arthrodesis or some other method, may make a short trek possible. One member of the successful Everest 1953 expedition who climbed to 8500 m had a fixed flexed elbow, the result of an accident as a child.

27.8 ENT CONDITIONS AND DENTAL PROBLEMS

Nasal polyps or a deflected nasal septum, which interferes with breathing, should be treated prior to ascent. Patients with perennial rhinitis and sinusitis should ensure supplies of their usual medication.

Dental problems theoretically are not made worse by altitude but in practice dental abscesses seem to be quite common. Anyone planning a holiday or expedition out of range of dental help on the mountains or anywhere else, is well advised to have a thorough dental check up and any suspect teeth dealt with before setting out.

A case of HAPE following root canal infection has been reported. This was successfully treated by descent, antibiotics and appropriate surgery (Finsterer 1999).

27.9 OBESITY

Obesity has been reported as being a risk factor for AMS (Chapter 18) and the overweight will have an increased oxygen uptake for a given task. At night obese individuals may suffer from a greater fall in arterial P_{O_2} as the weight of the abdomen interferes with normal lung expansion. The repeated episodes of hypoxemia lead to increased pulmonary hypertension. In addition, they are more likely to have sleep disorders with, in particular, obstructive sleep apnea during which the arterial P_{O_2} can fall precipitously. In residents at altitude this may cause an undue increase in red blood cells and may be implicated as a cause of chronic mountain sickness (Chapter 21).

27.10 NEUROLOGICAL PROBLEMS

27.10.1 Headache

Headaches are common on ascent to altitude, probably because of mild cerebral edema. These are features of AMS and resolve spontaneously in a few days. There is anecdotal evidence that altitude tends to trigger migraine attacks which can be severe. One sufferer had an attack of transient nominal aphasia at 5500 m. A history of migraine is a risk factor for AMS (Chapter 18).

27.10.2 Epilepsy

There is no evidence that epileptics are worse off or that fits are more frequent at altitude. However, the consequences of an epileptic attack need to be considered both on affected individuals and on their companions. Understanding this, it is probably reasonable for patients with well controlled epilepsy, who have not had a fit for 6 months, to go on a trek but not to undertake rock or ice climbing. Some antiepileptic preparations may affect breathing adversely during sleep, and others in high doses may affect coordination.

27.10.3 Sleep

Nightmares and vivid dreams are not unusual at altitude and sleep may be very disturbed. Those who take drugs at sea level to induce sleep should remember that these often depress respiration and can lead to severe transient hypoxia. In any event, sleep at altitude is usually lighter and often less refreshing than at sea level (Chapter 13).

27.11 MENTAL OUTLOOK

Mountaineering is a potentially dangerous sport with an appreciable mortality. It requires time and patience to master all the skills necessary to move safely in mountain country, which is no place for the danger-mystic with or without religious overtones.

Mental agility and emotional stability are important and the gregarious extrovert who can only be effective with constant activity and an impressionable audience is not so likely to function effectively as the more self-sufficient. Those who are obliged to live harmoniously in close proximity for long periods should be stable, loyal and have both a social and intellectual tolerance for their companions. Above all, a sense of humor and the ability to control and sublimate hostile and aggressive impulses are of great importance.

Considerable attention has been paid to the possible effects of emotional deprivation, with reference to sexual abstinence, in isolated single-sex communities. Most agree that sexual deprivation is usually of minor significance and, as a subject of conversation, ranks rather lower than food, drink or the task in hand. At high altitude reduction in libido has been reported in some lowlanders. High altitude residents do not appear to be affected. Instructions on the frequency of sexual intercourse are included in a work on traditional Tibetan medicine: 'During winter one can indulge in intercourse twice or thrice daily, since sperm increases in winter. In the autumn and spring there must be an interval of two days, and during the summer an interval of 15 days. Excessive intercourse affects the five sense organs' (Rinpoche 1973, pp. 54–5). Elderly, enfeebled Tibetans drank the urine of young boys to increase their sexual vigor (MacDonald 1929, p. 184).

For the majority of people, venturing into the high mountains is a wonderful experience even if, at times, the conditions are harsh and uncomfortable. Most have graduated via family trips into the hills, short camping trips near home, hill walking, etc. , but some suddenly get the idea that they want to embark on some big trek or expedition with no previous experience and have quite unrealistic ideas of their own performance. Sometimes all works out well and they adapt to what is a very different lifestyle with no problem, but others are clearly psychologically quite unsuited to it and become psychiatric casualties, to the distress of themselves and their companions.

28

Women, children and elderly people at altitude

SUMMARY

Women respond to altitude in very much the same way as men. They acclimatize in a similar way and are as likely to get acute mountain sickness (AMS). Their exercise performance is similarly affected by altitude. Recent studies into the effect of the menstrual cycle have failed to find significant differences in performance or susceptibility to AMS in different phases of the cycle. Women seem to have an advantage over men in that they lose less weight at altitude, probably because they suffer less loss of appetite. The risk of altitude in pregnancy is not known but in the present state of knowledge women in the early stages of pregnancy are advised not to go beyond moderate altitudes. This is because of the possible risk of hypoxia on organogenesis in the fetus and likely discomfort for the mother in later pregnancy. Oral contraceptives (the pill) are widely used for both contraception and for menstrual regulation by women at altitude. Although there is the theoretical risk that altitude and increased hematocrit may lead to thrombosis, there is no direct evidence that this is the case.

Children are at risk at altitude if they are too young to be able to voice their symptoms of AMS which then may not be diagnosed promptly. Any child who has recently ascended to altitude and becomes unwell must be assumed to be suffering from AMS unless there are clear signs of an alternative diagnosis. Children are as likely to get AMS, high altitude pulmonary edema (HAPE) and high altitude cerebral edema (HACE) as adults are. The management of all forms of AMS is similar to that in adults with appropriate adjustment of dosage of drugs. Children are more at risk of hypothermia and cold injury because of their larger surface to weight ratio and especially if they are being carried and not exercising. Infants are at risk of subacute mountain sickness if they remain at altitude for months. The justification for taking young children to altitude is questionable and is discussed.

Increasing numbers of elderly people are going on holidays to the mountains. If they are otherwise fit, age is no bar to enjoying such holidays. Their exercise capacity will be less than that of younger mountaineers and their goals must be adjusted accordingly. With age comes the likelihood of various medical conditions, especially heart and lung disease, which may interfere with performance at altitude. However, the risk from occult disease, specifically asymptomatic coronary artery disease, is very small. Elderly are no more likely to get AMS than young people, indeed in practice they seem to suffer less, perhaps because they are likely to gain altitude more slowly or they may be less susceptible.

28.1 INTRODUCTION

Until recently, studies of the effect of altitude on humans have used fit young men as their subjects. There have been few studies addressing the question of the effect of altitude specifically on women, children or elderly people. In the last few years this deficiency has been repaired to some extent in the case of women but we have very few hard data on children or elderly people. Such studies as have been published are reviewed in this chapter but in trying to provide answers to frequently asked questions we still have to rely often on anecdote or extrapolation from inadequate data. This chapter deals mainly with lowland women, children and elderly people going to altitude, highland populations being the subject of Chapter 17.

28.2 WOMEN

28.2.1 Introduction

In 1970 the Japanese climber Setuko Wanatabe was the first woman to climb Everest; since then, women of many nationalities have also made the ascent, some without the use of supplementary oxygen. Women have climbed other 8000 m peaks including K2 and Kangchenjunga without added oxygen, and it will probably not be long before someone claims the record of the first woman to climb all 14 8000-m peaks. By the end of 1999 there were 54 ascents of Everest by women (Unsworth, 2000).

Clearly women can acclimatize and perform at altitude as well as most men, even if there are fewer women in the elite category. In this section the differences in physiology between women and men will be discussed though, as women's achievements demonstrate, similarities are probably greater than differences.

28.2.2 Acclimatization

Women acclimatize in a similar way to men. In respect of respiratory acclimatization their increase in ventilation in response to chronic hypoxia was documented as long ago as 1911 by Mabel FitzGerald (FitzGerald 1913). She measured the alveolar P_{CO_2} of acclimatized men and women over a range of altitudes and showed that the PA_{CO_2} is about 2 mm Hg less in women than in men. Their P_{O_2} is correspondingly slightly higher. Others, including Hannon (1978), have confirmed this finding and Barry et al. (1995) found, using arterialized capillary blood, that P_{CO_2} fell more in women than in men during acclimatization, as did their bicarbonate. Women's greater ventilation at all altitudes is assumed to be due to the stimulatory effect of sex hormones and disappears after the menopause.

Women increase their hemoglobin concentration, hematocrit and red cell mass in the same way as men in general, though some women fail to do so because their iron stores are low as a consequence of their menstrual blood loss. Richalet et al. (1994) reported two such cases in their study on Samaja in Bolivia and documented their low iron stores. It was also shown that their erythropoietin response was good. In an early study on Pikes Peak (4300 m) in Colorado (Hannon et al. 1966) it was shown that women on iron supplements had rises in hemoglobin concentration similar to men whereas women not taking iron had a slower increase in hemoglobin concentration.

If susceptibility to AMS is seen as slow acclimatization then, again, there is probably no significant difference between men and women.

28.2.3 Performance and the menstrual cycle

Beidleman and colleagues (1999) tested the possibility that the effect of hormones in the midluteal phase of the menstrual cycle on exercise ventilation might improve oxygen transport especially at altitude. They undertook a chamber study at sea level and 4300 m equivalent in eight female subjects, testing them in their early follicular and midluteal phases. They found that there was no difference between the phases for peak and submaximal exercise ventilation. Sa_{O_2} was 3 per cent higher at altitude during the midluteal phase but $\dot{V}_{O_2 max}$ and time to exhaustion were no different between phases at sea level or altitude.

28.2.4 Weight loss

Women seem better able to maintain their weight on going to altitude than men do. In a group of women studied on Pikes Peak (4300 m) Hannon et al. (1976)

found that they lost only 1.49 per cent of their body weight compared with 4.86 per cent in a group of men. This was attributed to the fact that the women seemed to regain their appetites sooner than the men did. Collier *et al.* (1997b) also found less weight loss in a group of women trekkers to Everest Base Camp (5340 m). The women had no significant weight loss during their stay at this altitude, while the men lost an average of 0.11 kg m^{-2} day^{-1}. In seven men who climbed to altitudes of 7100–8848 m the weight loss averaged 0.15 kg m^{-2} day^{-1} whereas the one woman who climbed to above 8000 m lost no weight.

28.2.5 Catecholamines and carbohydrate metabolism

In a 12-day study on Pikes Peak (4200 m) Mazzeo *et al.* (1998) found no difference in catecholamine response between men and women or between the follicular and luteal phases of the menstrual cycle. However, for a given norepinephrine urinary excretion the heart rate and blood pressure response were lower in the follicular than in the luteal phase.

As mentioned in section 15.8, sensitivity to insulin appears to be increased at altitude in men. Braun *et al.* (1998) found that after 9 days at altitude (4300 m) the blood glucose response to a standard meal was reduced in women, possibly due to increased stimulation of peripheral glucose uptake or suppression of hepatic glucose production. They found that the glucose response was lower in the estrogen phase than in the estrogen plus progesterone phase of the menstrual cycle.

In a recent study Mawson *et al.* (2000) found that the total energy requirement of women at 4300 m was 6 per cent above sea level values. Although there was a transient rise in basal metabolic rate (BMR) this did not explain all the increase. Unlike men, blood glucose utilization rates in young women after 10 days at 4300 m were lower at rest and no different during submaximal exercise from those observed at sea level. There was no correlation with circulating estrogens or progesterone (Braun *et al.* 2000).

28.2.6 Pregnancy and oral contraceptives

The risk to a pregnancy of going to altitude is not known with confidence, but it seems wise to advise pregnant women against ascent to more than a modest altitude. In the early months of pregnancy, during organogenesis, there is the risk that hypoxia might result in fetal abnormalities. Later in pregnancy the increased bulk of the uterus and raised diaphragm will make for discomfort in the mother and interfere with her breathing.

There are no data on the risk of using oral contraceptives at altitude but it is well known that they increase the risk of thrombosis at sea level. However, the risk is less in current formulations and is even smaller in nonsmokers. The increased hematocrit at altitude and dehydration, should it occur, may increase this risk. After some weeks at altitude vascular episodes, some thrombotic in nature, have been reported, though not in women. A recent survey (Miller 1999) of 926 trekkers on the Everest Base Camp route found that of 316 women, 30 per cent were using an oral contraceptive, mostly for control of menstruation. A significant number did report irregularities of menstruation especially if pills were not taken regularly, but there were no medical complications. However, though reassuring, the numbers were too small to draw firm conclusions regarding safety. A discussion of this question can be found in the *International Society of Mountain Medicine Newsletter* (ISMM 1998). In earlier editions we advised against the use of the pill. Clearly women are using it, and the advice now should be that if used it should be taken regularly.

28.2.7 Women and cold

Cold injury, hypothermia, frostbite and immersion injury are seldom reported in women at altitude. A factor may be the relatively thicker layer of subcutaneous fat found in women. It is also possible that women are more meticulous in their preparation for cold conditions and so avoid cold injury through negligence.

28.3 CHILDREN

28.3.1 Introduction

The increased accessibility of the high altitude regions of the world to adults means that more children are now being taken on adventure holidays to these places. Even infants have been carried over 6000 m peaks in Nepal (Pollard *et al.* 1998). Are these children at risk from the effects of altitude? What advice should a doctor give to parents considering taking children to altitude?

28.3.2 Diagnosis of AMS in children

In older children, the diagnosis of AMS can be made on symptoms as in adults. The diagnostic problems are much the same. Those feeling cold, miserable and depressed may exaggerate while those (usually boys in a group) who consider it 'sissy' to admit to symptoms will minimize them. However, in younger children who cannot articulate their feelings the problems are worse. In them AMS symptoms cannot be distinguished from other causes of ill health. In the setting of a recent increase in altitude, the only safe course is to assume a young child's fractiousness is due to AMS unless there are signs clearly pointing to some other cause. Yaron *et al.* (1998) have proposed a 'fussiness score' in such preverbal children, analogous to the Lake Louise score for AMS (section 18.8). They studied 23 children aged 3–36 months in Colorado at Denver (1609 m), Fort Collins (1615 m) and Keystone Summit Lodge (3488 m), taking 4 days to reach there. There were 45 accompanying adults and 20 per cent of these had AMS at Keystone. Using their score, 21 per cent of the infants were diagnosed as having AMS. Fussiness is scored on a scale of 0 to 6 for both amount and intensity. This equates to the headache symptom. Other symptoms are then scored 0 to 3 for, 'How well has your child eaten?', 'How playful is your child today?' and 'How has the child napped today?'.

28.3.3 Incidence of AMS in children

There have been a few surveys of children at altitude. Wu (1994b) studied adults and children as they travelled the Qinghai–Tibet highway to Lhasa. He surveyed 5355 adults and 464 children at the overnight stop, Tuo-Tuo (4550 m). These people were lowland Han Chinese. The diagnosis was made on symptoms and on the response to oxygen breathing. HAPE was also diagnosed by chest radiograph. The incidences for AMS and HAPE respectively were 38.2 per cent and 1.27 per cent in adults and 34.1 per cent and 1.51 per cent in children. In

Colorado Theis *et al.* (1993) found an incidence of AMS of 28 per cent at an altitude of 2835 m for children aged 9–14 years, but there was no comparable figure for adults. This may seem rather high for this altitude but a control group at sea level had a 20 per cent incidence of these symptoms, so some may have been due to the travel itself. From these studies (including that of Yaron *et al.* (1998) above) it would seem that children probably have about the same susceptibility to AMS and HAPE as adults. One paper also suggests that, as in adults, respiratory infection predisposes to HAPE in children (Durmowicz *et al.* 1997).

28.3.4 Management of AMS in children

The management of AMS in children is the same as in adults (section 18.7). The crucial first step is to have a high index of suspicion in the setting of a recent gain in altitude. The essential step is to get the child down to a lower altitude. Only in the mildest cases is a 'wait and see' policy justified. If there is any suspicion of AMS further ascent is out of the question. There have been no formal trials of any drugs in children in this setting but it is assumed that the same medication can be used in children as in adults. The dosage suggested for drugs used in AMS is shown in Table 28.1.

The management of HAPE and HACE is similar to that in adults (Chapters 19 and 20). There is a report of the successful use of the Gamow bag in a 3.5-year-old child with severe AMS (Taber 1994).

28.3.5 Infants at altitude

There are some special considerations that apply to infants at altitude relating to the immaturity of their respiratory control mechanisms and the fact that their pulmonary arteries are undergoing involution of the thick muscular layers at this time.

In the neonate, hypoxia has a depressant effect on ventilation. Normally this reverses to the adult pattern of stimulation in the first few weeks of life, but a study by Parkins *et al.* (1998) found that even at 3 months infants responded to 15 per cent oxygen breathing by frequent periods of isolated and periodic apnea. The mean saturation on 15 per cent oxygen was 92 per cent in these infants. The responses were very variable, but some infants had

Table 28.1 *Dosage for drugs used in children for AMS, HAPE and HACE*

Drug	Dose	Route
Paracetamol	12 mg kg^{-1} dose 6 hourly	Oral
Dexamethasone	0.15 mg kg^{-1} dose 4 hourly	Oral or i.v.
Acetazolamide	5 mg kg^{-1} 8–12 hourly, max 350 mg	Oral
Nifedipine	0.5 mg kg^{-1} dose 8 hourly, max 20 mg for caps, 40 mg for tabs	Oral

Aspirin should be avoided because of the slight risk of Reye's syndrome.
Source: after Pollard and Murdoch (1997).

saturations which fell to less than 80 per cent for up to a minute (at which time the intervention was stopped). This response must be part of the mechanism of infantile subacute mountain sickness (Sui *et al.* 1988) described in Chapter 22.

The question of risk of sudden infant death syndrome (SIDS) at altitude has been addressed in one study. It might be thought that altitude could be an added risk factor for SIDS. Kohlendorfer *et al.* (1998) carried out a case control study in Austria of SIDS deaths. They found that higher altitude districts did have higher rates of SIDS but these districts also had higher rates for the practice of placing infants in the prone position for sleep. This effect largely accounted for the difference in rate of SIDS. The possibility that altitude has some risk for SIDS cannot be ruled out, especially at altitudes higher than in this study.

28.3.6 Children, cold and heat

Children are not only smaller than adults but have a larger surface to weight ratio, so as a result cool faster in cold and heat up more quickly in hot conditions (Kennedy 1995). Thermal balance is less efficient in children, and during exercise they generate more metabolic heat for a unit mass than adults, have lower cardiac output and gain heat more rapidly from the environment. They also acclimatize to heat more slowly in hot conditions. In addition to their larger surface to mass ratio, they have less subcutaneous fat and may have an underdeveloped shivering mechanism. For all these reasons, they are at greater risk than adults of hypothermia in a cold environment and of overheating in hot environments.

In cold or wet conditions a windproof and water-proof garment is essential, and particular attention should be paid to the head from which proportionally more heat is lost than in an adult. It should also be remembered that a child who is being carried is not generating heat in the way the adult carrier is and so needs more clothing.

Overheating can occur when on a glacier or snowfield in sunny conditions because of direct and reflected heat. Eyes must be protected by goggles and the exposed skin by sunblock cream. Adequate fluid must be given, especially in hot conditions, to prevent dehydration (Pollard and Murdoch 1997).

28.3.7 Conclusions

Although children are at no greater risk of AMS than adults at the same altitude, the fact that young children have difficulty in articulating their symptoms means that diagnosis is more difficult and may be delayed. The fact that in most cases an altitude holiday is also a holiday in a part of the world where medical help is far away and gastrointestinal infections and other diseases are common must be borne in mind. Also it is true that children with these problems can progress from being perfectly healthy to being seriously ill at an alarming rate. Finally, it is questionable if young children really appreciate the mountain environment in the way adults do, so the rewards of such a holiday, as compared with a more conventional bucket and spade or low altitude country holiday, are less. On the other hand family travel is undoubtedly a valuable experience. On balance we would concur with Pollard *et al.* (1998) in a cautious approach in advising families considering high altitude trips. They suggest that, with children under 2 years of age, parties should not sleep at over

2000 m and no higher than 3000 m for children of 2–10 years. The latter may be too conservative since children of say 6–10 years who can express their symptoms could well enjoy higher altitudes with probably little more risk than adults.

28.4 ELDERLY PEOPLE

28.4.1 Introduction

The increased numbers of people going to high altitude, mainly for recreation, include a large proportion of elderly people. Many retired men and women have both the money and time to enjoy treks to the great ranges, to ski and to attend conferences. Doctors are often asked questions about risks involved. In Chapter 27 specific pre-existing conditions are considered which are more frequently encountered in elderly patients. In this section we consider the apparently fit elderly person at altitude.

The effects of altitude on cardiovascular and pulmonary problems have been studied in elderly people, and a survey of over 1900 visitors to Keystone, Colorado (2783 m), revealed that 48 per cent were aged 40–60 years and 15 per cent were over 60. Approximately 10 per cent of trekkers in Nepal were 50 years of age or older (Hultgren 1992) and a few mountaineers of this age have climbed Everest using supplementary oxygen (Gillman 1993).

28.4.2 Performance

All bodily functions deteriorate with age and this includes the maximum oxygen uptake both at sea level and at altitude (Pugh *et al.* 1964). However, the effect of age on $V_{O_2 max}$ is very variable (Dill *et al.* 1964). West *et al.* (1983c) reported the results of measurements of $V_{O_2 max}$ on two subjects. There was only a moderate deterioration in performance over a 20-year period (aged 31–51 years). Ability to go to altitude depends more on an individual's degree of fitness than on age. Fit men of 75 years who normally live at sea level have spent months at 5000 m without difficulty and a peak of 6000 m has been climbed by an 80-year-old mountaineer. However, their ability to carry loads is reduced. No one should be discouraged from going to altitude on grounds of age alone,

but rapid ascent and undue exertion will place more strain on those in the older age group than on those who are younger. However, their greater experience will enable them to pace themselves so that given time they can often achieve worthwhile objectives. Levine *et al.* (1997) studied 20 subjects with a mean age of 68 years attending a veterans' reunion at a resort at 2500 m. They found the expected decrease in Pa_{O_2}, Sa_{O_2} and $V_{O_2 max}$ and increase in pulmonary artery pressure of 43 per cent associated with sympathetic activation. The induction of a 1 mm depression of the S-T segment occurred at a lower exercise rate at altitude but this returned to sea level values after 5 days at altitude. They conclude that elderly men acclimatize well at this altitude and retain sea level performance after 5 days.

28.4.3 Age and AMS

It might be assumed that older people would be more prone to AMS, but there is no evidence that this is the case. Anecdotal evidence suggests that older mountaineers do better than the young but this may be because they do not climb so fast and therefore are at lower risk of AMS. Also there could be selection bias – poor acclimatizers do not go back to the mountains later in life. Surveys such as that by Kayser (1991) find no significant age effect on the incidence of AMS. Although it is true that older people have more pre-existing disease, especially heart and lung disease, it seems that this does not increase the risk of AMS (Roach *et al.* 1995); nor does the fact that with age the sensitivity of the ventilatory response to carbon dioxide and to hypoxia decline (Kronenberg and Drage 1973, Poulin *et al.* 1993).

28.4.4 Conclusions and advice

The evidence that we have indicates that age alone is no bar to a fit person going to altitude. Exercise capacity is reduced in elderly people as in young people, and the itinerary planned accordingly, but the risk of AMS is no greater. However, 'age never comes alone' and the presence of pre-existing conditions which might reduce one's enjoyment of a holiday at best and be life threatening at worst should give pause for thought. Some of these conditions are considered in Chapter 27. However, anyone who can manage a full day walking on hills at low altitude without undue strain is likely to be able to enjoy a standard Himalayan trek. In a situation of having to go rapidly to altitude, for instance having to fly into an airport at high altitude, it is probably more important for elderly people than for young people that they should give themselves 2–3 days to acclimatize before undertaking any strenuous activity (Levine et al. 1997).

29

Commercial activities at altitude

SUMMARY

Increasingly, large numbers of people are commuting to high altitude for commercial and scientific activities. Several mines are now situated at altitudes of 4000–6000 m. In some cases, the miners live at sea level and are bussed up to the mine where they spend 7 days, then return to their families at sea level for a further 7 days, and the cycle is repeated indefinitely. This pattern raises interesting questions about acclimatization. In addition, studies are in progress to try to determine how best to select people for this work. Telescopes are being sited at an altitude of 4200 m in Mauna Kea (Hawaii), and even higher at 5000 m in Chajnantor in north Chile. In Mauna Kea, some of the workers commute daily from sea level. For the Chajnantor project, many workers will live at an altitude of 2400 m and commute to the telescope though some will sleep at 5000 m. An important innovation is the use of oxygen-enriched rooms at high altitude to reduce the equivalent altitude. Each 1 per cent increase of oxygen concentration reduces the equivalent altitude by 300 m. Oxygen enrichment has been shown to improve neuro-psychological function during the day and enhance sleep at night. The use of oxygen-enriched modules at the Chajnantor site shows great promise.

29.1 INTRODUCTION

Currently one of the most challenging and interesting topics in high altitude medicine and physiology relates to the increasing number of people who commute to high altitude for commercial or scientific activities. The two main areas are high altitude mining and high altitude astronomy. Mining at high altitude goes back several hundred years, although the modern practice of having miners commute from much lower altitudes, even sea level, is relatively recent. Siting telescopes at high altitudes, for example over 4000 m, is also a more recent activity. Some of the most interesting problems arise in connection with placing telescopes at an altitude of 5000 m in north Chile.

This chapter overlaps somewhat with two previous chapters. The value of oxygen enrichment of room air to improve sleep at high altitude was briefly discussed in Chapter 13. The improvement of neuro-psychological function at an altitude of 5000 m as a result of oxygen enrichment of room air was referred to in Chapter 16.

29.2 HISTORICAL

Mining activities at high altitude are very old. Gold has been mined in west Tibet for centuries. The open cast mines at Thok Jalung (Thok is Tibetan for gold) were investigated in 1867 by Nain Singh, one of the early pundits, secret native explorers of the Survey of India (Waller 1990). Chinese sources suggest that Tibetans worked at 6000 m in the Tanggula range of central Tibet mining quartz, and chromate mines are also found in central Tibet (Ward 1990). In several areas of the South American Andes, there is evidence that mining activities were carried out by the Incas before the Spanish conquest. The Spanish conquistadors founded the imperial city of Potosí (4060 m) in Bolivia, the site of an enormous silver mine, in the 1540s. According to one historian quoted by Monge, M. (1948) when the city was founded there were 100 000 natives and 20 000 Spaniards. However, little information remains about the actual mining activities.

A very informative account of the mining practices in Cerro de Pasco, Peru (4340 m), was given by Barcroft *et al.* (1923) in their account of the International High Altitude Expedition to Cerro de Pasco which took place in 1921–2. Although most of the studies carried out by the physiologists were on themselves, many interesting observations were made on the native miners. One mine was 250 ft (76 m) below the surface, and the staircase which led down to it was 600 ft (183 m) in length. The porters who carried up the loads of ore from the mine varied greatly in age and stature. One boy who was said to be 10 years of age carried a load of 40 lb (18 kg) (Figure 29.1). Another porter who was thought to be 19 years old brought up a load of about 100 lb (45 kg). The physiologists noted that the exercise was spasmodic. The climb was very slow and consisted of the ascent of a few steps, followed by a long pause during which the porter regained his breath. They noted that the panting of the porters could be heard far down the staircase, before they came into view. The miners enjoyed sports, for example soccer, when they were not working. Each period of the game was 15 min long.

More recently, the extraordinary physical activity of miners at the Aucanquilcha mine (5950 m) in north Chile has been described (McIntyre 1987). The photograph on page 455 of that article shows the miners shattering boulders of sulfur ore using sledgehammers. The caretakers of this mine lived indefinitely at this altitude, and they were probably the highest inhabitants in the world (West 1986a). The mine is no longer working.

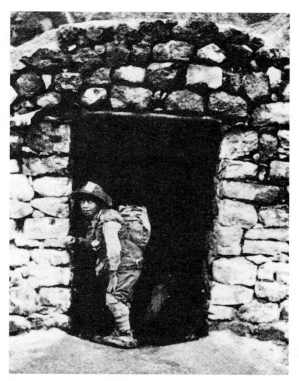

Figure 29.1 *Photograph from the report of the 1921–2 International High Altitude Expedition to Cerro de Pasco, Peru, showing a young boy, said to be 10 years old, carrying a load of 18 kg, which he has just brought up from the mine 250 ft (76 m) below the surface. (From Barcroft* et al. *1923.)*

29.3 MINING

Table 29.1 lists the altitudes of some of the most important commercial activities at high altitude. All of these are mines, except for two telescope sites. It can be seen that many of the mines are above 4000 m in altitude, with the highest being Aucanquilcha at 5950 m, although, as indicated earlier, this mine is no longer operating.

The mines fall into two categories. Many of the old mines, such as those at Cerro de Pasco and Morococha, have complete communities near the mine itself. This means that the families are located there and, in particular, the children are raised at these high altitudes. Many people question the wisdom of this because there is some evidence that children grow more slowly at high altitude (Frisancho and Baker 1970), although the issue is somewhat controversial. Certainly the central nervous system is

Table 29.1 *Examples of commercial and scientific activities at altitudes of 3500–6000 m*

	Facility	Altitude (m)	Latitude	Product or activity
Chile	Andina	3400–4200	33°S	Copper
	Aucanquilcha[a]	5950	21°S	Sulfur
	Choquelimpie	4500	20°S	Silver
	Collahuasi	4400–4600	21°S	Copper
	El Indio	3800–4000	30°S	Copper, gold, silver
	Quebrada Blanca	4400	21°S	Copper
	Chajnantor	5000	23°S	Telescope site
Peru	Cerro de Pasco	4330	11°S	Copper, gold, lead, zinc
	Morococha	4550	12°S	Copper
Bolivia	Potosí	4060	20°S	Silver, tin
Hawaii	Mauna Kea	4200	20°N	Telescope site
Colorado	Climax	4350	39°N	Molybdenum
	Summitville	4050	37°N	Gold

[a] This mine is not operating at present.

exquisitely sensitive to hypoxia, as discussed in Chapter 16, and, other things being equal, one would prefer to see children brought up in a more normal ambient P_{O_2}.

Another disadvantage of having whole communities at the site of the high altitude mine is that a large amount of infrastructure has to be provided. This includes schools, medical facilities and meeting halls, all of which increases the expenses of the mine. These considerations have led many modern mining operations to develop a commuting pattern where the families live at or near sea level and the miners commute to the mine itself where they spend a period of 7–10 days.

As an example of a modern mine based on the commuting pattern, the new mine at Collahuasi will be briefly described. This is a very large, open-cut copper mine in north Chile at a latitude of 21°S. Mining operations in this area were carried out in pre-Spanish times. It is interesting that Thomas H. Ravenhill (1881–1952), who gave the first accurate clinical descriptions of high altitude pulmonary edema (HAPE) and high altitude cerebral edema (HACE) (Ravenhill 1913), was the medical officer at this mine in 1909–11 (West 1996b). The working areas of the mine are at altitudes of 4400–4600 m, though the mining camp where the miners sleep is at an altitude of 3800 m. There are currently several thousand people working at the mine, which makes it one of the largest copper mines in the world. Copper is a major export of Chile.

The miners' families live in Iquique on the coast in accommodation supplied by the mining company. The miners are transported to the mine by special buses which take a few hours for the trip on a new road built by the mining company. A typical schedule is that the miners spend 7 days at the mine, where they work for up to 12 h per day, and then sleep in the mining camp at an altitude of 3800 m. At the end of 7 days they are bussed down to Iquique, where they spend the next 7 days with their families. The cycle is repeated indefinitely.

This pattern raises many questions for which answers are not presently available. For example, it is not clear to which altitude the miners will be acclimatized. Since they oscillate between sea level and 4400–4600 m every week, they presumably will not fully acclimatize to either altitude. In this respect, they have some similarities with the railway crews who shuttle between Lima and the high Andes (Hurtado *et al.* 1945). On the other hand, it is likely that the mine workers tolerate the altitude of the mine much better than would be the case if they came straight from sea level with no previous exposure to altitude. An interesting anecdotal fact is that when these miners return to their families at sea level, they complain of being very 'tired' for the first couple of days. A common joke has it that any children are conceived on the third night of return.

The 7 by 7-day schedule referred to above is not universally employed in the high altitude mines that use commuting. Periods at high altitude as long as 10–14 days have been tried. It clearly does not make much sense from a physiological point of view to have a period at high altitude of less than 7 days because there is evidence that the ventilatory acclimatization continues for at least this period of time (Lahiri 1972, Dempsey and Forster 1982). Other features of high altitude acclimatization, such as the development of polycythemia, take several weeks to reach a steady state. On the other hand, the physiological value of polycythemia is unclear (Winslow and Monge C. 1987).

Another important question is the rate of deacclimatization. Ideally, the workers should not lose all the acclimatization that they have developed at high altitude during their period with their families at sea level. Relatively little information about the rate of deacclimatization is available, although some measurements suggest that the rate of change of the ventilatory response during deacclimatization is slower than during acclimatization (Lahiri 1972). Deacclimatization is discussed further in section 4.4.4.

Finally, although the physiological aspects of scheduling are important, it may be that social factors will be dominant. Experience has shown that miners are reluctant to leave their homes for more than 7–10 days, and it is probable that a schedule of 7 days of high altitude followed by 7 days at sea level, or alternatively 10 by 10 days, will be the most acceptable.

Reference was made above to the miners at Aucanquilcha (5950 m) breaking large pieces of sulfur ore using sledgehammers. However, the activities at a modern mine such as Collahuasi are quite different. The ore is dislodged using explosives, and then it is picked up by enormous diesel electric front-end loaders that can scoop up 80 tons of ore at a time.

Three scoops are then placed in an gigantic diesel electric truck, which can carry 240 tons (Figure 29.2). Of course, considerable skill is necessary to operate these very large pieces of equipment, and substantial damage can be done to people or machines if the equipment is not operated correctly.

The highly skilled nature of modern mining is one reason why, in mines like Collahuasi, none of the miners are people indigenous to the high altitudes. Another reason is that there is not a large indigenous high altitude population in Chile. This is in contrast to the situation in many mines in Peru where, for example at Cerro de Pasco and Morococha, there are large indigenous populations who can provide relatively cheap, unskilled labor for the mines.

Another challenging problem of these high altitude mines is the selection of workers. Certainly not everybody is able to work effectively at altitudes of 4400–4500 m. There is considerable interest in possible medical tests that could predict who will be able to work well at altitude or, perhaps more important, who will be unable to tolerate the altitude. One possible test is the ventilatory response to hypoxia, during both rest and exercise (Rathat *et al.* 1992). As pointed out in Chapter 12, there is evidence that tolerance to extreme altitude requires a reasonable level of hypoxic ventilatory response in order to defend the alveolar P_{O_2} at a viable level. However, whether this will be a useful prognostic test for working at altitudes of 4000–5000 m is not clear. Probably the best predictor at the present time is whether a prospective worker has previously worked effectively at high altitude.

Even if workers have been shown to tolerate these

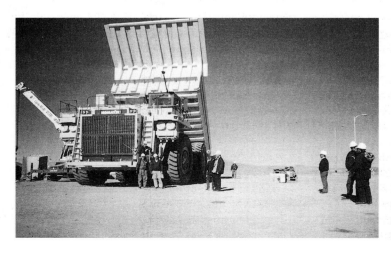

Figure 29.2 *Enormous diesel electric truck at the modern Collahuasi mine in north Chile. This can transport 240 tons of copper ore.*

Table 29.2 *Increase in mine equipment size at 3000 m and 4000 m to achieve the same output as at sea level*

Equipment	Output unit	Increase at altitude (%)	
		3000 m	4000 m
Diesel engines	Brake horsepower	40	55
Compressors	Airtool work	55	75
Vacuum filters	Tons solids h^{-1}	30	45
Vacuum pumps	Intake volume	30	40
Transmission lines	MVA km^{-1}	20	30
Transformers	MVA	15	25
Electrical machines	kW	15	25
Flotation	tons h^{-1}	35	50
Leach vessels	tons h^{-1}	50	85

Source: modified from Jimenez (1995).

high altitudes reasonably well, it should not be expected that they can accomplish the same amount of physical work as at sea level. The decline in maximal oxygen consumption with increasing altitude was discussed in Chapter 11, where it was pointed out that the $\dot{V}_{O_2 max}$ of an acclimatized subject at an altitude of 5000 m is only about 70 per cent of the sea level value. Another way of looking at this is that the work force would have to be increased by about 40 per cent at high altitude to accomplish the same amount of physical work. It is interesting that this inefficiency is not confined to human beings, but is also seen in mechanical equipment. Table 29.2 shows that, at an altitude of 4000 m, the amount of equipment to produce the same amount of work as at sea level has to be increased from 25 to 85 per cent (Jimenez 1995).

29.4 TELESCOPES

29.4.1 Mauna Kea

As indicated previously, there have been mines at altitudes over 4000 m in the South American Andes for many years, even before the Spanish invasion. However, the practice of siting telescopes at high altitude is much more recent, mostly within the last 50 years. There are several advantages in siting telescopes at high altitudes. One is that the instrument is then above much of the Earth's atmosphere, which otherwise absorbs some of the optical and radio waves. Another advantage is that in some areas, for

example Chajnantor (see below), the atmosphere is extremely dry and absorption of radio waves by water vapor is therefore much less. Finally, remote mountain sites tend to have little light or radio wave pollution, although this advantage can also be achieved in other remote areas at lower altitudes.

Two telescope sites will be considered here. One is the extinct volcano at Mauna Kea in the big island of Hawaii. The summit is at an altitude of 4200 m and at least 10 instruments are located either on the summit or not far below it. A feature of Mauna Kea is that it is close to the city of Hilo, which is at sea level, and it is possible to drive from one site to the other in a couple of hours. There is also an intermediate station with dormitories at 3000 m at Hale Pohaku, and some newcomers can spend a night there before going to the summit. However, the majority of the staff who operate the telescopes commute from sea level every day. The barometric pressure at the summit is about 465 mm Hg, so the P_{O_2} of moist inspired gas is only 87 mm Hg, as against 150 mm Hg at sea level. The hypoxic stress is therefore severe.

Forster (1986) has studied the incidence of acute mountain sickness (AMS) and the arterial blood gases of some of the workers on the United Kingdom Infrared Telescope (UKIRT) on the summit of Mauna Kea. These shift workers spent 40 days working at sea level at Hilo, followed by a 5-day shift at high altitude. The first night of the shift was spent in the dormitories at 3000 m, and following that 4 days were spent on the summit of Mauna Kea, with the workers returning to 3000 m for each night. It was found that 80 per cent of the shift workers had symptoms of AMS on their first day at the summit. Apart from breathlessness, headache was the most frequent complaint, and this affected 41 per cent of shift workers at the start of their high altitude shift. Other common symptoms were insomnia, lethargy, poor concentration, poor memory, and unsteadiness of gait. The frequency of symptoms decreased over the 5 days of the shift, and at the end 60 per cent of the workers were asymptomatic.

Arterial blood gases were measured in 27 UKIRT shift workers. On day 1 at 4200 m, the mean arterial P_{O_2} was 42 mm Hg, rising to 44 mm Hg on day 5. The arterial P_{CO_2} was 29 mm Hg on the first day, falling to 27 mm Hg on the fifth day. Arterial pH was 7.49 on day 1, falling to 7.48 on day 5.

It is interesting that there was no difference in the incidence of AMS between shift workers who worked at the summit after a brief sojourn at sea level (mean 4 days), compared to a protracted rest period (mean 37 days) at sea level. This suggests that in this group, the acclimatization to high altitude achieved during 5 days on Mauna Kea was lost within a few days of return to sea level. High altitude pulmonary edema (HAPE) was rarely seen at Mauna Kea, with only 1 case in 41 shift workers during a 2-year study period. Also only one worker on Mauna Kea had an episode of high altitude cerebral edema (HACE).

29.4.2 Chajnantor

The other telescope site that will be discussed here is Chajnantor in north Chile, southeast of San Pedro de Atacama, at a latitude of 23°S and an altitude of 5000 m. This is a remarkable site because it is fairly flat, covers a large area, and is easily accessible by road from San Pedro (altitude 2440 m). The first part of the road is an international highway leading from Chile to Bolivia and Argentina, and the final 15 km is now also paved. The drive from San Pedro to Chajnantor takes only about 1 h. There must be few places in the world where it is possible to reach an altitude of 5000 m so easily.

Several small radio telescopes have been sited at Chajnantor or nearby. At the time of writing, the California Institute of Technology has a radio telescope that is studying the cosmic microwave background radiation. However, part of the interest of Chajnantor is that it will be the site of an enormous multinational radio telescope, construction of which will start in 2004. When finished it will be the largest radio telescope in the world, with a cost of $400 million. Since the barometric pressure is 420 mm Hg, the inspired P_{O_2} is only 78 mm Hg, so the degree of hypoxic stress is substantial. The large amount of construction work required to complete the telescope, and the number of workers who will be at the site to run it, means that this is a particularly challenging problem in high altitude medicine.

29.5 OXYGEN ENRICHMENT OF ROOM AIR TO RELIEVE THE HYPOXIA OF HIGH ALTITUDE

Partly in response to the burgeoning of commercial and scientific activities at high altitude, considerable work has recently been done on the feasibility and value of raising the oxygen concentration of room air at high altitude in order to relieve the hypoxia. The possibility of doing this was suggested by Cudaback (1984) and, at one stage, plans were made to oxygen enrich the control room of the Keck telescope at Mauna Kea, although these never materialized.

The principle of oxygen enrichment is simple. Oxygen, either from a concentrator or a cryogenic source, is added to the ventilation of a room, thus increasing the oxygen concentration from 21 per cent to a higher value. The reason why oxygen enrichment is so powerful is that relatively small degrees of oxygen enrichment result in large reductions of equivalent altitude. The term 'equivalent altitude' refers to the altitude at which the moist inspired P_{O_2}, when a subject is breathing ambient air, is the same as the inspired P_{O_2} in the oxygen-enriched environment. Figure 29.3 shows that, between altitudes of 3000 and 6000 m, each 1 per cent of oxygen enrichment results in a reduction of equivalent altitude by about 300 m. In other words, if we oxygen enrich a room at the Chajnantor site, altitude 5000 m, by 6 per cent (that is, we increase the oxygen concentration from 21 to 27 per cent), the equivalent altitude is reduced by about 6 × 300 m, or 1800 m. Therefore we go from an altitude of 5000 m to one of 3200 m, which is much more easily tolerated.

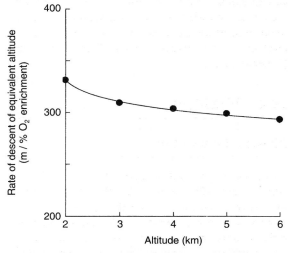

Figure 29.3 *Degree of reduction of equivalent altitude (meters of descent per 1 per cent oxygen enrichment) plotted against the altitude at which the enrichment is made. Note that at altitudes up to about 6000 m, each 1 per cent of oxygen enrichment results in an altitude reduction of more than 300 m. (From West 1995.)*

When this idea was originally proposed, some people argued that it would be impossible to maintain an enriched-oxygen atmosphere within the room because of inevitable leaks. However, in practice, oxygen enrichment is relatively simple and reliable. The room does not have to be gas tight. Large potential leaks such as window surrounds are taped, and a double door is provided so that there is an air lock. However, oxygen-enriched air is blown into the room and escapes through small leaks, and in practice it is easy to control the oxygen level within 0.25 per cent.

Oxygen enrichment of rooms has become feasible largely because large quantities of oxygen can now be produced relatively cheaply. The simplest way to do this is to use an oxygen concentrator; thousands of these are now used in homes to provide oxygen for patients with chronic lung disease. The principle is that air is pumped at high pressure through a non-flammable ceramic material such as synthetic zeolite which absorbs nitrogen from the air. The result is that the effluent gas has a high oxygen concentration, typically 90–95 per cent. After 20–30 s, the zeolite is unable to absorb more nitrogen and the compressed air is then switched to another cylinder containing the same material. The original cylinder is then purged of nitrogen by blowing air through it at normal pressures. In this way, a continuous supply of 90–95 per cent oxygen is available. A typical unit provides 5 L min^{-1} of nearly pure oxygen at a power consumption of 350 W. It is also possible to provide the oxygen from liquid oxygen tanks, but this is more expensive and less convenient because the tanks need to be replenished.

An important issue is what level of ventilation to use in the room. Clearly, the higher the ventilation, the larger the amount of oxygen that must be produced to maintain a given degree of oxygen enrichment. This topic has been discussed extensively elsewhere (West 1995). We use the 1975 American Society of Heating, Refrigeration and Air-Conditioning Engineers (ASHRAE) standard of 8.5 m^3 person^{-1} h^{-1}, which corresponds to 142 L min^{-1}. This is calculated to maintain the carbon dioxide concentration in the room below 0.24 per cent, based on a carbon dioxide production rate per person of 0.3 L min^{-1}. This concentration of carbon dioxide was chosen by ASHRAE as a measure of acceptable ventilation levels. Substantially higher concentrations of carbon dioxide can exist without

people being aware of them. However, the carbon dioxide concentration is a useful objective marker of adequacy of ventilation, and higher levels tend to be associated with awareness of body odor.

It should be added that in 1989, ASHRAE increased the minimum standard of ventilation by three to fourfold. This was a somewhat controversial decision, and was partially based on the facts that there may be smokers in the room, there are health variations among people, and some types of room furniture cause outgassing, which may be injurious. In designing a facility for use at high altitude, it can be assumed that people will not be allowed to smoke in the room, and it is also possible to choose furniture that does not provide outgassing hazards.

Figure 29.4 shows a sketch of a module that can be used for oxygen enrichment in the field. In this instance, a standard shipping container of dimensions 20 ft (6.1 m) long, 8 ft (2.44 m) wide and 8 ft high is fitted out as a living space with beds, or a laboratory or a machine shop. A larger laboratory can be housed in a standard shipping container of dimensions 40 ft (12.19 m) long by 8 ft wide by 8 ft high. Such containers are currently in use at the Chajnantor site, in connection with the CalTech radio telescope. The oxygen is provided from oxygen concentrators, and the concentrations of both oxygen and carbon dioxide are continually monitored inside the rooms.

The experience of the astronomers with oxygen enrichment has been very satisfactory. There have been no technical problems in maintaining the target oxygen concentration of 27 per cent, and the carbon dioxide concentration is typically less than 0.25 per cent. The CalTech project was a particularly valuable field test of oxygen enrichment because, for the first 2 weeks, the astronomers were working in ambient air conditions. They found this extremely tiring, despite the fact that they slept every night at San Pedro (altitude 2440 m). When the oxygen enrichment modules were set up, they noticed an immediate improvement in work productivity and efficiency. In fact, they soon instituted a rule that no one was allowed to control the telescope or use power tools unless using oxygen enrichment. When the astronomers were not in the oxygen-enriched modules, they used portable oxygen in order to provide oxygen enrichment. They also reported that it was feasible to sleep at the Chajnantor site in the oxygen-enriched rooms. This had not proved to be possible while breathing ambient air because of the poor quality of sleep.

Several studies have now been carried out on the physiological effects of oxygen enrichment of room air at high altitude. The first studies were performed at the Barcroft facility of the White Mountain Research Station (altitude 3800 m) in California, where the oxygen concentration of the test room was raised from 21 to 24 per cent (Luks *et al.* 1998). This reduced the equivalent altitude to about 2900 m. In a double-blind study, it was shown that oxygen enrichment during the night resulted in fewer apneas and less time spent in periodic breathing with apneas. Subjective assessments of sleep quality showed significant improvement. There was also a lower AMS score during the morning after oxygen-enriched

sleep. An unexpected finding was that there was a larger increase in arterial oxygen saturation from evening to morning after oxygen-enriched sleep than after sleeping in ambient air (Figure 29.5). Of course, both measurements of arterial oxygen saturation were made with the subject breathing ambient air.

In another study, the mechanism of the unexpected increase in arterial oxygen saturation the following morning was investigated (McElroy *et al.* 2000). Because this could have been caused by a change in the control of ventilation, the ventilatory responses to hypoxia and to carbon dioxide were measured in the evening and in the morning after sleeping both in the oxygen-enriched environment and in ambient air. No effect of oxygen enrichment on the control of ventilation was found. An

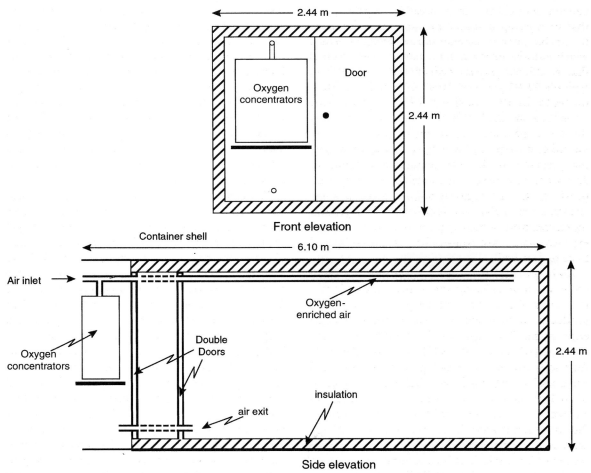

Figure 29.4 *A self-contained oxygen-enriched module suitable for field work at high altitude. The module uses a standard shipping container 20 ft (6.10 m) long and 8 ft (2.44 m) wide and high. These oxygen-enriched modules are being used at the California Institute of Technology radio telescope at Chajnantor, altitude 5050 m.*

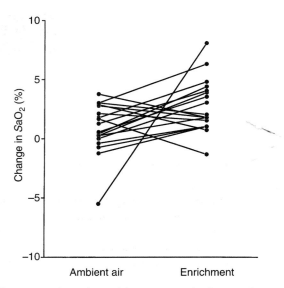

Figure 29.5 *Change in arterial oxygen saturation from evening to morning for subjects sleeping in ambient air, compared with the same subjects sleeping in 24 per cent oxygen enrichment, at an altitude of 3800 m. The measurements of oxygen saturation were made by pulse oximetry, with the subjects breathing ambient air. The increase was greater after sleep in oxygen enrichment (p < 0.05). (From Luks et al., 2000.)*

alternative explanation is that the increase in arterial oxygen saturation seen following sleep in the oxygen-enriched environment might have been the result of less subclinical pulmonary edema, compared with sleeping in ambient air. An interesting additional piece of information that might support this explanation was that the increase in arterial oxygen saturation was transient, so that by midday the difference between the oxygen-enriched and ambient air treatments on oxygen saturation was abolished.

A final study was carried out on the effects of oxygen enrichment on neuropsychological function at a simulated altitude of 5000 m, as referred to briefly in Chapter 16. Again, the Barcroft facility, at an altitude of 3800 m, was used, and the concentration of oxygen in the room was manipulated to simulate ambient air at an altitude of 5000 m, and an oxygen concentration of 27 per cent at an altitude of 5000 m. A large battery of neuropsychological tests was performed in a double-blinded manner, and it was found that there were significant improvements in reaction times, hand–eye coordination, and mood (Gerard *et al.* 2000). These findings are directly relevant to the project of oxygen enrichment at the Chajnantor site.

An important consideration when oxygen is added to air is whether the fire hazard is increased, compared with sea level. This has been analyzed carefully (West 1997) and it has been shown that, with the levels of oxygen enrichment considered here, the fire hazard is less than at sea level. The basic reason is that, although the P_{O_2} is increased by oxygen enrichment at high altitude, it is still far below the value at sea level. Although it is true that the reduction of P_{N_2} at altitude also increases the fire hazard to a small extent, because of the smaller extinguishing effect of this inert gas, it remains true that the fire hazard using the degrees of oxygen enrichment described here is less than at sea level. As an example, the National Fire Protection Association (NFPA 1993) defines an oxygen-enriched atmosphere as having an increased fire hazard, in the sense that it will support an increased burning rate of materials, if the percentage concentration of oxygen is greater than $23.45/(P_f)^{0.5}$, where P_f is the total barometric pressure expressed as a fraction of the sea level pressure. For the Chajnantor site, $P_f = 0.55$, so that if the oxygen concentration is greater than 31.6 per cent it would exceed the NFPA threshold. The oxygen concentration of 27 per cent is well below this value.

It could be argued that oxygen enrichment of room air represents a new attitude to living and working at high altitude. Until now, most people have accepted hypoxia as something that has to be endured. However, this proactive attitude of raising oxygen concentration of the rooms to reduce the equivalent altitude could represent a major advance.

30

Athletes and altitude

SUMMARY

It is only recently that athletes have used high altitude training to enhance sea level performance, but many remarkable feats of endurance have been recorded in mountains. One of the most remarkable was the first ascent of Everest without supplementary oxygen in 1978.

In athletic competitions at altitude, slower times are recorded in sprint events because of lowered air resistance, whilst in endurance events, because of a lower $V_{O_2 max}$, times are slower.

The paradox is that acclimatization to altitude results in central and peripheral adaptation that enhances oxygen delivery and utilization, but hypoxia decreases the intensity of training and may even cause detraining.

As polycythemia increases the $V_{O_2 max}$ and endurance performance, this might indicate that the higher the athlete goes to train the better, but this is not the case; an increased hematocrit carries its own disadvantages, as well as the problem of decreased exercise capacity resulting in decreased training intensity.

There is some evidence that athletes who live at moderate altitude (2500 m) and train at low altitude (1500 m) improve their endurance performance. However, there is considerable individual variation in the results of the 'live high – train low' method, and in one series, sea level $V_{O_2 max}$ did not improve, yet race times improved by about 6 per cent.

For maximal sea level performance it is still not clear how long or how high the athletes should live at altitude or how long they should remain at sea level before racing.

Unfortunately, few trials have adequate sea level controls to compare with altitude training. Until this is done much information will remain largely anecdotal.

30.1 INTRODUCTION

Pugh (1965) suggested that athlete performance at altitude would result in slower times in sprint events due to decreased air resistance, which parallels barometric pressure; by contrast, in distance events times would be increased because the maximum oxygen uptake falls with altitude.

Comparing the times of athletes in the 1965 Pan-American games held in Mexico (2250 m) with those of the Melbourne Olympics of 1956 at sea level, Pugh showed that there was an increase in time of 2.6 per cent in the 800 m and 14.9 per cent in the 10 000 m events. In the 100 m and 400 m, but not the 200 m, race times at altitude were faster than at sea level.

When the Olympic Games were held in Mexico City in 1968, several world records in short and sprint events were broken but in the longer endurance events times were slower than at sea level. This was due to the reduced $V_{O_2 max}$ which at this altitude is 84 per cent of sea level values. However, the times were not as slow as had been predicted.

Marathon performance at altitude is affected mainly by a lowered $V_{O_2 max}$, which decreases by about 1.5–3.5 per cent for every 300 m of ascent above 1500 m (Roi *et al.* 1999).

30.2   ALTITUDE AND TRAINING

To achieve optimum physical performance at altitude it is clear that adequate acclimatization to hypoxia is essential or, better still, being born and bred at altitude. Evidence that after a period at altitude returning to sea level improves performance is still equivocal and the timing for maximum sea level performance after altitude training is not clear. However, altitude training is frequently used by competition athletes to improve their sea level performance, despite lack of evidence that it is beneficial. On the one hand acclimatization to high altitude results in central and peripheral adaptations that improve oxygen delivery and utilization. Hypoxic exercise may increase the stimulus of training thus magnifying the effect of endurance training. On the other hand, the hypoxia of altitude limits the intensity of training and may result in detraining.

Numerous anecdotal reports suggest that endurance athletes benefit from altitude training; however, when appropriate controls have been included in studies, the benefit has been found to be no greater than equivalent training at sea level. Many results are equivocal. Using controls Roskamm *et al.* (1969) found that subjects who trained at 2250 m improved their $V_{O_2 max}$ by comparison with sea level subjects and those at 3450 m, but Hanson *et al.* (1967), also with sea level controls and starting with unfit subjects, ($V_{O_2 max} < 40$ mL min^{-1} kg^{-1}), found no advantage in training at an altitude of 4300 m. In well trained subjects too, the picture is not clear. A well controlled study by Adams *et al.* (1975) using a crossover design in experienced trained athletes ($V_{O_2 max}$ 73 mL min^{-1} kg^{-1}) showed no significant differences in performance between altitude (2300 m) and sea level training.

It is not clear which physiological parameters are important. Altitude training may result in a greater density of muscle capillaries, but this can also be achieved by training at low altitude. In addition, hypoxia over a long period in lowlanders causes loss of muscle mass and increased capillary density due mainly to a decrease in muscle fiber density. In any event lowland athletes, using altitude training, cannot in a few weeks or months achieve the effect of lifetime exposure.

Some of the best endurance runners have been born and bred in East Africa, living at an altitude of 1500–2000 m, and this upbringing will contribute to their continued success. Also, hypoxia increases hemoglobin concentration which is associated with an increased endurance performance. However, Weston *et al.* (1999) have compared elite African 10 km runners and their white counterparts, both of whom lived at sea level. The African runners had a greater resistance to fatigue, and higher oxidative enzyme activity, combined with a lower accumulation of lactate.

With the difference between winning and losing an event being often so small, the psychological effects of altitude training should not be discounted.

30.3   THE MOUNTAINEER AS AN ATHLETE

The first mountaineers who could be called athletes were Hebler and Messner (Messner 1979, pp. 178–82). In 1978, they made the first ascent of Everest without supplementary oxygen and this focused attention on their birth, upbringing and training at intermediate altitude in the European Alps. A number of high altitude natives have repeated this feat on Everest, but then so have mountaineers born and bred at sea level (Unsworth 2000).

Habler and Messner's training, which included long distance running and very rapid alpine ascents up to 4875 m and later rapid ascents in the Himalayas, played a major role in their exceptional fitness and subsequent success.

With training, outstanding feats of endurance have been recorded. In 1899, a Ghurka soldier born and bred at intermediate altitude in Nepal ascended and descended a 800 m peak in Scotland and crossed 4 miles of scree and bog in 55 min. This feat was repeated in 1999 by a trained athlete (a fell runner) in 53 min 45 s (*The Times* 1999b).

Other outstanding endurance feats at low and high altitude are recorded. For instance, a man in his fiftieth year ran 391 miles in 7 days 1 h 25 min over Lakeland hills up to 850 m in the UK. This involved a total ascent of 37 000 m, an average of over 5000 m per day (Brasher 1986). In June 1988, 76 summits in the same region were reached in 24 h involving an ascent and descent of 12 000 m (Brasher 1988). At intermediate altitude all 54 of the peaks over 4300 m in Colorado, USA, were climbed in 21 days (Boyer 1978) and the ascent of Mont Blanc (4807 m) in France from Chamonix (1050 m), with return to Chamonix, was made in 5.5 h (Smyth 1988). At high altitude, one ascent in the Karakoram Mountains was made from 4900 m to 8047 m with return to 4900 m in 22 h (Wielicki 1985) and on Mount McKinley in Alaska from 3000 m to 6000 m in 19 h (Rowell 1982).

In 1986 an ascent and descent of Everest (8848 m) in 2 days by a new route on the north face was completed from the head of the West Rongbuck glacier (5800 m); supplementary oxygen was not used (Everest 1987). In 1990, Marc Batard ascended from Base Camp to the summit of Everest in 22.5 h also without the use of supplementary oxygen (Gillman 1993, p. 200).

30.4 POLYCYTHEMIA AND INCREASED HEMATOCRIT

Up to about 2500 m polycythemia increases the $V_{O_2\,max}$ and endurance performance (Levine and Stray-Gundersen 1992). For this reason the use of erythropoietin by subcutaneous injection or autologous blood transfusion, both of which create a transient increase in red cell mass, has been banned for athletic events. The effect of autologous red cell infusion on exercise performance at high altitude (4300 m) was studied by Pandolf *et al.* (1998). No significant improvement in a 3.2 km run at sea level was found after infusion, and at altitude times were only slightly faster.

Hypoxia stimulates the release of erythropoietin and in turn the bone marrow is stimulated to produce more red cells. The process takes weeks rather than days, however, and the initial rise in hemoglobin and hematocrit on going to altitude is almost entirely due to a reduction in plasma volume

(Chapter 8). The increase in hematocrit is advantageous as it increases the oxygen-carrying capacity of the blood. However, the resulting reduction in blood volume may be part of the reason for the reduction in cardiac output found at an early stage of altitude exposure. For the sea level athletes training at altitude, this decrease in plasma volume on ascent is rapidly reversed on descent and any advantage in terms of hematocrit is quickly lost. In a person resident at altitude for many months or years, the red cell mass may be increased by as much as 50 per cent of its normal sea level value. On descent to sea level this increased cell mass is retained for some weeks which could be an advantage in endurance events.

It is still not clear what the optimum altitude is at which athletes should be taken to maximize their performance.

Considering the inverse relationship between P_{O_2} and hemoglobin concentration, it might be thought that the higher the athlete can go the better, but recent work (Gore *et al.* 1998) suggests that altitude training at 2650 m does not increase $V_{O_2\,max}$ or hemoglobin. Also when sea level dwellers spend long periods over 5000 m physical and mental deterioration occurs, associated with loss of appetite, loss of weight and reduction of muscle mass (Ward 1954). In addition a high hematocrit carries with it the danger of transient or permanent vascular episodes and possible death.

30.5 DETRAINING AND HYPOXIA

It has recently been seen that in elite endurance athletes, $V_{O_2\,max}$ can be reduced at altitudes as low as 610 m (Gore *et al.* 1996). This occurred in about 50 per cent of trained subjects with $V_{O_2\,max}$ above 65 mL min^{-1} kg^{-1} (Anselme *et al.* 1992), and they appeared to develop a more severe level of arterial hypoxemia during maximal and submaximal exercise than more sedentary controls under hypoxic and normoxic conditions (Lawler *et al.* 1988, Koistenen *et al.* 1995).

This might have been due to a detraining effect (Saltin 1967). However, it has also been suggested that intermittent exposure to altitudes of 2300–3300 m maximizes the balance between acclimatization and intensity of training (Daniels and Oldridge 1970). It is also possible that the intensity of training at sea level could produce as good a result as intermittent visits to altitude.

30.6 LIVING HIGH – TRAINING LOW

Levine and Stray-Gundersen (1997) suggested that if athletes were acclimatized to a moderate altitude (2500 m) and trained at lower altitude (1500 m) they could get the best of both worlds and improve their performance more than an equivalent control group at sea level or altitude. A 5000 m run time trial was the main measure of performance and in trained runners those who 'lived high – trained low' showed an increase in sea level performance. Sea level performance was not improved in those who lived and trained at moderate altitude or in those who lived and trained at sea level only.

There is, however, considerable individual variation in the response to altitude training and some do not respond to the 'live high – train low' regime (Chapman et al. 1998).

30.7 CRITICAL P_{O_2} FOR HEMATOLOGICAL ADAPTATION

In one study of elite cross-country skiers, 3 weeks' training at an altitude of 1900 m was sufficient to raise the hematocrit by 5 per cent (Ingier and Myhre 1992). However, the scarcity of similar studies does not allow any definite conclusion to be made.

It has been suggested that the longer the period at altitude the greater the hemopoietic response. However, during the Silver Hut Expedition 1960–1, when 3 months were spent at 5800 m and above, the hemoglobin concentration leveled off after about 6 weeks.

Obviously hypoxia increases the demand for iron and athletes training at altitude may prove to be iron deficient, particularly female athletes. Again few studies have been made but differences in iron status may explain differences in individual hematological response (Ingier and Myhre 1992).

On descent from altitude hemoglobin levels return to normal quite quickly. In Operation Everest III (COMEX) after 30 days in a chamber ascending to the equivalent height of the summit of Everest, the hemoglobin concentration was back to normal val-

ues after 4 days at sea level pressure (Richalet et al. 1999). Also after a long period at altitude individuals feel physically 'slack' and less energetic for the first few days. Most coaches therefore advise return to low altitude at least 2–3 days before an important race.

30.8 MEASUREMENT OF THE EFFECTS OF ALTITUDE TRAINING

Because so many hypoxic training studies have been completed without normoxic controls, it is difficult to determine whether the physiological changes noted are due to hypoxia alone or a training effect.

In one series with controls, 10 elite middle to long distance runners trained for 10 weeks at the same exercise rate at sea level and at a simulated altitude of 4000 m. There was no improvement in $V_{O_2 max}$, yet personal best times over 10 km improved by about 6 per cent (Asano et al. 1986). Is it possible that this was due to a psychological effect?

Anaerobic performance may also improve after returning to sea level, following a stay at altitude, but many studies have shown no improvement (Martin and Pyne 1998).

30.9 IMMUNE RESPONSE AT ALTITUDE

The question of immunity and training even at sea level is a hotly debated subject as is immunity and altitude. However, the possibility that training at altitude may cause some defect in the immune system is real. A defect in B cell function has been suggested but not proved (Meehan 1987). On Operation Everest II when individuals ascended to the 'summit' of Everest in a decompression chamber, results suggested that T-cell activation was blunted during exposure to severe hypoxia whereas B-cell function and mucosal immunity were not (Meehan et al. 1988).

Athletes frequently complain of recurrent minor infections, and mountaineers at high altitude find that cuts and infections seem to improve more rapidly on return to lower altitude. Bailey et al. (1998), in two studies with a total of 24 elite endurance athletes training at altitudes of 1500–2000 m, found a 50 per cent increase in the frequency of upper respiratory and gastrointestinal tract infections during the altitude period. They also recorded a reduction in plasma glutamine concentration at rest. Glutamine is important as a substrate for macrophages and lymphocytes and a reduction in its concentration might indicate impairment of immune defense against opportunistic infections.

30.10   IS ALTITUDE TRAINING WORTH IT?

Is it worthwhile for athletes to train at altitude? At present there is no clear answer to this question. The disadvantages are the risk of AMS and HAPE and HACE. The reduction of $\dot{V}_{O_2 max}$ and the earlier onset of fatigue mean that altitude training is less intense than at sea level. However, living high and training low has shown improved performance in a 5 km time trial.

On the strength of that one trial, it would seem that for distance events it would be better to live at 2500 m and train at 1500 m. Bailey and Davis (1997) reviewed the available evidence for the efficacy of altitude training for sea level events and concluded,

> Scientific evidence to support the claim that either continuous or intermittent hypoxic training will enhance sea level performance remains at present equivocal.

The optimum time of stay at altitude is still not clear, but to increase red cell mass at least 4 weeks at altitude may be necessary, but the associated reduction in training intensity would not be advantageous. To obtain maximum performance after the athlete descends to lower levels, the timing of the event is also not clear: a minimum of 2–3 days with a maximum of 14–21 days has been suggested (Suslov 1994).

31

Clinical lessons from high altitude

SUMMARY

The study of healthy subjects at altitude has given valuable insights into the effects of hypoxia on human physiology. In this chapter we consider the similarities and differences between humans at high altitude and patients at sea level with various medical conditions. Altitude acclimatized humans are a very good model for the hypoxia suffered by patients with lung diffusion limitation due to conditions such as fibrosing alveolitis and pneumoconiosis where there is little or no airways obstruction. Chronic obstructive lung diseases (chronic bronchitis, emphysema and chronic asthma) have many similarities to acclimatized humans but differ in that such patients have normal or raised P_{CO_2} whereas acclimatized humans have a low P_{CO_2}. Healthy subjects at altitude have some similarities to patients with cardiac conditions which limit the heart in its response to exercise. The sensation of fatigue in the working muscles is similar and is experienced by both. It is probably due to insufficient oxygen supply in both cases. Anemia gives rise to the same sensation due to oxygen lack though through different mechanisms. The problems of patients with cyanotic heart disease are also reflected in acclimatized humans.

At a more fundamental level altitude physiology has influenced clinical medicine through concepts such as

the importance of partial pressure of gases, especially of oxygen and carbon dioxide and, by extension, of anesthetic gases, and of acid–base and oxygen dissociation curves. Much early work was stimulated by interest in humans and animals at altitude. In hematology the very early work on polycythemia of altitude provided a stimulus to much work on erythropoiesis. In cardiology the raised pulmonary artery pressure found at altitude has stimulated work on the control of pressure in the lesser circulation.

31.1 INTRODUCTION

High altitude medicine and physiology constitute a legitimate subject for study in their own right and if, like any branch of science, such study casts light on other fields, including clinical medicine, that is a bonus.

However, it is often argued that a justification for human studies at high altitude is that the knowledge so gained may be applied in clinical medicine. Patients hypoxic because of pulmonary or cardiovascular disease present a complex picture in which hypoxia is only one of their many problems. In the study of humans at high altitude one can study the effects of hypoxia alone in otherwise healthy subjects. The stimulus, hypoxia, can be applied in a measurable controlled way at a time to suit the scientist, so that controlled measurements can be made before and after hypoxia.

The insight so gained can be applied to the more complicated uncontrolled situation of the hypoxic patient. This chapter discusses how good a model human subjects at high altitude are for the hypoxic patient, and the similarities and the differences between these two situations. It also reviews the extent to which high altitude physiology has illuminated clinical medicine.

31.2 CHRONIC OBSTRUCTIVE LUNG DISEASE

Probably the commonest cause of hypoxia in medicine is chronic obstructive lung disease (COLD). Within this category are included patients with chronic obstructive bronchitis, emphysema and chronic fixed asthma. Patients with long-standing severe deformity, such as kyphoscoliosis, also develop hypoxia in the later stages of their disease. Table 31.1 lists the similarities and differences between a patient with COLD and a subject at high altitude.

31.2.1 Symptoms

The similarities include the symptoms of dyspnea, especially on exertion, and the limitation of work capacity. Dyspnea is a difficult sensation to describe and probably the term includes more than one sort of sensation. Patients with asthma, for instance, say that the sensation during an attack is quite different from the breathlessness they feel at the end of a run when free of asthma. The dyspnea of an individual at high altitude is probably more like the latter; the sensation is of needing to hyperventilate and being quite free to do so. Patients with COLD, on the other hand, probably suffer a rather different sensation, akin to that of the asthmatic patient in an attack, which is described as a difficulty in 'getting the breath' or of suffocation.

The reduction in work or exercise capacity is very similar in both patients and high altitude subjects. In both, the dyspnea is felt to play a part but both also complain that work is limited by a sensation of the legs 'giving out' or 'feeling like lead'. This is for large muscle mass dynamic work such as walking, cycling, and climbing stairs. If the strength of a small muscle mass is tested (e.g. hand grip), it is found to be largely unimpaired in both cases. The possibility that the central nervous system may play a role in limiting exhaustive exercise fatigue at altitude has been proposed (Kayser et al. 1993b). Could this also apply to patients with COLD?

In the patient with COLD the work of breathing (per liter) is increased because of airways obstruction. The total ventilation may be increased as well, even if there is alveolar hypoventilation, because of the increased dead space; thus the total work of breathing is further increased. At high altitude, the

Table 31.1 *Comparison of clinical aspects of chronic obstructive lung disease with findings in people at high altitude*

Symptom/finding	At high altitude	Chronic obstructive lung disease
Dyspnea on exertion	Yes	Yes
Limited work capacity	Yes	Yes
Peripheral edema	Seen in AMS	Frequent
Polycythemia	Yes	Yes
Red cell mass	Increased	Increased
Arterial P_{O_2}	Reduced	Reduced
Arterial P_{CO_2}	Reduced	Normal or raised
Arterial pH	Raised	Normal or reduced
Bicarbonate level in blood, CSF	Reduced	Raised
Work of breathing L^{-1}	Reduced	Increased
Work of breathing, total	Increased	Increased
CO_2 ventilatory response	Shift to left and steepened	Shift to right and flattened
Cerebral blood flow	Increased/normal	Increased
Pulmonary arterial pressure	Raised	Raised

CSF, cerebrospinal fluid; AMS, acute mountain sickness.

work of breathing per liter is modestly decreased because of the reduction in air density at reduced barometric pressure; however, the total work of breathing is increased due to the marked hyperventilation especially on exercise (Chapter 11).

31.2.2 Blood gases and acid–base balance

Subjects at high altitude and patients with COLD both have reduced P_{O_2}. At high altitude this is due to low inspired P_{O_2} whereas in COLD patients it is caused by gas transfer problems due to ventilation/perfusion ratio inequalities. In both cases, the hypoxemia is made worse by exertion.

The P_{CO_2} level, however, is different. In patients with COLD the Pa_{CO_2} is either normal or, in more severe cases, raised. The pH is consequently lowered; respiratory acidosis and secondary renal compensation result in elevated blood bicarbonate concentration. The cerebrospinal fluid (CSF) bicarbonate concentration is also elevated and there follows a shift to the right of the ventilatory carbon dioxide response line and the response becomes flattened (i.e. blunted). In contrast, at high altitude the Pa_{CO_2} is reduced, pH elevated, blood and CSF bicarbonate concentration reduced, and the carbon dioxide response shifts to the left and becomes more brisk (Chapter 5).

31.2.3 Hematological changes

At high altitude and in COLD patients there is an increase in red cell mass. This invariably results in polycythemia at high altitude where it is accompanied at first by a reduced plasma volume (Chapter 8). In COLD the plasma volume is usually increased, for reasons which are unclear, so that polycythemia is often not seen until red cell mass is considerably increased by a more extreme hypoxia. In both cases the increase is due to more erythropoiesis, stimulated by increased levels of erythropoietin. After the first few days at a given high altitude, levels of erythropoietin fall to within the normal or control range (Chapter 8) and similarly, in over half the patients with polycythemia due to hypoxic lung disease, erythropoietin levels are within the normal range (Wedzicha *et al.* 1985).

Plasma volume, as already mentioned, is increased in COLD. Plasma volume is decreased on first going to altitude but returns towards normal after about 3 months (Chapter 8). In high altitude residents plasma volume is decreased by about 27 per cent compared with sea level residents (Sanchez *et al.* 1970).

31.2.4 Fluid balance and peripheral edema

Patients with COLD are at risk of developing peripheral edema, mainly dependent, and raised venous pressure. They have been shown to have a defect of sodium and water handling; they fail to excrete a water load at the normal rate if they have a high P_{CO_2} (Farber *et al.* 1975, Stewart *et al.* 1991a). COLD patients have a reduced effective renal plasma flow and urinary sodium excretion. They may have raised plasma renin activity and aldosterone levels. The development of peripheral edema may take place without increase in body weight (Campbell *et al.* 1975), suggesting a transfer of fluid from intracellular to extracellular compartments. This is in contrast to edema formation in cardiac failure when, as expected, it is associated with weight gain. How these findings can be fitted into a coherent account of the mechanism of this condition is still not clear.

The fluid balance in people at high altitude is also far from clear. It seems likely that the development of acute mountain sickness (AMS) is associated with fluid retention, whereas the healthy response on going to high altitude is a diuresis. Peripheral edema frequently occurs in AMS, often affecting the periorbital regions and hands as well as the ankles, whereas pulmonary edema and cerebral edema are the malignant forms of AMS (Chapters 18–20). In the acclimatized there is no evidence of any problem in fluid handling.

Whether there are analogies between the mechanisms of AMS and cor pulmonale are questions for future research in both fields. For instance, it is the COLD patients with high Pa_{CO_2} who are likely to develop cor pulmonale, and in subjects at altitude higher Pa_{CO_2} may be associated with AMS.

31.2.5 The circulation

The systemic circulation is not importantly affected by either COLD or altitude. There is often mild elevation of the blood pressure in both cases, but there are important changes in the pulmonary circulation. In both patients with COLD and those at high altitude there is increased pulmonary resistance, resulting in raised pulmonary artery and right ventricular pressures and similar electrocardiographic (ECG) changes (i.e. right axis deviation) (Chapter 7).

31.2.6 Cerebral blood flow (CBF)

In patients with COLD the CBF is increased due to the cerebral vasodilatory effects of both hypoxia and hypercarbia. On going to altitude the CBF is normally modestly increased at first, then tends to fall towards sea level values (Severinghaus et al. 1966b). This is due to the low Pa_{CO_2}, which tends to reduce CBF opposing the effect of hypoxia. Polycythemia, as it develops in both COLD patients and those at high altitude, will tend to reduce CBF. Very low CBF values have been inferred from the large arteriovenous cerebral oxygen difference in Andean altitude residents with marked polycythemia (Milledge and Sorensen 1972) whereas patients with COLD are to a degree protected from cerebral hypoxia by their hypercapnia, which causes increased CBF.

31.2.7 Alimentary system

There has been little work on the effect of hypoxia on bowel function in either patients or individuals at high altitude. Milledge (1972) showed that small bowel absorption, as measured by the xylose absorption test, was reduced in patients with either hypoxic lung disease or cyanotic heart disease, when the saturation fell below about 70 per cent. It was suggested that this finding might explain the loss of weight which often characterizes patients with severe emphysema towards the end of the course of their disease.

Subjects at high altitude tend to lose weight and, although much of this weight reduction is due to reduced energy intake, there has been uncontrolled evidence that at altitudes above about 5500 m there is continued weight loss even with adequate energy intake (Pugh 1962a). During the American Medical Research Expedition to Everest (AMREE) in 1981, there was a significant reduction in both fat and xylose absorption in subjects at 6300 m (Blume 1984). More recently Dinmore et al. (1994) found

that absorption of both D-xylose and 3-o-methyl-D-glucose was reduced in subjects at 6300 m, and Travis et al. (1993) also found a reduction in the ratio of these carbohydrates at 5400 m, indicating impairment of absorption (Chapter 14).

31.2.8 Mental effects

Patients with hypoxia due to COLD frequently have disturbance of mental function, especially during exacerbations, when their P_{O_2} falls to very low levels. In the milder stages these disturbances may be quite subtle but, as hypoxia becomes severe, patients become irritable, restless and confused. Motor function may become impaired with ataxia. These changes are very similar to those observed in healthy subjects exposed to acute hypoxia in decompression chambers. However, in acclimatized subjects, very low saturations may be seen, especially on exercise, with very little mental disturbance, though at extreme altitude and with AMS these mental problems may be seen (Chapter 16).

31.2.9 Summary

Table 31.1 summarizes the similarities and differences between patients with COLD and those at high altitude. Healthy people at altitude differ in a number of important respects from patients with hypoxia due to COLD. Most of these differences are attributable to the one being hypocapnic and the other hypercapnic. However, the hypoxia is, of course, similar and results in similar effects on a number of bodily systems, including erythropoiesis, muscles, the alimentary system and mental function. Providing the carbon dioxide effect is borne in mind, persons at high altitude can be considered as a model for the hypoxia of COLD.

31.3 INTERSTITIAL LUNG DISEASE

Within this category are included such conditions as sarcoidosis, fibrosing alveolitis, allergic alveolitis (farmer's lung, etc.), pneumoconiosis (including silicosis) and other causes of diffuse pulmonary fibrosis. Some types of pneumonia, for instance that due to *Pneumocystis pneumoniae*, which are diffuse rather than lobar, present similar pathophysiology. In all these conditions the main problem is an impairment of gas exchange. There usually develops some restriction of lung volumes as well but, unlike COLD, there is little or no airways obstruction. The result is that hypoxia develops without any rise in Pa_{CO_2}. Indeed, the Pa_{CO_2} is characteristically decreased as it is in subjects at high altitude.

The dominant symptom in these patients is breathlessness on exertion and, later, even at rest. The arterial desaturation becomes worse on exertion just as it does in those at extreme altitudes (Chapter 12). The cause of the hypoxemia in these patients is a defect of gas transfer. This is due to ventilation/perfusion ratio inhomogeneity and an increase in the diffusion path length, that is, a thickening of the alveolar capillary membrane by cellular infiltrate or fibrosis. In most cases the ventilation/perfusion mismatch problem is the more important. These conditions usually develop over a period of months and a subject well acclimatized to high altitude is a very good model for the hypoxia of a patient with interstitial lung disease.

31.4 CYANOTIC HEART DISEASE

Most patients in this group have congenital cardiac defects which result in right to left shunts and therefore in cyanosis. Diagnoses include tetralogy of Fallot, ventricular and atrial septal defects with reversed shunts, patent ductus arteriosus with reversed shunt, and most forms of anomalous venous drainage.

These patients, often hypoxic from birth, sometimes have most extreme cyanosis with severe polycythemia. Pa_{CO_2} is usually in the normal range but may be low as is found at high altitude. Those with extreme polycythemia, in whom the hematocrit can be up to 70 per cent, resemble cases of chronic mountain sickness and may suffer the same symptoms of lethargy, poor concentration, being easily fatigued, etc. (Chapter 21). Though they do get out of breath on exertion, dyspnea is not a prominent symptom, perhaps because the condition has been present since birth. Again, like chronic mountain sickness and the 'blue bloater' type of COLD patient, it may be due to a blunted respiratory drive. The histopathology of the pulmonary circulation of children with cyanotic heart

disease is comparable to that of high altitude residents (Heath and Williams 1995 pp. 121–39). The normal demuscularization of pulmonary arteries after birth is retarded so that the wall thickness, especially of the resistance arterioles, is increased compared with the normal pulmonary arterial tree (Chapter 17).

Children with cyanotic heart disease have retarded growth, as do children at altitude (Chapter 17). If their defect can be corrected by surgery, growth accelerates and they catch up with their peers. If their arterial saturation is below about 70 per cent they will have impaired small bowel absorption which may contribute to their growth retardation. Surgical repair of the defect relieves the cyanosis and the small bowel absorption improves (Milledge 1972). In this respect they resemble those at high altitude (Chapter 14).

31.5 LOW OUTPUT CARDIAC CONDITIONS

Ischemic heart disease and cardiomyopathy can result in low cardiac output. In milder forms of this condition the output at rest is normal but there is failure of the normal response to exercise of an increase in cardiac output. Patients are symptom free at rest but find that their exercise tolerance is markedly diminished; they can only walk slowly and the slightest uphill slope causes them to stop and rest. They are not limited by dyspnea but by fatigue in the leg muscles. In these patients the Pa_{O_2} is normal, but blood flow is limited, which reduces oxygen delivery and results in tissue hypoxia. The tissues most affected are those which have a high extraction of oxygen and which increase their oxygen demand on exercise, that is, the working muscles. The mixed venous Pa_{O_2} is very low but Pa_{CO_2} is normal.

The subject at high altitude is obviously not such a good model for this type of patient, but, especially at extreme altitude, there are physiological similarities. The maximum cardiac rate and output are limited to some degree (Chapter 12), so that, during large muscle mass dynamic exercise, oxygen delivery to the working muscles is limited. There is certainly tissue hypoxia, especially of these muscles, due to a reduction in delivery of oxygen and possibly also to limitation of oxygen diffusion at the tissue level (Chapter 12). As mentioned in section 31.2.1, the sensation of work being limited by 'the legs giving out' rather than dyspnea alone is common both to individuals at high altitude and to these patients.

31.6   CHRONIC ANEMIA

Patients with chronic anemia have a very similar pathophysiology to patients with low cardiac output. The oxygen delivery to the tissues is reduced in their case by the reduced oxygen capacity of the blood. Cardiac output increases, partly due to a decreased viscosity of the blood, and this partially compensates for the loss of oxygen-carrying capacity. Nevertheless, oxygen delivery is reduced, especially to the working muscles, during exercise. The resulting symptoms are similar to those of low cardiac output and have their analogy in those at extreme altitude.

31.7   HEMOGLOBINOPATHIES WITH ALTERED OXYGEN AFFINITY

The hemoglobinopathies are a rare, but interesting, group of conditions in which patients have a genetic defect resulting in minor changes to their hemoglobin. These changes result in their hemoglobin having either a greater or a reduced affinity for oxygen compared with normal hemoglobin. The oxygen dissociation curve is shifted either to the left (increased affinity) or to the right (decreased affinity).

Patients with increased affinity hemoglobin experience a degree of tissue hypoxia because oxygen is not readily unloaded in the tissues. This evidently stimulates erythropoietin production since these patients are typically polycythemic.

Conversely, patients with decreased affinity hemoglobin are anemic, presumably because their tissue P_{O_2} is higher than normal, as evidenced by the ease with which oxygen is unloaded there. At moderate altitude this may confer some advantage, though this has not been demonstrated, and on exercise the difficulty of oxygen loading in the lungs would probably outweigh any advantage in the tissues. At higher altitude the difficulty in loading oxygen into the blood in the lungs would certainly be a disadvantage.

Indeed, increased oxygen affinity is probably beneficial, since, at high altitude, the advantage in the lungs more than outweighs the disadvantage in the tissues. A study by Hebbel et al. (1978) of two sub-jects with Hb Andrews-Minneapolis, a high affinity hemoglobin ($P_{50} = 17$ mm Hg), found that they had less reduction in exercise capacity on going to altitude than their siblings with normal hemoglobin.

Normal subjects at high altitude, especially at extreme altitudes above 8000 m, have their oxygen dissociation curves shifted to the left by respiratory alkalosis; this is probably advantageous for the above reason (Chapters 9 and 11). Thus, those at high altitude can be a model for some aspects of hemoglobinopathies.

31.8   CONTRIBUTION OF HIGH ALTITUDE PHYSIOLOGY TO CLINICAL MEDICINE

31.8.1   Partial pressure of gases

The importance to clinical medicine of Paul Bert's work published in his landmark La Pression Barométrique (1878) is enormous. This work clearly showed that it is the partial pressure of oxygen, rather than the barometric pressure or oxygen percentage, that determines the effect of hypoxia in causing mountain sickness and death. Although he did not work at altitude himself he corresponded with and encouraged people who did, and used chambers to reduce the ambient pressure for both human and animal subjects. He can truly be claimed as a father figure for both altitude physiology and aviation medicine. Of course, other physiologists and clinicians after Paul Bert developed the idea of the partial pressure of gases and its importance, including such workers as Haldane, Douglas, FitzGerald, Henderson, Schneider, Bohr, Krogh and Barcroft, all of whose work was stimulated by the problems of altitude physiology.

The concept of the effect of gases on the body being due to their partial pressures (especially of oxygen and carbon dioxide) is fundamental to respiratory medicine and physiology, and to aviation and underwater medicine. In anesthesia the partial pressure of gases extends to all volatile agents.

31.8.2   Hematology

The polycythemia of high altitude was first documented by Viault (1890) and has been extensively studied ever since. As a tool in hematological research, this stimulus to erythropoiesis has been invaluable. Much of the early work on the oxygen dissociation curve, by Haldane, Barcroft and others, owes its stimulus to the question of human survival and acclimatization to high altitude. These 'lessons from high altitude' are amongst the foundation stones of modern hematology, open heart surgery, respiratory medicine, cardiology and anesthetics. More recently, research on 2,3-diphosphoglycerate and its influence on the position of the oxygen dissociation curve has been studied at altitude (Chapter 9) and the results incorporated into the body of hematological knowledge.

31.8.3 Respiratory medicine

Work on the effect of altitude acclimatization on the control of breathing (Chapter 5) has helped in the understanding of the changes in control of breathing in patients with COLD with hypercapnia. These patients 'acclimatize' to a high Pa_{CO_2} and their carbon dioxide ventilatory response becomes blunted, the opposite of altitude acclimatization. They are then dependent on hypoxia as a drive to ventilation and may have their breathing depressed if given high inspired oxygen mixtures to breathe.

In patients with asthma, as the condition worsens, their Pa_{O_2} falls. At first the Pa_{CO_2} is reduced because of the hypoxic drive to ventilation; then, with increasing airways resistance, Pa_{CO_2} rises to 'normal' and finally rises above normal. Cochrane et al. (1980) have pointed out that the Pa_{CO_2} in the middle of these three stages should be below 'normal', depending on the degree of hypoxia. Drawing on altitude data, Wolff (1980) gives a predicted value for Pa_{CO_2}, dependent on Pa_{O_2}. The patient should be considered to be in respiratory failure if the Pa_{CO_2} is above this value. For instance, a patient with a Pa_{O_2} of 60 mm Hg has a predicted Pa_{CO_2} of 30 mm Hg, assuming full acclimatization to this degree of hypoxia.

Study of the increasing arterial desaturation due to diffusion limitations found in climbers on exercise at altitude (Chapter 6) helps in the understanding of the similar problems in patients at sea level with interstitial lung disease and limited diffusing capacity.

31.8.4 Cardiology

The phenomenon of the hypoxic pulmonary pressor response has been studied at sea level and altitude in humans and animals, with results from altitude stimulating work at sea level and vice versa. The insights gained have helped in the understanding of patients with pulmonary hypertension due to hypoxia secondary to heart or lung disease.

31.8.5 Other areas of clinical medicine

High altitude physiology and medicine have lessons for other branches of clinical medicine, for example:

- small bowel function, which is impaired at altitude as well as in hypoxic patients (Chapter 14)
- metabolism, in the slower growth of children at altitude, and patients hypoxic due to congenital heart disease
- reproductive medicine, in the problem of fertility at altitude
- endocrinology, in the effect of hypoxia on various endocrine systems (Chapter 15), and their counterparts in patients with similar conditions.

However, these fields have been less thoroughly explored both by high altitude and by clinical scientists. No doubt high altitude has yet more lessons to teach clinical medicine in the future.

32

Practicalities of field studies

SUMMARY

The practical difficulties of carrying out good research at altitude in the mountains are obvious and are considered in this chapter. However, there are many compensations. The difficulties can be met by careful planning and by choosing projects and techniques that are appropriate for field work.

The advantages and disadvantage of field versus chamber studies, including cost, are discussed. There is a place for both types of study and they are complementary. Most of the techniques of classical cardiorespiratory and exercise physiology have been used at altitude. Blood urine and saliva samples can be taken, stored and brought back for biochemical and hormonal analysis. With the advance of electronics quite sophisticated techniques in sleep studies, audiometry, visual fields, psychometric testing and even Doppler echocardiography and near-infrared spectroscopy have been used in the field. Laptop computers have been used at great altitudes and can be used on line with the more sophisticated equipment.

In planning either a pure scientific expedition or one in which science is combined with mountaineering, it is important to ensure the support of all members for the scientific program. This is best done by communicating the objectives of the program to everyone in simple terms and giving all members (professional and lay) an active role in the science.

32.1 INTRODUCTION

The problems associated with field research in the great ranges are obvious and include cold, hypoxia, fatigue and lack of amenities of civilization such as piped hot and cold water, reliable electricity supplies, heating, etc. The lack of easy access to specialist advice from service engineers or colleagues can be a severe problem. However, there are compensations. Perhaps the greatest is the elimination of distractions from the work in hand. There is no commuting to work, no committees, no lectures to give or attend, no family commitments and little in the way of social events. If the site has been well chosen there is the added advantage of living for a while among the grandest and most beautiful scenery on Earth.

32.1.1 Planning, testing and practice

Many of the data referred to in this book have been collected on expeditions to the major mountain regions of the world. Good scientific work under these conditions can be difficult but is perfectly possible, providing adequate time, thought and effort are given to planning and preparation. The preparation time will be at least 3–6 months for a small expedition and 2 years or more for a major scientific expedition.

The techniques and apparatus to be used must be tested adequately beforehand. Many studies require control measurements at sea level and these are best carried out using the same equipment as will be used in the field. Not only are results more reliable if the same equipment is used, but problems and deficiencies are identified before leaving for the mountains. Practice with the equipment in the comfort of a standard laboratory is also highly desirable, though not absolutely essential. One of the authors of this book taught one of the others the technique of gas analysis using the Lloyd–Haldane apparatus during the course of their first Himalayan expedition at 5800 m. Even if study protocols do not demand control measurements before leaving, it is advisable to carry out a complete dummy run of the observations to be made, listing all the equipment needed, down to the last rubber band and needle.

32.1.2   Field versus chamber studies

Although this chapter is concerned with field studies at altitude, much valuable work has been done in decompression chambers. The advantages of chamber studies over field studies are:

- Rate of ascent and descent, and altitude can be controlled to suit the problem under study.
- Other factors such as temperature and humidity can be controlled.
- More invasive procedures can be justified since, in the event of some complication, help is readily available.

The disadvantages are perhaps not so obvious, especially to people who have not been involved with such work. Living for more than a few hours in a decompression chamber is not pleasant. The environment is usually noisy, confined and often smelly – though this is less true of large modern facilities such as the chamber at Natick, MA, operated by the US Army Institute of Environmental Medicine. However, even the largest chamber is cramped compared with being in the mountains and it is difficult and very boring to take much exercise. Acclimatization seems to be slower and less complete in chamber studies than on the mountain. Values for P_{CO_2} are consistently higher for the same altitude in chambers than on the mountain. This may be due to less exercise taken by subjects in chambers or due to other factors or stresses (Rahn and Otis 1949, Houston 1988–9, West 1988b). In studies lasting more than a few hours, boredom, and hence morale, is a problem. A limiting factor for chamber studies is the number of subjects that can be accommodated. This might be less of a drawback for most physiological studies but it would be important in studies of acute mountain sickness (AMS) where a large number of subjects is needed to ensure that some have symptoms and others are unaffected. Finally, chambers are built with specific tasks in mind; usually their use is geared to short-term experiments on acute hypoxia and so they may not be available to altitude scientists for prolonged experiments.

In comparing the results of studies carried out in the field with those done in low pressure chambers, it is useful to look at the results obtained from the Silver Hut Expedition and the American Medical Research Expedition to Everest (AMREE), and compare these with the two major simulation studies to date, Operation Everest I and II. In many areas, the results of the two types of studies have been very similar. For example, the measurements of maximal oxygen consumption for the inspired P_{O_2} on the summit of Mount Everest were almost identical in AMREE and Operation Everest II. However, the two types of studies have yielded quantitatively different information in some areas, presumably because of the different periods of acclimatization. The main differences are seen in three areas:

- Alveolar gas composition. The shorter period of acclimatization in the two low pressure chamber studies to date resulted in very different alveolar P_{O_2} and P_{CO_2} values at extreme altitudes compared with the results from the field studies (see Figure 12.4). The differences are particularly marked for Operation Everest I and are discussed in section 12.3.3.
- Blood lactate concentration. Blood lactate concentrations after maximal exercise were appreciably higher on Operation Everest II than on

the AMREE and extensive field measurements made by Cerretelli (1980). These are shown in Figure 12.5 and discussed in section 12.3.4. Again the differences are presumably due to the shorter period of acclimatization on Operation Everest II. This topic is discussed fully by West (1993b).

- Exercise ventilation at extreme altitude. As was pointed out in section 11.3, both the Silver Hut Expedition and AMREE found a decrease in ventilation at maximal exercise at extreme altitude (see Figure 11.3). By contrast, maximal exercise ventilation on Operation Everest II continued to increase with greater altitude. The reason for the differences is not clear; it is presumably related to the different degrees of acclimatization.

32.1.3 Cost

It is often assumed that chamber studies must be cheaper than field studies. This is not necessarily the case. Accounting in both cases is a very inexact science. The cost of a mountaineering expedition is clear, but in many cases the climbers are going to the mountains anyway and the scientific work can be carried out at very little extra cost. Chambers represent a huge capital cost but usually the altitude scientist is not called upon to contribute to this. However, even the running costs of a chamber are not inconsiderable. Apart from the subjects and scientists, chambers have to manned 24 h a day by teams of highly trained technicians whose salaries have to be met. If all expenses are charged realistically to the study, long-term chamber projects are very expensive.

In summary, chambers are very useful in studies of acute and subacute hypoxia lasting a few hours. Their advantage over field studies becomes less as the duration of the study and the number of subjects increase. Thus the two modes of research are complementary.

32.1.4 Personnel management

The psychodynamics of a mountaineering expedition are fascinating and of vital importance in achieving both climbing and scientific goals, but too great an emphasis on psychological factors may well be self-defeating. The essential aspect of leadership of a scientific expedition is to ensure that the whole team is as fully aware of the scientific program as possible and in sympathy with it. Climbers may be suspicious of scientists but can understand quite abstruse scientific argument providing terms and concepts are explained in everyday language. They are naturally interested in topics such as AMS, work performance at altitude and the effect of altitude on various biological systems and can become enthusiastic participants, providing the issues are clearly explained.

Time spent in presenting the scientific program to the whole team is well spent, as was evident from experience on the AMREE, where climbers as well as climbing scientists were enthusiastic about working on the scientific program as well as climbing the mountain. In a large party with a number of scientists it is equally important that the various scientific members understand the relevance of each other's projects and are in sympathy with them.

After presenting the program, the next essential is to delegate responsibility as widely as possible. It is highly desirable that every member of the expedition has a job to do in relation to the scientific program, for two reasons.

- The programs are usually overambitious in terms of what can be achieved in the time available and, by sharing the work out, the load on the main scientists is reduced.
- By having a designated job, each member feels he or she is personally committed to the scientific program, with consequent improvement in morale. This is particularly important if nonscientific members are expected to act as subjects. Having a job to do as well as being a subject avoids the feeling, 'they only want me as a guinea-pig'. There are many jobs which can be carried out perfectly well by expedition members who are not scientifically trained, such as measurement of urine volume or body weights, or clerking results as another member reads them off. Even the spinning and pipetting of blood samples can be quickly taught. A further important aspect of delegating work as widely as possible is that it helps to keep the work going should any of the scientific members be unable to function owing to illness or accident.

32.2 LABORATORY WORK IN THE FIELD

32.2.1 Laboratory accommodation

However small the expedition, some form of designated laboratory accommodation is recommended. For small expeditions this will be a tent; if at all possible it should be of the type high enough to stand up in, and have a folding table and chairs. Cold is a major problem in the mountains. Most types of scientific work cannot be carried out in temperatures below 5–10 °C, and certainly not below freezing. Battery operated instruments work poorly below freezing, plastic bags crack easily and venepuncture is difficult because of vasoconstriction. Under severe freezing conditions blood samples will freeze and hemolyse. If there is no space heating available, the time for scientific work will be limited to the warmest hours of the day. However, it must also be said that at high altitude the sun is strong and when it is shining on a tent the temperature rises rapidly inside, even though the outside shade temperature remains well below zero. On the recent Medical Research Expeditions to Kangchenjunga no less than five large tents, each 3 m × 5 m floor area, were set up at Base Camp (5100 m) in which up to 12 teams successfully worked on over 20 projects. There was also a large dome tent which was used for a mess tent, communications, battery and power control facility.

On a large expedition, good laboratory conditions can be achieved by using a modern 'tent', such as a Weatherport (Hansen Weatherport, Gunniston, CO). This is a tubular aluminium frame with padded plastic cover made in various sizes which proved very satisfactory in the Western Cwm in 1981 (West 1985a). Heating was provided by a propane stove of the type designed for mobile homes in which a heat exchanger heats the air, which is blown into the tent. In this way there is no possibility of carbon monoxide from the burning propane entering the tent. Carbon monoxide poisoning is a real danger from less sophisticated forms of heating.

The Silver Hut similarly provided almost ideal conditions in 1960–1, though at far greater expense. It was a prefabricated hut made from boxed-up marine plywood members with foam insulation within the box sections. A similar hut but using fiberglass sections was used at Base Camp on the AMREE and was also successful. Work surfaces, seating and lighting should also be provided. In such conditions, the working day can be prolonged into the night if necessary, allowing more work to be carried out than in an unheated laboratory, as well as avoiding the problem of cold as an interfering factor if one is studying the effects of chronic hypoxia.

32.2.2 Electrical supply

Early in the planning of an expedition the decision will have to be made about whether to use mains voltage apparatus or to restrict work to battery operated and nonelectrical equipment.

The advantages of mains voltage equipment are obvious, and certain types of equipment are only available as mains operated versions. It is possible to get petrol-powered generators that weigh not more than one porter load, and on a large expedition this is the chosen option. The disadvantages are not inconsiderable. In order to try to ensure that one generator is working, at least two must be taken; even then it is quite likely that both will break down. Extra spare parts must be taken and at least one expedition member should be a mechanic with knowledge of that particular generator. Altitude affects petrol engines as it does the animal organism and adjustments must be made to the fuel mix, usually by changing the jets in the carburetor. Some generators are available with variable jets, in which case the settings required for various altitudes should be ascertained before the expedition. The power output declines with altitude, as it does in humans, so a more powerful generator must be taken than would be needed for the same equipment at sea level. Petrol and oil must also be carried.

Alternative sources of electrical power have been used. In the Silver Hut Expedition much of the electricity used over the winter was derived from a wind generator and on the AMREE a battery of solar cells gave almost 30 A at 15 V. In both cases this power was fed into 12 V storage batteries and mains voltage was obtained by using converters. These introduced their own degree of inefficiency, as well as further expense and transport penalties. In 1998 on Kangchenjunga we were able to supply almost all our not inconsiderable power needs from solar cells because we were fortunate with the weather. However, this required discipline in the use of power especially in the morning to allow the batteries to charge up in the morning sun after they had been used at night often for communication by satellite phone. These alternative sources cannot be relied upon and petrol generators are needed for back up.

32.2.3 Water, reagents, etc.

Water at altitude is obtained either from melting snow or ice or from mountain streams. In either case it has a fairly high degree of purity so that for most chemical uses it will be adequate if water is passed through a deionizing column which will include a filter. If distilled water is essential it will have to be carried out from home.

Analytical balances are impractical in the field. Reagents should be weighed at the home institution into capped tubes. These can then be made up in the field as needed by dissolving in deionized water.

32.3 RESPIRATORY MEASUREMENTS

32.3.1 Classical methods

Classical measurements of ventilation and oxygen consumption using Douglas bags, taps and valves are as easy to carry out in the field as in the laboratory (providing all the bits are remembered, including the nose clip). The gas meter will be of the dry type or a Wright's respirometer (anemometer) can be used if care is taken not to empty the Douglas bag too fast through it (accuracy ± 2 per cent). The gas analysis is more of a problem for the physiologist used to using a mass spectrometer. If mains voltage is available (section 32.2.2) an infrared carbon dioxide meter and paramagnetic oxygen meter can be used, though calibrating gases will have to be carried. Paramagnetic oxygen analyzers are available as battery operated instruments but carbon dioxide meters are not. Alternatively, one can be really classical and use the Lloyd–Haldane or Scholander apparatus and analyze samples chemically.

Care should be taken with modern Douglas bags. The plastic that is used now for these bags is much less likely to become hard and brittle in the cold than was previously the case but care may be needed if overnight temperatures have been very low. A repair kit should be taken.

32.3.2 Alveolar gas sampling

Alveolar or end-tidal gas samples have been taken from subjects at altitude on a number of expeditions, in 1981 from the summit of Everest itself.

Glass ampoules were successfully used on a number of expeditions, including the Silver Hut Expedition, when samples were brought back from 7830 m. These were of 50 mL capacity and had a stem with two necks in it. The ampoules were pre-evacuated before leaving. In the field, a Haldane–Priestley sample was delivered down a tube with the ampoule attached to a side arm by a short length of pressure tubing. Surgical forceps were then used to break the glass within the pressure tube and the sample entered the ampoule. With the rubber tube clamped the ampoule was brought back to base where, with a suitable gas flame, the ampoule was sealed at the lower neck and transported back for analysis.

More recently, 20 mL aerosol cans of the type used in asthma inhalers have been successfully used. These cans, supplied by the pharmaceutical industry, had the metering device removed and were then pre-evacuated. They were shown to hold their vacuum for at least 6 months. In the field, the simplest apparatus involved merely a T-shaped piece of tubing into the stem of which the can was fitted with its nozzle resting on a shoulder. The subject delivered a Haldane–Priestley alveolar sample across the T to which was added a soft, widebore tube; the can was then depressed, which opened its valve, and the sample entered the can. Releasing the can sealed it again and it was then transported back for analysis.

The actual device used on the summit of Everest was rather more complicated (West 1985a); it held six pre-evacuated cans in a rotating cylinder to which two handles were attached. The subject blew across the top of the cylinder through two one-way valves and the end-tidal gas was caught between them. On squeezing the handles, one can was opened and a sample taken. On releasing the handles the can was closed; the cylinder rotated to present the next can for a second sample (Maret *et al.* 1984).

Analysis at the home institute was by mass spectrometry using a special inlet device which would accept the aerosol can. The sample volume at sea level pressure would be only 5–7 mL.

If rapid carbon dioxide and oxygen analyzers are taken, end-tidal gases can be measured over sufficient time to be sure of a steady state.

32.3.3 The Oxylog and electronic spirometers

The Oxylog is a portable electronic instrument giving a continuous read-out of minute ventilation and oxygen consumption (updated each minute), and the total ventilation and oxygen consumption since it was last reset. The subject wears a mask, into the inspiratory port of which is fitted an electronic spirometer or anemometer. It is normally supplied with rechargeable batteries but can be modified to take non-rechargeable batteries. The output (V and V_{O_2}) can be recorded for hours on a portable tape recorder. It is accurate for submaximal work rates (Milledge et al. 1983c) but is not suitable for $V_{O_2 max}$ measurements.

Ventilation alone can be recorded using one of a number of electronic spirometers such as that used in the Oxylog, though the resistance of most commercially available models is not well tolerated at the very high ventilation found in climbers exercising at altitude. Such an electronic spirometer was successfully used by Pizzo near the summit of Everest (West et al. 1983c).

32.3.4 Pulse oximetry

The pulse oximeter allows the easy measurement of arterial oxygen saturation with a very lightweight battery powered instrument. There are many models on the market now and most are accurate and reliable. They also read heart rate. Many also have data storage facilities and data can be downloaded into laptop computers. This allows them to be readily used for sleep studies. They are not suitable for ambulatory measurements, though they can be used during exercise on a cycle ergometer. The sensors are made for use either on the finger or earlobe, the former being usually preferred. It is essential for the finger to be warm in order to get a good signal.

32.4 CARDIOLOGICAL MEASUREMENTS

32.4.1 Electrocardiography (ECG)

The ECG is easy to record at altitude, either the classical 12-lead ECG at rest, or ambulatory recording over many hours. Such recordings have been made on Everest climbers (West et al. 1983c). The pulse

rate can be obtained from such recordings. Computer analysis can be carried out looking for arrhythmia and spectral analysis of R-R intervals, etc. Care is needed in the electrode placement and attachment (as at sea level).

32.4.2 Echocardiography

Until recently the size, weight and complexity of ultrasound machines for conducting echocardiography were such that there was no question of using this technique in the field. However, machines are getting smaller, lighter and more reliable and it can now be considered as a possibility. Such a machine was used by Dubowitz at the Himalayan Rescue Association Clinic at Pheriche (4243 m) to complete a study measuring pulmonary artery pressure by Doppler echocardiography in trekkers on their way to Everest Base Camp (Dubowitz and Peacock 1999). The same machine was taken to Kangchenjunga Base Camp (5100 m) but unfortunately developed a fatal electrical fault soon after the study started.

32.4.3 Cardiac catheterization

More invasive cardiac techniques, such as right heart and pulmonary artery catheterization, have been discussed and, though possible under field conditions with mains voltage electricity available, are probably not justified, though this is debatable. Catheterization has been carried out in chamber studies, most extensively in Operation Everest II (Houston et al. 1987); in skilled hands it carries very little risk.

32.5 SLEEP STUDIES

Sleep studies have been carried out on a number of expeditions where mains voltage was provided (Chapter 13). ECGs, electroencephalograms (EEGs), electro-oculograms, ear and pulse oximetry and respiratory movements have all been monitored simultaneously and recorded on tape and paper while the subject was asleep. Most of this monitoring can be carried out with battery operated instruments but it is important that some way of monitoring the signals during the recording is provided, even if the analysis from tape is left until after the expedition.

32.6 BLOOD SAMPLING AND STORAGE

32.6.1 Venepuncture

There is little problem in performing venepuncture in the field. Two physician climbers took samples from each other on the South Col of Everest the morning after climbing to the summit (Winslow *et al.* 1984). 'Vacutainer' systems using pre-evacuated tubes and double-ended needles are particularly convenient, as the sampling tubes are used for centrifuging. They fill (from the vein) perfectly well at altitude.

32.6.2 Centrifuging blood samples

If mains voltage is available, a small electrical centrifuge can be used and this presents no problem. Hand centrifuges can be used but require quite a lot of muscle power. They need to be spun very vigorously for 15–20 min; even then the cells are not as tightly packed as by even the lowest powered electrical centrifuge. This means that the yield of plasma is less, typically a maximum of 5 mL from 10 mL of blood. When subjects become polycythemic the problem becomes worse.

These hand centrifuges usually take four 10 mL tubes compared with six or eight in the small electrical centrifuges; they are really intended for spinning urine samples and are not designed for such vigorous spinning. Older designs with brass gears and cast metal casings stand up better than do modern models with nylon gears and plastic cases. A firm bench on which to clamp the centrifuge is essential. However, with all these drawbacks, hand centrifuging of blood is possible if mains voltage is unavailable. A dry battery centrifuge is not a viable possibility.

32.6.3 Arterial blood sampling and analysis

If the usual precautions are taken and if the doctor is experienced in the procedure, there should be no problem in arterial puncture. Arterial cannulation is more hazardous and probably not justified in the field. The measurement of arterial pH, P_{CO_2} and P_{O_2} is really not possible without mains voltage for the various meters and temperature control. Although there is no inherent reason why these electrodes could not be run from battery operated electronics, the market is not big enough for manufacturers to develop them commercially.

32.6.4 Sample storage

Plasma, serum and urine samples can be deep frozen, stored and transported back to the home laboratory by using liquid nitrogen in a suitable container. In previous editions of this book we described how a portable deep-freeze container could be made by using a 28 L liquid nitrogen flask (often called a Dewar flask) and packing it with dry ice (solid carbon dioxide). This gave up to 130 days of use. However, dry ice is no longer readily obtainable so this method has now been abandoned. There was also the disadvantage that although the necks of these flasks were quite narrow, they could not be tightly sealed because the nitrogen could not evolve and there would be danger of explosion. Therefore there was always the potential for spillage of liquid nitrogen and harm to porters, though I know of no such accident ever happening.

However, systems have now been developed for the safe transport of deep-frozen samples using liquid nitrogen trapped in an absorbent matrix inside a vacuum container. One such commercial system is called a Cryopak. Much of the capacity of the flask is taken up with the filler material and there is quite a small well for the samples. The makers supply a vial holder or canister, which slides into this well and takes sample vials. This allows vials to be removed, inspected, sampled and replaced but further reduces the capacity of the flask. Alternatively the canister can be dispensed with and vials just thrown into the well. This allows more samples, but at the risk of losing labels, and makes sorting more of a problem. There is a range of flask sizes with capacity ranging from 30 to 324 2 mL vials. The gross weight when charged with nitrogen ranges from 7.3 to 22.7 kg. The static holding time (full of liquid nitrogen) is 30 days but the working time (absorbed nitrogen only, empty well) is only 21 days. The flask, of course, can be topped up with liquid nitrogen. This system is safer than the previous one since once any excess liquid nitrogen has evolved, there is no risk of spillage. This means that they can be freighted on aircraft as normal instead of going as 'dangerous goods' and, of course, they are safer as porter loads. This system was used on the recent Kangchenjunga Expedition. The more limited time available is a disadvantage and without the benefit of helicopter freight and topping up we would have had difficulty in keeping our samples frozen until return to London.

Samples should be taken into PTFE tubes with good screw caps. Tubes should have a matt surface for labeling, which should be done in pencil; they should then be covered in low temperature adhesive tape. During transportation (if the canister or holder is dispensed with) these tubes are constantly chafed together, and unless the labels are firm they will come off or run and all will be lost. It was found that pencil under low temperature clear adhesive tape was safe.

For shorter periods of up to 1–2 weeks, it may be adequate to use polystyrene boxes of dry ice. Although the newer Cryopak flasks are not treated as 'dangerous goods', airline regulations are frequently changed and anyone planning to use these or other systems should check the current regulations with the airline they are using, including the container requirements in force. Airlines are usually familiar with handling 'medical samples' in this way but expect to deal with recognized shippers. The bureaucracy and expense of such a shipment are not inconsiderable; delays of a few days at each end can be anticipated and must be allowed for in calculating the time available at deep-freeze temperature.

32.7 HEMATOLOGY

Much hematology can be done with quite simple equipment in the field. Battery operated microcentrifuges for packed cell volume are available commercially. Hemoglobin can be measured by the cyanmethemoglobin method and a battery operated spectrometer. Cell count can be carried out by classical microscopy techniques. With mains voltage electricity and P_{O_2} electrodes, the oxygen dissociation curve and P_{50} can be measured (Winslow *et al.* 1984).

32.8 COMPUTERS

Laptop or notebook computers are now commonplace on expeditions. They are now reasonably reliable and robust and, compared with much scientific equipment, they are not expensive. Their power requirements are not great. If generators are being taken there is no problem; otherwise their batteries can be recharged from solar panels if necessary. Therefore there need be no hesitation in including computers in expedition equipment. Like all battery operated apparatus they work better at comfortable temperatures but are no more fussy than ECG machines, for instance. Computers have many applications, from writing reports to online control of other equipment. They are good for storing data, on or off line with backup on discs. If more than one computer is to be taken, as is likely, it is worth ensuring that the same programs are installed on all of them so that one can act as a backup for any other machine.

32.9 OTHER AREAS OF SCIENTIFIC STUDY

The areas of research mentioned are the classical ones for altitude research. As more workers from different fields have become interested in the effects of altitude hypoxia on other systems of the body, more techniques have been used in the mountains. Psychomotor testing equipment has changed from clipboard, stopwatch and pencil to computers. Visual field testing, audiometry and measurement of balance or sway have been made using computer based systems. Overnight cough frequency has been monitored with voice activated battery tape recorders and cough threshold measured with nebulized citric acid solutions. Even near-infrared spectroscopy has been used to measure brain oxygenation at altitude in the field (Morgan *et al.* 1999). All these applications of modern electronics, and others, show how the possibilities for research at altitude have expanded. The future of the subject is only limited by the imagination of researchers and should be bright indeed.

References

Acosta, I. de (1590) *Historia Natural y Moral de las Indias*, Lib 3, Cap. 9, Iuan de Leon, Seville. Section of English translation of 1604 (1604), Edward Blount and William Aspley, London. Reprinted in *High Altitude Physiology* (ed. J.B. West), Hutchinson Ross Publishing Company, Stroudsburg, PA, 1981.

Acute mountain sickness (1979) *Postgrad. Med. J.* **55**, 445–512.

Acute mountain sickness (1987) *Postgrad. Med. J.* **63**, 163–93.

Adam, J.M. and Goldsmith, R. (1965) Cold climates, in *Exploration Medicine* (eds. O.G. Edholm and A.L. Bacharach), Wright, Bristol, pp. 245–77.

Adams, W.C., Bernauer, E.M., Dill, D.B., Bowmar, J.B. Jr (1975) Effects of equivalent sea-level and altitude training on VO_2 max and running performance. *J. Appl. Physiol.* **39**, 262–6.

Adams, W.H. and Strang, L.J. (1975) Haemoglobin levels in persons of Tibetan ancestry living at high altitude. *Proc. Soc. Exp. Biol. Med.* **149**, 1036–9.

Adnot, S., Chabrier, P.E., Brun-Buisson, C., Voissat, I. and Braguet, P. (1988) Atrial natriuretic factor attenuates the pulmonary pressor response to hypoxia. *J. Appl. Physiol.* **65**, 1975–83.

Adzaku, F., Mohammed, S., Annobil, S. and Addae, S. (1993) Relevant laboratory findings in patients with sickle cell disease living at high altitude. *J. Wilderness Med.* **4**, 374–83.

Ahle, N.W., Buroni, J.R., Sharp, M.W. and Hamlet, M.P. (1990) Infrared thermographic measurement of circulatory compromise in trenchfoot-injured Argentine soldiers. *Aviat. Space Environ. Med.* **61**, 247–50.

Aigner, A., Berghold, F. and Muss, N. (1980) Investigations on the cardiovascular system at altitudes up to a height of 7,800 meters. *Z. Kardiol.* **69**, 604–10.

Albrecht, P.H. and Littell, J.K. (1972) Plasma erythro-poietin in men and mice during acclimatization to different altitudes. *J. Appl. Physiol.* **32**, 54–8.

Albutt, T.C. (1870) On the effect of exercise upon the body temperature. *Alpine J.* **5**, 212–18.

Albutt, T.C. (1876) On the health and training of mountaineers. *Alpine J.* **8**, 30–40.

Alexander, J.K., Hartley, L.H., Modelski, M. and Grover, R.F. (1967) Reduction of stroke volume during exercise in man following ascent to 3100 m altitude. *J. Appl. Physiol.* **23**, 849–58.

Alexander, L. (1945) *The Treatment of Shock from Prolonged Exposure to Cold Especially in Water*, Combined Intelligence Objective Sub-Committee, Item No. **24**, File No. 24–37.

Allegra, L., Cogo, A., Legnani, D., Diano, P.L., Fasano, V. and Negretto, G.G. (1995) High altitude exposure reduces bronchial responsiveness to hypo-osmolar aerosols in lowland asthmatics. *Eur. Respir. J.* **8**, 1842–6.

Anand, I.S., Chandrashekhar, Y., Rao, S.K. *et al.* (1993) Body fluid compartments, renal blood flow, and hormones at 6000 m in normal subjects. *J. Appl. Physiol.* **74**, 1234–9.

Anand, I.S., Malhotra, R.M., Chandrashekhar, Y. *et al.* (1990) Adult subacute mountain sickness – a syndrome of congestive heart failure in man at very high altitude. *Lancet* **335**, 561–5.

Anand, I.S., Prasad, B.A., Chugh, S.S. *et al.* (1998) Effect of inhaled nitric oxide and oxygen in high-altitude pulmonary edema. *Circulation* **98**, 2441–5.

Andersen, P. and Henriksson, J. (1977) Capillary supply of the quadriceps femoris muscle of man: adaptive response to exercise. *J. Physiol. (Lond.)* **270**, 677–90.

Anderson, J.V., Struthers, A.D., Payne, N.N., Slater, J. D. and Bloom, S. R. (1986) Atrial natriuretic peptide inhibits the aldosterone response to angiotensin II in man. *Clin. Sci.* **70**, 507–12.

Anderson, S., Herbring, B.G. and Widman, B. (1970) Accidental profound hypothermia (case report). *Br. J. Anaesth.* **42**, 653–5.

Andrew, H.G. (1963) Work in extreme cold. *Trans. Assoc. Indust. Med. Off.* **13**, 16–19.

Andrew, M., O'Brodovitch, H. and Sutton, J. (1987) Operation Everest II; coagulation system during prolonged decompression to 282 torr. *J. Appl. Physiol.* **63**, 1262–7.

Anholm, J.D., Milne, E.N., Stark, P., Bourne, J.C. and Friedman, P. (1999) Radiographic evidence of interstitial pulmonary edema after exercise at altitude. *J. Appl. Physiol.* **86**, 503–9.

Anooshiravani, M., Dumont, L., Mardirosoff, C., Soto-Debeuf, G. and Delavelle, J. (1999) Brain magnetic resonance imaging (MRI) and neurological changes after a single high altitude climb. *Med. Sci. Sports Exerc.* **31**, 969–72.

Another Ascent of the World's Highest Peak – Qomolangma (1975) Foreign Languages Press, Peking.

Anselme, F., Caillaud, C., Courret, I. and Prefaut, C. (1992) Exercise induced hypoxaemia and histamine excretion in extreme athletes. *Int. J. Sports Med.* **13**, 80–1.

Antezana, A-M., Richalet, J-P., Noriega, I., Galarza, M. and Antezana, G. (1995) Hormonal changes in normal and polycythemic high-altitude natives. *J. Appl. Physiol.* **79**, 795–800.

Antezana, G., Leguia, G., Guzman, A.M., Coudert, J. and Spielvogel, H. (1982) Hemodynamic study of high altitude pulmonary edema (12200 ft), in *High Altitude Physiology and Medicine* (eds. W. Brendel and R.A. Zink), Springer-Verlag, New York, pp. 232–41.

Anthony, A., Ackerman, E. and Strother, G.K. (1959) Effects of altitude acclimatization on rat myoglobin. Changes in myoglobin content of skeletal and cardiac muscle. *Am. J. Physiol.* **196**, 512–16.

Aoki, V.S. and Robinson, S.M. (1971) Body hydration and the incidence and severity of acute mountain sickness. *J. Appl. Physiol.* **31**, 363–7.

Appell, H.-J. (1978) Capillary density and patterns in skeletal muscle. III. Changes of the capillary pattern after hypoxia. *Pflügers Arch.* **377**, R53 (abstract).

Araki, T. (1891) Ueber die Bildung von Milchsäure und Glycose im Organismus bei Sauerstoffmangel. *Z. Physiol. Chem.* **15**, 335–70.

Archer, S.L., Tolins, J.P., Raij, L. and Weir, E.K. (1989) Hypoxic pulmonary vasoconstriction is enhanced by inhibition of the synthesis of an endothelium derived relaxing factor. *Biochem. Biophys. Res. Commun.* **164**, 1198–205.

Arias-Stella, J. (1969) Human carotid body at high altitudes (abstract). *Am. J. Pathol.* **55**, 82.

Arias-Stella, J. (1971) Chronic mountain sickness: pathology and definition, in *High Altitude Physiology: Cardiac and Respiratory Aspects,* Ciba Foundation Symposium (eds. R. Porter and J. Knight), Churchill Livingstone, Edinburgh, pp. 31–40.

Arias-Stella, J. and Kruger, H. (1963) Pathology of high altitude pulmonary edema. *Arch. Pathol.* **76**, 147–57.

Arias-Stella, J., Kruger, H. and Recavarren, S. (1973) Pathology of chronic mountain sickness. *Thorax* **28**, 701–8.

Arias-Stella, J. and Recavarren, S. (1962) Right ventricular hypertrophy in native children living at high altitude. *Am. J. Pathol.* **41**, 55–64.

Arias-Stella, J. and Saldaña, M. (1963) The terminal portion of the pulmonary arterial tree in people native to high altitudes. *Circulation* **28**, 915–25.

Arias-Stella, J. and Topilsky, M. (1971) Anatomy of the coronary circulation at high altitude, in *High Altitude Physiology: Cardiac and Respiratory Aspects* (eds. R. Porter and J. Knight), Churchill Livingstone, London, pp. 149–57.

Asaji, T., Sakurai, E., Tanizaki, Y. *et al.* (1984) Report on medical aspects of Mount Lhotse and Everest expedition in 1983: with special reference to a case of cerebral venous thrombosis in the altitude. *Jpn. J. Mount. Med.* **4**, 91–8.

Asano, K., Sub, S., Matsuzaka, A. *et al.* (1986) The influence of simulated high altitude training on work capacity and performance in middle and long distance runners. *Bull. Inst. Health Sports Med.* **9**, 1195–202.

Ashack, R., Farber, M.O., Weinberger, M.H., Robertson, G.L., Fineberg, N.S. and Manfredi, F. (1985) Renal and hormonal responses to acute hypoxia in normal individuals. *J. Lab. Clin. Med.* **106**, 12–16.

Asmussen, E. and Consolazio, F.C. (1941) The circulation in rest and work on Mount Evans (4,300 m). *Am. J. Physiol.* **132**, 555–63.

Aste-Salazar, H. and Hurtado, A. (1944) The affinity of hemoglobin for oxygen at sea level and at high altitudes. *Am. J. Physiol.* **142**, 733–43.

Astrup, P. and Severinghaus, J.W. (1986) *The History of Blood Gases, Acids and Bases*, Munksgaard, Copenhagen.

Atrial natriuretic peptide [editorial]. (1986) *Lancet* **2**, 371–2.

Au, J., Brown, J.E., Lee, M.R. and Boon, N.A. (1990) Effect of cardiac tamponade on atrial natriuretic peptide concentrations: influence of stretch and pressure. *Clin. Sci.* **79**, 377–80.

Ayton, J.M. (1993) Polar hands: spontaneous skin fissures closed with cyanoacrylate (Histoacryl Blue) tissue adhesive in Antarctica. *Arctic Med. Res.* **52**, 127–30.

Baddeley, A.D., Cuccaro, W.J., Egstrom, G.H. and Willis, M.A. (1975) Cognitive efficiency of divers working in cold water. *Hum. Factors* **17**, 446–54.

Baertschi, A.J., Hausmaninger, C., Walsh, R.S. *et al.* (1986) Hypoxia-induced release of atrial natriuretic factor (ANF) from isolated rat and rabbit heart. *Biochem. Biophys. Res. Commun.* **140**, 427–33.

Bailey, D.M. and Davies, B. (1997) Physiological implications of altitude training for endurance performance at sea level: a review. *Br. J. Sports Med.* **31**, 183–90.

Bailey, D.M., Davies, B., Milledge, J.S. *et al.* (2000) Elevated plasma cholecystokinin at high altitude: metabolic implications for the anorexia of acute mountain sickness. *High Alt. Med. Biol.* **1**, 9–23.

Bailey, D.M., Davies, B., Romer, L. *et al.* (1998) Implications of moderate altitude training for sea-level endurance in elite distance runners. *Eur. J. Appl. Physiol.* **78**, 360–8.

Bailey, F.M. (1957) *No Passport to Tibet.* Hart Davis, London, p. 261.

Baker, P.T. (1966) Microenvironment cold in a high altitude Peruvian population, in *Human Adaptability and Its Methodology* (eds. H. Yoshimura and J.S. Weiner), Japanese Society for the Promotion of Sciences, Tokyo, pp. 67–77.

Baker, P.T. (ed.) (1978) *The Biology of High Altitude Peoples,* Cambridge University Press, Cambridge.

Baker, P.T. (1978) The adaptive fitness of high-altitude populations, in *The Biology of High Altitude Peoples* (ed. P.T. Baker), Cambridge University Press, Cambridge, pp. 317–50.

Baker, P.T. and Dutt, J.S. (1972) Demographic variables as measures of biological adaptation: a case study of high altitude population, in *The Structure of Human Populations* (eds. G.A. Harrison and A.J. Boyce), Clarendon Press, Oxford, pp. 352–78.

Bakewell, S.E., Hart, N.D., Wilson, C.M. *et al.* (1999) A randomised, double blind placebo controlled trial of the effect of inhaled nedocromil sodium or slameterol xinafoate on the citric acid cough threshold in subjects travelling to high altitude (abstract), in *Hypoxia: Into the Next Millennium* (eds. R.C. Roach, P.D. Wagner and P.H. Hackett), Plenum/Kluwer Academic Publishing, New York, p. 362.

Banchero, N. (1982) Long term adaptation of skeletal muscle capillarity. *Physiologist* **25**, 385–9.

Bangham, C.R.M. and Hackett, P.H. (1978) Effects of high altitude on endocrine function in the Sherpas of Nepal. *J. Endocrinol.* **79**, 147–8.

Banner, A.S. (1988) Relationship between cough due to hypotonic aerosol and the ventilatory response to CO_2 in normal subjects. *Am. Rev. Respir. Dis.* **137**, 647–50.

Barber, S.G. (1978) Drugs and doctoring for trans-Saharan travellers. *BMJ* **2**, 404–6.

Barcroft, J. (1911) The effect of altitude on the dissociation curve of blood. *J. Physiol. (Lond.)* **42**, 44–63.

Barcroft, J. (1925) *The Respiratory Function of the Blood. Part I. Lessons from High Altitudes*, Cambridge University Press, Cambridge.

Barcroft, J. and King, W.O.R. (1909) The effect of temperature on the dissociation curve of blood. *J. Physiol. (Lond.),* **39**, 374–84.

Barcroft, J. and Orbeli, L. (1910) The influence of lactic acid upon the dissociation curve of blood. *J. Physiol. (Lond.).* **41**, 355–67.

Barcroft, J., Binger, C.A., Bock, A.V. *et al.* (1923) Observations upon the effect of high altitude on the physiological processes of the human body, carried out in the Peruvian Andes, chiefly at Cerro de Pasco. *Philos. Trans. R. Soc. Lond. Ser. B* **211,** 351–480.

Barcroft, J., Camis, M., Mathison, C.G., Roberts, F.F. and Ryffel, J.H. (1914) Report of the Monte Rosa Expedition of 1911. *Philos. Trans. R. Soc. Lond. Ser. B* **206,** 49–102.

Barcroft, J., Cooke, A., Hartridge, H., Parsons, T.R. and Parsons, W. (1920) The flow of oxygen through the pulmonary epithelium. *J. Physiol. (Lond.)* **53**, 450–72.

Barer, G.R., Howard, P. and Shaw, J.W. (1970) Stimulus–response curves for the pulmonary vascular bed to hypoxia and hypercapnia. *J. Physiol. (Lond.)* **211,** 139–55.

Barnard, P., Andronikou, S., Pokorski, M. *et al.* (1987) Time-dependent effect of hypoxia on carotid body chemosensory function. *J. Appl. Physiol.* **63,** 684–91.

Barry, P.B., Mason, N.M. and Collier, D.J. (1995) Sex differences in blood gases during acclimatization, in *Hypoxia and the Brain* (eds. J.R. Sutton, C. S Houston and G. Coates), Queen City Printers, Burlington, VA, p. 314.

Barry, P.W., Mason, N.P., Nicol, A. *et al.* (1997c) Cough receptor sensitivity and dynamic ventilatory response to carbon dioxide in man acclimatized to high altitude (Abstract), in *Women at Altitude* (eds. C.S.

Houston and G. Coates), Queens City Press, Burlington, VA, p. 303.

Barry, P.W., Mason, N.P. and O'Callaghan, C. (1997b) Nasal mucociliary transport is impaired at altitude. *Eur. Respir. J.* **10**, 35–7.

Barry, P.W., Mason, N.P., Riordan, M. and O'Callaghan, C. (1997a) Cough frequency and cough receptor sensitivity are increased in man at high altitude. *Clin. Sci.* **93**, 181–6.

Bartlett, D. Jr and Remmers, J.E. (1971) Effects of high altitude exposure on the lungs of young rats. *Respir. Physiol.* **13**, 116–25.

Bärtsch, P., Baumgartner, R.W., Waber, U., Maggiorini, M. and Oelz, O. (1990) Comparison of carbon dioxide enriched, oxygen enriched, and normal air in treatment of acute mountain sickness. *Lancet* **336**, 772–5.

Bärtsch, P., Lämmle, B., Huber, I. *et al.* (1989) Contact phase of blood coagulation is not activated in edema of high altitude. *J. Appl. Physiol.* **67**, 1336–40.

Bärtsch, P., Maggiorini, M., Ritter, M., Noti, C., Vock, P. and Oelz, O. (1991b) Prevention of high-altitude pulmonary edema by nifedipine. *N. Engl. J. Med.* **325**, 1284–9.

Bärtsch, P., Merki, B., Hofsetter, D., Maggiorini, M., Kayser, B. and Oelz, O. (1993) Treatment of acute mountain sickness by simulated descent: a randomised controlled trial. *BMJ* **306**, 1098–101.

Bärtsch, P., Pfluger, N., Audetat, M.S. *et al.* (1991a) Effects of slow ascent to 4559 m on fluid homeostasis. *Aviat. Space Environ. Med.* **62**, 105–10.

Bärtsch, P., Schmidt, E.K. and Straub, P.W. (1982) Fibrinopeptide A after strenuous physical exercise at high altitude. *J. Appl. Physiol.* **53**, 40–3.

Bärtsch, P., Shaw, S., Franciolli, M. *et al.* (1988) Atrial natriuretic peptide in acute mountain sickness. *J. Appl. Physiol.* **65**, 1929–37.

Bärtsch, P., Waber, U., Haeberli, A., Gnädinger, M.P. and Weidmann, P. (1987) Enhanced fibrin formation in high-altitude pulmonary edema. *J. Appl. Physiol.* **63**, 752–7.

Basnyat, B. (1997) Seizure and hemiparesis at high altitudes outside the setting of acute mountain sickness. *J. Wilderness Environ. Med.* **8**, 221–2.

Basnyat, B., Leomaster, J. and Litch, J.A. (1999) Everest or bust: a cross sectional, epidemiological survey of acute mountain sickness at 4234m in the Himalaya. *Aviat. Space Environ. Med.* **70**, 867–73.

Bauer, P. (ed.) (1938) *Himalayan Quest: the German Expeditions to Siniolchum and Nanga Parbat* (trans. E.G. Hall) Nicholson and Watson, London.

Baumgartner, R.W., Bärtsch, P., Maggiorini, M., Waber, U. and Oelz, O. (1994) Enhanced cerebral blood flow in acute mountain sickness. *Aviat. Space Environ. Med.* **65**, 726–9.

Baumgartner, R.W., Spyridopoulos, I., Bartsch, P., Maggiorini, M. and Oelz, O. (1999) Acute mountain sickness is not related to cerebral blood flow: a decompression chamber study. *J. Appl. Physiol.* **86**, 1578–82.

Bayliss, R.I.S. (1987) Endocrine manifestations of non-endocrine disease, in *Oxford Textbook of Medicine*, 2nd edn (eds. D.J. Weatherall, J.G.G. Leadingham and D.A. Warrell), Oxford University Press, Oxford, pp. 101–19.

Bazett, H.C. and McGlone, B. (1927) Temperature gradients in the tissues of man. *Am. J. Physiol.* **82**, 415–51.

Beall, C.M., Almasy, L.A., Blangero, J. *et al.* (1999) Percent of oxygen saturation of arterial hemoglobin among Bolivian Aymara at 3,990–4,000 m. *Am. J. Phys. Anthropol.* **108**, 41–51.

Beall, C.M., Blangero, J., Williams-Blangero, S. and Goldstein, M.C. (1994) Major gene for percent of oxygen saturation of arterial hemoglobin in Tibetan highlanders. *Am. J. Phys. Anthropol.* **95**, 271–6.

Beall C.M., Brittenham, G.M., Strohl, K.P. *et al.* (1998) Hemoglobin concentration of high-altitude Tibetans and Bolivian Aymara. *Am. J. Anthropol.* **106**, 385–400.

Beall, C.M., Goldstein, M.C. and the Tibetan Academy of Sciences (1987) Hemoglobin concentration of pastoral nomads permanently resident at 4850–5450 meters in Tibet. *Am. J. Phys. Anthropol.* **73**, 433–8.

Beall, C.M., Strohl, K.P., Blangero, J. *et al.* (1997a) Ventilation and hypoxic ventilatory response of Tibetan and Aymara high altitude natives. *Am. J. Anthropol.* **104**, 427–47.

Beall, C.M., Strohl, K.P., Blangero, J. *et al.* (1997b) Quantitative genetic analysis of arterial oxygen saturation in Tibetan highlanders. *Hum. Biol.* **69**, 597–604.

Beaumont, M., Goldenberg, F., Lejeune, D., Marotte, H., Horf, A. and Lofaso, F. (1996) Effect of zolpidem on sleep and ventilatory patterns at simulated altitude of 4,000 meters. *Am. J. Respir. Crit. Care Med.* **153**, 1864–9.

Beidleman, B.A., Rock, P.B., Muza, S.R. *et al.* (1999) Exercise VE and physical performance at altitude are not affected by menstrual cycle phase. *J. Appl. Physiol.* **86**, 1519–26.

Beidleman, B.A., Muza, S.R., Rock, P.B. *et al.* (1997)

Exercise responses after altitude acclimatization are retained during reintroduction to altitude. *Med. Sci. Sports Exerc.* **29**, 1588–95.

Bell, C. (1928) *The People of Tibet,* Oxford University Press, Oxford, p. 197.

Bellew, H.W. (1875) *Kashmir and Kashgar,* Trubner, London, pp. 163–4.

Bencowitz, H.Z., Wagner, P.D. and West, J.B. (1982) Effect of change in P_{50} on exercise tolerance at high altitude: a theoretical study. *J. Appl. Physiol.* **53**, 1487–95.

Bender, P.B., DeBehnke, D.J., Swart, G.L. and Hall, K.N. (1995) Serum potassium concentration as a predictor of resuscitation outcome in hypothermic cardiac arrest. *Wilderness Environ. Med.* **6**, 273–82.

Benesch, R. and Benesch, R.E. (1967) The effect of organic phosphates from the human erythrocyte on the allosteric properties of hemoglobin. *Biochem. Biophys. Res. Commun.* **26**, 162–7.

Benson, H., Lehmann, J.W., Malhotra, M.S. *et al.* (1982) Body temperature changes during the practice of g-tum-mo yoga. *Nature* **295**, 234–6.

Berg, J.T., Breen, E.C., Fu, Z., Mathieu-Costello, O. and West, J.B. (1998) Alveolar hypoxia causes increased gene expression of extracellular matrix proteins and platelet-derived growth factor B in lung parenchyma. *Am. J. Respir. Crit. Care Med.* **158**, 1920–8.

Berg, J.T., Fu, Z., Breen, E.C., Tran, H.-C., Mathieu-Costello, O. and West, J.B. (1997) High lung inflation increases mRNA levels of ECM components and growth factors in lung parenchyma. *J. Appl. Physiol.* **83**, 120–8.

Berlin, N.I., Reynafarje, C. and Lawrence, J.H. (1954) Red cell life span in the polycythemia of high altitude. *J. Appl. Physiol.* **7**, 271–2.

Berner, G., Froelicher, V.F. and West, J.B. (1988) Trekking in Nepal: safety after coronary artery bypass. *JAMA* **259**, 3184.

Bernhard, W.N., Schalick, I.M., Delaney, P.A. *et al.* (1998) Acetazolamide plus dexamethasone is better than acetazolamide alone to ameliorate symptoms of acute mountain sickness. *Aviat. Space Environ. Med* **69**, 883–6.

Berre, J., Vachiery, J.L., Moraine, J.J. and Naeije, R. (1999) Cerebral blood flow velocity responses to hypoxia in subjects who are susceptible to high-altitude pulmonary oedema. *Eur. J. Appl. Physiol.* **80**, 260–3.

Berssenbrugge, A., Dempsey, J., Iber, C., Skatral, J. and Wilson, P. (1983) Mechanisms of hypoxia-induced periodic breathing during sleep in humans. *J. Physiol. (Lond.)* **343**, 507–26.

Bert, P. (1878) *La Pression Barométrique.* Masson, Paris. English translation by M.A. Hitchcock and F.A. Hitchcock, College Book Co., Columbus, OH, 1943.

Bigard, A.X., Douce, P., Merino, D. *et al.* (1996a) Changes in dietary protein fail to prevent decrease in muscle growth induced by severe hypoxia in rats. *J. Appl. Physiol.* **80**, 208–15.

Bigard, A.X., Lavier, P., Ullman, L. *et al.* (1996b) Branched-chain amino acid supplementation during repeated prolonged skiing exercises at altitude. *Int. J. Sport Nutr.* **6**, 295–306.

Bircher, H.P., Eichenberger, U., Maggiorini, M., Oelz, O. and Bärtsch, P. (1993) Relationship of mountain sickness to physical fitness and exercise intensity during ascent. *J. Wilderness Med.* **5**, 302–11.

Birks, J.W., Klassen, L.W. and Curney, C.W. (1975) Hypoxia induced thrombocytopenia in mice. *J. Lab. Clin. Med.* **86**, 230–8.

Birmingham Medical Research Expeditionary Society Mountain Sickness Study Group (1981) Acetazolamide in control of acute mountain sickness. *Lancet* **1**, 180–3.

Biscoe, T.J. and Duchen, M.R. (1990) Cellular basis of transduction in carotid body chemoreceptors. *Am. J. Physiol.* **258**, L270–8.

Bisgard, G.E., Busch, M.A. and Forster, H.V. (1986) Ventilatory acclimatization to hypoxia is not dependent on cerebral hypocapnic alkalosis. *J. Appl. Physiol.* **60**, 1011–14.

Bishop, R.A., Litch, J.A. and Stanton, J.M. (2000) Ketamine anesthesia at high altitude. *High Alt. Med. Biol.* **1**, 111–14.

Bjurstrom, R.L. and Schoene, R.B. (1986) Ventilatory control in elite synchronized swimmers. *Am. Rev. Respir. Dis.* **133** (Suppl.), A134.

Black, C.P. and Tenney, S.M. (1980) Oxygen transport during progressive hypoxia in high-altitude and sea-level waterfowl. *Respir. Physiol.* **39**, 217–39.

Blauw, G.J., Westerterp, R.G., Srivastava, N. *et al.* (1995) Hypoxia induced arterial endothelin does not influence peripheral vascular tone. *J. Cardiol. Pharm.* **3**, S242–3.

Bledsoe, S.W. and Hornbein, T.F. (1981) Central chemosensors and the regulation of their chemical environment, in *Regulation of Breathing, Part I* (ed. T.F. Hornbein), Marcel Dekker, New York, pp. 347–428.

Bligh, J. and Chauca, D. (1978) The effects of intracerebroventricular injections of carbachol and noradrenaline in cold induced pulmonary artery hypertension in sheep. *J. Physiol.* **284**, 53P.

Bligh, J. and Chauca, D. (1982) Effects of hypoxia, cold exposure and fever on pulmonary artery pressure and their significance for Arctic residents, in *Circum Polar Health 1981* (eds. B. Harvald and J.B. Hart Hansen), Report **32**, Nordic Council for Arctic Medical Research, Copenhagen, pp. 606–7.

Blows from the winter wind (editorial) (1980) *BMJ* **1**, 137–8.

Blume, F.D. (1984) Metabolic and endocrine changes at altitude, in *High Altitude and Man* (eds. J.B. West and S. Lahiri), American Physiological Society, Bethesda, MD, pp. 37–45.

Blume, F.D., Boyer, S.J., Braverman, L.E. and Cohen, A. (1984) Impaired osmoregulation at high altitude. *JAMA* **252,** 524–6.

Blume, F.D. and Pace, N. (1967) Effect of translocation to 3800 m altitude on glycolysis in mice. *J. Appl. Physiol.* **23**, 75–9.

Blume, F.D. and Pace, N. (1971) The utilisation of ^{14}C-labelled palmitic acid, alanine and aspartic acid at high altitude. *Environ. Physiol.* **1**, 30–6.

Bohn, D.J. (1987) Treatment of hypothermia in hospital, in *Hypothermia and Cold* (eds. J.R. Sutton, C.S. Houston and G. Coates), Prager, New York, pp. 286–305.

Bohr, C. (1885) *Experimentale Untersuchungen über die Sauerstoffaufnahme des Blutfarbstoffes*, O.C. Olsen, Copenhagen.

Bohr, C. (1891) Über die Lungenatmung. *Skand. Arch. Physiol.* **2**, 236–68. English translation in *Translations in Respiratory Physiology* (ed. J.B. West), Hutchinson Ross, Stroudsburg, PA, 1981.

Bohr, C. (1909) Über die spezifische Tätigkeit der Lungen bei der respiratorischen Gasaufnahmne und ihr Verhalten zu der durch die Alveolarwand stattfindenden Gasdiffusion. *Skand. Arch. Physiol.* **22**, 221–80. English translation in *Translations in Respiratory Physiology* (ed. J.B. West), Hutchinson Ross, Stroudsburg, PA, 1981.

Bohr, C., Hasselbalch, C.B.K. and Krogh, A. (1904) Ueber einen in biologischer Beziehung wichtigen Einfluss, den die Kohlensäurespannuny des Blutes auf dessen Sauerstoffbinding übt. *Skand. Arch. Physiol.* **16**, 402–12.

Bonavia, D., Leon-Velarde, F., Monge, C.C., Sanchez-Griñan, M.I. and Wittembury, J. (1985) Acute mountain sickness: critical appraisal of the Pariacaca story and on-site study. *Respir. Physiol.* **62**, 125–34.

Bonelli, J., Waldhausl, W., Magometschnigg, D. *et al.* (1977) Effect of exercise and of prolonged administration of propranolol on haemodynamic variables, plasma renin concentration, plasma aldosterone and c-AMP. *Eur. J. Clin. Invest.* **7**, 337–43.

Bonvalot, G. (1891) *Across Thibet,* Cassell, London.

Borgström, L., Johannsson, H. and Siesjö, B.K. (1975) The relationship between arterial P_{O_2} and cerebral blood flow in hypoxic hypoxia. *Acta Physiol. Scand.* **93**, 423–32.

Bouissou, P., Guezennec, C.Y., Galen, F.X. *et al.* (1988) Dissociated response of aldosterone from plasma renin activity during prolonged exercise under hypoxia. *Horm. Metab. Res.* **20**, 517–21.

Bouissou, P., Peronnet, F., Brisson, C. *et al.* (1986) Metabolic and endocrine responses to graded exercise under acute hypoxia. *Eur. J. Appl. Physiol.* **55**, 290–4.

Bouissou, P., Richalet, J.-P., Galen, F.X., Lartigue, M., Larmignet, P., Devaux, F. *et al.* (1989) Effect of β-adrenoreceptor blockade on renin–aldosterone and α-ANF during exercise at altitude. *J. Appl. Physiol.* **67**, 141–6.

Boutellier, U., Howald, H., di Prampero, P.E., Giezendanner, D. and Cerretelli, P. (1983) Human muscle adaptations to chronic hypoxia. *Prog. Clin. Biol. Res.* **136**, 273–85.

Bower, H. (1893) *Diary of a Journey across Tibet,* Office of the Superintendent of Government Printing, Calcutta, India, p. 5.

Boycott, A.E. and Haldane, J.S. (1908) The effects of low atmospheric pressures on respiration. *J. Physiol. (Lond.)* **37**, 355–77.

Boyer, S.J. (1978) Endurance test on Colorado's 14,000 ft peaks. *Summit Magazine* **24**, 30–5.

Boyer, S.J. and Blume, F.D. (1984) Weight loss and changes in body composition at high altitude. *J. Appl. Physiol.* **57,** 1580–5.

Boyle, R. (1662) *New Experiments Physico-Mechanical, Touching the Air: Whereunto is Added a Defence of the Authors Explication of the Experiments, Against the Objections of Franciscus Linus, and, Thomas Hobbes.* H. Hall for T. Robinson, Oxford. Relevant pages reprinted in *High Altitude Physiology* (ed. J.B. West), Hutchinson Ross, Stroudsburg, PA, 1981.

Bradwell, A.R. and Delamere, J.P. (1982) The effect of acetazolamide on the proteinuria of altitude. *Aviat. Space Environ. Med.* **53**, 40–3.

Bradwell, A.R., Dykes, P.W., Coote, J.H. *et al.* (1986) Effect of acetazolamide on exercise performance and muscle mass at high altitude. *Lancet* **1**, 1001–5.

Bradwell, A.R., Winterbourn, M., Wright, A.D. *et al.* (1988) Acetazolamide treatment in acute mountain sickness. *Clin. Sci.* 74 (Suppl. 18), 62P.

Brasher, C. (1986) Wizard of the peaks. *Observer* (London) 29 June.

Brasher, C. (1988) Ascent of superman. *Observer* (London) 26 June.

Braun, B., Butterfield, G.E., Dominick, S.B. *et al.* (1998) Women at altitude: changes in carbohydrate metabolism at 4,300m elevation and across the menstrual cycle. *J. Appl. Physiol.* **85**, 1966–73.

Braun, B., Mawson, J.T., Muza, S.R. *et al.* (2000) Women at altitude: carbohydrate utilization during exercise at 4300m. *J. Appl. Physiol.* **88**, 246–56.

Braun, P. (1985) Pathophysiology and treatment of hypothermia, in *High Altitude Deterioration* (eds. J. Rivolier, P. Cerretelli, J. Foray and P. Segantini), Karger, Basel, pp. 140–8.

Brendel, W. (1956) Anpassung von Atmung, Hämoglobin, Körpertemperatur und Kreislauf bei langfristigem Aufenthalt in grossen Höhen (Himalaya). *Pflügers Arch.* **263**, 227–52.

Brendel, W. and Zink, R.A. (eds.) (1982) *High Altitude Physiology and Medicine,* Springer-Verlag, New York.

Brennan, P.J., Greenberg, G., Miall, W.E. and Thompson, S.G. (1982) Seasonal variation in arterial blood pressure. *BMJ* **2**, 919–23.

Brenner, I.K.M., Castellani, J.W., Gabaree, C. *et al.* (1999) Immune changes in humans during cold exposure: effects of prior heating and exercise. *J. Appl. Physiol.* **87**, 699–710.

Brent, P. (1974) *Captain Scott and the Antarctic Tragedy,* Weidenfeld and Nicolson, London.

Brodal, P., Ingjer, F. and Hermansen, L. (1977) Capillary supply of skeletal muscle fibers in untrained and endurance-trained men. *Am. J. Physiol.* **232**, H705–12.

Brooks, G.A., Butterfield, G.E., Wolfe, R.R. *et al.* (1991) Increased dependence on blood glucose after acclimatization to 4300 m. *J. Appl. Physiol.* **70**, 919-27.

Brooks, G.A., Wolfel, E.E., Butterfield, G.E. *et al.* (1998) Poor relationship between arterial [lactate] and leg net release during exercise at 4,300 m altitude. *Am. J. Physiol.* **275**, R1192–201.

Broom, J.R., Stoneham, M.D., Beeley, J.M., Milledge, J.S. and Hughes, A.S. (1994) High altitude headache: treatment with ibuprofen. *Aviat. Space Environ. Med.* **65**, 19–20.

Brown, J.M. and Page, J. (1952) The effect of chronic exposure to cold or temperature and blood flow of the hands. *J. Appl. Physiol.* **5**, 221–7.

Bruce, C.G. (1923) *The Assault on Mount Everest,* Arnold, London.

Brunt, D. (1952) *Physical and Dynamical Meteorology*, 2nd edn, Cambridge University Press, Cambridge, p. 379.

Budd, G.M. (1984) Daily fluid balance. International Biomedical Expedition to the Antarctic. *6th International Symposium on Circum Polar Health,* Anchorage, May 1984, pp. 59–60.

Buettner, K.J.K. (1969) The effect of natural sunlight on human skin, in *The Biologic Effects of Ultraviolet Radiation, with Special Emphasis on the Skin* (ed. F. Urbach), Pergamon Press, Oxford, pp. 237–49.

Buguet, A.G.C., Livingstone, S.D. and Reed, L.D. (1979) Skin temperature changes in paradoxical sleep in man in the cold. *Aviat. Space Environ. Med.* **50**, 567–70.

Buick, F., Gledhill, N., Froese, A. *et al.* (1980) Effects of induced erythrocythemia on aerobic work capacity. *J. Appl. Physiol.* **48**, 636–42.

Bulow, K. (1963) Respiration and wakefulness in man. *Acta Physiol. Scand.* **59** (Suppl. 209), 1–110.

Burnett, C.S.F. (1983) High altitude mountaineering 1600 years ago. *Alpine J.* **88**, 127.

Burr, R.E. (1993) Trench foot. *J. Wilderness Med.* **4**, 348–52.

Burri, P.H. and Weibel, E.R. (1971) Morphometric estimation of pulmonary diffusion capacity. II. Effect of P_{O_2} on the growing lung; adaption of the growing rat lung to hypoxia and hyperoxia. *Respir. Physiol.* **11**, 247–64.

Burton, A.C. and Edholm, O.G. (1955) *Man in a Cold Environment,* Arnold, London.

Burtscher, M.B., Likar, R., Nachbauer, W. and Philadelphy, M. (1998) Aspirin for prophylaxis against headache at high altitudes: randomised, double blind, placebo controlled trial. *BMJ* **316**, 1057–8.

Burtscher, M.B., Philadelphy, M., Likar, R. and Nachbauer, W. (1999) Aspirin versus diamox plus aspirin for headache during physical activity at high altitude (abstract), in *Hypoxia: Into the Next Millennium* (eds. R.C. Roach, P.D. Wagner and P.H. Hackett), Plenum/Kluwer, New York, p. 133.

Buschke, H. (1973) Selective reminding for analysis of memory and learning. *J. Verb. Learn. Verb. Behav.* **13**, 543–50.

Buskirk, E.R. (1977) Temperature regulation with exercise. *Exerc. Sport Sci. Rev.* **5**, 45–88.

Buskirk, E.R. (1978) Work capacity of high-altitude natives, in *The Biology of High Altitude Peoples* (ed. P.T. Baker), Cambridge University Press, Cambridge, pp. 173–87.

Butson, A.R.C. (1949) Acclimatization to cold in Antarctica (Letter). *Nature* **163**, 132–3.

Butson, A.R.C. (1975) Effects and prevention of frostbite in wound healing. *Can. J. Surg.* **18**, 145–8.

Butterfield, G.E., Gates, J., Fleming, S. *et al.* (1992) Increased energy intake minimizes weight loss in men at high altitude. *J. Appl. Physiol.* **72**, 1741–8.

Byrne-Quinn, E., Weil, J.V., Sodal, I.E. *et al.* (1971) Ventilatory control in the athlete. *J. Appl. Physiol.* **30**, 91–8.

Cabanac, M. and LeBlanc, J. (1983) Physiological conflict in humans: fatigue vs. cold discomfort. *Am. J. Physiol.* **244**, R621–8.

Cahoon, R.L. (1972) Simple decision making at high altitude. *Ergonomics* **15**, 157–63.

Cain, S.M. and Dunn, J.E. (1965) Increase of arterial oxygen tension at altitude by carbonic anhydrase inhibition. *J. Appl. Physiol.* **20**, 882–4.

Campbell, R.H.A., Brand, H.L., Cox, J.R. and Howard, P. (1975) Body weight and body water in chronic cor pulmonale. *Clin. Sci. Mol. Med.* **49**, 323–35.

Caplan, C.E. (1999) The big chill: diseases exacerbated by exposure to cold. *Can. Med. Assoc. J.* **160**, 88.

Cargill, R.I., Kiely, D.G., Clark, R.A. and Lipworth, B.J. (1995) Hypoxaemia and release of endothelin-1. *Thorax* **50**, 1308–10.

Carpenter, T.C., Reeves, J.T. and Durmowicz, A.G. (1998) Viral respiratory infection increases susceptibility of young rats to hypoxia-induced pulmonary edema. *J. Appl. Physiol.* **84**, 1048–54.

Carrillo, C. (1996) Pregnancy at high altitude (abstract). *Acta Andina* **5**(2), 67.

Cassin, S.R., Gilbert, R.D., Bunnell, C.E. and Johnson, E.M. (1971) Capillary development during exposure to chronic hypoxia. *Am. J. Physiol.* **220**, 448–51.

Castellani, J.W., Young, A.J., Sawka, M.W. *et al.* (1998) Amnesia during cold water immersion. A case report. *Wilderness Environ. Med.* **9**, 153–5.

Castellani, J.W., Young, A.J., Kain, J.E. and Sawka, M.W. (1999a) Thermo regulatory responses to cold water at different times of day. *J. Appl. Physiol.* **87**, 243–6.

Castellani, J.W., Young, A.J., Kain, J.E. *et al.* (1999b) Thermoregulation during cold exposure: effects of prior exercise. *J. Appl. Physiol.* **87**, 247–52.

Castellini, M.A. and Somero, G.N. (1981) Buffering capacity of vertebrate muscle – correlations with potentials for anaerobic function. *J. Comp. Physiol.* **143**, 191–8.

Castilla, E.E., Lopez-Camelo, J.S. and Campana, H. (1999) Altitude as a risk factor for congenital anomalies. *Am. J. Med. Genet.* **86**, 9–14.

Cattermole, T.J. (1999) The epidemiology of cold injury in Antarctica. *Aviat. Space Environ. Med.* **70**, 135–40.

Cavaletti, G., Moroni, R., Garavaglia, P. and Tredici, G. (1987) Brain damage after high-altitude climbs without oxygen. *Lancet* **1**, 101.

Cavaletti, G. and Tredici, G. (1993) Long-lasting neuropsychological changes after a single high altitude climb. *Acta Neurol. Scand.* **87**, 103–5.

Cerretelli, P. (1976a) Limiting factors to oxygen transport on Mount Everest. *J. Appl. Physiol.* **40**, 658–67.

Cerretelli, P. (1976b) Metabolismo ossidativo ed anaerobico nel soggetto acclimatato all'altitudine. Rilievi sperimentali nel corso della spedizione italiana all'Everest. *Minerva Med.* **67**, 2331–46.

Cerretelli, P. (1980) Gas exchange at high altitude, in *Pulmonary Gas Exchange,* Vol. II (ed. J.B. West), Academic Press, New York, pp. 97–147.

Cerretelli, P. (1987) Extreme hypoxia in air breathers: some problems, in *Comparative Physiology of Environmental Adaptations,* Vol. 2: *Adapatations to Extreme Environments* (ed. P. Dejours), Karger, Basel.

Cerretelli, P. (1992) Energy sources for muscular exercise. *Int. J. Sports Med.* **13** (Suppl. 1), S106–10.

Cerretelli, P. and Hoppeler, H. (1996) Morphologic and metabolic response to chronic hypoxia: the muscle system, in *Handbook of Physiology*, Section 4: *Environmental Physiology,* Vol. II (eds. M.J. Fregly and C.M. Blatteis), American Physiological Society, New York, pp. 1155–81.

Cerretelli, P., Marconi, C., Dériaz, O. and Giezendanner, D. (1984) After effects of chronic hypoxia on cardiac output and muscle blood flow at rest and exercise. *Eur. J. Appl. Physiol.* **53**, 92–6.

Cerretelli, P. and Whipp, B.J. (1980) *Exercise Bioenergetics and Gas Exchange*, Elsevier/North-Holland, Amsterdam.

Chance, B. (1957) Cellular oxygen requirements. *Fed. Proc.* **16**, 671–80.

Chance, B., Cohen, P., Jobsis, F. and Schoener, B. (1962) Intracellular oxidation-reduction states *in vivo. Science* **137**, 499–508.

Chandrashekhar, Y., Anand, I.S., Rao, K.S. and Malhotra, R.M. (1992) Continuous ambulatory electrocardiographic changes after rapid ascent to extreme altitudes. *Indian Heart J.* **44**, 403–5.

Chang, C., Chen, N., Coward, M.P. *et al.* (1986) Preliminary conclusions of the Royal Society and Academia Sinica 1985 Geotraverse of Tibet. *Nature* **323**, 501–7.

Chanutin, A. and Curnish, R.R. (1967) Effect of organic and inorganic phosphates on the oxygen equilibrium of human erythrocytes. *Arch. Biochem. Biophys.* **121**, 96–102.

Chapman, F.S. (1938) *Lhasa. The Holy City,* Chatto and Windus, London, p. 241.

Chapman, J.A., Grant, I.S., Taylor, G. *et al.* (1972) Endemic goitre in the Gilgit Agency, West Pakistan. *Philos. Trans. R. Soc. Lond. Ser. B* **263**, 459–91.

Chapman, K.R. and Cherniack, N.S. (1986) Aging effects on the interaction of hypercapnia and hypoxia as ventilatory stimuli. *Am. Rev. Respir. Dis.* **133** (Suppl. A), 137.

Chapman, R.F., Stray-Gundersen, J. and Levine, B.D. (1998) Individual response to altitude training. *J. Appl. Physiol.* **85**, 1448–56.

Chatterji, J.C., Ohri, V.C., Das, B.K. *et al.* (1982) Platelet count, platelet aggregation and fibrinogen levels following acute induction to high altitude (3200 and 3771 metres). *Thromb. Res.* **26**, 177–82.

Chen, Q.H., Ge, R.L., Wang, X.Z. *et al.* (1997) Exercise performance of Tibetan and Han adolescents at altitudes of 3,417 and 4,300 m. *J. Appl. Physiol.* **83**, 661–7.

Chernow, B., Lake, C.R., Zaritsky, A. *et al.* (1983) Sympathetic nervous system 'switch off' with severe hypothermia. *Crit. Care Med.* **11**, 677–80.

Chesner, I.M., Small, N.A. and Dykes, P.W. (1987) Intestinal absorption at high altitude. *Postgrad. Med. J.* **63**, 173–5.

Cheyne, J. (1818) A case of apoplexy in which the fleshy part of the heart was converted into fat. *Dublin Hosp. Rep.* **2**, 216–23.

Chiodi, H. (1957) Respiratory adaptations to chronic high altitude hypoxia. *J. Appl. Physiol.* **10**, 81–7.

Chrenko, F.A. and Pugh, L.G.C.E. (1961) The contribution of solar radiation to the thermal environment of man in Antarctica. *Proc. R. Soc. Lond. Ser. B* **155**, 243–65.

Christensen, E.H. (1937) Sauerstoffaufnahme und Respiratorische Funktionen in Grossen Höhen. *Skand. Arch. Physiol.* **76**, 88–100.

Christensen, E.H. and Forbes, W.H. (1937) Der Kreislauf in grossen Höhen. *Skand. Arch. Physiol.* **76**, 75–87.

Cibella, F., Cuttitta, G., Romano, S., Grassi, B., Bonsignore, G. and Milic-Emili, J. (1999) Respiratory energetics during exercise at high altitude. *J. Appl. Physiol.* **86**, 1785–92.

Clark, C.F., Heaton, R.K. and Wiens, A.N. (1983) Neuropsychological functioning after prolonged high altitude exposure in mountaineering. *Aviat. Space Environ. Med.* **54**, 202–7.

Clark, I.M., Awburn, M.M., Cowden, W.B. and Rockett, K.A. (1999) Can excessive iNOS induction explain much of the illness of acute mountain sickness, in *Hypoxia: Into the Next Millennium* (eds. R.C. Roach, P.D. Wagner and P.H. Hackett), Plenum/Kluwer, New York, p. 373.

Clark, R.T., Criscuolo, D. and Coulson, D.K. (1952) Effects of 20,000 feet simulated altitude on myoglobin content of animals with and without exercise. *Fed. Proc.* **11**, 25.

Clarke, C. and Duff, J. (1976) Mountain sickness, retinal haemorrhages, and acclimatization on Mount Everest in 1975. *BMJ* **2**, 495–7.

Clarke, C.R.A. (1983) Cerebral infarction at extreme altitude, in *Hypoxia, Exercise and Altitude* (eds. J.R. Sutton, C.S. Houston and N.L. Jones), Liss, New York, pp. 453–4.

Claybaugh, J.R., Wade, C.E., Sato, A.K. *et al.* (1982) Antidiuretic hormone responses to eucapnic and hypocapnic hypoxia in humans. *J. Appl. Physiol. Respir. Environ. Exerc. Physiol.* **53**, 815–23.

Clegg, E.J. (1978) Fertility and early growth, in *The Biology of High Altitude Peoples* (ed. P.T. Baker), Cambridge University Press, Cambridge, pp. 65–115.

Cochrane, G.M., Prior, J.G. and Wolff, C.B. (1980) Chronic stable asthma and the normal arterial pressure of carbon dioxide in hypoxia. *BMJ* **301**, 705–7.

Cold hypersensitivity (editorial) (1975) *BMJ* **1**, 643–4.

Colice, C.L. and Ramirez, C. (1986) Aldosterone response to angiotensin II during hypoxemia. *J. Appl. Physiol.* **61**, 150–4.

Collier, D.J., Collier, C.J., Dubowitz, G., and Rosenberg, M. (1997b) Gender and weight loss at altitude (abstract), in *Hypoxia: Women at Altitude* (eds. C.S. Houston and G. Coates), Queen City Printers, Burlington, VA, p. 308.

Collier, D.J., Nickol, A., Milledge, J.S. *et al.* (1995) Dynamic chemosensitivity to carbon dioxide increases with acclimatisation to chronic hypoxia in man. *J. Physiol. (Lond.)* **487**, 109P.

Collier, D., Wolff, C.B., Nathan, J. *et al.* (1997a) Benzolamide, acidosis and acute mountain sickness, in *Hypoxia: women at altitude* (eds. C.S. Houston and G. Coates), Queen City Printers, Burlington, VA. p. 307.

Colquohoun, W.P. (1984) Effects of personality on body temperature and mental efficiency following transmeridian flight. *Aviat. Space Environ. Med.* **55**, 493–6.

Comroe, J.H. (1938) The location and function of the chemoreceptors of the aorta. *Am. J. Physiol.* **127**, 176–91.

Connaughton, J.J., Douglas, N.J., Morgan, A.D. *et al.* (1985) Almitrine improves oxygenation when both awake and asleep in patients with hypoxia and carbon dioxide retention caused by chronic bronchitis and emphysema. *Am. Rev. Respir. Dis.* **132,** 206–10.

Consolazio, C.F., Johnson, H.L., Krzywicki, H.J. and Daws, T.A. (1972) Metabolic aspects of acute altitude exposure (4300m) in adequately nourished humans. *Am. J. Clin. Nutr.* **25**, 23–9.

Consolazio, C.F., Matoush, L.O., Johnson, H.L. and Daws, T.A. (1968) Protein and water balances of young adults during prolonged exposure to high altitude (4300m). *Am. J. Clin. Nutr.* **21**, 134–61.

Consolazio, C.F., Matoush, L.O., Johnson, H.L. *et al.* (1969) Effects of high carbohydrate diets on performance and clinical symptomatology after rapid ascent to high altitude. *Fed. Proc.* **28**, 937–43.

Coppin, E.G., Livingstone, S.P. and Kuehn, L.A. (1978) Effects on hand grip strength due to arm immersion in a 10°C water bath. *Aviat. Space Environ. Med.* **49**, 1319–26.

Cosby, R.L., Sophocles, A.M., Durr, J.A. *et al.* (1988) Elevated plasma atrial natriuretic factor and vasopressin in high-altitude pulmonary edema. *Ann. Intern. Med.* **109**, 796–9.

Costello, M.L., Mathieu-Costello, O. and West, J.B. (1992) Stress failure of alveolar epithelial cells studied by scanning electron microscopy. *Am. Rev. Respir. Dis.* **145**, 1446–55.

Costil, D.L., Coyle, E., Dalsky, G. *et al.* (1977) Effect of elevated plasma FFA and insulin on muscle glycogen usage during exercise. *J. Appl. Physiol.* **43**, 695–9.

Cotes, J.E. (1954) Ventilatory capacity at altitude and its relation to mask design. *Proc. R. Soc. Lond. Ser. B* **143**, 32–9.

Coward, W.A. (1991) Measurement of energy expenditure: the doubly labelled water method in clinical practice. *Proc. Nutr. Soc.* **50**, 227–37.

Crawford, J.P. (1979) Endogenous anxiety and circadian rhythms. *BMJ* **1**, 662.

Crawford, R.D. and Severinghaus, J.W. (1978) CSF pH and ventilatory acclimatization to altitude. *J. Appl. Physiol.* **44**, 274–83.

Cruden, N.L.M., Newby, D.E., Ross, J.A., Johnston, N.R. and Webb, D.J. (1998) Effect of high altitude, cold and exercise on plasma endothelin-1 and markers of endothelial function in man. (Abstract) *Clin. Sci.* **94**, p. 20.

Cruden, N.L.M., Newby, D.E., Ross, J.A. *et al.* (1999) Effect of cold exposure, exercise and high altitude on plasma endothelin-1 and endothelial cell markers in man. *Scott. Med. J.* **44**, 143–6.

Cruz, J.C., Diaz, C., Marticorena, E. and Hilario, V. (1979) Phlebotomy improves pulmonary gas exchange in chronic mountain polycythemia. *Respiration* **38**, 305–13.

Cruz, J.C., Reeves, J.T., Grover, R.F. *et al.* (1980) Ventilatory acclimatization to high altitude is prevented by CO_2 breathing. *Respiration* **39**, 121–30.

Cudaback, D.M. (1984) Four-km altitude effects on performance and health. *Publ. Astronom. Soc. Pacif.* **96**, 463–77.

Cummings, P. and Lysgaard, M. (1981) Cardiac arrhythmia at high altitude. *West. J. Med.* **135**, 66–8.

Cunningham, D.J.C., Patrick, J.M. and Lloyd, B.B. (1964) The respiratory response of man to hypoxia, in *Oxygen in the Animal Organism* (eds. F. Dickens and E. Niel), Pergamon, Oxford, pp. 277–93.

Cunningham, W.L., Becker, E.J. and Kreuzer, F. (1965) Catecholamine in plasma and urine at high altitude. *J. Appl. Physiol.* **20**, 607–10.

Curran, L.S., Zhuang, J., Droma, T. *et al.* (1995) Hypoxic ventilatory response in Tibetan residents of 4400 m compared with 3658 m. *Respir. Physiol.* **100**, 223–30.

Curran, L.S., Zhuang, J., Sun, S.F. and Moore, L.G. (1997) Ventilation and hypoxic ventilatory responsiveness in Chinese-Tibetan residents at 3,658m. *J. Appl. Physiol.* **83**, 2098–104.

Currie, T.T., Carter, P.H., Champion, W.L. *et al.* (1976) Spironolactone and acute mountain sickness. *Med. J. Aust.* **2**, 168–70.

Daniels, J. and Oldridge, N. (1970) The effects of alternate exposure to altitude and sea level on world class middle distance runners. *Med. Sci. Sports Exerc.* **2**, 107–112.

Danielsson, U. (1996) Windchill and the risk of tissue freezing. *J. Appl. Physiol.* **81**, 2666–73.

Danzl, D.F., Pozos, R.S. and Hamlet, M.P. (1995) Accidental hypothermia, in *Wilderness Medicine* (ed. P.S. Auerbach), Mosby, St Louis, MO, pp. 51–103.

Das, B.K., Tewari, S.C., Parashar, S.K. *et al.* (1983) Electrocardiographic changes at high altitude. *Indian Heart J.* **35**, 30–3.

Das, S.C. (1902) *Journey to Lhasa and Central Tibet,* John Murray, London, pp. 257–60.

Datta, A.K. and Nickol, A. (1995) Dynamic chemo-receptiveness studied in man during moderate exercise breath by breath, in *Modeling and Control of Ventilation* (eds. S.J.G. Semple, L. Adams, and B.J. Whipp), Plenum Press, New York, pp. 235–8.

Davies, R.O., Edwards, M.W. Jr and Lahiri, S. (1982) Halothane depresses the response of carotid body chemoreceptors to hypoxia and hypercapnia in the cat. *Anesthesiology* **57**, 153–9.

Dawson, A. (1972) Regional lung function during early acclimatization to 3,100 m altitude. *J. Appl. Physiol.* **33**, 218–23.

De Angelis, C., Ferri, C., Urbani, L. and Ferrace, S. (1996) Effect of acute exposure to hypoxia on electrolyes and water metabolism regulatory hormones. *Aviat. Space Environ. Med.* **67**, 746–50.

De Jong, G.F. (ed.) (1968) *Demography of High Altitude Populations,* WHO/PAHO/IBP Meeting of Investigators on Population Biology of Altitude, Pan American Health Organization, Washington DC.

de Meer, K., Heymans, H.S. and Zijlstra, W.G. (1995) Physical adaptation of children to life at high altitude. *Eur. J. Ped.* **154**, 263–72.

De Pay, A.W. (1982) Medical treatment of hypothermic victims, in *Unterkuhlung im Seenotfall,* 2nd Symposium Deutsche Gesellschaft zur Rettung Schiffbruchiger (eds. P. Koch and M. Kohfahl), Cuxhaven, Germany pp. 146–53.

de Saussure, H.-B. (1786–7) *Voyages Dans Les Alpes*, 4 volumes, Barde, Manget, Geneva.

Deasy, H.H.P. (1901) *In Tibet and Chinese Turkestan,* T. Fisher Unwin, London, pp. 2–73.

DeGraff, A.C., Jr, Grover, R.F., Johnson, R.L., Jr, Hammond, J.W., Jr and Miller, J.M. (1970) Diffusing capacity of the lung in Caucasians native to 3,100m. *J. Appl. Physiol.* **29**, 71–6.

Dempsey, J.A. (1983) Ventilatory regulation in hypoxic sleep: introduction, in *Hypoxia, Exercise, and Altitude* (eds. J.R. Sutton, C.S. Houston and N.L. Jones), Liss, New York, pp. 61–3.

Dempsey, J.A. and Forster, H.V. (1982) Mediation of ventilatory adaptations. *Physiol. Rev.* **62**, 262–346.

Dempsey, J.A., Forster, H.V., Bisgard, G.E. *et al.* (1979) Role of cerebrospinal fluid [H⁺] in ventilatory deacclimatization from chronic hypoxia. *J. Clin. Invest.* **64**, 199–204.

Dempsey, J.A., Forster, H.V., Chosy, L.W., Hanson, P.G. and Reddan, W.G. (1978) Regulation of CSF [HCO₃⁻] during long-term hypoxic hypocapnia in man. *J. Appl. Physiol.* **44**, 175–82.

Dempsey, J.A., Reddan, W.G., Birnbaum, M.L. *et al.* (1971) Effects of acute through life-long hypoxic exposure on exercise pulmonary gas exchange. *Respir. Physiol.* **13**, 62–89.

Denison, D.M., Ledwith, F. and Poulton, E.C. (1966) Complex reaction times at simulated cabin altitudes of 5,000 feet and 8,000 feet. *Aerosp. Med.* **37**, 1010–13.

Desideri, L. (1712–27) Journey across the great desert of Nguari Giongar, and assistance rendered by a Tartar princess and her followers, in *An Account of Tibet* (ed. F. de Filippi), Routledge, London, 1932, p. 87.

Desplanches, D., Hoppeler, H., Linossier, M.T. *et al.* (1993) Effects of training in normoxia and normobaric hypoxia on human muscle structure. *Pflügers Arch.* **425**, 263–7.

Dickinson, J., Heath, D., Gosney, J. and Williams, D. (1983) Altitude related deaths in seven trekkers in the Himalayas. *Thorax* **38**, 646–56.

Dickinson, J.G. (1979) Severe acute mountain sickness. *Postgrad. Med. J.* **55**, 454–8.

Dickinson, J.G. (1982) Terminology and classification of acute mountain sickness. *BMJ* **285**, 720–1.

Dill, D.B. (1938) *Life, Heat and Altitude,* Harvard University Press, Cambridge, MA, pp. 144–74.

Dill, D.B., Edwards, H.T., Fölling, A., Oberg, S.A., Pappenheimer, A.M. Jr and Talbott, J.H. (1931) Adaptations of the organism to changes in oxygen pressure. *J. Physiol. (Lond.)* **71**, 47–63.

Dill, D.B., Robinson, S., Balke, B. and Newton, J.L. (1964) Work tolerance: age and altitude. *J. Appl. Physiol.* **19**, 483–8.

Dill, D.B., Talbott, J.H. and Consolazio, W.V. (1937) Blood as a physiochemical system. XII. Man at high altitudes. *J. Biol. Chem.* **118**, 649–66.

Dinmore, A.J., Edwards, J.S.A., Menzies, I.S. and Travis, S.P.L. (1994) Intestinal carbohydrate absorption and permeability at high altitude (5730 m). *J. Appl. Physiol.* **76**, 1903–7.

Dittert, R., Chevalley, G. and Lambert, R. (1954) *Forerunners to Everest,* Allen and Unwin, London, pp. 141–53.

Dombret, M.C., Rouby, J.J., Smeijan, J.M. *et al.* (1987) Pulmonary oedema during pulmonary embolism. *Br. J. Dis. Chest,* **81**, 407–10.

Donaldson, G.C., Ermakov, S.P., Komarov, Y. *et al.* (1998b) Cold related mortalities and protection against cold in Yakutsk, eastern Siberia: observation and interview study. *BMJ* **317**, 978–82.

Donaldson, G.C., Tchernjavski, V.E., Ermakov, S.P. *et al.* (1998a) Winter mortality and cold stress in Yekaterinburg, Russia: interview survey. *BMJ* **316**, 514–18.

Dong-Sheng, L. (ed.) (1981) *Proceedings of Symposium on Qinghai-Xizang (Tibet) Plateau,* Vols. 1 and 2, Beijing Science Press/Gordon and Breach, New York.

Douglas, C.G. and Haldane, J.S. (1909) The causes of periodic or Cheyne–Stokes breathing. *J. Physiol. (Lond.)* **38**, 401–19.

Douglas, C.G., Haldane, J.S., Henderson, Y. and Schneider, E.C. (1913) Physiological observations made on Pike's Peak, Colorado, with special reference to adaptation to low barometric pressures. *Philas Trans. R. Soc. Lond. Ser. B* **203**, 185–381.

Drinking and drowning (editorial) (1979) *BMJ* **1**, 70–1.

Droma, Y., Ge, R.L., Tanaka, M. *et al.* (1996b) Acute hypoxic pulmonary vascular response does not accompany plasma endothelin-1 elevation in subjects susceptible to high altitude pulmonary edema. *Int. Med.* **35**, 257–60.

Droma, Y., Hayano, T., Takabayashi, Y. *et al.* (1996a) Endothelin-1 and interleukin-8 in high altitude pulmonary oedema. *Eur. Respir. J.* **9**, 1947–9.

Dubas, F. (1980) Aspects de medicaux de l'accident par avalanche. Hypotherme et gelure. *Z. Unfallmed. Berfskr.* **73**, 164–7.

Dubas, F., Henzwlin, R. and Michelet, J. (1991a) Avalanche prevention and rescue, in *A Colour Atlas of Mountain Medicine* (eds. J. Vallotten and F. Dubas), Wolfe, London, pp. 104–12.

Dubas, F., Henzwlin, R. and Michelet, J. (1991b) Rescue in crevasses, in *A Colour Atlas of Mountain Medicine* (eds. J. Vallotten and F. Dubas), Wolfe, London, pp. 112–16.

Dubowitz, G. (1998) Effect of temazepam on oxygen saturation and sleep quality at high altitude: randomised placebo controlled crossover trial. *BMJ* **21**, 587–9.

Dubowitz, G. and Peacock, A.J. (1999) Pulmonary artery pressure variation measured by Doppler echocardiography in healthy subjects at 4250m (abstract), in *Hypoxia: Into the Next Millennium* (eds. R.C. Roach, P.D. Wagner and P.H. Hackett), Plenum/Kluwer, New York, p. 378.

Dudley, G.A., Tullson, P.C. and Terjung, R.L. (1987) Influence of mitochondrial content on the sensitivity of respiratory control. *J. Biol. Chem.* **262**, 9109–14.

Duff, J. (1999) Observations while treating altitude illness (Letter). *Wilderness Environ. Med.* **10**, 274.

Duff, J. (1999) The Tibetan tuck: a dry land cold condition survival position equivalent to that used in cold water. *Wilderness Environ. Med.* **10**, 206–7.

Duke, H.N. (1954) Site of action of anoxia on the pulmonary blood vessels of the cat. *J. Physiol. (Lond.)* **125**, 373–82.

Duplain, H., Lepori, M., Sartori, C. *et al.* (1999b) Inflammation does not contribute to high altitude pulmonary edema. *Am. J. Respir. Crit. Care* **159**, A345 (abstract).

Duplain, H., Vollenweider, L., Delabeys, A. *et al.* (1999a) Augmented sympathetic activation during short-term hypoxia and high-altitude exposure in subjects susceptible to high-altitude pulmonary edema. *Circulation* **99**, 1713–18.

Durand, J. and Martineaud, J.P. (1971) Resistance and capacitance vessels of the skin in permanent and temporary residents at high altitude, in *High Altitude Physiology: Cardiac and Respiratory Aspects,* Ciba Foundation (eds. R. Porter and J. Knight), Churchill Livingstone, London, pp. 159–70.

Durand, J. and Raynaud, J. (1987) Limb blood and heat exchange at altitude, in *Hypoxia and Cold* (eds. J.R. Sutton, C.S. Houston and G. Coates), Praeger, New York, pp. 100–13.

Durig, A. (1911) Ergebnisse der Monte Rosa Expedition vom Jahre 1906 von Prof. Dr. A. Durig. Über den Gaswechsel beim Gehen. *Denkschr. d. Mathem. - Naturw. Kl.* **86**, 293–347.

Durmowicz, A.G., Noordeweir, E., Nicholas, R. and Reeves, J.T. (1997) Inflammatory processes may predispose children to high altitude pulmonary edema. *J. Pediatr.* **130**, 838–40.

Eady, R.A.J., Bentley-Phillips, C.B., Keahey, T.M. and Greaves, M.W. (1978) Cold urticaria vasculitis. *Br. J. Dermatol.* **99** (Suppl. 16), 9–10.

Eaton, J.W., Skelton, T.D. and Berger, E. (1974) Survival at extreme altitude: protective effect of increased hemoglobin-oxygen affinity. *Science* **183**, 743–4.

Echevarria, E. (1968) The South American Indian as a pioneer alpinist. *Alpine J.* **73**, 81–8.

Echevarria, E. (1979) Note on objects found on Andean summits. *Am. Alpine J.* **23**, 588.

Echevarria, E. (1983) Legends of the high Andes. *Alpine J.* **88**, 85–91.

Eckardt, K., Boutellier, U., Kurtz, A. *et al.* (1989) Rate of erythropoietin formation in humans in response to acute hypobaric hypoxia. *J. Appl. Physiol.* **66**, 1785–8.

Edwards, H.T. (1936) Lactic acid in rest and work at high altitude. *Am. J. Physiol.* **116**, 367–75.

Eger, E.I., Kellogg, R.H., Mines, A.H. *et al.* (1968) Influence of CO_2 on ventilatory acclimatization to altitude. *J. Appl. Physiol.* **24**, 607–14.

Egli-Sinclair. (1891–2) Ueber die Bergkrankheit. *Jahrbuch des Schweizer Alpen Klub* **27**, 308–26.

Egli-Sinclair. (1894) Le mal de montagne. *Rev. Sci. (Revue Rose) (Paris)* (4) **1**, 172–80.

Eichenberger, U., Weiss, E., Riemann, D., Oelz, O. and Bartsch, P. (1996) Nocturnal periodic breathing and the development of acute high altitude illness. *Am. J. Respir. Crit. Care Med.* **154**, 1748–54.

Ekelund, L.G. (1967) Circulatory and respiratory adaptation during prolonged exercise. *Acta Physiol. Scand.* (Suppl.) **292**, 1–38.

Eldridge, M.W., Podolsky, A., Richardson, R.S. *et al.* (1996) Pulmonary haemodynamic response to exercise in subjects with prior high-altitude pulmonary edema. *J. Appl. Physiol.* **81**, 911–21.

Eldridge, W.E., Braun, R.K., Yoneda, K.Y. *et al.* (1998) Lung injury after heavy exercise at altitude. *Chest* **114**, 66S–67S.

Elias, N. and Ross, E.D. (1898) *A History of the Moghuls of Central Asia, Being the Tarikh-I-Rashidi of Mirza Muhammed Haidar, Dughlat,* Sampson, Low, London, pp. 412–13.

Elliott, A.R., Fu, Z., Tsukimoto, K. *et al.* (1992) Short-term reversibility of ultrastructural changes in pulmonary capillaries caused by stress failure. *J. Appl. Physiol.* **73**, 1150–8.

Elliott, M.E. and Goodfriend, T.L. (1986) Inhibition of aldosterone synthesis by atrial natriuretic factor. *Fed. Proc.* **45**, 2376–81.

Ellsworth, A.J., Meyer, E.F. and Larson, E.B. (1991) Acetazolamide or dexamethasone use versus placebo to prevent acute mountain sickness on Mount Rainier. *West. J. Med.* **154**, 289–93.

Elterman, L. (1964) *Atmospheric Attenuation Model, 1964, in the Ultraviolet, Visible, and Infrared Regions for Altitudes to 50 km*, Environmental Research Papers No. **46**, L.G. Hanscom Field, MA, Air Force Cambridge Research Laboratories, Office of Aerospace Research, AFCRL-64-740.

Enander, A. (1984) Performance and sensory aspects of work in cold environments – a review. *Ergonomics* **27**, 365–78.

English, J.S.C. (1987) High altitude and the skin, in *Abstracts of the UIAA Mountain Medicine Conference*, Mountain Medicine Data Centre, St Bartholomew's Hospital, London, p. 20.

Engwall, M.J.A. and Bisgard, G.E. (1990) Ventilatory response to chemoreceptor stimulation after hypoxic acclimatization in awake goats. *J. Appl. Physiol.* **69**, 1236–43.

Ennemoser, O., Ambach, W. and Flora, G. (1988) Physical assessment of heat insulation of rescue foils. *Int. J. Sports Med.* **9**, 179–82.

Erdman, J., Sun, K.T., Masar, P. and Niederhauser, H. (1998) Effects of exposure to altitude on men with coronary artery disease and impaired left ventricular function. *Am. J. Cardiol.* **81**, 266–70.

Erslev, A. (1987) Erythropoietin coming of age. *N. Engl. J. Med.* **316**, 101–3.

Evans, R.C. (1956) *Kanchenjunga. The Untrodden Peak,* Hodder and Stoughton, London.

Everest: the Hornbein Couloir direct from Tibet. (1987) *Am. Alpine J.* **29**, 302–4.

Eversman, T., Gottsman, M., Uhlich, E. *et al.* (1978) Increased secretion of growth hormone, prolactin, antidiuretic hormone and cortisol induced by the stress of motion sickness. *Aviat. Space Environ. Med.* **49**, 53–7.

Fâ-Hien (399–414) *A Record of Buddhistic Kingdoms, Being an Account by the Chinese Monk Fâ-Hien of his Travels in India and Ceylon (AD 399–414) in Search of the Buddhist Books of Discipline.* Translated and annotated with a Corean recension of the Chinese text by J. Legge, Dover Publications, New York (1965), pp. 40–1 (p. 12 of the Korean text).

Falk, B., Bar-Or, J., Smolander, J. and Frost, G. (1994) Response to rest and exercise in the cold: the effect of age and aerobic fitness. *J. Appl. Physiol.* **76**, 72–8.

Farber, M.O., Bright, T.P., Strawbridge, R.A. *et al.* (1975) Impaired water handling in chronic obstructive lung disease. *J. Lab. Clin. Med.* **85**, 41–9.

Feldman, K.W. and Herndon, S.P. (1977) Positive expiratory pressure for the treatment of high altitude edema. *Lancet* **1**, 1036–7.

Fencl, V., Gabel, R.A. and Wolfe, D. (1979) Composition of cerebral fluids in goats adapted to high altitude. *J. Appl. Physiol.* **47**, 408–13.

Fencl, V., Miller, T.B. and Pappenheimer, J.R. (1966) Studies on the respiratory response to disturbances of acid–base balance, with deductions concerning ionic composition of cerebral interstitial fluid. *Am. J. Physiol.* **210**, 449–72.

Ferrazzini, G., Maggiorini, M., Kriemler, S., Bärtsch, P. and Oelz, O. (1987) Successful treatment of acute mountain sickness with dexamethasone. *BMJ* **294**, 1380–2.

Ferri, C., Bellini, C., De Angelis, C. *et al.* (1995) Circulating endothelin-1 concentrations in patients with chronic hypoxia. *J. Clin. Path.* **48**, 519–24.

Ferrus, L., Commenges, D., Gire, J. and Varene, P. (1984) Respiratory water loss. *Respir. Physiol.* **56**, 11–20.

Filippi, F. de (1912) *Karakoram and Western Himalaya 1909,* Constable, London.

Fineman, J.R., Heymann, M.A. and Soifer, S.J. (1991) N^{ω}-nitro-L-arginine attenuates endothelium-dependent pulmonary vasodilation in lambs. *Am. J. Physiol.* **260**, H1299–306.

Finisterer, J. (1999) High altitude illness induced by tooth root infection. *Postgrad. Med. J.* **75**, 227–9.

Fiorenzano, G., Papalia, M.A., Parrivicini, M. *et al.* (1997) Prolonged ECG abnormalities in a subject with high altitude pulmonary edema (HAPE). *J. Sports Med. Phys. Fitness* **37**, 292–6.

Fischer, A.P., Stumpe, F. and Vallotton, J. (1991) Hypothermia in an avalanche: a case report, in *A Colour Atlas of Mountain Medicine* (eds. J. Vallotton and F. Du Bas), Wolfe, London, pp. 96–7.

Fisher, J.W. and Langston, J.W. (1967) The influence of hypoxia and cobalt on erythropoietin production in the isolated perfused dog kidney. *Blood* **29**, 114–25.

Fishman, A.P. (1985) Pulmonary circulation, in *Handbook of Physiology,* Section 3: *The Respiratory System,* Vol. 1: *Circulation and Nonrespiratory Functions* (eds. A.P. Fishman and A.B. Fisher), American Physiological Society, Bethesda, MD, pp. 93–165.

Fishman, R.A. (1975) Brain edema. *N. Engl. J. Med.* **293**, 706–11.

Fitch, R.F. (1964) Mountain sickness: a cerebral form. *Ann. Intern. Med.* **60**, 871–6.

Fitzgerald, F.T. and Jessop, C. (1982) Accidental hypothermia. A report of 22 cases and review of the literature. *Adv. Intern. Med.* **27**, 127–50.

FitzGerald, M.P. (1913) The changes in the breathing and the blood at various altitudes. *Philos. Trans. R. Soc. Lond. Ser. B* **203**, 351–71.

Flora, G. (1985) Secondary treatment of frostbite, in *High Altitude Deterioration* (eds. J. Rivolier, P. Cerretelli, J. Foray and P. Segantini), Karger, Basel, pp. 159–69.

Foray, J. and Cahen, C. (1981) Les hypothermies de montagne. *Chirurgie* **107**, 255–310.

Foray, J. and Salon, F. (1985) Casualties with cold injuries: primary treatment, in *High Altitude Deterioration* (eds. J. Rivolier, P. Cerretelli, J. Foray and P. Segantini), Karger, Basel, pp. 149–58.

Forbes, C.B. and Drenick, E.J. (1979) Loss of body nitrogen of fasting. *Am. J. Clin. Nutr.* **32**, 1370–4.

Forsling, M.L. and Milledge, J.S. (1977) Effect of hypoxia on vasopressin release in man. *J. Physiol.* **267**, 22–23P.

Forsling, M.L. and Milledge, J.S. (1980) The effect of simulated altitude (4000 m) on plasma cortisol and vasopressin concentration in man. *Proc. Int. Union Physiol. Sci.* **14**, 414.

Forster, H.V., Bisgard, G.E. and Klein, J.P. (1981) Effect of peripheral chemoreceptor denervation on acclimatization of goats during hypoxia. *J. Appl. Physiol.* **40**, 392–8.

Forster, H.V., Dempsey, J.A. and Chosy, L.W. (1974) Incomplete compensation of CSF [H+] in man during acclimatization to high altitude (4300 m). *J. Appl. Physiol.* **38**, 1067–72.

Forster, P. (1984) Reproducibility of individual response to exposure to high altitude. *BMJ* **289**, 1269.

Forster, P. (1986) Telescopes in high places, in *Aspects of Hypoxia* (ed. D. Heath), Liverpool University Press, Liverpool, pp. 217–33.

Forsyth, T.D. (1875) *Report of a Mission to Yarkund in 1873.* Foreign Department Press, Calcutta, pp. 66–9.

Forwand, S.A., Landowne, M., Follansbee, J.N. and Hansen, J.E. (1968) Effect of acetazolamide on acute mountain sickness. *N. Engl. J. Med.* **279**, 839–45.

Fox, V.F. (1967) Human performance in the cold. *Hum. Factors* **9**, 203–90.

Francis, T.J.R. and Golden, F. St C. (1985) Non-freezing cold injury: the pathogenesis. *J. R. Nav. Med. Serv.* **71**, 3–8.

Franz, D.R., Berberich, J.J., Blake, S. and Mills, W.J. (1978) Evaluation of fasciotomy and vasodilators for the treatment of frostbite in the dog. *Cryobiology* **15**, 659–69.

Fraser, J.B. (1820) *Journal of a Tour Through Part of the Snowy Range of the Himala Mountains, and to the Sources of the Rivers Jumna and Ganges,* Rodwell and Martin, London, p. 349.

Frayser, R., Houston, C.S., Bryan, A.C., Rennie, I.D. and Gray, G. (1970) Retinal hemorrhage at high altitude. *N. Engl. J. Med.* **282**, 1183–4.

Frayser, R., Rennie, I.D., Gray, G.W. and Houston, C.S. (1975) Hormonal and electrolyte response to exposure to 17,500 ft. *J. Appl. Physiol.* **38**, 636–42.

Fred, H.L., Schmidt, A.M., Bates, T. and Hecht, H.H. (1962) Acute pulmonary edema of altitude. Clinical and physiologic observations. *Circulation* **25**, 929–37.

Freshfield, D.W. (1903) Appendix C. The narratives of the pundits, in *Round Kangchenjunga,* Arnold, London.

Freund, B.J., O'Brien, C. and Young, A.J. (1994) Alcohol ingestion and temperature regulation during cold exposure. *J. Wilderness Med.* **5**, 88–98.

Friedman, N.B. (1945) The pathology of trench foot. *Am. J. Pathol.* **21**, 387–433.

Frisancho, A.R. (1978) Human growth and development among high-altitude populations, in *The Biology of High Altitude Peoples* (ed. P.T. Baker), Cambridge University Press, Cambridge, pp. 117–71.

Frisancho, A.R. (1988) Origins of differences in hemoglobin concentration between Himalayan and Andean populations. *Respir. Physiol.* **72**, 13–18.

Frisancho, A.R. and Baker, P.T. (1970) Altitude and growth: a study of the patterns of physical growth of a high altitude Peruvian Quechua population. *Am. J. Phys. Anthropol.* **32**, 279–92.

Froese, G. and Burton, A.C. (1957) Heat loss from the human head. *J. Appl. Physiol.* **10**, 235–41.

Frostell, C.G., Blomqvist, H., Hedenstierna, G., Lundberg, J. and Zapol, W.M. (1993) Inhaled nitric oxide selectively reverses human hypoxic pulmonary vasoconstriction without causing systemic vasodilation. *Anesthesiology* **78**, 427–35.

Fu, Z., Costello, M.L., Tsukimoto, K. *et al.* (1992) High lung volume increases stress failure in pulmonary capillaries. *J. Appl. Physiol.* **73**, 123–33.

Fuhrer-Haimendorf, C. von (1964) *The Sherpas of Nepal: Bhuddist Highlanders*, John Murray, London.

Fujimaki, T., Matsutani, M. Asai, A., Kohno, T. and Koike, M. (1986) Cerebral venous thrombosis due to high altitude polycythemia. Case report. *J. Neurosurg.* **64**, 148–50.

Fukushima, M., Yasaki, K., Shibamoto, T. *et al.* (1983) Findings of brain computed tomography in patients with high altitude pulmonary edema, in *Hypoxia, Exercise and Altitude* (eds. J.R. Sutton, C.S. Houston and N.L. Jones), Liss, New York, pp. 456–7.

Gale, G.E., Torre-Bueno, J.R., Moon, R.E. *et al.* (1985) Ventilation–perfusion inequality in normal humans during exercise at sea level and simulated altitude. *J. Appl. Physiol.* **58**, 978–88.

Galeotti, G. (1904) Les variations de l'alcalinité du sang sur le sommet du Mont Rosa. *Arch. Ital. Biol.* **41**, 80–92.

Galileo, G. (1638) *Dialogues Concerning Two New Sciences.* English translation of relevant pages in *High Altitude Physiology* (ed. J.B. West), Hutchinson Ross, Stroudsburg, PA, 1981.

Galton, V.A. (1978) Environmental effects, in *The Thyroid*, 4th edn (eds. S.C. Werner and S.H. Ingbar), Harper Row, New York, pp. 247–52.

Ganfornina, M.D. and Lopez-Barneo, J. (1991) Single K channels in membrane patches of arterial chemoreceptor cells are modulated by O_2 tension. *Proc. Natl. Acad. Sci. USA* **88**, 2927–30.

Garcia, N., Hopkins, S.R. and Powell, F.L. (1999) Effects of intermittent vs. continuous hypoxia on the isocapnic ventilatory hypoxic response in man. *Am. J. Crit. Care Respir. Med.* **159**, A44.

Garrido, E., Castello, A., Ventura, J.L., Capdevila, A. and Rodriguez, F.A. (1993) Cortical atrophy and other brain magnetic resonance imaging (MRI) changes after extremely high-altitude climbs without oxygen. *Int. J. Sports Med.* **14**, 232–4.

Garrod, E., Rodas, G., Javieere, C. *et al.* (1997) Cardiovascular response to exercise in elite Sherpa climbers transferred to sea level. *Med. Sci. Sports Exerc.* **29**, 937–42.

Garrow, J.S. (1987) Are liquid diets (VLCD) safe or necessary? in *Recent Advances in Obesity Research, V* (eds. E.M. Berry, S.H. Blondheim, H.E. Eliahou and E. Shafrir), Food and Nutrition Press, Westport, CT, pp. 312–16.

Gautier, H., Bonora, M., Schultz, S.A. and Remmers, J.E. (1987) Hypoxia induced changes in shivering and body temperature. *J. Appl. Physiol.* **62**, 2577–81.

Gautier, H., Peslin, R., Grassino, A. *et al.* (1982) Mechanical properties of the lungs during acclimatization to altitude. *J. Appl. Physiol.* **52**, 1407–15.

Gazenko, O.G. (1987) *Physiology of Man at High Altitude* [in Russian], Nauka, Moscow.

Ge, R.L., Matsuzawa, Y., Takeoka, M., Kubo, K., Sekiguchi, M. and Kobayashi, T. (1997) Low pulmonary diffusing capacity in subjects with acute mountain sickness. *Chest* **111**, 58–64.

Gehr, P., Bachofen, M. and Weibel, E.R. (1978) The normal human lung: ultrastructure and morphometric estimation of diffusion capacity. *Respir. Physiol.* **32**, 121–40.

Gerard, A.B., McElroy, M.D., Taylor M.J. *et al.* (2000) Six percent oxygen enrichment of room air at simulated 5000 m altitude improves neuropsychological function. *High Alt. Med. Biol.* **1**, 51–61.

Gerlach, H., Clauss, M., Ogawa, S. and Stern, D.M. (1992) Modulation of endothelial coagulant properties and barrier function by factors in the vascular microenvironment, in *Endothelial Cell Dysfunctions* (ed. N. Simoniescu and M. Simoniescu), Plenum, New York, pp. 525–45.

Giesbrecht, G.E., Goheen, M.S.L., Johnston, C.E. *et al.* (1997) Inhibition of shivering increases core temperature after drop and attenuates rewarming in hypothermic humans. *J. Appl. Physiol.* **83**, 1630–4.

Gilbert, D.L. (1983a) The first documented report of mountain sickness: the China or Headache Mountain story. *Respir. Physiol.* **52**, 315–26.

Gilbert, D.L. (1983b) The first documented report of mountain sickness: the Andean or Pariacaca story. *Respir. Physiol.* **52**, 327–47.

Gilbert, D.L. (1988) Mountain sickness at Pariacaca: what's in a name? (abstract). FASEB J.2, A318.

Gill, M.B., Milledge, J.S., Pugh, L.G.C.E. and West, J.B. (1962) Alveolar gas composition at 21,000 to 25,700 ft (6400–7830 m). *J. Physiol. (Lond.)* **163,** 373–7.

Gill, M.B., Poulton, E.C., Carpenter, A., Woodhead, M.M. and Gregory, M.H.P. (1964) Falling efficiency at sorting cards during acclimatization at 19,000 ft. *Nature* **203,** 436.

Gill, M.B. and Pugh, L.G.C.E. (1964) Basal metabolism and respiration in men living at 5,800 m (19000 ft). *J. Appl. Physiol.* **19**, 949–54.

Gillman, P. (1993) *Everest,* Little Brown, Boston.

Gippenreiter, E. (1983) Biomedical experiences on the first Soviet expedition to Mount Everest, in *Hypoxia, Exercise and Altitude* (eds. J.R. Sutton, C.S. Houston and N.L. Jones), Proceedings of the 3rd Banff Symposium, Liss, New York, pp. 183–7.

Glaisher, J., Flammarion, C., de Fonvielle, W. and Tissandier, G. (1871) Ascents from Wolverhampton, in *Travels in the Air* (ed. J. Glaisher), Lippincott, Philadelphia, pp. 50–8.

Glazier, J.B., Hughes, J.M.B., Maloney, J.E. and West, J.B. (1969) Measurements of capillary dimensions and blood volume in rapidly frozen lungs. *J. Appl. Physiol.* **26**, 65–76.

Glazier, J.B. and Murray, J.F. (1971) Sites of pulmonary vasomotor reactivity in the dog during alveolar hypoxia and serotonin and histamine infusion. *J. Clin. Invest.* **50**, 2550–8.

Goldberg, S.V., Schoene, R.B., Haynor, D. *et al.* (1992) Brain tissue pH and ventilatory acclimatization to high altitude. *J. Appl. Physiol.* **72**, 58–63.

Golden, F. St C. (1973) Recognition and treatment of immersion hypothermia. *Proc. R. Soc. Med.* **66**, 1058–61.

Golden, F. St C. (1983) Rewarming, in *The Nature and Treatment of Hypothermia* (eds. R.S. Pozos and L.E. Wittmers), Croom Helm, London/University of Minnesota Press, Minneapolis, pp. 194–208.

Golden, F. St C. and Hervey, G.R. (1981) The 'after drop' and death after rescue from immersion in cold water, in *Hypothermia Ashore and Afloat* (ed. J.N. Adams), Aberdeen University Press, Aberdeen, pp. 37–56.

Goldsmith, R. and Minard, D. (1976) Cold, cold work, in *Occupational Health and Safety,* Vol. 1, International Labour Office, Geneva, pp. 319–20.

Goldstein, M.C. and Beall, C.M. (1989) *Nomads of Western Tibet,* Serindia, London.

Gollnick, P.D. and Saltin, B. (1982) Significance of skeletal muscle oxidative enzyme enhancement with endurance training. *Clin. Physiol.* **2**, 1–12.

Goñez, C., Villena, A. and Gonzales, G.F. (1993) Serum levels of adrenal androgens up to adrenarche in Peruvian children living at sea level and at high altitude. *J. Endocrinol.* **136**, 517–23.

Gonzales, G.F., Villena, A., Escuderl, F and Coyotupa, J. (1996) Reproduction in the Andes (Abstract). *Acta Andina* **5**(2), 68–9.

Gonzalez, N.C., Albrecht, T., Sullivan, L.P. and Clancy, R.L. (1990) Compensation of respiratory alkalosis induced after acclimation to simulated altitude. *J. Appl. Physiol.* **69**, 1380–6.

Goodenough, R.D., Royle, G.T., Nadel, E.R. *et al.* (1982) Leucine and urea metabolism in acute human cold exposure. *J. Appl. Physiol.* **53**, 367–72.

Goodman, L. (1964) Oscillatory behavior of ventilation in resting man. *IEEE Trans. Biomed. Elec.* **11**, 82–93.

Gore, C., Craig, N., Hahn, A. *et al.* (1998) Altitude training at 2690 m does not increase total haemoglobin mass or sea level VO$_2$ max in world champion track cyclists. *J. Sci. Med. Sport.* **1**, 156–70.

Gore, C.J., Hahn, A.G., Watson, D.B. *et al.* (1996) VO$_2$ max and arterial oxygen saturation at sea level and 610 m. *Med. Sci. Sports Exerc.* **27**, Abstract 42.

Gorlin, R. (1966) Physiology of the coronary circulation, in *The Heart* (eds. J.W. Hurst and R.B. Logan), McGraw-Hill, New York, pp. 653–8.

Gosney, J. (1986) Histopathology of the endocrine organs in hypoxia, in *Aspects of Hypoxia* (ed. D. Heath), Liverpool University Press, Liverpool, pp. 131–45.

Gosney, J., Heath, D., Williams, D. and Rios-Dalenz, J. (1991) Morphological changes in the pituitary–adrenocortical axis in natives of La Paz. *Int. J. Biometeorol.* **35**, 1–5.

Grahn, D. and Kratchman, J. (1963) Variations in neonatal death rate and birth weight in the United States and possible relations to environmental radiation, geology and altitude. *Am. J. Hum. Genet.* **15**, 329–52.

Gray, D. (1987) Survival after burial in an avalanche. *BMJ* **294**, 611–12.

Gray, G.W. (1983) High altitude pulmonary edema. *Semin. Respir. Med.* **5**, 141–50.

Green, H.J., Sutton, J.R., Cymerman, A., Young, P.M. and Houston, C.S. (1989) Operation Everest II: adaptations in human skeletal muscle. *J. Appl. Physiol.* **66**, 2454–61.

Green, S.P.T. (1992) The 1991 Everest marathon and the Namche Bazaar dental clinic. *J. R. Nav. Med. Serv.* **78**, 165–71.

Greene, R. (1934) Observations on the composition of alveolar air on Mt. Everest. *J. Physiol. (Lond.)* **32**, 481–5.

Greene, R. (1943) The immediate vascular changes in true frostbite. *J. Pathol. Bacteriol.* **55**, 259–68.

Gregory, I.C. (1974) The oxygen and carbon monoxide capacities of foetal and adult blood. *J. Physiol.* **236**, 625–34.

Grenard, F. (1904) *Tibet,* Hutchinson, London.

Grissom, C.K., Albertinae, K.H. and Elstsda, M.R. (2000) Alveolar haemorrhage in a case of high altitude pulmonary oedema. *Thorax* **55,** 167–9.

Grissom, C.K., Roach, R.C., Sarnquist, F.H. and Hackett, P.H. (1992) Acetazolamide in the treatment of acute mountain sickness: clinical effect on gas exchange. *Ann. Intern. Med.* **116,** 461–5.

Groechenig, E. (1994) Treatment of frostbite with iloprost. *Lancet* **394,** 1152–3.

Grollman, A. (1930) Physiological variations of the cardiac output of man. VII. The effect of high altitude on the cardiac output and its related functions: an account of experiments conducted on the summit of Pikes Peak, Colorado. *Am. J. Physiol.* **93,** 19–40.

Gronbeck, C. (1984) Chronic mountain sickness at an elevation of 2000 metres. *Chest* **85,** 577–8.

Grover, R.F. (1980) Speculations on the pathogenesis of high-altitude pulmonary edema. *Adv. Cardiol.* **27,** 1–5.

Grover, R.F., Lufschanowski, R. and Alexander, J.K. (1970) Decreased coronary blood flow in man following ascent to high altitude. *Adv. Cardiol.* **5,** 72–9.

Groves, B.M., Droma, T., Sutton, J.R. *et al.* (1993) Minimal hypoxic pulmonary hypertension in normal Tibetans at 3,658 m. *J. Appl. Physiol.* **74,** 312–18.

Groves, B.M., Reeves, J.T., Sutton, J.R. *et al.* (1987) Operation Everest II: elevated high-altitude pulmonary resistance unresponsive to oxygen. *J. Appl. Physiol.* **63,** 521–30.

Guerra-Garcia, R. (1971) Testosterone metabolism in men exposed to high altitude. *Acta Endocrinol. Panama* **2,** 55–9.

Guezennec, C.Y. and Pesquies, P.C. (1985) Biochemical basis for physical exercise fatigue, in *High Altitude Deterioration* (eds. J. Rivolier, P. Cerretelli, J. Foray and P. Segantini), Karger, Basel, pp. 79–89.

Guilleminault, C., Connolly, S., Winkle, R., Melvin, K. and Tilkian, A. (1984) Cyclical variation of the heart rate in sleep apnoea syndrome. Mechanisms, and usefulness of 24 h electrocardiography as a screening technique. *Lancet* **1,** 126–31.

Gulatee, B.L. (1954) *The Height of Mt Everest. A New Determination (1952–54),* Survey of India, Technical Paper No. 8, Dehra Dun, India.

Guleria, J.S., Pande, J.N. and Khanna, P.K. (1969) Pulmonary function in convalescents of high altitude pulmonary edema. *Dis. Chest* **55,** 434–7.

Guleria, J.S., Pande, J.N., Sethi, P.K. and Roy, S.B. (1971) Pulmonary diffusing capacity at high altitude. *J. Appl. Physiol.* **31,** 536–43.

Gunga, H-C., Kirsch, K., Rocker, L., and Schobersberger, W. (1994) Time course of erythropoietin, triiodothyronine, thyroxin, and thyroid-stimulating hormone at 2315 m. *J. Appl. Physiol.* **76,** 1068–72.

Gupta, M.L., Rao, K.S., Andand, I.S., Banerjee, A.K. and Boparai, M.S. (1992) Lack of smooth muscle in the small pulmonary arteries of the native Ladakhi. *Am. Rev. Respir. Dis.* **145,** 1201–4.

Guttman, R. and Gross, M.M. (1956) Relationship between electrical and mechanical changes in muscle caused by cooling. *J. Coll. Comp. Physiol.* **48,** 421–30.

Guyton, A.C., Jones, C.E. and Coleman, T.C. (1973) *Cardiac Output and its Regulation,* 2nd edn, Saunders, Philadelphia, p. 396.

Haab, P., Perret, C. and Piiper, J. (1965) La capacité de diffusion pulmonaire pour l'oxygène chez l'homme normal jeune. *Helv. Physiol. Acta* **23,** C23–5.

Haas, J.D. (1976) Prenatal and infant growth and development, in *Man in the Andes* (eds. P.T. Baker and M.A. Little), Dowden, Hutchinson & Ross, Stroudsburg, PA, pp. 161–78.

Habeler, P. (1979) *Everest: Impossible Victory,* Arlington, London.

Haberman, S., Capildeo, R. and Rose, F. (1981) The seasonal variation in mortality from cerebro-vascular disease. *J. Neurol. Sci.* **52,** 25–36.

Hackett, P.H. (1999) The cerebral etiology of high-altitude cerebral edema and acute mountain sickness. *Wilderness Environ. Med.* **10,** 97–109.

Hackett, P.H., Bertman, J. and Rodriguez, G. (1986) Pulmonary edema fluid protein in high-altitude pulmonary edema. *JAMA* **256,** 36.

Hackett, P.H., Creagh, C.E., Grover, R.F. *et al.* (1980a) High altitude pulmonary edema in persons without the right pulmonary artery. *N. Engl. J. Med.* **302,** 1070–3.

Hackett, P.H., Forsling, M.L., Milledge, J. and Rennie, D. (1978) Release of vasopressin in man at altitude. *Horm. Metab. Res.* **10,** 571.

Hackett, P.H., Hollingshead, K.F., Roach, R.B. *et al.* (1987b) Arterial saturation during ascent predicts subsequent acute mountain sickness (abstract), in *Hypoxia and Cold* (eds. J.R. Sutton, C.S. Houston and G. Coates), Praeger, New York, p. 544.

Hackett, P.H., Hollingshead, K.F., Roach, R.B. *et al.* (1987c) Cortical blindness in high altitude climbers and trekkers – a report of six cases (abstract), in *Hypoxia, and Cold* (eds. J.R. Sutton, C.S. Houston and G. Coates), Praeger, New York, p. 536.

Hackett, P.H. and Rennie, D. (1976) The incidence, importance and prophylaxis of acute mountain sickness. *Lancet* **2**, 1149–54.

Hackett, P.H. and Rennie, D. (1979) Râles, peripheral edema, retinal hemorrhage and acute mountain sickness. *Am. J. Med.* **67**, 214–18.

Hackett, P.H. and Rennie, D. (1982) Cotton wool spots: a new addition to high altitude retinopathy, in *High Altitude Physiology and Medicine* (eds. W. Brendel and R.A. Zink), Springer-Verlag, New York, pp. 215–16.

Hackett, P.H., Rennie, D. and Levine, H.D. (1976) The incidence, importance and prophylaxis of acute mountain sickness. *Lancet* **2**, 1149–54.

Hackett, P.H., Reeves, J.T., Reeves, C.D. *et al.* (1980b) Control of breathing in Sherpas at low and high altitude. *J. Appl. Physiol.* **49**, 374–9.

Hackett, P.H., Rennie, D., Grover, R.F. and Reeves, J.T. (1981) Acute mountain sickness and the edemas of high altitude: a common pathogenesis? *Respir. Physiol.* **46**, 383–90.

Hackett, P.H., Rennie, D., Hofmeister, S.E., Grover, R.F., Grover, E.B. and Reeves, J.T. (1982) Fluid retention and relative hypoventilation in acute mountain sickness. *Respiration* **43**, 321–9.

Hackett, P.H., Roach, R.C., Harrison, C.L., Schoene, R.B. and Miles, W.J., Jr (1987a) Respiratory stimulants and sleep periodic breathing at high altitude. Almitrine versus acetazolamide. *Am. Rev. Respir. Dis.* **135**, 896–8.

Hackett, P.H., Swenson, E.R., Roach, R.C. *et al.* (1988a) 250 mg acetazolamide intravenously does not increase cerebral blood flow at high altitude (abstract), in *Hypoxia the Tolerable Limits* (eds. J.R. Sutton, C.S. Houston and G. Cotes), Benchmark Press, Indianapolis, p. 383.

Hackett, P.H., Roach, R.C., Schoene, R.B. *et al.* (1988b) Abnormal control of ventilation in high-altitude pulmonary edema. *J. Appl. Physiol.* **64**, 1268–72.

Hackett, P.H., Roach, R.C., Hartig, G.S. *et al.* (1992) The effect of vasodilators on pulmonary hemodynamics in high altitude pulmonary edema: a comparison. *Int. J. Sports Med.* **13**, S68–S71.

Hackett, P.H., Yarnell, P.R., Hill, R. *et al.* (1998) High-altitude cerebral edema evaluated with magnetic resonance imaging. *JAMA* **280**, 1920–5.

Haddad, G.G. and Jiang, C. (1993) O_2 deprivation in the central nervous system: on mechanisms of neuronal response, differential sensitivity and injury. *Progr. Neurobiol.* **40**, 277–318.

Haight, J.S.J. and Keatinge, W.R. (1973) Failure of thermoregulation in the cold during hypoglycaemia induced by exercise and ethanol. *J. Physiol. (Lond).* **229**, 87–97.

Haldane, J.S., Kellas, A.M., and Kennaway, E.L. (1919) Experiments on acclimatisation to reduced atmospheric pressure. *J. Physiol. (Lond.)* **53**, 181–206.

Haldane, J.S. and Priestley, J.G. (1935) Oxygen secretion in the lungs, in *Respiration,* 2nd edn, Yale University Press, New Haven, CT, pp. 250–96.

Haldane, J.S. and Priestley, J.G. (1935) *Respiration*, 2nd edn, Yale University Press, New Haven, CT.

Haldane, J. and Smith, J. Lorrain (1897) The absorption of oxygen by the lungs. *J. Physiol. (Lond.)* **22**, 231–58.

Halhuber, M.J., Humpeler, E., Inama, A.K. and Jungmann, H. (1985) Does altitude cause exhaustion of the heart and circulatory system? Indications and contra-indications for cardiac patients in altitudes, in *High Altitude Deterioration* (eds. R.J. Rivolier, P. Cerretelli, J. Foray and P. Segantini), Karger, Basel, pp. 192–202.

Hall, F.G. (1936) The effect of altitude on the affinity of hemoglobin for oxygen. *J. Biol. Chem.* **115,** 485–90.

Hall, F.G., Dill, D.B. and Guzman-Barron, E.S. (1936) Comparative physiology in high altitudes. *J. Cell. Comp. Physiol.* **8**, 301–13.

Halperin, B.D., Sun, S., Zhuang, J., Droma, T. and Moore, L.G. (1998) ECG observations in Tibetan and Han residents of Lhasa. *J. Electrocardiol.* **31**, 237–43.

Hamilton, R.S. and Paton, B.C. (1996) The diagnosis and treatment of hypothermia by mountain rescue teams: a survey. *Wilderness Environ. Med.* **7**, 28–37.

Hamilton, S.J.C. (1980) Hypothermia and unawareness of mental impairment. *BMJ* **1**, 565.

Hamlet, M.P. (1983) Fluid shifts in hypothermia, in *The Nature and Treatment of Hypothermia* (eds. R.S. Pozos and L.E. Wittmers), Croom Helm, London/ University of Minnesota Press, Minneapolis, pp. 94–9.

Hamlet, M.P., Veghte, J., Bowers, W.D. and Boyce, J. (1977) Thermographic evaluation of experimentally produced frostbite of rabbit feet. *Cryobiology* **14**, 197–204.

Hammel, H.T. (1964) Terrestrial animals in the cold. Recent studies in primitive man, in *Handbook of Physiology: Adaptation to the Environment,* American Physiological Society, Washington DC, pp. 413–34.

Hammond, M.D., Gale, G.E., Kapitan, K.S., Ries, A. and Wagner, P.D. (1986) Pulmonary gas exchange in humans during normobaric hypoxic exercise. *J. Appl. Physiol.* **61**, 1749–57.

Han, J.L., Chen, D.X. and Chen, G.I. (1985) The investigation of nail fold microcirculation in 1–13 year old healthy children at different altitudes, in *Abstracts of the Second High Altitude Medicine Symposium,* Department of High Altitude Science, Xining, Quinghai, China, p. 44.

Handley, A.J., Golden, F. St C., Keatinge, W.R. *et al.* (1993) *Report of the Working Party on Out of Hospital Management of Hypothermia,* Medical Commission on Accident Prevention, UK.

Hann, J. von (1901) *Lehrbuch der Meteorologie,* Tauchnitz, Leipzig. English translation by R.D.C. Ward, MacMillan, New York, 1903, p. 222.

Hannon, J. (1966) High altitude acclimatization in women, in *The Effects of Altitude on Physical Performance* (ed. R. Goddard), Athletic Institute, Chicago, pp. 37–44.

Hannon, J. (1978) Comparative adaptability of young men and women, in *Environmental Stress: Individual Human Adaptation* (eds. L. Folinsby, J. Wagner, J. Borgia *et al.*) Academic Press, New York, pp. 335–60.

Hannon, J.P., Klain, G.J., Sudman, D.M. and Sullivan, F.J. (1976) Nutritional aspects of high-altitude exposure in women. *Am. J. Clin. Nutr.* **29**, 604–13.

Hanoka, M., Kubo, K., Yamazaki, Y. *et al.* (1998) Association of high altitude pulmonary edema with the major histocompatibility complex. *Circulation* **97**, 1124–8.

Hansen, J.E. and Evans, W.O. (1970) A hypothesis regarding the pathophysiology of acute mountain sickness. *Arch. Environ. Health* **21**, 666–9.

Hanson, J.E., Vogel, J.A., Stelter, G.P. and Consolazio, F. (1967) Oxygen uptake in man during exhaustive work at sea level and high altitude. *J. Appl. Physiol.* **23**, 511–22.

Harber, M.J., Williams, J.D. and Morton, J.J. (1981) Antidiuretic hormone excretion at high altitude. *Aviat. Space Environ. Med.* **52**, 38–40.

Harbinson, M.J. (1999) William Harvey, hypothermia and battle injuries. *BMJ* **319**, 1561.

Harnett, R.M., Pruitt, J.R. and Sias, F.R. (1983) A review of the literature concerning resuscitation from hypothermia, Part II. Selected rewarming protocols. *Aviat. Space Environ. Med.* **54**, 487–95.

Harper, A.M. and Glass, H.I. (1965) Effect of alterations in the arterial carbon dioxide tension on the blood flow through the cerebral cortex at normal and low arterial blood pressures. *J. Neurol. Neurosurg. Psychiatry* **28**, 449–52.

Harris, P. (1986) Evolution, hypoxia and high altitude, in *Aspects of Hypoxia* (ed. D. Heath), Liverpool University Press, Liverpool, pp. 207–16.

Harris, P., Castillo, Y., Gibson, K. *et al.* (1970) Succinic and lactic dehydrogenase activity in myocardial homogenates from animals at high and low altitude. *J. Mol. Cell. Cardiol.* **1**, 189–93.

Harrison, G.A., Kuchemann, C.F., Moore, M.A.S. *et al.* (1969) The effects of altitudinal variation in Ethiopian populations. *Philos. Trans. R. Soc. Lond. Ser. B* **256**, 147–82.

Harrison, M.H. (1985) Effects of thermal stress and exercise on blood volume in humans. *Physiol. Rev.* **65**, 149–208.

Hartmann, H., Hepp, G. and Luft, U.C. (1942) Physiologische Beobachtungen am Nanga Parbat. 1937/1938. *Lufthahrtmedizin* **6**, 10–44.

Hartung, G.H., Myhre, L.G., Nunnerly, S.A. and Tucker, D.M. (1984) Plasma substrate response in men and women during marathon running. *Aviat. Space. Environ. Med.* **55**, 128–31.

Harvey, T.C., Raichle, M.E., Winterborn, M.H. *et al.* (1988) Effect of carbon dioxide in acute mountain sickness: a rediscovery. *Lancet* **2**, 639–41.

Hashmi, M.A., Bokjari, S.A.H., Rashid, M. *et al.* (1998) Frostbite: epidemiology at high altitude in the Karakoram mountains, *Ann. R. Coll. Surg.* **80**, 91–5.

Hatcher, J.D. (1965) Acute anoxic anoxia, in *The Physiology of Human Survival* (eds. O.G. Edholm and A.L. Bacharach), Academic Press, London, pp. 81–120.

Hathorn, M.K.S. (1971) The influence of hypoxia on iron absorption in the rat. *Gastroenterology,* **60**, 76–81.

Hayward, J.S. (1997) Inhibition of shivering increases core temperature after-drop and attenuates rewarming in hypothermic humans. *J. Appl. Physiol.* **83**, 1030–4.

Hayward, J.S., Eckerson, J.D. and Kemna, D. (1984) Thermal and cardiovascular changes during three methods of resuscitation from mild hypothermia. *Resuscitation* **11**, 21–33.

Hayward, M.G. and Keatinge, W.R. (1979) Progressive symptomless hypothermia in water. Possible cause of diving accidents. *BMJ* **1**, 1222.

Heath, D. (1986) Carotid body hyperplasia, in *Aspects of Hypoxia* (ed. D. Heath), Liverpool University Press, Liverpool, pp. 61–74.

Heath, D., Edwards, C., Winson, M. and Smith, P. (1973) Effects on the right ventricle, pulmonary vasculature, and carotid bodies of the rat of exposure to, and recovery from, simulated high altitude. *Thorax* **28**, 24–8.

Heath, D. and Williams, D.R. (1995) *High-Altitude Medicine and Pathology,* 4th edn, Oxford University Press, Oxford.

Heaton, J.M. (1972) The distribution of brown adipose tissue in the human. *J. Anat.* **112**, 35–9.

Hebbel, R.P., Eaton, J.W., Kronenberg, R.S., Zanjani, E.D., Moore, L.G. and Berger, E.M. (1978) Human llamas: adaptation to altitude in subjects with high hemoglobin oxygen affinity. *J. Clin. Invest.* **62**, 593–600.

Hecht, H.H., Kuida, H., Lange, R.L., Horne, J.L. and Brown, A.M. (1962) Brisket disease. III. Clinical features and hemodynamic observations in altitude-dependent right heart failure of cattle. *Am. J. Med.* **32**, 171–83.

Hecht, H.H., Lang, R.L., Carnes, W.H. *et al.* (1959) Brisket disease. I. General aspects of pulmonary hypertensive heart disease in cattle. *Trans. Assoc. Am. Physiol.* **72**, 157–72.

Hedin, S. (1903a) *Central Asia and Tibet,* Hurst and Blackett, London.

Hedin, S. (1913) *Trans-Himalaya,* Macmillan, London, vol. 3, pp. 123–8.

Heggers, J.P., Phillips, L.G., McAuley, R.L. and Robson, M.C. (1990) Frostbite: experimental and clinical evaluation of treatment. *J. Wilderness Med.* **1**, 27–32.

Henderson, Y. (1919) The physiology of the aviator. *Science* **49**, 431–41.

Hepburn, M.L. (1901) The influence of high altitude in mountaineering. *Alpine J.* **20**, 368–93.

Hepburn, M.L. (1902) Some reasons why the science of altitude illness is still in its infancy. *Alpine J.* **21**, 161–79.

Hepple, R.T., Agey, P.J., Szewczak, J.M. *et al.* (1998) Increased capillarity in leg muscle of finches living at altitude. *J. Appl. Physiol.* **85**, 1871–6.

Hepple, R.T., Hogan, M.C., Stary, C., Bebout, D.E., Mathieu-Costello, O. and Wagner, P.D. (2000) Structural basis of muscle O_2 diffusing capacity: evidence from muscle function *in situ. J. Appl. Physiol.* **88**, 560–6.

Hernandez, M.J. (1983) Cerebral circulation during hypothermia, in *The Nature and Treatment of Hypothermia* (eds. R.S. Pozos and L.E. Wittmers), Croom Helm, London/University of Minnesota, Minneapolis, pp. 61–8.

Herschkowitz, M. (1977) Penile frostbite: an unforeseen hazard of jogging (letter). *N. Engl. J. Med.* **296**, 178.

Hertzman, A.B. (1957) Individual differences in regional sweating patterns. *J. Appl. Physiol.* **10**, 242–8.

Hervey, G.R. (1973) Physiological changes encountered in hypothermia. *Proc. R. Soc. Med.* **66**, 1053–7.

Hervey, G.R. and Tobin, G. (1983) Luxuskonsumption. Diet-induced thermogenesis and brown fat: a critical review. *Clin. Sci.* **64**, 7–22.

Hetzel, B.S. (1989) *The Story of Iodine Deficiency,* Oxford Medical Publications, Oxford.

Heyman, A., Patterson, J.L. and Duke, T.W. (1952) Cerebral circulation and metabolism in sickle cell and other chronic anemias, with observations on the effects of oxygen inhalation. *J. Clin. Invest.* **31**, 824–8.

Heymans, J.-F. and Heymans, C. (1925) Sur le mécanisme de l'apnée réflexe ou pneumogastrique. *Comptes Rendus Soc. Biol.* **92**, 1335–8.

Heymans, J.-F. and Heymans, C. (1927) Sur les modifications directes et sur la regulation reflexe de l'activité du centre respiratoire de la tête isolée du chien. *Arch. Intern. Pharmacodyn.* **33**, 273–370.

Hill, A.V. (1928) The diffusion of oxygen and lactic acid through tissues. *Proc. R. Soc. Lond. Ser. B* **104**, 39–96.

Hill, L. (1934) Foreword, in *Oxygen and Carbon Dioxide Therapy* (eds A. Campbell and E.P. Poulton), Oxford University Press, London.

Hillary, E.P. (1954) Everest 1953: (4) The last lap. *Alpine J.* **59**, 235–8.

Hinchliff, T.W. (1876) *Over the Sea and Far Away,* Longmans Green, London.

Hingston, R.W.G. (1914) Records of the survey of India, Vol. VI. Completion of the link connecting the triangulation of India and Russia 1913. Prepared under the direction of Col. Sir S.G. Burrard FRS, Dehra Dun. Printed at the office of the Trigonometrical Survey, 1914. Blood observations at high altitude and some conclusions drawn from this enquiry in relation to mountain distress, pp. 88–91.

Hirata, K., Matsuyama, S. and Saito, A. (1989) Obesity as a risk factor for acute mountain sickness. *Lancet* **2**, 1040–1.

Hirvonen, J. (1982) Accidental hypothermia, in *Report* **30**, Nordic Council for Arctic Medical Research, Copenhagen, pp. 15–19.

Hochachka, P.W., Clark, C.M., Stanley, C., Uqurbil, K. and Menon, R.S. (1996) 31P Magnetic resonance spectroscopy of the Sherpa heart: a phosphocreatine/adenosine defence against hypobaric hypoxia. *Proc. Natl. Acad. Sci. USA* **93**, 1215–20.

Hoff, C.J. and Abelson, A.E. (1976) Fertility, in *Man in The Andes, A Multidisciplinary Study of High-Altitude Quechua* (eds. P.T. Baker and M.A. Little), Dowden, Hutchinson & Ross, Stroudsburg, PA, pp. 128–46.

Hoffman, R.C. and Wittmers, L.E. (1990) Cold vasodilatation, pain and acclimatization in Arctic explorers. *J. Wilderness Med.* **1**, 225–34.

Hogan, M.C., Bebout, D.E. and Wagner, P.D. (1991) Effect of increased Hb-O_2 affinity on $\dot{V}_{O_2 max}$ at constant O_2

delivery in dog muscle in situ. *J. Appl. Physiol.* **70**, 2656–62.

Hogan, R.P., Kotchen, T.A., Boyd, A.E. and Hartley, L.H. (1973) Effect of altitude on the renin–aldosterone system and metabolism of water and electrolytes. *J. Appl. Physiol.* **35**, 385–90.

Hogan, M.C., Roca, J., Wagner, P.D. and West, J.B. (1988a) Limitation of maximal oxygen uptake and performance by acute hypoxia in dog muscle *in situ*. *J. Appl. Physiol.* **65**, 815–21.

Hogan, M.C., Roca, J., West, J.B. and Wagner, P.D. (1988b) Dissociation of maximal O_2 uptake from O_2 delivery in canine gastrocnemius *in situ*. *J. Appl. Physiol.* **66**, 1219–26.

Hohenhaus, E., Niroomand, F.G., Goerre, S., *et al.* (1994) Nifedipine does not prevent acute mountain sickness. *Am. J. Respir. Crit. Care* **150**, 857–60.

Hohenhaus, E., Paul, A., McCullough, R.E. *et al.* (1995) Ventilatory and pulmonary vascular response to hypoxia and susceptibility to high altitude pulmonary oedema. *Eur. Respir. J.* **8**, 1825–33.

Holditch, T. (1907) *Tibet the Mysterious*, Alston Rivers, London, pp. 242–3.

Holloszy, J.O. and Coyle, E.F. (1984) Adaptations of skeletal muscle to endurance exercise and their metabolic consequences. *J. Appl. Physiol.* **56**, 831–8.

Holm, P. (1997) Endothelin in the pulmonary circulation with special reference to hypoxic pulmonary vasoconstriction. *Scand. Cardiovasc. J.* Suppl. **46**, 1–40.

Homik, L.A., Bshouty, Z., Light, R.B. and Younes, M. (1988) Effect of alveolar hypoxia on pulmonary fluid filtration in *in-situ* dog lungs. *J. Appl. Physiol.* **65**, 46–52.

Hong, S.I. and Nadel, E.R. (1979) Thermogenic control during exercise in a cold environment. *J. Appl. Physiol.* **47**, 1084–9.

Hong, S.K. (1973) Pattern of cold adaptation in women divers of Korea. *Fed. Proc.* **32**, 1414–22.

Honig, A. (1983) Role of arterial chemoreceptors in the reflex control of renal function and body fluid volumes in acute arterial hypoxia, in *Physiology of the Peripheral Arterial Chemoreceptors* (eds. H. Acher and R.C. O'Regan), Elsevier, Amsterdam, pp. 395–429.

Honig, A. (1989) Peripheral arterial chemoreceptors and reflex control of sodium and water homeostasis. *Am. J. Physiol.* **257**, R1282–302.

Honig, C.R., Gayeski, T.E.J. and Groebe, K. (1991) Myoglobin and oxygen gradients, in *The Lung: Scientific Foundations* (eds. R.G. Crystal and J.B. West), Raven Press, New York, pp. 1489–96.

Honig, C.R. and Tenney, S.M. (1957) Determinants of the circulatory response to hypoxia and hypercapnia. *Am. Heart J.* **53**, 687–98.

Honigman, B., Thesis, M.K., Koziol-McLain, J. *et al.* (1993) Acute mountain sickness in a general tourist population at moderate altitude. *Ann. Intern. Med.* **118**, 587–92.

Hoon, R.S., Sharma, S.C., Balasubramanian, V. and Chadha, K.S. (1977) Urinary catecholamine excretion on induction to high altitude (3658 m) by air and road. *J. Appl. Physiol.* **42**, 728–30.

Hoppeler, H., Howald, H. and Cerretelli, P. (1990) Human muscle structure after exposure to extreme altitude. *Experientia* **46**, 1185–7.

Hoppeler, H., Kayar, S.R., Claassen, H., Uhlmann, E. and Karas, R.H. (1987) Adaptive variation in the mammalian respiratory system in relation to energetic demand: III. Skeletal muscles: setting the demand for oxygen. *Respir. Physiol.* **69**, 27–46.

Horio, T., Kohno, M., Yokokawa, K. *et al.* (1991) Effect of hypoxia on plasma immunoreactive endothelin-1 concentration in anaesthetized rats. *Metabolism* **40**, 999–1001.

Hornbein, T.F., Townes, B.D., Schoene, R.B. *et al.* (1989) The cost to the central nervous system of climbing to extremely high altitude. *N. Engl. J. Med.* **321**, 1714–19.

Horton, B.T. and Brown, G.E. (1929) Systemic histamine like reactions in allergy due to cold. *Am. J. Med. Sci.* **198**, 191–202.

Horvath, S.M. (1981) Exercise in a cold environment. *Exercise Sports Sci. Rev.* **9**, 191–263.

Hossmann, K.A. (1999) The hypoxic brain. Insights from ischemia research. *Adv. Exp. Med. Biol.* **474**, 155–69.

Houk, V.N. (1959) Transient pulmonary insufficiency caused by cold. *US Armed Forces Med. J.* **10**, 1354–7.

Houston, C.S. (1960) Acute pulmonary edema of high altitude. *N. Engl. J. Med.* **263**, 478–80.

Houston, C.S. (ed.) (1980) *High Altitude Physiology Study*. Collected Papers, Arctic Institute of North America, Arlington, Virginia/Calgary, Alberta.

Houston, C.S. (1987) Transient visual disturbance at high altitude (abstract), in *Hypoxia and Cold* (eds. J.R. Sutton, C.S. Houston and G. Coates), Praeger, New York, p. 536.

Houston, C.S. (1988–9) Operation Everest II – 1985. *Alpine J.* **93**, 196–200.

Houston, C.S. and Bates, R. (1979) K2, *The Savage Mountain*. McGraw-Hill, New York, pp. 180–99.

Houston, C.S. and Dickinson, J. (1975) Cerebral form of high-altitude illness. *Lancet* **2**, 758–61.

Houston, C.S. and Riley, R.L. (1947) Respiratory and

circulatory changes during acclimatization to high altitude. *Am. J. Physiol.* **149**, 565–88.

Houston, C.S., Sutton, J.R., Cymerman, A. and Reeves, J.T. (1987) Operation Everest II: man at extreme altitude. *J. Appl. Physiol.* **63**, 877–82.

Howald, H., Pette, D., Simoneau, J.A., Uber, A., Hoppler, H. and Cerretelli, P. (1990) Effect of chronic hypoxia on muscle enzyme activities. *Int. J. Sports Med.* **11** (Suppl. 1), S10–14.

Howard, L.S.G.E. and Robbins, P.A. (1995) Alterations in respiratory control during 8 h of isocapnic and poikilocapnic hypoxia in humans. *J. Appl. Physiol.* **78**, 1089–107.

Howard-Bury, C.K. (1922) *Mt. Everest: The Reconnaissance, 1921*, Arnold, London.

Howarth, M. (1999) High altitude cerebral oedema – a rescue. *ISMM Newsletter* **9**(4), 15–17.

Hu, S.T. (1983) Hypoxia research in China: an overview, in *Hypoxia, Exercise and Altitude* (eds. J.R. Sutton, C.S. Houston and N.L. Jones), Proceedings of the 3rd Banff Symposium, Liss, New York, pp. 157–71.

Hu, S.T., Huang, W.Y., Chu, S.C. and Pa, C.F. (1982) Chemoreflexive ventilatory response at sea level in subjects with past history of good acclimatization and severe acute mountain sickness, in *High Altitude Physiology and Medicine* (eds. W. Brendel and R.A. Zink), Springer-Verlag, New York, pp. 28–32.

Huang, S.Y., Moore, L.G., McCullough, R.E. *et al.* (1987) Internal carotid and vertebral arterial flow velocity in men at high altitude. *J. Appl. Physiol.* **63**, 395–400.

Huang, S.Y., Ning, X.H., Zhou, Z.N. *et al.* (1984) Ventilatory function in adaptation to high altitude: studies in Tibet, in *High Altitude and Man* (eds. J.B. West and S. Lahiri), American Physiological Society, Bethesda, MD, pp. 173–7.

Huang, S.Y., Sun, S., Droma, T. *et al.* (1992) Internal carotid arterial flow velocity during exercise in Tibetan and Han residents of Lhasa (3,658 m). *J. Appl. Physiol.* **73**, 2638–42.

Huang, S.Y., Tawney, K.W., Bender, P.R. *et al.* (1991) Internal carotid flow velocity with exercise before and after acclimatization to 4300 m. *J. Appl. Physiol.* **71**, 1469–76.

Hubbard, R.W., Gaffin, S.L. and Squire, D.L. (1995) Heat related illness, in *Wilderness Medicine* (ed. P.S. Auerbach), Mosby, St Louis, pp. 167–212.

Hüfner, C.G. (1890) Uber das Gesetz der Dissociation des Oxyhamoglobins und über einige daran sich knupfende wichtige Fragen aus der Biologie. *Arch. Pathol. Anat. Physiol.* 1–27.

Hultgren, H., Spickard, W. and Lopez, C. (1962) Further studies of high altitude pulmonary edema. *Br. Heart J.* **24**, 95–102.

Hultgren, H.N. (1969) High altitude pulmonary edema, in *Biomedicine Problems of High Terrestrial Altitude* (ed. A.H. Hegnauer), Springer-Verlag, New York, pp. 131–41.

Hultgren, H.N. (1978) High altitude pulmonary edema, in *Lung Water and Solute Exchange* (ed. N.C. Staub), Dekker, New York, pp. 437–69.

Hultgren, H.N. (1992) Effect of altitude on cardio-vascular diseases. *J. Wilderness Med.* **3**, 301–8.

Hultgren, H.N. (1997) *High Altitude Medicine,* Hultgren Publications, Stanford, CA, p. 12.

Hultgren, H.N., Grover, R.F. and Hartley, L.H. (1971) Abnormal circulatory responses to high altitude in subjects with a previous history of high-altitude pulmonary edema. *Circulation* **44**, 759–70.

Hultgren, H.N., Lopez, C.E., Lundberg, E. and Miller, H. (1964) Physiologic studies of pulmonary edema at high altitude. *Circulation* **29**, 393–408.

Hultgren, H.N. and Marticorena, E.A. (1978) High altitude pulmonary edema. Epidemiologic observations in Peru. *Chest* **74**, 372–6.

Hultgren, H.N., Robison, M.C. and Wuerflein, R.D. (1966) Over perfusion pulmonary edema. *Circulation* **34** (Suppl. 3), 132–3.

Hultgren, H.N. and Spickard, W. (1960) Medical experiences in Peru. *Stanford Med. Bull.* **18**, 76–95.

Hunt, J. (1953) *The Ascent of Everest*, Hodder and Stoughton, London.

Hunter, J. (1781) *Original Cases*, Library of Royal College of Surgeons of England, London.

Hunter, J., Kerr, E.H. and Whillans, M.G. (1952) The relation between joint stiffness upon exposure to cold and the characteristics of synovial fluid. *J. Can. Med. Sci.* **39**, 367–77.

Huonker, M., Schmidt-Trucksass, A., Sorichter, S. *et al.* (1997) Highland mountain hiking and coronary artery disease: exercise tolerance and effects on left ventricular function. *Med. Sci. Sports Exerc.* **29**, 1554–60.

Hurtado, A. (1937) *Aspectos fisiológicos y Patologicos de la Vida en la Altura*. Rimac, Lima.

Hurtado, A. (1942) Chronic mountain sickness. *JAMA* **120**, 1278–82.

Hurtado, A. (1964) Animals in high altitudes: resident man, in *Handbook of Physiology, Section IV, Adaptation to the Environment* (ed. D.B. Dill), American Physiological Society, Washington DC, pp. 843–60.

Hurtado, A. (1971) The influence of high altitude on physiology, in *High Altitude Physiology* (eds. R. Porter and J. Knight), Ciba Foundation Symposium, Churchill Livingstone, Edinburgh, pp. 3–13.

Hurtado, A., Merino, C. and Delgado, E. (1945) Influence of anoxemia on the hemopoietic activity. *Arch. Intern. Med.* **75**, 284–323.

Hurtado, A., Rotta, A., Merino, C. and Pons, J. (1937) Studies of myohemoglobin at high altitude. *Am. J. Med. Sci.* **194**, 708–13.

Hutchinson, S.J. and Litch, J.A. (1997) Acute myocardial infarction at high altitude. *JAMA* **278**, 1661–2.

Hyde, R.W., Forster, R.E., Power, G.G. *et al.* (1966) Measurement of O_2 diffusing capacity of the lungs with a stable O_2 isotope. *J. Clin. Invest.* **45**, 1178–93.

Hyers, T.M., Scoggin, C.H., Will, D.H. *et al.* (1979) Accentuated hypoxemia at high altitude in subjects susceptible to high-altitude pulmonary edema. *J. Appl. Physiol. Respir. Environ. Exercise Physiol.* **46**, 41–6.

Ibbertson, H.K., Tair, J.M., Pearl, M. *et al.* (1972) Himalayan cretinism. *Adv. Exp. Med. Biol.* **30**, 51–69.

ICAO (1964) *Manual of the ICAO Standard Atmosphere*, 2nd edn, International Civil Aviation Organization, Montreal, Canada.

Ignarro, L.J., Buga, GM., Wood, K.S. *et al.* (1987) Endothelium-derived relaxing factor produced and released from artery and vein is nitric oxide. *Proc. Natl. Acad. Sci. USA* **84**, 9265–9.

Ikawa, G., Dos Santos, P.A.L., Yamaguchi, K.T. *et al.* (1986) Frostbite and bone scanning: the use of [99]m-labelled phosphates in demarcating the line of viability in frostbite victims. *Orthopaedics* **9**, 1257–61.

Iliff, L.D. (1971) Extra-alveolar vessels and edema development in excised dog lungs. *Circ. Res.* **28**, 524–32.

Imray, C.H., Brearey, S., Clarke, T. *et al.* (2000) Cerebral oxygenation at high altitude and the response to carbon dioxide, hyperventilation and oxygen. *Clin. Sci.* **98**, 159–64.

Imray, C.H., Chesner, I., Winterbourn, M. *et al.* (1992) Fat absorption at altitude: a reappraisal (abstract). *Int. J. Sports Med.* **13**, 87.

Ind, P.W., Maxwell, D.L., Causon, R.C. *et al.* (1984) Hypoxia and catecholamine secretion in normal man. *Clin. Sci.* **67**, 58–59P.

Ingjer, F. and Brodal, P. (1978) Capillary supply of skeletal muscle fibers in untrained and endurance-trained women. *Eur. J. Appl. Physiol.* **38**, 291–9.

Ingjer, F. and Myhre, K. (1992) Physiological effects of altitude training on elite male cross-country skiers. *J. Sports Sci.* **10**, 37–47.

Irwin, M.S., Sanders, R., Gren, C.J. and Terenghi, G. (1997) Neuropathy in non-freezing injuries (trench foot). *J. R. Soc. Med.* **90**, 433–8.

Irwin, M.S., Thorniley, M.S. and Green, C.J. (1994) An investigation into the aetiology of non-freezing cold injury using infrared spectroscopy. *Biochem. Soc. Trans.* **22**, 418S.

ISMM Newsletter (1998) The combined oral contraceptive (COC) at altitude – is it safe? (10 discussants) *ISMM Newsletter* **8**(2), 11–13.

Itskovitz, J., LaCamma, E.F. and Rudolph, A.M. (1987) Effects of cord compression on fetal blood flow distribution and O_2 delivery. *Am. J. Physiol. (Heart Circ. Physiol.)* **21**, H100–9.

Jackson, F. and Davies, H. (1960) The electrocardiogram of the mountaineer at high altitude. *Br. Heart J.* **22**, 671–85.

Jackson, F.S. (1968) The heart at high altitude. *Br. Heart J.* **30**, 291–4.

Jackson, F.S., Turner, R.W.D. and Ward, M.P. (1966) *Report on IBP Expedition to North Bhutan*, Royal Society, London.

Jackson, J.A. (1975) Avoidance of cold injury. Outline of basic principles, in *Mountain Medicine and Physiology* (eds. C. Clarke, M.P. Ward and E.S. Williams), Alpine Club, London, pp. 28–30.

Jain, S.C., Bardhan, J., Swamy, Y.V. *et al.* (1980) Body fluid compartments in humans during acute high-altitude exposure. *Aviat. Space Environ. Med.* **51**, 234–6.

Jain, S.C., Singh, M.V., Sharma, V.M. *et al.* (1986) Amelioration of acute mountain sickness: comparative study of acetazolamide and spironolactone. *Int. J. Biometeorol.* **30**, 293–300.

Jansen, G.F., Krins, A. and Basnyat, B. (1999) Cerebral vasomotor reactivity at high altitude in humans. *J. Appl. Physiol.* **86**, 681–6.

Jansson, E., Sylven, C. and Nordevang, E. (1982) Myoglobin in the quadriceps femoris muscle of competitive cyclists and untrained men. *Acta Physiol. Scand.* **114**, 627–9.

Jensen, G.M. and Moore, L.G. (1997) The effect of high altitude and other risk factors on birthweight: independent or interactive effect. *Am. J. Public Health* **87**, 1003–7.

Jensen, J.B., Wright, A.D., Lassen, N.A. *et al.* (1990) Cerebral blood flow in acute mountain sickness. *J. Appl. Physiol.* **69**, 430–3.

Jenzer, G. and Bärtsch, P. (1993) Migraine with aura at

high altitude: case report. *J. Wilderness Med.* **4**, 412–15.

Jequier, E., Gygax, P-H., Pittet, P. and Vannotti, A. (1974) Increased thermal body insulation: relationship to the development of obesity. *J. Appl. Physiol.* **36**, 674–8.

Jessen, K. and Hagelstein, J.O. (1978) Peritoneal dialysis in the treatment of profound accidental hypothermia. *Aviat. Space Environ. Med.* **49**, 424–9.

Jiménez, D. (1995) High altitude intermittent chronic exposure: Andean miners, in *Hypoxia and the Brain* (eds. J.R. Sutton, C.S. Houston and G. Coates), Queen City Printers, Burlington, VT, pp. 284–91.

Johnson, T.S., Rock, P.B., Fulco, C.S. *et al.* (1984) Prevention of acute mountain sickness by dexamethasone. *N. Engl. J. Med.* **310**, 683–6.

Josephson, M.E. and Wellens, H.J. (eds.) (1984) *Tachycardia: Mechanisms, Diagnosis, Treatment,* Lea and Febiger, Philadelphia, PA.

Jourdanet, D. (1875) *Influence de la Pression de l'Air sur la Vie de l'Homme*, Masson, Paris.

Kacimi, R., Richalet, J.-P., Corsin, A. *et al.* (1992) Hypoxia-induced downregulation of β-adrenergic receptors in rat heart. *J. Appl. Physiol.* **73**, 1377–82.

Kapanci, Y., Assimacopoulos, A., Irle, C. *et al.* (1974) 'Contractile interstitial cells' in pulmonary alveolar septa: a possible regulator of ventilation–perfusion ratio? Ultrastructural, immunofluorescence, and in vitro studies. *J. Cell Biol.* **60**, 375–92.

Kaplan, L.A. (1992) Suntan, sunburn and sun protection. *J. Wilderness Med.* **3**, 173–96.

Kapoor, S.C. (1984) Changes in electrocardiogram among temporary residents at high altitude. *Defence Sci. J.* **34**, 389–95.

Kappes, B.W. and Mills, W.J. (1984) Thermal biofeedback training with frostbite patients (abstract). *Sixth International Symposium on Circumpolar Health,* 13–18 May, Anchorage, Alaska, p. 100.

Karliner, J., Sarnquist, F.H., Graber, D.J., Peters, R.M. Jr and West, J.B. (1985) The electrocardiogram at extreme altitude: experience on Mt. Everest. *Am. Heart J.* **109**, 505–13.

Kato, M. and Staub, N.C. (1966) Response of small pulmonary arteries to unilobar hypoxia and hypercapnia. *Circ. Res.* **19**, 426–40.

Kawashima, A., Kubo, K., Kobayashi, T. and Sekiguchi, M. (1989) Hemodynamic response to acute hypoxia, hypobaria and exercise in subjects susceptible to high-altitude pulmonary edema. *J. Appl. Physiol.* **67**, 1982–9.

Kawashima, A., Kubo, K., Matsuwara, Y. *et al.* (1992)

Hypoxia-induced ANP secretion in subjects susceptible to high-altitude pulmonary edema. *Respir. Physiol.* **89**, 309–17.

Kay, J.M. and Edwards, F.R. (1973) Ultrastructure of the alveolar-capillary wall in mitral stenosis. *J. Pathol.* **111**, 239–45.

Kay, J.M., Waymire, J.C. and Grover, R.F. (1974) Lung mast cell hyperplasia and pulmonary histamine-forming capacity in hypoxic rats. *Am. J. Physiol.* **226**, 178–84.

Kayser, B. (1991) Acute mountain sickness in western tourists around the Thorong pass (5400 m) in Nepal. *J. Wilderness Med.* **2**, 110–17.

Kayser, B., Acheson, K., Decombaz, J., Fern E. and Carretelli, P. (1992) Protein absorption and energy digestibility at high altitude. *J. Appl. Physiol.* **73**, 2425–31.

Kayser, B., Binzoni, T., Hoppeler, H. *et al.* (1993a) A case of severe frostbite on Mt Blanc: a multi-technique approach. *J. Wilderness Med.* **4**, 167–74.

Kayser, B., Narici, M.V. and Cibella, F. (1993b) Fatigue and performance at high altitude, in *Hypoxia and Molecular Medicine* (eds. J.R. Sutton, C.S. Houston and G. Coates), Queen City Printers, Burlington, VA, pp. 222–34.

Kearney, M.S. (1973) Ultrastructural changes in the heart at high altitude. *Pathol. Microbiol.* **39**, 258–65.

Keatinge, W.R. and Cannon, P. (1960) Freezing point of human skin. *Lancet* **1**, 11–14.

Keatinge, W.R., Coleshaw, S.R.K., Cotter, F. *et al.* (1984) Increases in platelet and red cell counts, blood viscosity and arterial pressure during mild surface cooling: factors in mortality from coronary and cerebral thrombosis in winter. *BMJ* **2**, 1405–8.

Keatinge, W.R., Coleshaw, S.R.K., Millard, C.E. and Axelsson, J. (1986) Exceptional case of survival in cold water. *BMJ* **292**, 171–2.

Keatinge, W.R., Hayward, M.G. and McIver, N.K.I. (1980) Hypothermia during saturation diving in the North Sea. *BMJ* **1**, 291.

Keighley, J.H. and Steele, G. (1981) The functional and design requirements of clothing. *Alpine J.* **86**, 138–45.

Kellas, A.M. (1917) A consideration of the possibility of ascending the loftier Himalaya. *Geogr. J.* **49**, 26–47.

Kellas A.M. (1921) Expedition to Kamet, in 1920. *Alpine J.* **33**, 313–19.

Kellas, A.M. (1921) Sur les possibilités de faire l'ascension du Mount Everest. *Congrès de l'Alpinisme, Monaco, 1920. Comptes Rendus des Seances* (Paris) **1**, 451–521.

Keller, H.-R., Maggiorini, M., Bärtsch, P. and Oelz, O. (1995) Simulated descent v dexamethasone in treatment of acute mountain sickness: a randomized trial. *BMJ* **310**, 1232–5.

Kellogg, R.H. (1963) The role of CO_2 in altitude acclimatization, in *The Regulation of Human Respiration* (eds. D.J.C. Cunningham and B.B. Lloyd), Blackwell Scientific Publications, Oxford, pp. 379–94.

Kellogg, R.H. (1978) La Pression Barométrique: Paul Bert's hypoxia theory and its critics. *Respir. Physiol.* **34**, 1–28.

Kellogg, R.H. (1980) Acid–base balance in high altitude: historical perspective, in *Environmental Physiology: Aging, Heat and Altitude* (eds. S.M. Horvath and M.K. Yousef), Elsevier, New York, pp. 295–308.

Kelman, C.R. (1966a) Digital computer subroutine for the conversion of oxygen tension into saturation. *J. Appl. Physiol.* **21**, 1375–6.

Kelman, C.R. (1966b) Calculation of certain indices of cardio-pulmonary function using a digital computer. *Respir. Physiol.* **1**, 335–43.

Kelman, C.R. (1967) Digital computer procedure for the conversion of P_{CO_2} into blood CO_2 content. *Respir. Physiol.* **3**, 335–43.

Kennedy, B.C. and Gentle, D.A. (1995) Children in the wilderness, in *Wilderness Medicine* (ed. P.S. Auerbach), Mosby, St Louis, pp. 466–89.

Kety, S.S. (1950) Circulation and metabolism of the human brain in health and disease. *Am. J. Med.* **8**, 205–17.

Keynes, R.J., Smith, G.W., Slater, J.D.H. *et al.* (1982) Renin and aldosterone at high altitude in man. *J. Endocrinol.* **92**, 131–40.

Keys, A. (1936) The physiology of life at high altitude: the International High Altitude Expedition to Chile 1935. *Sci. Mon.* **43**, 289–312.

Keys, A., Hall, F.G. and Guzman Barron, E.S. (1936) The position of the oxygen dissociation curve of human blood at high altitude. *Am. J. Physiol.* **115**, 292–307.

Keys, A., Stapp, J.P. and Violante, A. (1943) Responses in size, output and efficiency of the human heart to acute alteration in the composition of inspired air. *Am. J. Physiol.* **138**, 763–71.

Khoo, M.C., Anholm, J.D., Ko, S.W. *et al.* (1996) Dynamics of periodic breathing and arousal during sleep at extreme altitude. *Respir. Physiol.* **103**, 33–43.

Khoo, M.C.K., Kronauer, R.E., Strohl, K.P. and Slutsky, A.S. (1982) Factors inducing periodic breathing in humans: a general model. *J. Appl. Physiol.* **53**, 644–59.

King, A.B. and Robinson, S.M. (1972) Ventilation response to hypoxia and acute mountain sickness. *Aerospace Med.* **43**, 419–21.

Klausen, K. (1966) Cardiac output in man in rest and work during and after acclimatization to 3800 m. *J. Appl. Physiol.* **21**, 609–16.

Kleger, G.-R., Bärtsch, P., Vock, P. *et al.* (1996) Evidence against an increase in capillary permeability in subjects exposed to high altitude. *J. Appl. Physiol.* **81**, 1917–23.

Klokker, M., Kharazmi, A., Galbo, H. *et al.* (1993) Influence of *in vivo* hypobaric hypoxia on function of lymphocytes, natural killer cells, and cytokines. *J. Appl. Physiol.* **74**, 1100–6.

Knaupp, W., Khilnani, S., Sherwood, J. *et al.* (1992) Erythropoietin response to acute normobaric hypoxia in humans. *J. Appl. Physiol.* **73**, 837–40.

Knill, R.L. and Celb, A.W. (1978) Ventilatory responses to hypoxia and hypercapnia during halothane sedation and anaesthesia in man. *Anesthesiology* **49**, 244–51.

Kobrick, J.L. (1972) Effects of hypoxia on voluntary response time to peripheral stimuli during central target monitoring. *Ergonomics* **15**, 147–56.

Kobrick, J.L. (1975) Effects of hypoxia on peripheral visual response to dim stimuli. *Percept. Mot. Skills* **41**, 467–74.

Kohlendorfer, U., Kiechl, S. and Sperl, W (1998) Living at high altitude and risk of sudden infant death syndrome. *Arch. Dis. Child.* **79**, 506–9.

Koistenen, P., Takala, T., Martikkala, V. and Leppalouto, J. (1995) Aerobic fitness influences the response of maximal oxygen uptake and lactate threshold in acute hypobaric hypoxia. *Int. J. Sports Med.* **26**, 78–81.

Kontos, H.A., Levasseur, J.E., Richardson, D.W. *et al.* (1967) Comparative circulatory responses to systemic hypoxia in man and in unanesthetized dog. *J. Appl. Physiol.* **23**, 381–6.

Kontos, H.A. and Lower, R.R. (1963) Role of beta-adrenergic receptors in the circulatory response to high altitude hypoxia. *Am. J. Physiol.* **217**, 756–63.

Kosunen, K.J. and Pakarinen, A.J. (1976) Plasma renin, angiotensin II, and plasma and urinary aldosterone in running exercise. *J. Appl. Physiol.* **41**, 26–9.

Kotchen, T.A., Mougey, E.H., Hogan, R.P. *et al.* (1973) Thyroid responses to simulated altitude. *J. Appl. Physiol.* **34**, 145–8.

Koyama, S., Kobayashi, T., Kubo, K. *et al.* (1984) Catecholamine metabolism in patients with high altitude pulmonary edema (HAPE). *Jpn. J. Mount. Med.* **4**, 119.

Krakauer, J. (1997) *Into Thin Air*, Macmillan, London, pp. 189–284.

Krarup, N. and Larsen, J.A. (1972) The effect of slight hypothermia on liver function as measured by the elimination rate of ethanol, the hepatic uptake and excretion of indocyanine green and bile formation. *Acta Physiol. Scand.* **84**, 396–407.

Kreuzer, F. and van Lookeren Campagne, P. (1965) Resting pulmonary diffusing capacity for CO and O_2 at high altitude. *J. Appl. Physiol.* **20**, 519–24.

Kristensen, C., Drenk, N.E. and Jordening, H. (1986) Simple system for central rewarming of hypothermic patients. *Lancet* **2**, 1467–8.

Krogh, A. (1910) On the mechanism of the gas-exchange in the lungs. *Skand. Arch. Physiol.* **23**, 248–78.

Krogh, A. (1919) Number and distribution of capillaries in muscles with calculations of the oxygen pressure head necessary to supplying the tissue. *J. Physiol. (Lond.)* **52**, 409–15.

Krogh, A. (1929) *The Anatomy and Physiology of Capillaries*, Yale University Press, New Haven, CT.

Krogh, A. and Krogh, M. (1910) On the tensions of gases in the arterial blood. *Skand. Archiv. Physiol.* **23**, 179–92.

Krogh, M. (1915) The diffusion of gases through the lungs of man. *J. Physiol. (Lond.)* **49**, 271–96.

Kronecker, H. (1903) *Die Bergkrankheit,* Urban & Schwarzenberg, Berlin.

Kronenberg, R.S. and Drage, C.W. (1973) Attenuation of the ventilatory and heart rate responses to hypoxia and hypercapnia with ageing in normal men. *J. Clin. Invest.* **52**, 1812–19.

Kronenberg, R.S., Safar, P., Lee, J. *et al.* (1971) Pulmonary artery pressure and alveolar gas exchange in man during acclimatization to 12,470 ft. *J. Clin. Invest.* **50**, 827–37.

Kryger, M., McCullough, R.E., Collins, D., Scoggin, C.H., Weil, J.V. and Grover, R.F. (1978b) Treatment of excessive polycythemia of high altitude with respiratory stimulant drugs. *Am. Rev. Respir. Dis.* **117**, 455–64.

Kryger, M., McCullough, R., Doekel, R., Collins, D., Weil, J.V. and Grover, R.F. (1978a) Excessive polycythemia of high altitude: role of ventilatory drive and lung disease. *Am. Rev. Respir. Dis.* **118**, 659–66.

Kubo, K., Hanaoka, M., Hayano, T. *et al.* (1998) Inflammatory cytokines in BAL fluid and pulmonary hemodynamics in high-altitude pulmonary edema. *Respir. Physiol.* **111**, 301–10.

Kuepper, T. Hoefer, M., Gieseler, U. and Netzer, N. (1999) Prevention of acute mountain sickness with theophylline (abstract), in *Hypoxia: Into the Next Millennium* (eds. R.C. Roach, P.D. Wagner and P.H. Hackett), Plenum/Kluwer, New York, p. 400.

Kumar, V.N. (1982) Intractable foot pain following frostbite. *Arch. Phys. Med. Rehabil.* **63**, 284–5.

Lahiri, S. (1972) Dynamic aspects of regulation of ventilation in man during acclimatization to high altitude. *Respir. Physiol.* **16**, 245–58.

Lahiri, S. (1977) Physiological responses and adaptations to high altitude, in *International Review of Physiology Environmental Physiology II vol.* 14 (ed. D. Robertshaw), University Park Press, Baltimore, MD, pp. 217–51.

Lahiri, S. and Barnard, P. (1983) Role of arterial chemoreflexes in breathing during sleep at high altitude, in *Hypoxia, Exercise and Altitude* (eds. J.S. Sutton, C.S. Houston and N.L. Jones), Liss, New York, pp. 75–85.

Lahiri, S. and Delaney, R.G. (1975) Stimulus interaction in the response of carotid body chemoreceptor single afferent fibres. *Respir. Physiol.* **24**, 267–86.

Lahiri, S., Delaney, R.G., Brody, J.S. *et al.* (1976) Relative role of environmental and genetic factors in respiratory adaptation to high altitude. *Nature* **261**, 133–5.

Lahiri, S., Edelman, N.H., Cherniack, N.S. and Fishman, A.P. (1981) Role of carotid chemoreflex in respiratory acclimatization to hypoxemia in goat and sheep. *Respir. Physiol.* **46**, 367–82.

Lahiri, S., Kao, F.F., Velasquez, T. *et al.* (1969) Irreversible blunted sensitivity to hypoxia in high altitude natives. *Respir. Physiol.* **6**, 360–7.

Lahiri, S., Maret, K. and Sherpa, M.G. (1983) Dependence of high altitude sleep apnea on ventilatory sensitivity to hypoxia. *Respir. Physiol.* **52**, 281–301.

Lahiri, S., Maret, K.H., Sherpa, M.G. and Peters, R.M. Jr (1984) Sleep and periodic breathing at high altitude: Sherpa natives versus sojourners, in *High Altitude and Man* (eds. J.B. West and S. Lahiri), American Physiological Society, Bethesda, MD, pp. 73–90.

Lahiri, S. and Milledge, J.S. (1967) Acid–base in Sherpa altitude residents and lowlanders at 4880m. *Respir. Physiol.* **2**, 323–34.

Lahiri, S., Milledge, J.S., Chattopadhyay, H.P. *et al.* (1967) Respiration and heart rate of Sherpa highlanders during exercise. *J. Appl. Physiol.* **23**, 545–54.

Lahti, A. (1982) Cutaneous reactions to cold, in *Report* **30**, Nordic Council for Arctic Medical Research, Copenhagen, pp. 32–5.

Lakshminarayan, S. and Pierson, D.J. (1975) Recurrent high altitude pulmonary edema with blunted chemosensitivity. *Am. Rev. Respir. Dis.* **111**, 869–72.

Landon, P. (1905) *Lhasa,* vol. 2, Hurst and Blackett, London, p. 39.

Lang, S.D.R. and Lang, A. (1971) The Kunde Hospital and a demographic survey of the Upper Khumbu, Nepal. *N.Z. Med. J.* **74**, 1–8.

Laragh, J.H. (1985) Atrial natriuretic hormone, the renin–aldosterone axis, and blood pressure–electrolyte homeostasis. *N. Engl. J. Med.* **313**, 1330–40.

Larsen, E.B., Roach, R.C., Schoene, R.B. and Hornbein, T.F. (1982) Acute mountain sickness and acetazolamide. Clinical efficacy and effect on ventilation. *JAMA* **248**, 328–32.

Larsen, G.L., Webster, R.O., Worthen, G.S. *et al.* (1985) Additive effect of intravascular complement activation and brief episodes of hypoxia in producing increased permeability in the rabbit lung. *J. Clin. Invest.* **75**, 902–10.

Laufmann, H. (1951) Profound accidental hypothermia. *JAMA* **147**, 1201–12.

Lawler, J., Powers, S.K., Thompson, D. *et al.* (1988) Linear relationship between VO_2 max and VO_2 maximum decrement during exposure to acute hypoxia. *J. Appl. Physiol.* **64**, 1486–92.

Lawrence, D.L. and Shenker, Y. (1991) Effect of hypoxic exercise on atrial natriuretic factor and aldosterone regulation. *Am. J. Hypertens.* **4**, 341–7.

Lawrence, D.L., Skatrud, J.B. and Shenker, Y. (1990) Effect of hypoxia on atrial natriuretic factor and aldosterone regulation in humans. *Am. J. Physiol.* **258**, E243–8.

Lawrie, R.A. (1953) Effect of enforced exercise on myoglobin concentration in muscle. *Nature* **171**, 1069–70.

Lechner, A.J., Grimes, M.J., Aquin, L. and Banchero, N. (1982) Adapative lung growth during chronic cold plus hypoxia is age-dependent. *J. Exp. Zool.* **219**, 285–91.

Ledingham, I. McA. (1983) Clinical management of elderly hypothermic patients, in *The Nature and Treatment of Hypothermia* (eds. R.S. Pozos and L.E. Wittmers), Croom Helm, London/University of Minnesota Press, Minneapolis, pp. 165–81.

Ledingham, I. McA. and Mone, J.G. (1980) Treatment of accidental hypothermia: a prospective clinical study. *BMJ* **1**, 1102–5.

Lehmann, J.F. (1971) Diathermy, in *Handbook of Physical Medicine and Rehabilitation,* 2nd edn, Saunders, Philadelphia, pp. 1397–442.

Lehmuskallio, E. (1999) Cold protecting ointment and frostbite: a questionnaire study of 830 conscripts in Finland. *Acta Dermato-veneredlogica* **79**, 67–70.

Lehmuskallio, E. and Anttonen, H. (1999) Thermal physical effects of ointments in cold: an experimental study with a skin model. *Acta Dermato-veneredlogica* **79**, 33–6.

Lehmuskallio, E., Linholm, H., Koskenvvo, K. *et al.* (1995) Frostbite of the face and ears: an epidemiological study of risk factors in Finnish conscripts. *BMJ* **311**, 1661–3.

Lenfant, C. (1967) Time-dependent variations of pulmonary gas exchange in normal men at rest. *J. Appl. Physiol.* **22**, 675–84.

Lenfant, C. and Sullivan, K. (1971) Adaptation to high altitude. *N. Engl. J. Med.* **284**, 1298–309.

Lenfant, C., Torrance, J., English, E. *et al.* (1968) Effect of altitude on oxygen binding by hemoglobin and on organic phosphate levels. *J. Clin. Invest.* **47**, 2652–6.

Lenfant, C., Torrance, J.D. and Reynafarje, C. (1971) Shift of the O_2–Hb dissociation curve at altitude: mechanism and effect. *J. Appl. Physiol.* **30**, 625–31.

Lenfant, C., Ways, P., Aucutt, C. and Cruz, J. (1969) Effect of chronic hypoxic hypoxia on the O_2–Hb dissociation curve and respiratory gas transport in man. *Respir. Physiol.* **7**, 7–29.

Leonard, W.R., DeWalt, K.M., Stansbury, J.P. and McCaston, M.K. (1995) Growth differences between children of highland and coastal Equador. *Am. J. Phys. Anthropol.* **98**, 47–57.

Leon-Velarde, F. (1998) First International Group on Chronic Mountain Sickness (CMS) in Matsumoto, in *Progress in Mountain Medicine and High Altitude* (eds. H. Ohno, T. Kobayashi, S. Masuyama and M. Nakashima), Press Committee of the 3rd Congress on Mountain Medicine and High Altitude Physiology, Matsumoto, p. 166.

Léon-Velarde, F. and Arregui, A. (1993) Hipoxia: Investigacionas Basicas y Clinicias. *Homenaije a Carlos Monge Cassinelli*, Instituto Frances de Estudios Andinos Universidad Peruana Cayetano Heredia, Lima, Peru.

Leon-Velarde, F., Arregui, A., Monge C.C. and Ruiz, H. (1993) Ageing at high altitude and the risk of chronic mountain sickness. *J. Wilderness Med.* **4**, 183–8.

Leon-Velarde, F., Arregui, A., Vargas, M. *et al.* (1994) Chronic mountain sickness and chronic lower respiratory tract disorders. *Chest* **106**, 151–5.

Leon-Velarde, F., Monge, C.C., Vidal, A. *et al.* (1991) Serum immunoreactive erythropoietin in high altitude natives with and without excessive erythrocytosis. *Exp. Hematol.* **19**, 257–60.

Leon-Velarde, F., Ramos, M.A., Hermandez, J.A. *et al.* (1997) The role of menopause in the development of chronic mountain sickness. *Am. J. Physiol.* **272**, R90–4.

Lepori, M., Hummler, E., Feihl, F. *et al.* (1999) Amiloride sensitive sodium transport dysfunction augments susceptibility to hypoxia induced lung edema (abstract), in *Hypoxia: Into the Next Millennium* (eds. R.C. Roach, P.D. Wagner and P.H. Hackett), Plenum/Kluwer, New York, p. 403.

Leuthold, E., Hartmann, G., Buhlman, R. *et al.* (1975) Medical and physiological investigations on mountaineers. A field study during a winter climb in the Bernese Oberland, in *Mountain Medicine and Physiology* (eds. C. Clarke, M. Ward and E. Williams), Alpine Club, London, pp. 32–7.

Levin, E.R. (1995) Endothelins. *N. Engl. J. Med.* **333**, 356–61.

Levine, B.D. and Stray-Gundersen, J. (1992) A practical approach to altitude training: where to live and train for optimal performance enhancement. *Int. J. Sports Med.* **13**, S209–12.

Levine, B.D. and Stray-Gundersen, J. (1997) 'Living high–training low': effect of moderate altitude acclimatization with low altitude training on performance. *J. Appl. Physiol.* **83**(1), 102–12.

Levine, B.D., Yoshimura, K., Kobayashi, T. *et al.* (1989) Dexamethasone in the treatment of acute mountain sickness. *N. Engl. J. Med.* **321**, 1707–13.

Levine, B.D., Zuckerman, J.H. and deFilipps, C.R. (1997) Effect of high altitude exposure in the elderly: the Tenth Mountain Division Study. *Circulation* **96**, 1224–32.

Lewin, S., Brittman, L.R. and Holzman, R.S. (1981) Infections in hypothermic patients. *Arch. Intern. Med.* **141**, 920–5.

Lewis, R.B. and Moen, P.W. (1952) Further studies on the pathogenesis of cold induced muscle necrosis. *Surg. Gynecol. Obstet.* **95**, 543–51.

Lewis, R.F. and Rennick, P.M. (1979) *Manual for the Repeatable Cognitive–Perceptual–Motor Battery,* Axon, Grosse Pointe Park, MI.

Lexow, K. (1991) Severe accidental hypothermia: survival after 6 hrs 30 min of cardio-pulmonary resuscitation. *Arctic Med. Res.* **50**, Suppl. 6, 112–14.

Li, Y.Z. (1985) The birth weight, distribution of new born (in percentile) in high altitude (abstract), 2nd High Altitude Symposium, Qinghai, China (unpublished proceedings).

Lichty, J.A., Ting, R.Y., Bruns, P.D. and Dyar, E. (1957) Studies of babies born at high altitude. *Am. Med. Assoc. J. Dis. Child.* **93**, 666–7.

Lilja, G.P. (1983) Emergency treatment of hypothermia, in *The Nature and Treatment of Hypothermia* (eds. R.S.

Pozos and L.E. Wittmers), Croom Helm, London/ University of Minnesota Press, Minneapolis, pp. 143–51.

Lim, T.P.K. (1960) Central and peripheral control mechanisms of shivering and its effect on respiration. *J. Appl. Physiol.* **15**, 567–74.

Litch, J.A. and Bishop, R.A. (1999) Transient global amnesia at high altitude. *N. Engl. J. Med.* **340**, 1444.

Litch, J.A. and Bishop, R.A. (2000) High altitude global amnesia. *Wilderness Exp. Med.* **11**, 25–8.

Little, M.A. and Hanna, J.M. (1978) The responses of high altitude populations to cold and other stresses, in *The Biology of High Altitude Peoples* (ed. P.T. Baker), Cambridge University Press, Cambridge, pp. 251–98.

Liu, L., Cheng, H., Chin, W. *et al.* (1989) Atrial natriuretic peptide lowers pulmonary arterial pressure in patients with high altitude disease. *Am. J. Med. Sci.* **298**, 397–401.

Liu, L.S. (1986) Highlights from the national meeting on hypertension: held by the Chinese Medical Association. *Chin. J. Cardiol.* **14**, 2–3.

Lizárraga, L. (1955) Soroche agudo: edema agudo del pulmón. *An. Fac. Med. Lima* **38**, 244–74.

Lloyd, B.B., Jukes, M.G.M. and Cunningham, D.J.C. (1958) The relation of alveolar oxygen pressure and the respiratory response to carbon dioxide in man. *Q. J. Exp. Physiol.* **42**, 214–27.

Lloyd, E.L. (1972) Diagnostic problems and hypothermia. *BMJ* **3**, 417.

Lloyd, E.L. (1973) Accidental hypothermia treated by central re-warming through the airway. *Br. J. Anaesth.* **45**, 41–8.

Lloyd, E.L. (1979) Temperature sensations in veins. *Anaesthesia* **34**, 919.

Lloyd, E.L. (1986) *Hypothermia and Cold Stress,* Croom Helm, London.

Lloyd, E.L. (1996) Accidental hypothermia. *Resuscitation* **32**, 111–24.

Lloyd, E.L. and Mitchell, B. (1974) Factors affecting the onset of ventricular fibrillation in hypothermia: a hypothesis. *Lancet* **2**, 1294–6.

Lloyd, T.C. (1965) Pulmonary vasoconstriction during histotoxic hypoxia. *J. Appl. Physiol.* **20**, 488–90.

Lobenhoffer, H.P., Zink, R.A. and Brendel, W. (1982) High altitude pulmonary edema: analysis of 166 cases, in *High Altitude Physiology and Medicine* (eds. W. Brendel and R.A. Zink), Springer-Verlag, New York, pp. 219–31.

Lockhart, A., Zelter, M., Mensch-Dechene, M. *et al.* (1976) Pressure–flow–volume relationships in pulmonary circulation of normal highlanders. *J. Appl. Physiol.* **41**, 449–56.

Lomax, P., Thinney, R. and Mondino, B.J. (1991) The effects of solar radiation, in *A Colour Atlas of Mountain Medicine* (eds. J. Vallotton and F. Dubas), Wolfe, London, pp. 67–71.

Longmuir, I.S. and Betts, W. (1987) Tissue acclimation to altitude. *Fed. Proc.* **46**, 794.

Longstaff, T.G. (1906) *Mountain Sickness and its Probable Causes.* Spottiswode, London, p. 54.

Longstaff, T.G. (1908) A mountaineering expedition to the Himalaya of Garhwal. *Geogr. J.* **31**, 361–95.

Lugaresi, E., Coccagna, G., Cirignotta, R. *et al.* (1978) Breathing during sleep in man in normal and pathological conditions, in *The Regulation of Respiration during Sleep and Anesthesia* (eds. R.S. Fitzgerald, H. Cautier and S. Lahiri), Plenum, New York, pp. 35–45.

Luks, A.M., van Melick, H., Batarse, R. *et al.* (1998) Room oxygen enrichment improves sleep and subsequent day-time performance at high altitude. *Respir. Physiol.* **113**, 247–58.

Lundberg, E. (1952) Edema agudo del pulmon en el soroche. Conferencia sustentada en la ascociacion medica de Yauli, Oroya. (Quoted in Hultgren, H.N., Spickard, W.B., Hellriegel, K. and Houston, C.S. (1961) High altitude pulmonary edema. *Medicine,* **40**, 289–313.)

Lyons, T.P., Muza, S.R., Rock, P.B. and Cymerman, A. (1995) The effect of altitude pre-acclimatization on acute mountain sickness during reexposure. *Aviat. Space Environ. Med.* **66**, 957–62.

MacDonald, D. (1929) *The Land of the Lama,* Seeley Service, London.

MacDougall, J.D., Green, H., Sutton, J.R. *et al.* (1991) Operation Everest II: structural adaptations in skeletal muscle in response to extreme altitude. *Acta Physiol. Scand.* **142**, 421–7.

MacInnes, C. (1971) Steroids in mountain rescue. *Lancet* **1**, 599.

MacInnes, C. (1979) Treatment of accidental hypo-thermia. *BMJ* **1**, 130–1.

MacIntyre, B. (1994) Ice-cream comforts girl who survived big freeze. *The Times* (London), 4 March, p. 15.

MacKinnon, P.C.B., Monk-Jones, M.E. and Fotherby, K. (1963) A study of various indices of adrenocortical activity during 23 days at high altitude. *J. Endocrinol.* **26**, 555–6.

MacNeish, R.S. (1971) Early man in the Andes. *Sci. Am.* **224**, 36–46.

MacPhee, G.C. (1936) *Ben Nevis,* Scottish Mountaineering Club, Edinburgh, pp. 6–9.

Mader, T.H., Blanton, C.L., Gilbert, R.N. *et al.* (1996) Refractive changes during 72-hour exposure to high altitude after refractive surgery. *Ophthalmology* **103**, 1188–95.

Mader, T.H. and White, L.J. (1995) Refractive changes at extreme altitude after radial keratotomy. *Am. J. Ophthalmol.* **119**, 733–7.

Maggilivary, N. (1853) *The Travels and Researches of Alexander Von Humboldt,* Nelson, London, p. 285.

Maggiorini, M., Bärtsch, P. and Oelz, O. (1997) Association between body temperature and acute mountain sickness: cross sectional study. *BMJ* **315**, 403–4.

Maggiorini, M., Buhler, B., Walter, M. and Oelz, O. (1990) Prevalence of acute mountain sickness in the Swiss Alps. *BMJ* **301**, 853–5.

Maggiorini, M., Muller, A., Hofstetter, D. *et al.* (1998) Assessment of acute mountain sickness by different score protocols in the Swiss Alps. *Aviat. Space Environ. Med.* **69**, 1186–92.

Maher, J.T., Cymerman, A., Reeves, J.T. *et al.* (1975c) Acute mountain sickness: increased severity in eucapnic hypoxia. *Aviat. Space Environ. Med.* **46**, 826–9.

Maher, J.T., Denniston, J.C., Wolfe, D.L. and Cymerman, A. (1978) Mechanism of the attenuated cardiac response to β-adrenergic stimulation in chronic hypoxia. *J. Appl. Physiol. Respir. Environ. Exerc. Physiol.* **44**, 647–51.

Maher, J.T., Jones, L.G., Hartley, L.H., Williams, G.H. and Rose, L.I. (1975a) Aldosterone dynamics during graded exercise at sea level and high altitude. *J. Appl. Physiol.* **39**, 18–22.

Maher, J.T., Levine, P.H. and Cymerman, A. (1976) Human coagulation abnormalities during acute exposure to hypobaric hypoxia. *J. Appl. Physiol.* **41**, 702–7.

Maher, J.T., Manchanda, S.C., Cymerman, A. *et al.* (1975b) Cardiovascular responsiveness to β-adrenergic stimulation and blockade in chronic hypoxia. *Am. J. Physiol.* **228**, 477–81.

Malconian, M.K., Rock, P.B., Hultgren, H.N. *et al.* (1990) The electrocardiogram at rest and exercise during a simulated ascent of Mt. Everest (Operation Everest II). *Am. J. Cardiol.* **65**, 1475–80.

Malconian, M.K., Rock, P.B., Reeves, J.T. and Houston, C.S. (1993) Operation Everest II: gas tensions in expired air and arterial blood at extreme altitude. *Aviat. Space Environ. Med.* **64**, 37–42.

Manier, C., Guenard, H., Castaing, Y. *et al.* (1988) Pulmonary gas exchange in Andean natives with excessive polycythemia – effect of hemodilution. *J. Appl. Physiol.* **65**, 2107–17.

Mansell, A., Powles, A. and Sutton, J. (1980) Changes in

pulmonary PV characteristics of human subjects at an altitude of 5366m. *J. Appl. Physiol.* **49**, 79–83.

Marcet, W. (1886–88a) Climbing and breathing at high altitude. *Alpine J.* **13**, 1–13.

Marcet, W. (1886–88b) On the use of alcoholic stimulants in mountaineering. *Alpine J.* **13**, 319–27.

Marcus, P. (1979) The treatment of acute accidental hypothermia. Proceedings of a Symposium held at the RAF Institute of Aviation Medicine. *Aviat. Space Environ. Med.* **50**, 834–43.

Maret, K.H., Billups, J.O., Peters, R.M. and West, J.B. (1984) Automatic mechanical alveolar gas sampler for multiple sample collection in the field. *J. Appl. Physiol.* **56**, 1435–8.

Margaria, R. (1957) The contribution of hemoglobin to acid-base equilibrium of the blood in health and disease. *Clin. Chem.* **3**, 306–18.

Margaria, R. (ed.) (1967) *Exercise at Altitude,* Excerpta Medica Foundation, Amsterdam.

Marine, D. and Kimball, O.P. (1920) Prevention of simple goiter in man. *Arch. Intern. Med.* **25**, 661–72.

Marinelli, M., Roi, G.S., Giacometti, M., Bonini, P. and Banfi, G. (1994) Cortisol, testosterone and free testosterone in athletes performing a marathon at 4,000 m altitude. *Horm. Res.* **41**, 225–9.

Marsh, A.R. (1983) A short but distant war: the Falklands Campaign. *J. R. Soc. Med.* **76**, 972–82.

Marshall, H.C. and Goldman, R.F. (1976) Electrical response of nerve to freezing injury, in *Circumpolar Health* (eds. R.J. Shephard and S. Itoh), University Press, Toronto, p. 77.

Marsigny, B. (1998) Mountain frostbite. *ISSM Newsletter* **8**, 8–10.

Marsigny, B. (2000) A case of serious frostbite in the Mt. Blanc Massif. *ISSM Newsletter* **10**, 13–16.

Marticorena, E., Ruiz, L., Severino, J., Galvez, J. and Penaloza, D. (1969) Systemic blood pressure in white men born at sea level: changes after long residence in high altitudes. *Am. J. Cardiol.* **23**, 364–8.

Marticorena, E., Severino, J., Peñaloza, A.D. and Neuriegel, K. (1959) Influencia de las grandes alturas en la determinacion de la persistencia del canal arterial. Observaciones realizadas en 3500 escolares de altura a 4300m. Sombre el niuel dez mar. Primeros resultados operatorios. *Rev. Asoc. Med. Prov. Yauli* Nos 1–2, La Oroya.

Marticorena, E., Tapia, F.A., Dyer, J. *et al.* (1964) Pulmonary edema by ascending to high altitudes. *Dis. Chest* **45**, 273–83.

Martin, B.J., Wiel, J.V., Sparks, K.E. *et al.* (1978) Exercise ventilation corresponds positively with ventilatory chemoresponsiveness. *J. Appl. Physiol.* **44**, 447–84.

Martin, D. and Pyne, D. (1998) Altitude training at 2690m does not increase total haemoglobin mass or sea level VO$_2$max in world champion track cyclists. *J. Sci. Med. Sport* **1**, 156–70.

Mason, N.P., Barry, P.W., Despiau, G. *et al.* (1999) Cough frequency and cough receptor sensitivity to citric acid challenge during a simulated ascent to extreme altitude. *Eur. Respir. J.* **13**, 508–13.

Masuda, A., Kobayashi, T., Honda, Y. *et al.* (1992) Effect of high altitude on respiratory chemosensitivity. *Jpn. J. Mount. Med.* **12**, 177–81.

Mathews, C.E. (1898) *Annals of Mont Blanc,* T. Fisher Unwin, London, p. 82.

Mathieu-Costello, O. (1987) Capillary tortuosity and degree of contraction or extension of skeletal muscle. *Microvasc. Res.* **33**, 98–117.

Mathieu-Costello, O. (1989) Muscle capillary tortuosity in high altitude mice depends on sarcomere length. *Respir. Physiol.* **76**, 289–302.

Mathieu-Costello, O., Agey, P.J., Wu, L. *et al.* (1998) Increased fiber capillarization in flight muscle of finch at altitude. *Respir. Physiol.* **111,** 189–99.

Matsuyama, S., Kimura, H., Sugita, T. *et al.* (1986) Control of ventilation in extreme altitude climbers. *J. Appl. Physiol.* **61**, 400–6.

Matsuyama, S., Kohchiyama, S., Shinozaki, T. *et al.* (1989) Periodic breathing at high altitude and ventilatory responses to O$_2$ and CO$_2$. *Jpn. J. Physiol.* **39**, 523–35.

Matsuzawa, Y., Fujimoto, K., Kobayashi, T. *et al.* (1989) Blunted hypoxic ventilatory drive in subjects susceptible to high-altitude pulmonary edema. *J. Appl. Physiol.* **66**, 1152–7.

Matthews, B.H.C. (1932–3) Loss of heat at high altitudes. *J. Physiol.* **77**, 28–9P.

Matthews, B. (1954) Discussion on physiology of man at high altitudes; limiting factors at high altitude. *Proc. R. Soc. Lond. Ser. B* **143**, 1–4.

Maugham, R.J. (1984) Temperature regulation during marathon competition. *Br. J. Sports Med.* **22**, 257–60.

Mawson, J.T., Braun, B., Rock, P.B. *et al.* (2000) Women at altitude: energy requirements. *J. Appl. Physiol.* **88**, 272–81.

Mayhew, T. (1986) Morphometric diffusing capacity for oxygen of the human term placenta at high altitude, in *Aspects of Hypoxia* (ed. D. Heath), Liverpool University Press, Liverpool, pp. 181–90.

Mayhew, T.M. (1991) Scaling placental oxygen diffusion to

birthweight: studies on placentae from low- and high-altitude pregnancies. *J. Anat.* **175**, 187–94.

Mazzeo, R.S., Bender, P.R., Brooks, G.A. *et al.* (1991) Arterial catecholamine responses during exercise with acute and chronic high-altitude exposure. *Am. J. Physiol.* **261**, E419–24.

Mazzeo, R.S., Child, A., Butterfield, G.E. *et al.* (1998) Catecholamine response during 12 days of high-altitude exposure (4,300 m) in women. *J. Appl. Physiol.* **84**, 1151–7.

McCarrison, R. (1908) Observations on endemic cretinism in the Chitral and Gilgit valleys. *Lancet* **2**, 1275–80.

McCarrison, R. (1913) *The Pathology of Endemic Goitre (Milroy Lectures 1913),* Bale Sons and Danielson, London.

McCauley, R.C., Smith, D.J., Robson, M.C. and Heggers, J.P. (1995) Frostbite and other cold related injuries, in *Wilderness Medicine* (ed. P.S. Auerbach), Mosby, St Louis, MO, pp. 129–40.

McClung, J.P. (1969) *Effects of High Altitude on Human Birth,* Harvard University Press, Cambridge, MA.

McCormack, P.D., Thomas, J., Malik, M. and Staschen, C. (1998) Cold stress, reverse T3 and lymphocyte function. *Alaska Med.* **40**, 55–62.

McElroy, M.K., Gerard, A., Powell, F.L. *et al.* (2000) Nocturnal O_2 enrichment of room air at high altitude increases daytime O_2 saturation without changing control of ventilation. *High Alt. Med. Biol.* **1**.

McFarland, R.A. (1937a) Psycho-physiological studies at high altitude in the Andes. I. The effects of rapid ascents by aeroplane and train. *Comp. Psychol.* **23**, 191–225.

McFarland, R.A. (1937b) Psycho-physiological studies at high altitude. II. Sensory and motor responses during acclimatization. *Comp. Psychol.* **23**, 227–58.

McFarland, R.A. (1938a) Psycho-physiological studies at high altitude in the Andes. III. Mental and psycho-somatic responses during gradual adaptation. *Comp. Psychol.* **24**, 147–88.

McFarland, R.A. (1938b) Psycho-physiological studies at high altitude. IV. Sensory and circulatory responses of the Andean residents at 17 500 feet. *Comp. Psychol.* **24**, 189–220.

McIntyre, L. (1987) The high Andes. *Natl. Geogr.* **171**, 422–59.

McKendry, R.J.R. (1981) Frostbite arthritis. *Can. Med. Assoc. J.* **125**, 1128–30.

Mecham, R.P., Whitehouse, L.A., Wrenn, D.S. *et al.* (1987) Smooth muscle-mediated connective tissue remodeling in pulmonary hypertension. *Science* **237**, 423–6.

Meehan, R.T. (1987) Immune suppression at high altitude. *Ann. Emerg. Med.* **16**, 974–9.

Meehan, R., Duncan, U., Neal, L. *et al.* (1988) Operation Everest II: alterations in the immune system at high altitudes. *J. Clin. Immunol.* **8**, 397–406.

Megirian, D.A., Ryan, A.T. and Sherrey, J.H. (1980) An electrophysiological analysis of sleep and respiration of rats breathing different gas mixtures: diaphragmatic muscle function. *Electroencephalogr. Clin. Neurophysiol.* **50**, 303–13.

Menon, N.D. (1965) High altitude pulmonary edema: a clinical study. *N. Engl. J. Med.* **273**, 66–73.

Menzies, I.S. (1984) Transmucosal passage of inert molecules in health and disease, in *Intestinal Absorption and Secretion,* Falk Symposium 36 (eds. E. Skadhauge and K. Heintze), MTP Press, Lancaster, pp. 527–43.

Mercker, H. and Schneider, M. (1949) Uber capillarveranderungen des gehirns bei hohenanpassung. *Pflügers Arch.* **251**, 49–55.

Merino, C.F. (1950) Studies on blood formation and destruction in the polycythaemia of high altitude. *Blood* **5**, 1–31.

Messner, R. (1979) *Everest: Expedition to the Ultimate*, Kaye & Ward, London.

Messner, R. (1981) At my limit. *Natl. Geogr.* **160**, 553–66.

Meyrick, B. and Reid, L. (1978) The effect of continued hypoxia on rat pulmonary arterial circulation. An ultrastructural study. *Lab. Invest.* **38**, 188–200.

Meyrick, B. and Reid, L. (1980) Hypoxia-induced structural changes in the media and adventitia of the rat hilar pulmonary artery and their regression. *Am. J. Pathol.* **100**, 151–78.

Michel, C.C. and Milledge, J.S. (1963) Respiratory regulation in man during acclimatization to high altitude. *J. Physiol.* **168**, 631–43.

Milledge, J.S. (1963) Electrocardiographic changes at high altitude. *Br. Heart J.* **25**, 291–8.

Milledge, J.S. (1968) The control of breathing at high altitude, MD thesis, University of Birmingham.

Milledge, J.S. (1972) Arterial oxygen desaturation and intestinal absorption of xylose. *BMJ* **2**, 557–8.

Milledge, J.S. (1984) Renin aldosterone system, in *High Altitude and Man* (eds. J.B. West and S. Lahiri), American Physiological Society, Bethesda, MD, pp. 47–57.

Milledge, J.S. (1985) The great oxygen secretion controversy. *Lancet* **2**, 1408–11.

Milledge, J.S. (1992) Respiratory water loss at altitude. *ISMM Newsletter* **2**(3), 5–7.

Milledge, J.S., Beeley, J.M., Broom, J. *et al.* (1991a) Acute mountain sickness susceptibility, fitness and hypoxic ventilatory response. *Eur. Respir. J.* **4**, 1000–3.

Milledge, J.S., Beeley, J.M., McArthur, S. and Morice, A.H. (1989) Atrial natriuretic peptide, altitude and acute mountain sickness. *Clin. Sci.* **77**, 509–14.

Milledge, J.S., Bryson E.I., Catley, D.M. *et al.* (1982) Sodium balance, fluid homeostasis and the renin–aldosterone system during the prolonged exercise of hill walking. *Clin. Sci.* **62**, 595–604.

Milledge, J.S. and Catley, D.M. (1982) Renin, aldosterone and converting enzyme during exercise and acute hypoxia in humans. *J. Appl. Physiol.* **52**, 320–3.

Milledge, J.S. and Catley, D.M. (1987) Angiotensin converting enzyme activity and hypoxia. *Clin. Sci.* **72**, 149.

Milledge, J.S., Catley, D.M., Blume, F.D. and West, J.B. (1983b) Renin, angiotensin-converting enzyme, and aldosterone in humans on Mount Everest. *J. Appl. Physiol.* **55**, 1109–12.

Milledge, J.S., Catley, D.M., Ward, M.P. *et al.* (1983a) Renin–aldosterone and angiotensin-converting enzyme during prolonged altitude exposure. *J. Appl. Physiol.* **55**, 699–702.

Milledge, J.S., Ward, M.P., Williams, E.S. and Clarke, C.R.A. (1983c) Cardiorespiratory response to exercise in men repeatedly exposed to extreme altitude. *J. Appl. Physiol.* **55**, 1379–854.

Milledge, J.S., Catley, D.M., Williams, E.S. *et al.* (1983d) Effect of prolonged exercise at altitude on the renin–aldosterone system. *J. Appl. Physiol.* **55**, 413–18.

Milledge, J.S. and Cotes, P.M. (1985) Serum erythropoietin in humans at high altitude and its relation to plasma renin. *J. Appl. Physiol.* **59**, 360–4.

Milledge, J.S., Halliday, D., Pope, C. *et al.* (1977) The effects of hypoxia on muscle glycogen resynthesis in man. *Q. J. Exp. Physiol.* **62**, 237–45.

Milledge, J.S., Iliff, L.D. and Severinghaus, J.W. (1968) The site of vascular leakage in hypoxic pulmonary edema, in *Proceedings of the International Union of Physiological Sciences, Abstracts,* vol. 44, *International Congress,* p. 883.

Milledge, J.S. and Lahiri, S. (1967) Respiratory control in lowlanders and Sherpa highlanders at altitude. *Respir. Physiol.* **2**, 310–22.

Milledge, J.S., McArthur, S., Morice, A. *et al.* (1991b) Atrial natriuretic peptide and exercise-induced fluid retention in man. *J. Wilderness Med.* **2**, 94–101.

Milledge, J.S. and Sorensen, S.C. (1972) Cerebral arteriovenous oxygen difference in man native to high altitude. *J. Appl. Physiol.* **32**, 687–9.

Milledge, J.S., Thomas, P.S., Beeley, J.M. and English, J.S.C. (1988) Hypoxic ventilatory response and acute mountain sickness. *Eur. Respir. J.* **1**, 948–51.

Miller, D. (1999) Menstrual cycle abnormalities and the oral contraceptive pill at high altitude (abstract), in *Hypoxia: Into the Next Millennium* (eds. R.C. Roach, P.D. Wagner and P.H. Hackett), Plenum/Kluwer, New York, p. 412.

Mills, W.J. (1973a) Frostbite and hypothermia. Current concepts. *Alaska Med.* **15**, 26–59.

Mills, W.J. (1973b) Frostbite. A discussion of the problem and a review of an Alaskan experience. *Alaska Med.* **15**, 27–47.

Mills, W.J. (1983) General hypothermia. *Alaska Med.* **25**, 29–32.

Mills, W.J. (1983) Frostbite. *Alaska Med.* **25**, 33–8.

Mills, W.J. and Rau, D. (1983) University of Alaska, Anchorage. Section of high latitude study, and the Mount McKinley Project. *Alaska Med.* **25**, 21–8.

Mills, W.J. and Whaley, R. (1960, 1961) Frostbite: experience with rapid rewarming and ultrasonic therapy. *Alaska Med.* Part I **2**(1) March 1960, 1–4; with Fish, W. Part II **2**(4) December 1960, 114–22; with Fish, W. Part III **3**(2) June 1961, 28–36.

Mines, A.H. (1981) *Respiratory Physiology,* Raven Press, New York.

Mirrakhimov, M.M. (1978) Biological and physiological characteristics of high altitude natives of Tien Shan and the Pamirs, in *The Biology of High Altitude Peoples* (ed. P.T. Baker), Cambridge University Press, Cambridge, p. 313.

Mirrakhimov, M., Brimkulov, N., Cieslick, J. *et al.* (1993) Effect of acetazolamide on overnight oxygenation and acute mountain sickness in patients with asthma. *Eur. Respir. J.* **6**, 536–40.

Mitchell, R.A. (1963) The role of the medullary chemoreceptors in acclimatization to high altitude, in *Proceedings: International Symposium Cardiovascular Respiration*, Karger, Basel, pp. 124–44.

Molnar, G.W., Hughes, A.L., Wilson, O. and Goldman, R.F. (1973) Effect of wetting skin on finger cooling and freezing. *J. Appl. Physiol.* **35**, 205–7.

Moncada, S.R., Palmer, M.J. and Higgs, E.A. (1991) Nitric oxide physiology, pathophysiology, and pharmacology. *Pharmacol. Rev.* **43**, 109–42.

Moncloa, F., Donayre, J., Sobrevilla, L.A. and Guerra-Garcia, R. (1965) Endocrine studies at high altitude: I. Adrenal cortical function in sea level natives exposed to high altitudes (4300m) for two weeks. *J. Clin. Endocrinol. Metab.* **25**, 1640–2.

Monge C.C., Bonavia, D., Leon-Velard, F. and Arregui, A. (1990) High altitude populations in Nepal and the Andes, in *Hypoxia: the Adaptations* (eds. J.R. Sutton, G. Coates and J.E. Remmers), Decker, Toronto, pp. 53–8.

Monge C.C. and Whittembury, J. (1976) Chronic mountain sickness. *Johns Hopkins Med. J.* **139**, 87–9.

Monge M.C. (1925) Sobre el primer caso del policitemia encontrado en el Peru. *Bull. Acad. Méd. Lima.*

Monge M.C. (1948) *Acclimatization in the Andes: Historical Confirmations of 'Climatic Aggression' in the Development of Andean Man*, Johns Hopkins University Press, Baltimore, MD.

Monro, C.C. (1893) Mountain sickness. *Alpine J.* **16**, 446–55.

Mooi, W., Smith, P. and Heath, D. (1978) The ultrastructural effects of acute decompression on the lung of rats: the influence of frusemide. *J. Pathol.* **126**, 189–96.

Moorcroft, W. and Trebeck, G. (1841) Travels in the Himalayan provinces of Hindustan and the Punjab; in Ladakh and Kashmir; in Peshawar, Kabul, Kuduz and Bokhara, in *William Moorcroft, George Trebeck from 1819 to 1825* (ed. H.H. Wilson), vols. 1 and 2, John Murray, London.

Moore, L.G., Asmus, I. and Curran, L. (1998b) Chronic mountain sickness: gender and geographical variation, in *Progress in Mountain Medicine and High Altitude* (eds. H. Ohno, T. Kobayashi, S. Masuyama and M. Nakashima), Press Committee of the 3rd Congress on Mountain Medicine and High Altitude Physiology, Matsumoto, p. 114–19.

Moore, L.G., Cymerman, A., Huang, S.Y. *et al.* (1987) Propranolol blocks the metabolic rate increase but not ventilatory acclimatization to 4300 m. *Respir. Physiol.* **70**, 195–204.

Moore, L.G., Harrison, G.L., McCullough, R.E. *et al.* (1986) Low acute hypoxic ventilatory response and hypoxic depression in acute mountain sickness. *J. Appl. Physiol.* **60**, 1407–12.

Moore, L.G., Niermeyer, S. and Zamudio, S. (1998a) Human adaptation to high altitude: regional and life cycle perspectives. *Am. J. Physical. Anthropol. Ybk.* **41**, 25–64.

Mordes, J.P., Blume, F.D., Boyer, S., Zheng, M. and Braverman, L.E. (1983) High-altitude pituitary–thyroid dysfunction on Mount Everest. *N. Engl. J. Med.* **308**, 1135–8.

Moret, P.R. (1971) Coronary blood flow and myocardial metabolism in man at high altitude, in *High Altitude Physiology: Cardiac and Respiratory Aspects* (eds. R. Porter and J. Knight), Churchill Livingstone, Edinburgh, pp. 131–44.

Morgan, J., Wright, A., Hoar, H., Hale, D. and Imray, C. (1999) Near-infrared spectroscopy to assess cerebral oxygenation at high altitude (abstract), in *Hypoxia: Into the Next Millennium* (eds. R.C. Roach, P.D. Wagner and P.H. Hackett), Plenum/Kluwer, New York, p. 413.

Morganti, A., Giussani, M., Sala, C. *et al.* (1995) Effects of exposure to high altitude on plasma endothelin-1 levels in normal subjects. *J. Hyperten.* **13**, 859–65.

Morice, A., Pepke-Zaba, J., Loysen, E. *et al.* (1988) Low dose infusion of atrial natriuretic peptide causes salt and water excretion in normal man. *Clin. Sci.* **74**, 359–63.

Moro, P.L., Checkley, W., Gilmon, R.H. *et al.* (1999) Gallstone disease in high altitude Peruvian rural populations. *Am. J. Gastroenterol.* **94**, 153–8.

Morpurgo, G., Arese, P., Bosia, A. *et al.* (1976) Sherpas living permanently at high altitude: a new pattern of adaptation. *Proc. Natl. Acad. Sci. USA* **73**, 747–51.

Morrell, N.W., Sarybaev, A.S., Alikhan, A. *et al.* (1999) ACE genotype and risk of high altitude pulmonary hypertension in Kyrghyz highlanders. *Lancet* **353**, 814.

Morshead, H.T. (1921) Report of the expedition to Kamet, 1920. *Geogr. J.* **57**, 213–19.

Mortola, J.P., Rezzonico, R., Fisher, J.T. *et al.* (1990) Compliance of the respiratory system in infants born at high altitude. *Am. Rev. Respir. Dis.* **142**, 43–8.

Mosso, A. (1898) *Life of Man on the High Alps.* T. Fisher Unwin, London.

Motley, H.L., Cournand, A., Werko, L. *et al.* (1947) Influence of short periods of induced acute anoxia upon pulmonary artery pressure in man. *Am. J. Physiol.* **150**, 315–20.

Mountain (1988) News item, **121**, 11.

Mountains of Central Asia (1987) Compiled by the Royal Geographical Society and Mount Everest Foundation, London.

Muelleman, R.L., Grandstaff, P.M. and Robinson, W.A. (1997) The use of pegorgotein in the treatment of frostbite. *Wilderness Environ. Med.* **8**, 17–19.

Mulligan, E., Lahiri, S. and Storey, B.T. (1981) Carotid body O_2 chemoreception and mitochondrial oxidative phosphorylation. *J. Appl. Physiol.* **51**, 438–46.

Murdoch, D. (1995) Altitude illness among tourists flying to 3740 meters elevation in the Nepal Himalayas. *J. Travel Med.* **2**, 255–6.

Murdoch, D.R. (1994) Diplopia at high altitude *J. West. Med.* **5**, 179–81.

Murdoch, D.R. (1996) Focal neurological deficits associated with high altitude. *Wilderness Environ Med.* **7**, 79–82.

Murdoch, D.R. (1999) How fast is too fast? Attempts to define a recommended ascent rate to prevent acute mountain sickness. *ISMM Newsletter* **9**, 3–6.

Nair, C.S., Malhotra, M.S. and Gopinarth, P.M. (1971) Effect of altitude and cold acclimatization on the basal metabolism in man. *Aerosp. Med.* **42**, 1056–9.

Nakashima, M. (1983) High altitude medical research in Japan. *Jpn. J. Mount. Med.* **3**, 19–27.

Napier, J. (1972) *Big Foot: the Yeti and Sasquatch in Myth and Reality,* Cape, London.

National Fire Protection Association (1993) *Standard for Hypobaric Facilities,* Quincy, MA, NFPA Code 99B.

National Oceanic and Atmospheric Administration (1976) *US Standard Atmosphere,* 1976, NOAA, Washington, DC.

Nayak, N.C., Roy, S. and Narayanan, T.K. (1964) Pathologic features of altitude sickness. *Am. J. Pathol.* **45**, 381–7.

Needham, J. (1954) *Science and Civilisation in China,* Cambridge University Press, Cambridge, p. 195.

NHS (1974) *Accidental Hypothermia.* NHS Memorandum No. 1974 (Gen.) 7, Scottish Home and Health Department.

Niazi, S.A. and Lewis, F.J. (1958) Profound hypothermia in man: report of a case. *Ann. Surg.* **147**, 254–6.

Niermeyer, S., Yang, P., Shanmina, D. *et al.* (1995) Arterial oxygen saturation in Tibetan and Han infants born in Lhasa, Tibet. *N. Engl. J. Med.* **333**, 1248–52.

Norton, E.F. (1925) *The Fight for Everest, 1924.* Arnold, London.

Nugent, S.K. and Rogers, M.C. (1980) Resuscitation and intensive care monitoring following immersion hypothermia. *J. Trauma,* **20**, 814–15.

Nukada, H., Pollock, M. and Allpress, S. (1981) Experimental cold injury to nerve. *Brain* **104**, 779–813.

Nunn, J.F. (1961) Portable anaesthetic apparatus for use in the Antarctic. *BMJ* **1**, 1139–43.

Nusshag, W. (1954) *Hygiene der Haustiere,* Hirzel, Leipzig, p. 86.

Nygaard, E. and Nielsen, E. (1978) Skeletal muscle fibre capillarization with extreme endurance training in man, in *Swimming Medicine IV* (eds. B. Eriksson and B. Furberg), University Park Press, Baltimore, MD.

Oades, P.L., Buchdahl, R.M. and Bush, A. (1994) Prediction of hypoxaemia at high altitude in children with cystic fibrosis. *BMJ* **308**, 15–18.

O'Brien, C., Young, A.J. and Sawka, M.N. (1998) Hypothermia and thermoregulation in cold air. *J. Appl. Physiol.* **83**, 185–9.

Oelz, O., Howald, H., di Prampero, P.E. *et al.* (1986) Physiological profile of world-class high-altitude climbers. *J. Appl. Physiol.* **60**, 1734–42.

Oelz, O., Maggiorini, M., Ritter, M. *et al.* (1989) Nifedipine for high altitude pulmonary oedema. *Lancet* **2**, 1241–4.

Ogilvie, J. (1977) Exhaustion and exposure. *Climber and Rambler,* Sept., 34–9; Oct., 52–5.

Ohkuda, K., Nakahara, K., Weidner, W.J. *et al.* (1978) Lung fluid exchange after uneven pulmonary artery obstruction in sheep. *Circ. Res.* **43**, 152–61.

Olsen, N.V., Hansen, J.-M., Kanstrup, I., Richalet, J.-P. and Leyssac, P.P. (1993) Renal hemodynamics, tubular function, and the response to low-dose dopamine during acute hypoxia in humans. *J. Appl. Physiol.* **74**, 2166–73.

Oort, A.H. and Rasmusson, E.M. (1971) *Atmospheric Circulation Statistics,* US Department of Commerce, NOAA, Rockville, MD, pp. 84–5.

Opitz, E. (1951) Increased vascularization of the tissue due to acclimatization to high altitude and its significance of oxygen transport. *Exp. Med. Surg.* **9**, 389–403.

Orr, K.D. and Fainer, D.C. (1951) *Cold Injuries in Korea During Winter 1950–51,* Army Medical Research Laboratory, Fort Knox, KY.

Osborne, J.J. (1953) Experimental hypothermia: respiratory and blood pH changes in relation to cardiac function. *Am. J. Physiol.* **175**, 389–98.

Ou, L.C. and Tenney, S.M. (1970) Properties of mitochondria from hearts of cattle acclimatized to high altitude. *Respir. Physiol.* **8**, 151–9.

Pace, N., Griswold, R.L. and Grunbaum, B.W. (1964) Increase in urinary norepinephrine excretion during 14 days sojourn at 3800 m elevation (abstract). *Fed. Proc.* **23**, 521.

Pandolf, K.B., Young, A.J., Sawka, M.N. *et al.* (1998) Does erythrocyte infusion improve 3.2 km run performance at high altitude? *Eur. J. Appl. Physiol.* **79**, 1–6.

Pappenheimer, J. (1988) Physiological regulation of transepithelial impedance in the intestinal mucosa of rats and hamsters. *J. Membr. Biol.* **100**, 137–48.

Pappenheimer, J.R. (1977) Sleep and respiration of rats during hypoxia. *J. Physiol. (Lond.)* **266**, 191–207.

Pappenheimer, J.R. (1984) Hypoxic insomnia: effects of carbon monoxide and acclimatization. *J. Appl. Physiol.* **57**, 1696–1703.

Pappenheimer, J.R., Fencl, V., Heisey, S.R. and Held, D. (1964) Role of cerebral fluids in control of respiration as studied in unanesthetized goats. *Am. J. Physiol.* **208**, 436–40.

Pappenheimer, J.R. and Maes, J.P. (1942) A quantitative measure of the vasomotor tone in the hind limb muscles of the dog. *Am. J. Physiol.* **137**, 187–99.

Parfionovitch, Y., Dorge, C. and Meyer, F. (1992) *Tibetan Medical Paintings: Illustrations to the* Blue Beryl *Treatise of Sangye Gyamtso (1653–1705)*, Serindia, London, p. 103.

Parker, J.C., Breen, E.C. and West, J.B. (1997) High vascular and airway pressures increase interstitial protein mRNA expression in isolated rat lungs. *J. Appl. Physiol.* **83**, 1697–705.

Parkins, K.J., Poets, C.F., O'Brien, L.M. *et al.* (1998) Effect of exposure to 15% oxygen on breathing patterns and oxygen saturation in infants: interventional study. *BMJ* **316**, 887–94.

Pascal, B. (1648) *Story of the Great Experiment on the Equilibrium of Fluids*. English translation of relevant pages in *High Altitude Physiology* (ed. J.B. West), Hutchinson Ross, Stroudsburg, PA, 1981.

Paschen, W. (1996) Disturbances of calcium homeostasis within the endoplasmic reticulum may contribute to the development of ischemic cell damage. *Med. Hypotheses* **47**, 283–8.

Passino, C., Bernardi, L., Spadacini, G. *et al.* (1996) Autonomic regulation of heart rate and peripheral circulation: comparison of high altitude and sea level residents. *Clin. Sci.* **91**, 81–3.

Paton, B.C. (1983) Accidental hypothermia. *Pharmacol. Ther.* **22**, 331–77.

Paton, B.C. (1987) Pathophysiology of frostbite, in *Hypoxia and Cold* (eds. J.R. Sutton, C.S. Houston and G. Coates), Praeger, New York, pp. 329–39.

Paton, B.C. (1991) Hypothermia, in *A Colour Atlas of Mountain Medicine* (eds. J. Vallotton and F. Dubas), Wolfe, London, pp. 92–6.

Paton, B.C. (1999) Paul Siple and the origin of the wind chill – a commentary. *Wilderness Environ. Med.* **10**, 174–5.

Pattengale, P.K. and Holloszy, J.O. (1967) Augmentation of skeletal muscle myoglobin by a program of treadmill running. *Am. J. Physiol.* **213**, 783–5.

Patton, J.F. and Doolittle, W.H. (1972) Core rewarming by peritoneal dialysis following induced hypothermia in the dog. *J. Appl. Physiol.* **33**, 800–4.

Payot, A. (1881) *Du mal des Montagnes*, thèse pour le Doctorat en Médecine, Alphonse Derenne, Paris.

Peacock, A.J. and Jones, P.L. (1997) Gas exchange at extreme altitude: results from the British 40th Anniversary Everest Expedition. *Eur. Respir. J.* **10**, 1439–44.

Pearn, J.H. (1982) Cold injury complicating trauma in sub-zero environments. *Med. J. Aust.* **1**, 505–7.

Pederson, L. and Benumof, J. (1993) Incidence and management of hypothermia in a rural African hospital. *Anaesthesia* **48**, 67–9.

Pei, S.X., Chen, X.J., Si Ren, B.Z. *et al.* (1989) Chronic mountain sickness in Tibet. *Q. J. Med.* **71**, 555–74.

Pelliot, P. (ed.) (1928) Huc and Gabet. *Travels in Tartary, Thibet and China 1844–1846*, Routledge, London,

Peñaloza, D. (1971) Discussion, in *High Altitude Physiology: Cardiac and Respiratory Aspects* (eds. R. Porter and J. Knight), Churchill Livingstone, Edinburgh, p. 169.

Peñaloza, D., Arias-Stella, J., Sime, F., Recavarren, S. and Marticorena, E. (1964) The heart and pulmonary circulation in children at high altitudes: physiological, anatomical, and clinical observations. *Pediatrics* **34**, 568–82.

Peñaloza, D. and Echevarria, M. (1957) Electro-cardiographic observations on ten subjects at sea level and during one year of residence at high altitudes. *Am. Heart J.* **54**, 811–22.

Peñaloza, D. and Sime, F. (1969) Circulatory dynamics during high altitude pulmonary edema. *Am. J. Cardiol.* **23**, 369–78.

Peñaloza, D. and Sime, F. (1971) Chronic cor pulmonale due to loss of altitude acclimatization (chronic mountain sickness). *Am. J. Med.* **50**, 728–43.

Peñaloza, D., Sime, F., Banchero, N. and Gamboa, R. (1962) Pulmonary hypertension in healthy man born and living at high altitudes. *Med. Thorac.* **19**, 449–60.

Peñaloza, D., Sime, F., Banchero, N. *et al.* (1963) Pulmonary hypertension in healthy men born and living at high altitudes. *Am. J. Cardiol.* **11**, 150–7.

Peñaloza, D., Sime, F. and Ruiz, L. (1971) Cor pulmonale in chronic mountain sickness: present concept of Monge's disease, in *High Altitude Physiology: Cardiac and Respiratory Aspects*, Ciba Foundation Symposium (eds. R. Porter and J. Knight), Churchill Livingstone, Edinburgh, pp. 41–60.

Petetin, D. (1991) Eye protection at high altitude, in *A Colour Atlas of Mountain Medicine* (eds. J. Vallotton and F. Dubas), Wolfe, London, pp. 71–2.

Petit, J.M., Milic-Emili, J. and Troquet, J. (1963) Travail dynamique pulmonaire et altitude. *Rev. Med. Aerosp.* **2**, 276–9.

Peyronnard, J.M., Pednault, M. and Aquayo, A.J. (1977) Neuropathies due to cold. Quantitative studies of structural changes in human and animal nerves, in *Proceedings of the 11th World Congress of Neurology*, Amsterdam, pp. 308–29.

Phillipson, E.A., Sullivan, C.E., Read, D.J.C. *et al.* (1978) Ventilatory and waking responses to hypoxia in sleeping dogs. *J. Appl. Physiol. Respir. Environ. Exerc. Physiol.* **44**, 512–20.

Pickering, B.G., Bristow, G.K. and Craig, D.B. (1977) Core rewarming by peritoneal irrigation in accidental hypothermia. *Anesth. Analg.* **56**, 574–7.

Picon-Reategui, E. (1961) Basal metabolic rate and body composition at high altitudes. *J. Appl. Physiol.* **16**, 431–4.

Pierre, B. and Aulard, C. (1985) *Escalades et Randonnés du Hoggar et dans les Tassilis,* Arthaud, Paris, p. 153.

Piiper, J. and Scheid, P. (1980) Blood–gas equilibration in lungs, in *Pulmonary Gas Exchange,* vol. 1, *Ventilation, Blood Flow, and Diffusion* (ed. J.B. West), Academic Press, New York, pp. 131–71.

Piiper, J. and Scheid, P. (1986) Cross-sectional P_{O_2} distributions in Krogh cylinder and solid cylinder models. *Respir. Physiol.* **64**, 241–51.

Pines, A. (1978) High altitude acclimatization and proteinuria in East Africa. *Br. J. Dis. Chest* **72**, 196–8.

Pines, A., Slater, J.D.H. and Jowett, T.P. (1977) The kidney and aldosterone in acclimatization at altitude. *Br. J. Dis. Chest,* **71**, 203–7.

Pison, U., López, F.A., Heidelmeyer, C.F. *et al.* (1993) Inhaled nitric oxide reverses hypoxic pulmonary vasoconstriction without impairing gas exchange. *J. Appl. Physiol.* **74**, 1287–92.

Pitt, P. (1970) *Surgeon in Nepal,* Murray, London, p. 135.

Plutarch (46–120) Alexander and Caesar. *Loeb Classics,* vol. 7. (1971) Heinemann, London, p. 389.

Podolsky, A., Eldridge, M.W., Richardson, R.S. *et al.* (1996) Exercise-induced VA/Q inequality in subjects with prior high-altitude pulmonary edema. *J. Appl. Physiol.* **81**, 922–32.

Poiani, G.J., Tozzi, C.A., Yohn, S.E. *et al.* (1990) Collagen and elastin metabolism in hypertensive pulmonary arteries of rats. *Circ. Res.* **66**, 968–78.

Pollard, A.J., Barry, P.W., Mason, N.P. *et al.* (1997) Hypoxia, hypocapnia and spirometry at altitude. *Clin. Sci.* **92**, 593–8.

Pollard, A.J. and Murdoch, D.R. (1997) Children at altitude, in *The High Altitude Medicine Handbook*, 2nd edn, Radcliffe Medical Press, Oxford, pp. 39–49.

Pollard, A.J., Murdoch, D.R. and Bärtsch, P. (1998) Children at altitude. *BMJ* **316**, 874–5.

Poole, D.C. and Mathieu-Costello, O. (1990) Effects of hypoxia on capillary orientation in anterior tibialis muscle of highly active mice. *Respir. Physiol.* **82**, 1–10.

Potter, R.F. and Groom, A.C. (1983) Capillary diameter

and geometry in cardiac and skeletal muscle studied by means of corrosion casts. *Microvasc. Res.* **25**, 68–84.

Poulin, M.J., Cunningham, D.A., Paterson, D.H. *et al.* (1993) Ventilatory sensitivity to CO_2 in hyperoxia and hypoxia in older humans. *J. Appl. Physiol.* **75**, 2209–16.

Poulsen, T.D., Klausen, T., Richalet, J.P. *et al.* (1998) Plasma volume in acute hypoxia: comparison of a carbon monoxide rebreathing method and dye dilution with Evans' blue. *Eur. J. Appl. Physiol.* **77**, 457–61.

Prejavalski, A. (1876) *Mongolia, the Tangut Country and the Solitudes of Northern Tibet*, vol. 2, Samson Low, Marston, Searie and Rivington, London, p. 178.

Prescott, W.H. (1891) *History of Mexico,* Swan Sonnerschein & Son, London, p. 253.

Pretorius, H.A. (1970) Effect of oxygen on night vision. *Aerospace Med.* **41**, 560–2.

Priban, I. (1963) An analysis of some short term patterns of breathing in man at rest. *J. Physiol. (Lond.)* **166**, 425–34.

Pritchard, J.S. and Lane, D.J. (1974) Intestinal absorption studied in patients with chronic obstructive airways disease. *Thorax* **29**, 609.

Pugh, L.G.C.E. (1950) Physiological studies on HMS Vengence: Royal Navy cold weather cruise 1994, *MRC Royal Naval Personnel Research Committee RNP* 49/561.

Pugh, L.G.C.E. (1952) *Report on Cho Oyu Expedition,* Medical Research Council, London.

Pugh, L.G.C.E. (1954) Scientific aspects of the expedition to Mount Everest. *Geogr. J.* **120**(2), 183–92.

Pugh, L.G.C.E. (1955a) Acute pulmonary oedema and mountaineering. *Practitioner* **174**, 108–9.

Pugh, L.G.C.E. (1955b) Report on Cho Oyu 1952 and Everest 1953 expeditions. (Unpublished archival material held in the Archival Collection in High Altitude Medicine and Physiology at University of California, San Diego, USA.)

Pugh, L.G.C.E. (1957) Resting ventilation and alveolar air on Mount Everest: with remarks on the relation of barometric pressure to altitude in mountains. *J. Physiol. (Lond.)* **135**, 590–610.

Pugh, L.G.C.E. (1958) Muscular exercise on Mt. Everest. *J. Physiol. (Lond.)* **141**, 233–61.

Pugh, L.G.C.E. (1959) Carbon monoxide hazard in Antarctica. *BMJ* **1**, 192–6.

Pugh, L.G.C.E. (1962a) Physiological and medical aspects of the Himalayan Scientific and Mountaineering Expedition, 1960–61. *BMJ* **2**, 621–33.

Pugh, L.G.C.E. (1962b) Solar heat gain by man in the high

Himalaya: UNESCO Symposium on Environmental Physiology and Psychology, Lucknow, India, pp. 325–9.

Pugh, L.G.C.E. (1963) Tolerance to extreme cold at altitude in a Nepalese pilgrim. *J. Appl. Physiol.* **18**, 1234–8.

Pugh, L.G.C.E. (1964a) Man at high altitude. *Scientific Basis of Medicine, Annual Review* 32–54.

Pugh, L.G.C.E. (1964b) Blood volume and haemoglobin concentration at altitudes above 18000ft (5500m). *J. Physiol.* **170**, 344–54.

Pugh, L.G.C.E. (1964c) Animals in high altitudes: man above 5000m mountain exploration, in *Handbook of Physiology, Adaptation to the Environment,* section 4 (eds. D.B. Dill, E.F. Adolph and C.C. Wilber), Washington, DC, pp. 861–8.

Pugh, L.G.C.E. (1964d) Cardiac output in muscular exercise at 5800 m (19,000 ft). *J. Appl. Physiol.* **19**, 441–7.

Pugh, L.G.C.E. (1965) Altitude and athletic performance *Nature* **207**, 1397–8.

Pugh, L.G.C.E. (1966) Clothing insulation and accidental hypothermia in youth. *Nature* **209**, 1281–6.

Pugh, L.G.C.E. (1967) Cold stress and muscular exercise with special reference to accidental hypothermia. *BMJ* **2**, 333–7.

Pugh, L.G.C.E. (1969) Blood volume changes in outdoor exercise of 8–10h duration. *J. Physiol. (Lond.),* **200**, 345–51.

Pugh, L.G.C.E. and Band, G. (1953) Appendix VI: Diet, in *The Ascent of Everest* (ed. J. Hunt), Hodder and Stoughton, London, pp. 263–9.

Pugh, L.G.C.E., Gill, M.B., Lahiri, S., Milledge, J.S., Ward, M.P. and West, J.B. (1964) Muscular exercise at great altitudes. *J. Appl. Physiol.* **19**, 431–40.

Pugh, L.G.C.E. and Ward, M.P. (1956) Some effects of high altitude on man. *Lancet* **2**, 1115–21.

Pulfery, S.M. and Jones, P.L. (1996) Energy expenditure and requirement while climbing above 6,000 m. *J. Appl. Physiol.* **81**, 1306–11.

Radomski, M.N. and Boutelier, C. (1982) Hormone response of normal and intermittent cold pre-adapted humans to continuous cold. *J. Appl. Physiol.* **53**, 610–16.

Raff, H., Jankowski, B.M., Engeland, W.C. and Oaks, M.K. (1996) Hypoxia *in vivo* inhibits aldosterone and aldosterone synthase mRNA in rats. *J. Appl. Physiol.* **81**, 604–10.

Raff, H. and Kohandarvish, S. (1990) The effect of oxygen on aldosterone release from bovine adrenocortical cells *in vitro. Endocrinology,* **127**, 682–7.

Rahn, H. and Fenn, W.O. (1955) *A Graphical Analysis of the Respiratory Gas Exchange,* American Physiological Society, Washington, DC.

Rahn, H. and Otis, A.B. (1949) Man's respiratory response during and after acclimatization to high altitude. *Am. J. Physiol.* **157**, 445–62.

Rai, R.M., Malhotra, M.S., Dimri, G.P. and Sampathkumar, T. (1975) Utilization of different quantities of fat at high altitude. *Am. J. Clin. Nutr.* **28**, 242–5.

Raifman, M.A., Berant, M. and Levarsky, C. (1978) Cold weather and rhabdomyolysis. *J. Paediatr.* **93**, 970–1.

Raja, K.B., Pippard, M.J., Simpson, R.J. and Peters, T.J. (1986) Relationship between erythropoiesis and the enhanced intestinal uptake of ferric iron in hypoxia in the mouse. *Br. J. Haematol.* **64**, 587–93.

Ramirez, G., Bittle, P.A., Hammond, M. *et al.* (1988) Regulation of aldosterone secretion during hypoxemia at sea level and moderately high altitude. *J. Clin. Endocrinol. Metab.* **67**, 1162–5.

Ramirez, G., Hammon, M., Agousti, S.J. *et al.* (1992) Effects of hypoxemia at sea level and high altitude on sodium excretion and hormonal levels. *Aviat. Space Environ. Med.* **63**, 891–8.

Ramirez, G., Herrera, R., Pineda, D. *et al.* (1995) The effects of high altitude on hypothalamic–pituitary secretory dynamics in men. *Clin. Endocrinol.* **43**, 11–18.

Ramirez, G., Pineda, D., Bittle, P.A. *et al.* (1998) Partial renal resistance to arginine vasopressin as an adaptation to high altitude living. *Aviat. Space Environ. Med.* **69**, 58–65.

Ramos, D.A., Kruger, H., Muro, M. and Arias-Stella, J. (1967) Patologica del hombre nativo de las grande alturas: investigacion de las causes de muerte en 300 autopsias. *Bon. Sanit. Panam.* **62**, 497–507.

Rastogi, C.K., Malholtra, M.S., Srivastava, M.C. *et al.* (1977) Study of the pituitary–thyroid functions at high altitude in man. *J. Clin. Endocrinol. Metab.* **44**, 447–52.

Rathat, C., Richalet, J.-P., Herry, J.-P. and Largmighat, P. (1992) Detection of high-risk subjects for high altitude diseases. *Int. J. Sports Med.* **13**, S76–8.

Rathat, C., Richalet, J.-P., Larmignat, P. and Herry, J.-P. (1993) Neck irradiation by cobalt therapy and susceptibility to acute mountain sickness. *J. Wilderness Med.* **4**, 231–2.

Ravenhill, T.H. (1913) Some experience of mountain sickness in the Andes. *J. Trop. Med. Hyg.* **16**, 313–20.

Raynaud, J., Drouet. L., Martineaud, J.P. *et al.* (1981) Time course of plasma growth hormone during exercise in humans at altitude. *J. Appl. Physiol.* **50**, 229–33.

Read, J. and Fowler, K.T. (1964) Effect of exercise on zonal distribution of pulmonary blood flow. *J. Appl. Physiol.* **19**, 672–8.

RCP (1966) *Report of Committee on Accidental Hypothermia,* Royal College of Physicians, London.

Rebuck, A.S. and Campbell, E.J.M. (1974) A clinical method for assessing the ventilatory response to hypoxia. *Am. Rev. Respir. Dis.* **109**, 345–50.

Recavarren, S. and Arias-Stella, J. (1964) Right ventricular hypertrophy in people born and living at high altitudes. *Br. Heart J.* **26**, 806–12.

Reed, D.J.C. (1967) A clinical method of assessing the ventilatory response to carbon dioxide. *Australas. Ann. Med.* **16**, 20–32.

Reeves, J.T. and Grover, R.F. (1975) High-altitude pulmonary hypertension and pulmonary edema. *Prog. Cardiol.* **4**, 99–118.

Reeves, J.T., Groves, B.M., Sutton, J.T. *et al.* (1987) Operation Everest II: preservation of cardiac function at extreme altitude. *J. Appl. Physiol.* **63**, 531–9.

Reeves, J.T., Moore, L.G., McCullough, R.E. *et al.* (1985) Headache at high altitude is not related to internal carotid arterial blood velocity. *J. Appl. Physiol.* **59**, 909–15.

Regard, M., Oelz, O., Brugger, P. and Landis, T. (1989) Persistent cognitive impairment in climbers after repeated exposure to extreme altitude. *Neurology* **39**, 210–13.

Reichl, M. (1987) Neuropathy of the feet due to running on cold surfaces. *BMJ* **294**, 348–9.

Reinhard, J. (1983) High altitude archaeology and Andean mountain gods. *Am. Alpine J.* **25**, 54–67.

Reinhart, W.H., Kayser, B., Singh, A., Waber, U., Oelz, O. and Bärtsch, P. (1991) Blood rheology and acute mountain sickness and high-altitude pulmonary edema. *J. Appl. Physiol.* **71**, 934–8.

Reitan, R.M. and Davison, L.A. (eds.) (1974) *Clinical Neuropsychology: Current Status and Applications,* Winston, Washington, DC.

Reite, M., Jackson, D., Cahoon, R.L. and Weil, J.V. (1975) Sleep physiology at high altitude. *Electroencephalogr. Clin. Neurophysiol.* **38**, 463–71.

Remmers, J.E. and Mithoefer, J.C. (1969) The carbon monoxide diffusing capacity in permanent residents at high altitudes. *Respir. Physiol.* **6**, 233–44.

Ren, X. and Robbins, P.A. (1999) Ventilatory responses to hypercapnia and hypoxia after 6 h passive hyperventilation in humans. *J. Physiol. (Lond.)* **514**(3), 885–94.

Rennie, D. (1973) Field studies in hypoxia and the kidney,
in *Cornell Seminars in Nephrology* (ed. E.L. Becker), Wiley, New York, pp. 193–206.

Rennie, D. (1989) Will mountain trekkers have heart attacks? *JAMA* **261**, 1045–6.

Rennie, D., Frayser, R., Gray, G. and Houston, C. (1972) Urine and plasma proteins in men at 5,400 m. *J. Appl. Physiol.* **32**, 369–73.

Rennie, D., Lozano, R., Monge, C. *et al.* (1971a). Renal oxygenation in male Peruvian natives living permanently at high altitude. *J. Appl. Physiol.* **30**, 450–6.

Rennie, D., Marticorena, E., Monge, C. and Sirotzky, L. (1971b) Urinary protein excretion in high altitude residents. *J. Appl. Physiol.* **31**, 257–9.

Rennie, D. and Morrissey, J. (1975) Retinal changes in Himalayan climbers. *Arch. Ophthalmol.* **93**, 395–400.

Rennie, D. and Wilson, R. (1982) Who should not go high, in *Hypoxia: Man at Altitude* (eds. J.R. Sutton, N.L. Jones, and C.S. Houston), Thieme-Stratton, New York, pp. 186–90.

Rennie, I.D.B. and Joseph, B.L. (1970) Urinary protein excretion in climbers at high altitude. *Lancet* **1**, 1247–51.

Rennie, M.J., Babij, P., Sutton, J.R. *et al.* (1983) Effects of acute hypoxia on forearm leucine metabolism, in *Hypoxia, Exercise and Altitude* (eds. J.R. Sutton, C.S. Houston and N.L. Jones), Liss, New York, pp. 317–24.

Reshetnikova, O.S., Burton, G.J. and Milovanov, A.P. (1994) Effects of hypobaric hypoxia on the fetoplacental unit: the morphometric diffusing capacity of the villous membrane at high altitude. *Am. J. Obstet. Gynecol.* **171**, 1560–5.

Reynafarje, B. (1962) Myoglobin content and enzymatic activity of muscle and altitude adaptation. *J. Appl. Physiol.* **17**, 301–5.

Reynolds, R.D., Lickteig, J.A., Deuster, P.A. *et al.* (1999) Energy metabolism increases and regional body fat decreases while regional muscle mass is spared in humans climbing Mt. Everest. *J. Nutr.* **129**, 1307–14.

Reynolds, R.D., Lickteig, J.A., Howard, M.P. and Deuster, P.A. (1998) Intake of high fat and high carbohydrate foods by humans increased with exposure to increasing altitude during an expedition to Mt. Everest. *J. Nutr.* **128**, 50–5.

Richalet, J.-P. (1984) *Medicine de l'Alpinisme,* Masson, Paris.

Richalet, J.-P. (1990) The heart and adrenergic system, in *Hypoxia: the Adaptations* (eds. J.R. Sutton, G. Coates and J.E. Remmers), Dekker, Philadelphia, pp. 231–40.

Richalet, J.-P., Keromes, A., Dersch, B. *et al.* (1988) Caractéristiques physiologiques des alpinistes de haute altitude. *Sci. Sports* **3**, 89–108.

Richalet, J.-P., Bittel, J., Merry, J.P. *et al.* (1992) Pre-acclimatization to high altitude in a hypobaric chamber: Everest turbo, in *Hypoxia and Mountain Medicine* (eds. J.R. Sutton, J. Coates and C.S. Houston), Queen City Printers, Burlington, VT, pp. 202–12.

Richalet, J.-P., Dechaux, M., Bienvenu, A. *et al.* (1995) Erythropoiesis and renal function at the altitude of 6,542 m. *Jpn. J. Mount. Med.* **15**, 135–50.

Richalet, J.-P., Hornych, A., Rathat, C., Aumont, J., Lormignat, P. and Rémy, P. (1991) Plasma prostaglandins, leukotrienes and thromboxane in acute high altitude hypoxia. *Respir. Physiol.* **85**, 205–15.

Richalet, J.-P., Robach, S., Jarrot, J.C. *et al.* (1999) Operation Everest III (COMEX '97), in *Hypoxia: Into the Next Millennium* (eds. R.C. Roach, P.D. Wagner and P.H. Hackett), Plenum/Kluwer, New York, pp. 297–317.

Richalet, J.-P., Rutgers, V., Bouchet, P. *et al.* (1989) Diurnal variation of acute mountain sickness, colour vision, and plasma cortisol and ACTH at high altitude. *Aviat. Space Environ. Med.* **60**, 105–11.

Richalet, J.-P., Souberbielle, J.C., Antezana, A.M. *et al.* (1994) Control of erythropoiesis in humans during prolonged exposure to the altitude of 6542 m. *Am. J. Physiol.* **266**, R756–64.

Richardson, R.S., Tagore, K., Haseler, L.J. *et al.* (1998) Increased $\dot{V}_{O_2 max}$ with right-shifted Hb–O_2 dissociation curve at a constant O_2 delivery in dog muscle in situ. *J. Appl. Physiol.* **84**, 995–1002.

Richardson, T.Q. and Guyton, A.C. (1959) Effects of polycythemia and anemia on cardiac output and other circulatory factors. *Am. J. Physiol.* **197**, 1167–79.

Riley, D.J. (1991) Vascular remodeling, in *The Lung: Scientific Foundations* (eds. R.C. Crystal and J.B. West), Raven Press, New York, pp. 1189–98.

Riley, R.L. and Houston, C.S. (1951) Composition of alveolar air and volume of pulmonary ventilation during long exposure to high altitude. *J. Appl. Physiol.* **3**, 526–34.

Riley, R.L., Shephard, R.H., Cohn, J.E., Carroll, D.G. and Armstrong, B.W. (1954) Maximal diffusing capacity of the lungs. *J. Appl. Physiol.* **6**, 573–87.

Rinpoche, R. (1973) *Tibetan Medicine,* Wellcome Institute of the History of Medicine, London.

Rivolier, J. (1959) *Expéditions Francaises à l'Himalaya: Aspect Médical,* Hermann, Paris.

Rivolier, J. (ed.) (1976) *Colloque Médicine et Haute Montagne,* Fédération Française et de la Montagne, Grenoble, Juin 11–12.

Roach, R. and Hackett, P.H. (1992) Hyperbaria and high altitude illness, in *Hypoxia and Mountain Medicine* (eds. J.R. Sutton, C.S. Houston and G. Coates), Queen City Printers, Burlington, VT, pp. 266–73.

Roach, R.C., Bärtsch, P., Hackett, P.H. and Oelz, O. (1993) The Lake Louise acute mountain sickness scoring system, in *Hypoxia and Mountain Medicine* (eds. J.R. Sutton, C.S. Houston and G. Coates), Queen City Printers, Burlington, VT, pp. 272–4.

Roach, R.C., Greene, E.R., Schoene, R.B. and Hackett, P.H. (1998) Arterial oxygen saturation for prediction of acute mountain sickness. *Aviat. Space Environ. Med* **69**, 1182–5.

Roach, R.C., Houston, C.S., Hogigman, B. *et al.* (1995) How do older persons tolerate moderate altitude? *West. J. Med.* **162**, 32–6.

Roach, R.C., Maes, D., Sandoval, D. *et al.* (2000) Exercise exacerbates acute mountain sickness at simulated high altitude. *J. Appl. Physiol.* **88**, 581–5.

Roach, J.M., Muza, S.R., Rock, P.B. *et al.* (1996) Urinary leukotriene E4 levels increase upon exposure to hypobaric hypoxia. *Chest* **110**, 946–51.

Roberts, A.C., Butterfield, G.E., Cymerman, A., Reeves, J.T., Wolfel, E.E. and Brooks, G.A. (1996) Acclimatization to 4,300 m altitude decreases reliance on fat as a substrate. *J. Appl. Physiol.* **81**, 1762–71.

Robertson, J.A. and Shlim, D.R. (1991) Treatment of moderate acute mountain sickness with pressurization in a portable hyperbaric (Gamow) bag. *J. Wilderness Med.* **2**, 268–73.

Robin, E.D. and Gardner, F.H. (1953) Cerebral metabolism and hemodynamics in pernicious anemia. *J. Clin. Invest.* **32**, 598.

Roborovsky (1896) The Central Asian Expedition of Capt. Roborovsky and Lt. Kozloff. *Geogr. J.* **8**, 161.

Roca, J.M., Hogan, M.C., Storey, D. *et al.* (1989) Evidence for tissue limitation of $\dot{V}_{O_2 max}$ in normal man. *J. Appl. Physiol.* **67**, 291–9.

Rock, P.B., Johnson, T.S., Larsen, R.F. *et al.* (1989) Dexamethasone prophylaxis for acute mountain sickness. Effect of dose level. *Chest* **95**, 568–73.

Rockhill, W.W. (1891) *The Land of the Lamas,* Longmans Green, London.

Rogers, T.A. (1971) The clinical course of survival in the Arctic. *Hawaii Med. J.* **30**, 31–4.

Röggla, G., Moser, B. and Röggla, M. (2000) Effect of

temazepam on ventilatory response at moderate altitude (letter). *BMJ* **320**, 56.

Röggla, G., Röggla, M., Podolsky, A. *et al.* (1996) How can acute mountain sickness be quantified at moderate altitude? *J. R. Soc. Med.* **89**, 141–3.

Röggla, G., Röggla, M., Wagner, A. *et al.* (1994) Effect of low dose sedation with diazepam on ventilatory response at moderate altitude. *Wien Klin. Woch.* **106**, 649–51.

Roi, G.S., Giacometti, M. and Von Duvillard, S.P. (1999) Marathons in altitude. *Med. Sci. Sports Exerc.* **31**, 723–8.

Roncin, J.P., Schwartz, F. and D'Arbigny, P. (1996) EGb 761 in control of acute mountain sickness and vascular reactivity to cold exposure. *Aviat. Space Environ. Med* **67**, 445–52.

Rose, M.S., Houston, C.S., Fulco, C.S. *et al.* (1988) Operation Everest II: nutrition and body composition. *J. Appl. Physiol.* **65**, 2545–51.

Roskamm, F., Londry, F.K., Samek, L.L., Schlager, M., Weidermann, H. and Reindelch, H. (1969) Effects of standardised ergometer training produced at three different altitudes. *J. Appl. Physiol.* **27**, 840–7.

Ross, J.H. and Attwood, E.C. (1984) Severe repetitive exercise and haematological status. *Postgrad. Med. J.* **60**, 454–7.

Rossis, C.G., Yiacoumettis, A.M. and Elemenoglou, J. (1982) Squamous cell carcinoma of the heel developing at site of previous frostbite. *J. R. Soc. Med.* **75**, 715–18.

Rothwell, N.J. and Stock, M.J. (1983) Luxuskonsumption. Diet-induced thermogenesis and brown fat: the case in favour. *Clin. Sci.* **64**, 19–23.

Rotta, A., Canepa, A., Hurtado, A., Velásquez, T. and Chávez, R. (1956) Pulmonary circulation at sea level and at high altitudes. *J. Appl. Physiol.* **9**, 328–36.

Roughton, F.J. (1945) Average time spent by blood in human lung capillary and its relation to the rates of CO uptake and elimination in man. *Am. J. Physiol.* **143**, 621–33.

Roughton, F.J.W. (1964) Transport of oxygen and carbon dioxide, in *Handbook of Physiology*, Section 3, *Respiration*, Vol. 1 (eds. W.O. Fenn and H. Rahn), American Physiological Society, Washington, DC, pp. 767–825.

Roughton, F.J.W. and Forster, R.E. (1957) Relative importance of diffusion and chemical reaction rates in determining rate of exchange of gases in the human lung, with special reference to true diffusing capacity of pulmonary membrane and volume of blood in the lung capillaries. *J. Appl. Physiol.* **11**, 291–302.

Roussel, B., Dittmar, A., Delhomm, C. *et al.* (1982) Normal and pathological aspects of skin blood flow measurements by thermal clearance method, in *Biomedical Thermology* (eds. M. Guthrie, E. Albert and R. Alar), Liss, New York, pp. 421–9.

Rowell, G. (1982) High altitude pulmonary oedema during rapid ascent, in *Hypoxia: Man at High Altitude* (eds. J.R. Sutton, N.L. Jones and C.S. Houston), Thieme Stratton, New York, pp. 168–71.

Roy, C.S. (1894) Mountain sickness: maps and scientific reports, in *Climbing and Exploration in the Karakoram Himalayas* (ed. W.M. Conway), T. Fisher Unwin, London, pp. 117–27.

Roy, S.B., Guleria, J.S., Khanna, P.K., Manchanda, S.C., Pande, J.N. and Subba, P.S. (1969) Haemodynamic studies in high altitude pulmonary oedema. *Br. Heart J.* **31**, 52–8.

Ruiz, L. and Peñaloza, D. (1977) Altitude and hypertension. *Mayo Clin. Proc.* **52**, 442–5.

Russel, H. (1871) On mountains and mountaineering in general. *Alpine J.* **5**, 241–8.

Russell, E. (1975) A multiple scoring method for the assessment of complex memory functions. *J. Consult. Clin. Psychol.* **43**, 800–9.

Ruttledge, H. (1934) *Everest 1933.* Hodder and Stoughton, London, p. 78.

Ruttledge, H. (1937) *Everest: the Unfinished Adventure*, Hodder and Stoughton, London, p. 212.

Ryn, Z. (1970) Mental disorders in alpinists under conditions of stress at high altitudes, Doctoral thesis, University of Cracow, Poland.

Ryn, Z. (1971) Psychopathology in alpinism. *Acta Med. Pol.* **12**, 453–67.

Sadikali, F. and Owor, R. (1974) Hypothermia in the tropics. A review of 24 cases. *Trop. Geogr. Med.* **26**, 265–70.

Sahn, S.A., Lakshminarayan, S., Pierson, D.J. and Weil, J.V. (1974) Effect of ethanol on the ventilatory responses to oxygen and carbon dioxide in man. *Clin. Sci. Mol. Med.* **49**, 33–8.

Sakaguchi, E. and Yurugi, R. (1983) Retinal haemorrhages at simulated high altitude. *Jpn. J. Mount. Med.* **3**, 107–8.

Saldana, M. and Arias-Stella, J. (1963a) Studies on the structure of the pulmonary trunk. I. Normal changes in the elastic configuration of the human pulmonary trunk at different ages. *Circulation* **27**, 1086–93.

Saldana, M. and Arias-Stella, J. (1963b) Studies on the structure of the pulmonary trunk. II. The evolution of the elastic configuration of the pulmonary trunk in people native to high altitudes. *Circulation* **27**, 1094–100.

Saldana, M. and Arias-Stella, J. (1963c) Studies on the structure of the pulmonary trunk. III. The thickness of the media of the pulmonary trunk and ascending aorta in high altitude natives. *Circulation,* **27**, 1101–4.

Saldana, M.J., Salem, L.E. and Travezan, R. (1973) High altitude hypoxia and chemodectoma. *Hum. Pathol.* **4**, 251–63.

Saldeen, T. (1976) The microembolism syndrome. *Microvasc. Res.* **11**, 187–259.

Salimi, Z. (1985) Assessment of tissue viability by scintigraphy. *Postgrad. Med.* **17**, 133–4.

Saltin, B. (1967) Aerobic and anaerobic work capacity at 2300m. *Med. Thorac.* **24**, 205–10.

Saltin, B. and Gollnick, P.D. (1983) Skeletal muscle adaptability: significance for metabolism and performance, in *Handbook of Physiology*, Section 10 (ed. L.D. Peachey), American Physiological Society, Bethesda, MD, pp. 555–631.

Salvaggio, A., Insalaco, G., Marrone, O. *et al.* (1998) Effects of high-altitude periodic breathing on sleep and arterial oxyhaemoglobin saturation. *Eur. Respir. J.* **12**, 408–13.

Samaja, M., Mariani, C., Prestini, A. and Cerretelli, P. (1997) Acid–base balance and O_2 transport at high altitude. *Acta Physiol. Scand.* **159**, 249–56.

Samaja, M., Veicsteinas, A. and Cerretelli, P. (1979) Oxygen affinity of blood in altitude Sherpas. *J. Appl. Physiol.* **47**, 337–41.

Sampson, J.B., Cymerman, A., Burse, R.J. *et al.* (1983) Procedures for the measurement of acute mountain sickness. *Aviat. Space Environ. Med.* **54**, 1063–73.

Sanchez, C., Merino, C. and Figallo, M. (1970) Simultaneous measurement of plasma volume and cell mass in polycythemia of high altitude. *J. Appl. Physiol.* **30**, 775–8.

Santolaya, R.B., Lahiri, S., Alfaro, R.T. and Schoene, R.B. (1989) Respiratory adaptation in the highest inhabitants and highest Sherpa mountaineers. *Respir. Physiol.* **77**, 253–62.

Sarnquist, F.H., Schoene, R.B., Hackett, P.H. and Townes, B.D. (1986) Hemodilution of polycythemic mountaineers: effect on exercise and mental function. *Aviat. Space Environ. Med.* **57**, 313–17.

Sartori, C., Allemann, Y., Trueb, L. *et al.* (1999) Augmented vaso-reactivity in adult life associated with perinatal vascular insult. *Lancet* **353**, 2205–7.

Sato, M., Severinghaus, J.W. and Bickler, P. (1994) Time course of augmentation and depression of hypoxic ventilatory response at altitude. *J. Appl. Physiol.* **77**, 313–16.

Sato, M., Severinghaus, J.W., Powel, F.L. *et al.*(1992) Augmented hypoxic ventilatory response in men at altitude. *J. Appl. Physiol.* **73**, 101–7.

Saunders, R. (1789) Some account of the vegetable and mineral productions of Boutan and Tibet. *Philos. Trans. R. Soc.* **79**, 79–111.

Savard, G.K., Cooper, K.E., Veal, W.L. and Malkinson, T.J. (1985) Peripheral blood flow during rewarming from mild hypothermia in humans. *J. Appl. Physiol.* **58**, 4–13.

Savonitto, S., Cardellino, G., Doveri, G. *et al.* (1992) Effects of acute exposure to altitude (3460 m) on blood pressure response to dynamic and isometric exercise in men with systemic hypertension. *Am. J. Cardiol.* **70**, 1493–7.

Savourey, G., Garcia, N., Caravel, C. *et al.* (1998) Pre-adaptation, adaptation and de-adaptation to high altitude in humans: hormonal and biochemical changes at sea level. *Eur. J. Appl. Physiol.* **77**, 37–43.

Savourey, G., Moirant, C., Eterradossi, J. and Bittel, J. (1995) Acute mountain sickness relates to sea-level partial pressure of oxygen. *Eur. J. Appl. Physiol.* **70**, 469–76.

Sawhney, R.C., Chabra, P.C., Malhotra, A.S. *et al.* (1985) Hormone profiles at high altitude in man. *Andrologia* **17**, 178–84.

Sawhney, R.C. and Malhotra, A.S. (1991) Thyroid function in sojourners and acclimatized low landers at high altitude in man. *Horm. Metab. Res.* **23**, 81–4.

Sawhney, R.C., Malhotra, A.S., Singh, T. *et al.* (1986) Insulin secretion at high altitude in man. *Int. J. Biometeorol.* **30**, 23–8.

Schaefer, O., Eaton, R.D.P., Timmermans, F.J.W. and Hildes, J.A. (1980) Respiratory function impairment and cardiopulmonary consequences in long term residents of the Canadian Arctic. *Can. Med. Assoc. J.* **119**, 997–1004.

Schaller, G.B. (1998) *Wildlife of the Tibetan Steppe*, University of Chicago Press, Chicago.

Scherrer, U., Vollenweider, L., Delabays, A. *et al.* (1996) Inhaled nitric oxide for high-altitude pulmonary edema. *N. Engl. J. Med.* **334**, 624–9.

Schmid-Schonbein, H. and Neumann, F.J. (1985) Pathophysiology of cutaneous frost injury: disturbed microcirculation as a consequence of abnormal flow behaviour of the blood. Application of new concepts of blood rheology, in *High Altitude Deterioration* (eds. J. Rivolier, P. Cerretelli, J. Foray and P. Segantini), Karger, Basel, pp. 20–38.

Schmidt, W., Brabant, C., Kröger, C. *et al.* (1990) Atrial natriuretic peptide during and after maximal and submaximal exercise under normoxic and hypoxic conditions. *Eur. J. Appl. Phsyiol.* **61**, 398–407.

Schoeller, D.A. and Van Santen, E. (1982) Measurement of energy expenditure in humans by doubly labelled water method. *J. Appl. Physiol.* **53**, 955–9.

Schoene, R.B. (1982) Control of ventilation in climbers to extreme altitude. *J. Appl. Physiol.* **43**, 886–90.

Schoene, R.B., Hackett, P.H., Henderson, W.R. *et al.* (1986) High altitude pulmonary edema. Characteristics of lung lavage fluid. *JAMA* **256**, 63–9.

Schoene, R.B., Hackett, P.H. and Roach, R.C. (1987) Blunted hypoxic chemosensitivity at altitude and sea level in an elite high altitude climber, in *Hypoxia and Cold* (eds. J.R. Sutton, C.S. Houston and G. Coates), Praeger, New York, p. 532 (abstract).

Schoene, R.B., Lahiri, S., Hackett, P.H. *et al.* (1984) Relationship of hypoxic ventilatory response to exercise performance on Mount Everest. *J. Appl. Physiol.* **56**, 1478–83.

Schoene, R.B., Roach, R.C., Hackett, P.H. *et al.* (1985) High altitude pulmonary edema and exercise at 4400 m on Mount McKinley. Effect of expiratory positive airway pressure. *Chest* **87**, 330–3.

Schoene, R.B., Swenson, E.R., Pizzo, C.J. *et al.* (1988) The lung at high altitude: bronchoalveolar lavage in acute mountain sickness and pulmonary edema. *J. Appl. Physiol.* **64**, 2605–13.

Scholander, P. (1960) Oxygen transport through hemoglobin solution. *Science* **131**, 585–90.

Selkon, J. and Gould, J.C. (1966) Bacteriology, in *Report on IBP Expedition to North Bhutan* (eds. F.S. Jackson, R.W.D. Turner and M.P. Ward), Royal Society, London, pp. 88–98.

Selland, M.A., Stelzner, T.J., Stevens, T. *et al.* (1993) Pulmonary function and hypoxic ventilatory response in subjects susceptible to high altitude pulmonary edema. *Chest* **103**, 111–16.

Sellassie, S.H. (1972) *Ancient and Medieval Ethiopian History to 1270,* United Printers, Addis Ababa, Ethiopia.

Semenza, G.L., Agani, F., Iyer, N. *et al.* (1998) Hypoxia-inducible factor-1: from molecular biology to cardiopulmonary physiology. *Chest* **114**, 40S–45S.

Semple, P. d'A. (1986) The clinical endocrinology of hypoxia, in *Aspects of Hypoxia* (ed. D. Heath), Liverpool University Press, Liverpool, pp. 147–61.

Serebrovskaya, T.V. and Ivashkevich, A.A. (1992) Effects of a 1-yr stay at altitude on ventilation, metabolism and work capacity. *J. Appl. Physiol.* **73**, 1749–55.

Severinghaus, J.W. (1977) Pulmonary vascular function. *Am. Rev. Respir. Dis.* **115** (Suppl.), 149–58.

Severinghaus, J.W. (1995) Hypothetical roles of angiogenesis, osmotic swelling, and ischemia in high-altitude cerebral edema. *J. Appl. Physiol.* **79**, 375–9.

Severinghaus, J.W., Bainton, C.K. and Carcelen, A. (1966a) Respiratory insensitivity to hypoxia in chronically hypoxic man. *Respir. Physiol.* **1**, 308–34.

Severinghaus, J.W. and Carcelen, A. (1964) Cerebrospinal fluid in man native to high altitude. *J. Appl. Physiol.* **19**, 319–21.

Severinghaus, J.W., Chiodi, H., Eger, E.I. *et al.* (1966b) Cerebral blood flow in man at high altitude. *Circ. Res.* **19**, 274–302.

Severinghaus, J.W., Mitchell, R.A., Richardson, B.W. and Singer, M.M. (1963) Respiratory control at high altitude suggesting active transport regulation of CSF pH. *J. Appl. Physiol.* **18**, 1155–66.

Shapiro, C.M., Goll, C.C., Cohen, G.R. and Oswald, I. (1984) Heat production during sleep. *J. Appl. Physiol.* **56**, 671–7.

Sharma, A., Sharma, P.D., Malhotra, H.S. *et al.* (1990) Hemiplegia as a manifestation of acute mountain sickness. *J. Assoc. Physicians India* **38**, 662–4.

Sharma, S.C. (1980) Platelet count on acute induction to high altitude. *Thromb. Haemost.* **43**, 24.

Sharma, S.C. (1981) Platelet adhesiveness in temporary residents of high altitude. *Thromb. Res.* **21**, 685–7.

Sharma, S.C. (1982) Platelet count and adhesiveness on induction to high altitude by air and road. *Int. J. Biometeorol.* **26**, 219–24.

Sharma, S.C., Balasubramanian, V. and Chadha, K.S. (1980) Platelet adhesiveness in permanent residents of high altitude. *Thromb. Haemost.* **42**, 1508–12.

Sharma, V.M. and Malhotra, M.S. (1976) Ethnic variations in psychological performance under altitude stress. *Aviat. Space Environ. Med.* **47**, 248–51.

Sharma, V.M., Malhotra, M.S. and Baskaran, A.S. (1975) Variations in psychomotor efficiency during prolonged stay at high altitude. *Ergonomics* **18**, 511–16.

Sharp, C.R. (1978) Hypoxia and hyperventilation, in *Aviation Medicine Physiology and Human Factors* (ed. J. Ernsting), Tir-Med Books, London, p. 78.

Shepard, R.H., Varnauskas, E., Martin, H.B. *et al.* (1958) Relationship between cardiac output and apparent diffusing capacity of the lung in normal men during treadmill exercise. *J. Appl. Physiol.* **13**, 205–10.

Shephard, R.J. (1985) Adaptation to exercise in the cold. *Sports Med.* **2**, 59–71.

Shi, Z.Y., Ning, X.H., Huang, P.G. *et al.* (1979) Comparison of physiological responses to hypoxia at high altitudes between highlanders and lowlanders. *Sci. Sin.* **22**, 1446–69.

Shi, Z.Y., Ning, X.H., Zhu, S.C. *et al.* (1980) Electrocardiogram made on ascending the Mount Everest from 50m a. s. l. *Sci. Sin.* **23**, 1316–25.

Shigeoka, J.W., Colice, G.L. and Ramirez, G. (1985) Effect of normoxemic and hypoxemic exercise on renin and aldosterone. *J. Appl. Physiol.* **59**, 142–8.

Shih, W.J., Riley, C., Magoun, S. and Ryo, U.Y. (1988) Intense bone imaging agent uptake in the soft tissues of the lower legs and feet relating to ischemia and cold exposure. *Eur. J. Nucl. Med.* **14**, 419–21.

Shipton, E. (1938) *Blank on the Map,* Hodder and Stoughton, London, p. 265.

Shipton, E. (1943) *Upon That Mountain,* Hodder and Stoughton, London, pp. 129–30.

Shlim, D.R. and Houston, R. (1989) Helicopter rescues and deaths among trekkers in Nepal. *JAMA* **261**, 1017–19.

Shlim, D.R. and Meijer, H.J. (1991) Suddenly symptomatic brain tumours at altitude. *Ann. Emerg. Med.* **20**, 315–16.

Shukitt-Hale, B., Banderet, L.E. and Lieberman, H.R. (1991) Relationships between symptoms, moods, performance, and acute mountain sickness at 4700 meters. *Aviat. Space Environ. Med.* **62**, 865–9.

Siebkhe, H., Breivik, H., Rod, T. and Lind, B. (1975) Survival after 40 minutes' submersion without cerebral sequelae. *Lancet* **1**, 1275–9.

Siesjo, B.K. (1992a) Pathophysiology and treatment of focal cerebral ischemia. Part I. Pathophysiology. *J. Neurosurg.* **77**, 169–84.

Siesjo, B.K. (1992b) Pathophysiology and treatment of focal cerebral ischemia. Part II. Mechanisms of damage and treatment. *J. Neurosurg.* **77**, 337–54.

Siesjo, B.K. and Kjallquist, A. (1969) A new theory for the regulation of extra-cellular pH in the brain. *Scand. J. Clin. Lab. Invest.* **24**, 1–9.

Sime, F., Peñaloza, D., Ruiz, L. *et al.* (1974) Hypoxemia, pulmonary hypertension, and low cardiac output in newcomers at low altitude. *J. Appl. Physiol.* **36**, 561–5.

Simon-Schnass, I. and Korniszewski, L. (1990) The influence of vitamin E on rheological parameters in high altitude mountaineers. *Int. J. Vitam. Nutr. Res.* **60**, 26–34.

Singh, I., Chohan, J.S., Lal, M. *et al.* (1977) Effects of high altitude stay on the incidence of common diseases in man. *Int. J. Biometeorol.* **21**, 93–122.

Singh, I. and Chohan, I.S. (1972a) Abnormalities of blood coagulation at high altitude. *Int. J. Biometerol.* **16**, 283.

Singh, I. and Chohan, I.S. (1972b) Blood coagulation at high altitude predisposing to pulmonary hypertension. *Br. Heart J.* **34**, 611–17.

Singh, I., Chohan, I.S. and Mathew, N.T. (1969a) Fibrinolytic activity in high altitude pulmonary oedema. *Ind. J. Med. Res.* **57**, 210–17.

Singh, I., Kapila, C.C., Khanna, P.K., Nanda, R.B. and Rao, B.D.P. (1965) High-altitude pulmonary oedema. *Lancet* **1**, 229–34.

Singh, I., Khanna, P.K., Srivastava, M.C., Lal, M., Roy, S.B. and Subramanyam, C.S.V. (1969b) Acute mountain sickness. *N. Engl. J. Med.* **280**, 175–84.

Singh, I., Malhotra, M.S., Khanna, P.K. *et al.* (1974) Changes in plasma cortisol, blood antidiuretic hormone and urinary catecholamine in high altitude pulmonary oedema. *Int. J. Biometeorol.* **18**, 211–21.

Singh, M.V., Rawal, S.B. and Tyagi, A.K. (1990) Body fluid status on induction, reinduction and prolonged stay at high altitude on human volunteers. *Int. J. Biometeorol.* **34**, 93–7.

Siple, P.A. and Passel, C.F. (1945) Measurement of dry atmospheric cooling in sub-freezing temperatures. *Proc. Am. Philos. Soc.* **89**, 177–99.

Siri, W.E., Cleveland, A.S. and Blanche, P. (1969) Adrenal gland activity in Mount Everest climbers. *Fed. Proc.* **28**, 1251–6.

Siri, W.E., Van Dyke, D.C., Winchell, H.S. *et al.* (1966) Early erythropoietin, blood, and physiological responses to severe hypoxia in man. *J. Appl. Physiol.* **21**, 73–80.

Slater, J.D.H., Tuffley, R.E., Williams, E.S. *et al.* (1969) Control of aldosterone secretion during acclimatization to hypoxia in man. *Clin. Sci.* **37**, 327–41.

Slutsky, A.S. and Strohl, K.P. (1980) Quantification of oxygen saturation during episodic hypoxemia. *Am. Rev. Respir. Dis.* **121**, 893–5.

Smith, C.A., Bisgard, G.E., Nielsen, A.M. *et al.* (1986) Carotid bodies are required for ventilatory acclimatization to chronic hypoxia. *J. Appl. Physiol.* **60**, 1003–10.

Smyth, R. (1988) Alpine runners racing danger. *Observer* (London), 7 August.

Snellgrove, D. (1961) *Himalayan Pilgrimage,* Cassirer, Oxford.

Snodgrass, A.M. (1993) The early history of the Alps. *Alpine J.* **98**, 213–22.

Snyder, L.R.G., Born, S. and Lechner, A.L. (1982) Blood oxygen affinity in high- and low-altitude populations of the deer mouse. *Respir. Physiol.* **48**, 89–105.

Sobrevilla, L.A., Romero, L., Moncloa, F. *et al.* (1967)

Endocrine studies of high altitude. III. Urinary gonadotrophins in subjects native to and living at 14 000 feet and during acute exposure of men living at sea level to high altitude. *Acta Endocrinol.* **56**, 369–75.

Somers, V.K., Anderson, J.V., Conway, J. *et al.* (1986) Atrial natriuretic peptide is released by dynamic exercise in man. *Horm. Metab. Res.* **18**, 871–2.

Somervell, T.H. (1925) Note on the composition of alveolar air at extreme heights. *J. Physiol. (Lond.)* **60**, 282–5.

Somervell, T.H. (1936) *After Everest,* Hodder and Stoughton, London, p. 132.

Son, Y.A. (1979) Quantitative estimation of haemoglobin and its fractions in permanent mountain dwellers in the Tyan'-Shan' and Pamir. *Hum. Physiol.* **5**, 208–10.

Song, S.Y., Asaji, T., Tanizaki, Y. *et al.* (1986) Cerebral thrombosis at altitude. Its pathogenesis and the problems of prevention and treatment. *Aviat. Space Environ. Med.* **57**, 71–6.

Sorensen, S.C. (1970) Ventilatory acclimatization to hypoxia in rabbits after denervation of peripheral chemoreceptors. *J. Appl. Physiol.* **28**, 836–9.

Sorensen, S.C. and Milledge, J.S. (1971) Cerebrospinal fluid acid–base composition at high altitude. *J. Appl. Physiol.* **31**, 28–30.

Sorensen, S.C. and Mines, A.H. (1970) Ventilatory responses to acute and chronic hypoxia in goats after sinus nerve section. *J. Appl. Physiol.* **28**, 832–4.

Sorensen, S.C. and Severinghaus, J.W. (1968) Respiratory sensitivity to acute hypoxia in man at sea level and at high altitude. *J. Appl. Physiol.* **24**, 211–16.

Specht, H. and Fruhmann, G. (1972) Incidence of periodic breathing in 2000 subjects without pulmonary or neurological disease. *Bull. Physio-Pathol. Respir.* **98**, 1075–83.

Speechley-Dick, M.E., Rimmer, S.J. and Hodson, M.E. (1992) Exacerbation's of cystic fibrosis after holidays at high altitude – a cautionary tale. *Respir. Med.* **86**, 55–6.

Spriet, L.L., Cledhill, N., Froese, A.B. and Wilkes, D.L. (1986) Effect of graded erythrocythemia on cardiovascular and metabolic responses to exercise. *J. Appl. Physiol.* **61**, 1942–8.

Staub, N.C. (1986) The hemodynamics of pulmonary edema. *Clin. Respir. Physiol.* **22**, 319–22.

Steele, P. (1971) Medicine on Mount Everest. *Lancet* **ii**, 32–9.

Stein, R.A. (1972) *Tibetan Civilization,* Faber, London, pp. 26–37.

Steinacker, J.M., Tobias, P., Menold, E. *et al.* (1998) Lung diffusing capacity and exercise in subjects with

previous high altitude pulmonary edema. *Eur. Respir. J.* **11**, 643–50.

Steinbrook, R.A., Donovan, J.C., Gabel, R.A. *et al.* (1983) Acclimatization to high altitude in goats with ablated carotid bodies. *J. Appl. Physiol.* **44**, 16–21.

Stephens, D.H. (1982) Sleeping snugly in damp bedrooms. *J. R. Soc. Health* **6**, 272–5.

Stewart, A.G., Bardsley, P.A., Baudouin, S.V. *et al.* (1991a) Changes in atrial natriuretic peptide concentrations during intravenous saline infusion in hypoxic cor pulmonale. *Thorax* **46**, 829–34.

Stewart, A.G., Thompson, J.S., Rogers, T.K. and Morice, A.H. (1991b) Atrial natriuretic peptide-induced relaxation of pre-constricted isolated rat perfused lungs: a comparison in control and hypoxia-adapted animals. *Clin. Sci.* **81**, 201–8.

Stock, M.J., Chapman, C., Stirling, J.L. and Campbell, I.T. (1978b) Effects of exercise, altitude, and food on blood hormone and metabolite levels. *J. Appl. Physiol: Respir. Environ. Exerc. Physiol.* **45**, 350–4.

Stock, M.J., Norgan, N.G., Ferro-Luzzi, A. and Evans, E. (1978a) Effect of altitude on dietary-induced thermogenesis at rest and during light exercise in man. *J. Appl. Physiol. Respir. Environ. Exerc. Physiol.* **45**, 345–9.

Stokes, W. (1854) *The Diseases of the Heart and Aorta,* Hodges and Smith, Dublin, p. 320.

Stoneham, M.D. (1995) Anaesthesia and resuscitation at altitude. *Eur. J. Anaesthesiol.* **12**, 249–57.

Strauss, R.H., McFadden, E.R., Ingram, R.H. *et al.* (1978) Influence of heat and humidity on the airway obstruction induced by exercise in asthma. *J. Clin. Invest.* **61**, 433–40.

Strong, L.H., Gin, G.K. and Goldman, R.F. (1985) Metabolic and vasomotor insulative responses occurring on immersion in cold water. *J. Appl. Physiol.* **58**, 964–77.

Suarez, J., Alexander, J.K. and Houston, C.S. (1987) Enhanced left ventricular systolic performance at high altitude during Operation Everest II. *Am. J. Cardiol.* **60**, 137–42.

Sui, G.J., Lui, Y.H., Cheng, X.S. *et al.* (1988) Subacute infantile mountain sickness. *J. Pathol.* **155**, 161–70.

Sumner, D.S., Boswick, J.A. and Doolittle, W.H. (1971) Prediction of tissue loss in human frostbite with xenon-133. *Surgery* **69**, 899–903.

Sumner, D.S., Criblez, T. and Doolittle, W. (1974) Host factors in human frostbite. *Mil. Med.* **139**, 454–61.

Sun, J.H., Lin, Z.P. and Hu, X.L. (1985) An observation on the development of normal children age between 7–17 years at three elevations (abstract), 2nd High

Altitude Symposium, Qinghai, China (unpublished proceedings).

Sun, S., Oliver-Pickett, C., Ping, Y. *et al.* (1996) Breathing and brain blood flow during sleep in patients with chronic mountain sickness. *J. Appl. Physiol.* **81**, 611–18.

Sun, S.F. (1985) Epidemiology of hypertension of the Tibetan plateau (abstract), 2nd High Altitude Symposium, Qinghai, China (unpublished proceedings).

Sun, S.F. (1986) Epidemiology of hypertension on the Tibetan plateau. *Hum. Biol.* **58**, 507–15.

Sun, S.F., Droma, T.S., Zhang, J.G. *et al.* (1990) Greater maximal O_2 uptake and vital capacities in Tibetan than Han residents of Lhasa. *Respir. Physiol.* **79**, 151–62.

Suri, M.L., Vijayan, G.P., Puri, H.C. *et al.* (1978) Neurological manifestations of frostbite. *Indian J. Med. Res.* **67**, 292–9.

Surks, M.I. (1966) Elevated PBI, free thyroxine, and plasma protein concentration in man at high altitude. *J. Appl. Physiol.* **21**, 1185–90.

Suslov, F.P. (1994) Basic principles of training at high altitude. *New Studies in Athletes IAAF Quart. Mag.* **2**, 45–9.

Sutton, J.R. (1977) Effect of acute hypoxia on the hormonal response to exercise. *J. Appl. Physiol. Respir. Environ. Exerc. Physiol.* **42**, 587–92.

Sutton, J.R. (1987) Energy substrates and hypoglycaemia, in *Hypoxia and Cold* (eds. J.R. Sutton, C.S. Houston and G. Coates), Prager, New York, pp. 487–92.

Sutton, J.R., Bryan, A.C., Gray, G.W. *et al.* (1976) Pulmonary gas exchange in acute mountain sickness. *Aviat. Space Environ. Med.* **47**, 1032–7.

Sutton, J.R., Houston, C.S. and Coates, G. (1988) *Hypoxia: the Tolerable Limits,* Benchmark Press, Indianapolis.

Sutton, J.R., Houston, C.S. and Jones, N.L. (1983) *Hypoxia, Exercise, and Altitude,* Liss, New York.

Sutton, J.R., Houston, C.S., Mansell, A.L. *et al.* (1979) Effect of acetazolamide on hypoxemia during sleep at high altitude. *N. Engl. J. Med.* **301**, 1329–31.

Sutton, J.R., Reeves, J.T., Wagner, P.D. *et al.* (1988) Operation Everest II: oxygen transport during exercise at extreme simulated altitude. *J. Appl. Physiol.* **64**, 1309–21.

Sutton, J.R., Viol, G.W., Gray, G.W. *et al.* (1977) Renin, aldosterone, electrolyte, and cortisol responses to hypoxic decompression. *J. Appl. Physiol. Respir. Environ. Exerc. Physiol.* **43**, 421–4.

Svedenhag, J., Henriksson, J. and Sylven, C. (1983) Dissociation of training effects on skeletal muscle mitochondrial enzymes and myoglobin in man. *Acta Physiol. Scand.* **117**, 213–18.

Swenson, E.R., Duncan, T.B., Goldberg, S.V. *et al.* (1995) Diuretic effect of acute hypoxia in humans: relationship to hypoxic ventilatory responsiveness and renal hormones. *J. Appl. Physiol.* **78**, 377–83.

Swenson, E.R. and Hughes, J.M.B. (1993) Effects of acute and chronic acetazolamide on resting ventilation and ventilatory responses in men. *J. Appl. Physiol.* **74**, 230–7.

Swenson, E.R., Leatham, K.L., Roach, R.C. *et al.* (1991) Renal carbonic anhydrase inhibition reduces high altitude sleep periodic breathing. *Respir. Physiol.* **86**, 333–43.

Swenson, E.R., MacDonald, A., Vatheuer, M. *et al.* (1997) Acute mountain sickness is not altered by a high carbohydrate diet nor associated with elevated circulating cytokines. *Aviat. Space Environ. Med* **68**, 499–503.

Swenson, E.R., Mongovin, S., Gibbs, S. *et al.* (2000) Stress failure in high altitude pulmonary edema (HAPE). *Am. J. Respir. Crit. Care Med.* **161**, A418.

Symposium (Indian) (1962) *International Symposium on Problems of High Altitude at Darjeeling,* Armed Forces Medical Services. Gulabons Offset Works, Delhi.

Taber, R. (1994) A child in the pressure bag: a case. *ISMM Newsletter* **4**(1), 4–5.

Talbott, J.H. and Dill, D.B. (1936) Clinical observations at high altitude. *Am. J. Med. Sci.* **192**, 626–39.

Tansey, W.A. (1973) Medical aspects of cold water immersion: a review. *US Navy Submarine Medical Research Laboratory Report* NSMRL, 763, NTIS Document AD-775–687.

Tansley, J.G., Fatman, M., Howard, L.S.G.E. *et al.* (1998) Changes in respiratory control during and after 48 h of isocapnic and poikilocapnic hypoxia in humans. *J. Appl. Physiol.* **85**, 2125–34.

Tappan, D.V. and Reynafarje, B.D. (1957) Tissue pigment manifestation of adaptation to high altitude. *Am. J. Physiol.* **190**, 99–103.

Taring, R.D. (1970) *Daughter of Tibet,* Murray, London, p. 170.

Tasker, J. (1981) *Everest the Cruel Way*, Eyre Methuen, London.

Tatsumi, K., Pickett, C.K. and Weil, J.V. (1991) Attenuated carotid body hypoxic sensitivity after prolonged hypoxic exposure. *J. Appl. Physiol.* **70**, 748–55.

Taylor, M.S. (1999) Lumbar sympathectomy for frostbite injuries of the foot. *Mil. Med.* **164**, 566–7.

Tek, D. and Mackey, S. (1993) Non-freezing cold injury in a marine infantry battalion. *J. Wilderness Med.* **4**, 353–7.

Tenney, S.M. and Ou, L.C. (1970) Physiological evidence for increased tissue capillarity in rats acclimatized to high altitude. *Respir. Physiol.* **8**, 137–50.

Tenney, S.M. and Ou, L.C. (1977) Ventilatory response of decorticate and decerebrate cats to hypoxia and CO_2. *Respir. Physiol.* **29**, 81–2.

Tewari, S.C., Jayaswal, R., Kasturi, A.S. *et al.* (1991) Excessive polycythaemia of high altitude. Pulmonary function studies including carbon monoxide diffusion capacity. *J. Assoc. Physicians India* **39**, 453–5.

The Times (1999a) Mount Everest poses an even greater challenge, 13 November, p. 17.

The Times (1999b) Queen Victoria's Gurkha was a trailblazer extraordinary, 8 July, p. 50.

Theis, M.K., Honigman, B., Yip, R., McBride, D., Houston, C.S. and Moore, L.G. (1993) Acute mountain sickness in children at 2835 metres. *Am. J. Dis. Child.* **147**, 143–5.

Thomas, D.J., Marshall, J., Ross Russell, R.W. *et al.* (1977) Cerebral blood-flow in polycythaemia. *Lancet* **2**, 161–3.

Thomas, P.W. (1894) Rocky Mountain sickness. *Alpine J.* **17**, 140–9.

Thompson, D.G., Richelson, E. and Malagelada, J.R. (1983) A perturbation of upper gastro-intestinal function by cold stress. *Gut* **24**, 277–83.

Thompson, R.L. and Hayward, J.S. (1996) Wet cold exposure and hypothermia: thermal and metabolic responses to prolonged exercise in rain. *J. Appl. Physiol.* **81**, 1128–37.

Thompson, W.O., Thompson, P.K. and Dailey, M.M. (1928) The effect of posture on the composition and volume of the blood in man. *J. Clin. Invest.* **5**, 573–604.

Tierman, C.J. (1999) Splenic crisis at high altitude in two white men with sickle cell trait. *Ann. Emerg. Med.* **33**, 230–3.

Tikusis, P., Ducharme, M.B., Moroz, D. and Jacobs, I. (1999) Physiological responses on exercise fatigued individuals exposed to wet cold conditions. *J. Appl. Physiol.* **86**, 1319–25.

Tilman, H.W. (1948) *Mount Everest 1938,* Cambridge University Press, Cambridge, pp. 93–4.

Tilman, H.W. (1952) *Nepal Himalaya*, Cambridge University Press, Cambridge, p. 79.

Tilman, H.W. (1975) Practical problems of nutrition, in *Mountain Medicine and Physiology* (eds. C. Clarke, M. Ward and E. Williams), Alpine Club, London, pp. 62–6.

Timmons, B.A., Ararujo, J. and Thomas, T.R. (1985) Fat utilization in a cold environment. *Med. Sci. Sports Exerc.* **17**, 673–8.

Ting, S. (1984) Cold induced urticaria in infancy. *Pediatrics* **73**, 105–6.

Tissandier, G. (1875) Le voyage à grande hauteur du ballon 'Le Zenith'. *La Nature Paris* **3**, 337–44.

Tolman, K.G. and Cohen, A. (1970) Accidental hypothermia. *Can. Med. Assoc. J.* **103**, 1357–61.

Torricelli, E. (1644) Letter of Torricelli to Michelangelo Ricci. English translation of relevant pages in *High Altitude Physiology* (ed. J.B. West), Hutchinson Ross, Stroudsburg, PA, 1981.

Townes, B.D., Hornbein, T.F., Schoene, R.B., Sarnquist, F.H. and Grant, I. (1984) Human cerebral function at extreme altitude, in *High Altitude and Man* (eds. J.B. West and S. Lahiri), American Physiological Society, Bethesda, MD, pp. 32–6.

Tozzi, C.A., Poiani, G.J., Harangozo, A.M., Boyd, C.D. and Riley, D.J. (1989) Pressure-induced connective tissue synthesis in pulmonary artery segments is dependent on intact endothelium. *J. Clin. Invest.* **84**, 1005–12.

Travis, S.P.L., A'Court, C., Menzies, I.S. *et al.* (1993) Intestinal function at altitudes above 5000m (abstract). *Gut* **34**, T165.

Travis, S.P.L. and Menzies, I.S. (1992) Intestinal permeability: functional assessment and significance. *Clin. Sci.* **82**, 471–88.

Treating accidental hypothermia (editorial). (1978) *BMJ* **2**, 1383–4.

Treatment of Hypothermia (eds. R.S. Pozos and L.E. Wittmers), Croom Helm, London/University of Minnesota Press, Minneapolis, pp. 143–51.

Tschop, M., Strasburger, C.J., Hartmann, G. *et al.* (1998) Raised leptin concentration at high altitude associated with loss of appetite (letter). *Lancet* **352**, 1119–20.

Tsukimoto, K., Mathieu-Costello, O., Prediletto, R., Elliott, A.E. and West, J.B. (1991) Ultrastructural appearances of pulmonary capillaries at high transmural pressures. *J. Appl. Physiol.* **71**, 573–82.

Tsukimoto, K., Yoshimura, N., Ichioka, M. *et al.* (1994) Protein, cell, and leukotriene B4 concentrations of lung edema fluid produced by high capillary transmural pressures in rabbit. *J. Appl. Physiol.* **76**, 321–67.

Tuffley, R.E., Rubenstein, D., Slater, J.D.H. and Williams, E.S. (1970) Serum renin activity during exposure to hypoxia. *J. Endocrinol.* **48**, 497–510.

Turek, Z., Kreuzer, F. and Hoofd, L.J.C. (1973) Advantage or disadvantage of a decrease of blood oxygen affinity for tissue oxygen supply at hypoxia; a theoretical study comparing man and rat. *Pflügers Arch.* **342**, 185–97.

Turek, Z., Kreuzer, F. and Ringnalda, B.E.M. (1978) Blood gases at several levels of oxygenation in rats with a left shifted blood oxygen dissociation curve. *Pflügers Arch.* **376**, 7–13.

Turino, C.M., Bergofsky, E.H., Goldring, R.M. and Fishman, A.P. (1963) Effect of exercise on pulmonary diffusing capacity. *J. Appl. Physiol.* **18**, 447–56.

Tyndall, J. (1860) *The Glaciers of the Alps*, Murray, London, p. 80.

Ueda, G., Reeves, J.T. and Sekiguchi, M. (1992) *High Altitude Medicine*, Shinshu University, Matsumoto, Japan.

Unger, C., Weiser, J.K., McCullough, R.E. *et al.* (1988) Altitude, low birth weight, and infant mortality in Colorado. *JAMA* **259**, 3427–32.

Ungley, G.G., Channell, G.D. and Richards, R.L. (1945) The immersion foot syndrome. *Br. J. Surg.* **33**, 17–31.

Unna, P.J.H. (1921–2) The oxygen equipment of the 1922 Everest expedition. *Alpine J.* **34**, 235–50.

Unsworth, W. (2000) *Everest. A Mountaineering History (3rd edn)*. Baton Wicks.

Utiger, D., Bernasch, D., Eichenberger, U. and Bärtsch, P. (1999) Transient improvement in high altitude headache by sumatriptan in a placebo controlled trial (abstract), in *Hypoxia: Into the Next Millennium* (eds. R.C. Roach, P.D. Wagner and P.H. Hackett), Plenum/Kluwer, New York, p. 435.

Vachiery, J.L., McDonald, T., Moraine, J.J. *et al.* (1995) Doppler assessment of hypoxic pulmonary vasoconstriction and susceptibility to high altitude pulmonary oedema. *Thorax* **50**, 22–7.

Valdivia, E. (1958) Total capillary bed in striated muscle of guinea pigs native to the Peruvian mountains. *Am. J. Physiol.* **194**, 585–9.

Van Ruiten, H.J.A. and Daanen, H.A.M. (1999) Cold induced vasodilatation at altitude (abstract), in *Hypoxia: Into the Next Millennium* (eds. R.C. Roach, P.D. Wagner and P.H. Hackett), Plenum/Kluwer, New York, p. 436.

Vargas, M., Leon-Velarde, F., Monge, C.C. *et al.* (1998) Similar hypoxic ventilatory response in sea-level natives and Andean natives living at sea level. *J. Appl. Physiol.* **84**, 1024–9.

Vaughan, B.E. and Pace, N. (1956) Changes in myoglobin content of the high altitude acclimatized rat. *Am. J. Physiol.* **185**, 549–56.

Vaughn, P.B. (1942) Local cold injury – menace to military operations. A review. *Mil. Med.* **145**, 305–11.

Velásquez, M.T. (1956) *Maximal Diffusing Capacity of the Lungs at High Altitudes.* Report 56–108, USAF School of Aviation Medicine, Randolph Air Force Base, TX.

Velasquez, T. (1976) Pulmonary function and oxygen transport, in *Man in the Andes: a Multidisciplinary Study of High-altitude Quechua* (eds. P.T. Baker and M.A. Little), Dowden, Hutchinson & Ross, Stroudsburg PA, pp. 237–60.

Vella, M.A., Jenner, C., Betteridge, D.J. and Jowett, N.I. (1988) Hypothermia induced thrombocytopenia. *J. R. Soc. Med.* **81**, 228–9.

Viault, F. (1890) Sur l'augmentation considerable de nombre des globules rouges dans le sang chez les habitants des haut plateaux de l'Amérique du Sud. *Comptes Rendus, Hebdomaire Des Seances de l'Academie Des Sciences (Paris)*, **III**, 917–18. English translation (1981) in *High Altitude Physiology* (ed. J.B. West), Hutchinson Ross, Stroudsburg PA, 1981, pp. 333–4.

Viault, F. (1891) Sur la quantité d'oxygène contenue dans le sang des animaux des hauts plateaux de l'Amérique du Sud. *C. R. Acad. Sci. (Paris)* **112**, 295–8.

Virokannas, H. and Anttonen, H. (1993) Risk of frostbite in vibration-induced finger cases. *Arctic Med. Res.* **52**, 69–72.

Viswanathan, R., Subramanian, S. and Radha, T.C. (1979) Effect of hypoxia on regional lung perfusion, by scanning. *Respiration* **37**, 142–7.

Vizek, M., Picket, C.K. and Weil, J.V. (1987) Increased carotid body sensitivity during acclimatization to hypobaric hypoxia. *J. Appl. Physiol.* **63**, 2403–10.

Voelkel, N.F., Hegstrand, L., Reeves, J.T., McMurty, I.F. and Molinoff, P.B. (1981) Effects of hypoxia on density of β-adrenergic receptors. *J. Appl. Physiol.* **50**, 363–6.

Vogel, J.A., Hansen, J.E. and Harris, C.W. (1967) Cardiovascular responses in man during exhaustive work at sea level and high altitude. *J. Appl. Physiol.* **23**, 531–9.

Vogel, J.A. and Harris, C.W. (1967) Cardiopulmonary responses of resting man during early exposure to high altitude. *J. Appl. Physiol.* **22**, 1124–8.

Vogel, J.A., Hartley, L.H. and Cruz, J.C. (1974) Cardiac output during exercise in altitude natives at sea level and high altitude. *J. Appl. Physiol.* **36**, 173–6.

Von Euler, U.S. and Liljestrand, G. (1946) Observations on the pulmonary arterial blood pressure in the cat. *Acta Physiol.* **22**, 1115–23.

Von Schlagintweit, A.H. and Von Schlagintweit, R. (1862) *Results of a Scientific Mission to India and High Asia*, vol. I, Trubner, London, p. 18.

Vonmoos, S., Nussberger, J., Waeber, J. *et al.* (1990) Effect of metoclopramide on angiotensin, aldosterone and atrial peptide during hypoxia. *J. Appl. Physiol.* **69**, 2072–9.

Vorstrup, S., Henriksen, L. and Paulson, O.B. (1984) Effect of acetazolamide on cerebral blood flow and cerebral metabolic rate for oxygen. *J. Clin. Invest.* **74**, 1634–9.

Vuolteenaho, O., Koistinen, P., Martikkala, V. *et al.* (1992) Effect of physical exercise in hypobaric conditions on atrial natriuretic peptide secretion. *Am. J. Physiol.* **263**, R647–52.

Waddell, L.A. (1899) *Among the Himalayas,* Constable, London, pp. 261–2.

Waddell, L.A. (1905) *Lhasa and its Mysteries,* Murray, London, p. 144.

Wagenvoort, C.A. and Wagenvoort, N. (1973) Hypoxic pulmonary vascular lesions in man at high altitude and in patients with chronic respiratory disease. *Pathol. Microbiol.* **39**, 276–82.

Wagenvoort, C.A. and Wagenvoort, N. (1976) Pulmonary venous changes in chronic hypoxia. *Virchows Arch. [A]* **372**, 51–6.

Waggener, T.B., Brusil, P.J., Kronauer, R.E. *et al.* (1984) Strength and cycle time of high-altitude ventilatory patterns in unacclimatized humans. *J. Appl. Physiol.* **56**, 576–81.

Wagner, P.D. (1988) An integrated view of the determinants of maximum oxygen uptake, in *Oxygen Transfer from Atmosphere to Tissues,* vol. 227 (eds. N.C. Gonzalez and M.R. Fedde), Plenum, New York, pp. 246–56.

Wagner, P.D. (1996) A theoretical analysis of factors determining $\dot{V}_{O_2\,max}$ at sea level and altitude. *Respir. Physiol.* **106**, 329–43.

Wagner, P.D., Hedenstierna, G. and Rodriguez-Roisin, R. (1996) Gas exchange, expiratory flow obstruction and the clinical spectrum of asthma. *Eur. Respir. J.* **9**, 1278–82.

Wagner, P.D., Saltzman, H.A. and West, J.B. (1974) Measurement of continuous distributions of ventilation–perfusion ratios: theory. *J. Appl. Physiol.* **36**, 588–99.

Wagner, P.D., Sutton, J.R., Reeves, J.T., Cymerman, A., Groves, B.M. and Malconian, M.K. (1987) Operation Everest II. Pulmonary gas exchange during a simulated ascent of Mt. Everest. *J. Appl. Physiol.* **63**, 2348–59.

Wagner, P.D. and West, J.B. (1972) Effects of diffusion impairment of O_2 and CO_2 time courses in pulmonary capillaries. *J. Appl. Physiol.* **33**, 62–71.

Walker, J.T. (1885) Four years journeyings through great Tibet by one of the trans-Himalayan explorers of the Survey of India. *Proc. R. Geogr. Soc.* **7**, 65–92.

Waller, D. (1990) *The Pundits: British Exploration of Tibet and Central Asia,* University Press of Kentucky, Lexington, KY.

Wanderer, A.A. (1979) An 'allergy' to cold. *Hosp. Pract.* **14**, 136–7.

Wang, L.C.H. (1978) Factors limiting maximum cold induced heat production. *Life Sci.* **23**, 2089–98.

Ward, M.P. (1954) High altitude deterioration, in: A discussion on the physiology of man at high altitude. *Proc. R. Soc., Series B, London* **143**, 40–2.

Ward, M.P. (1968) Diseases occurring at altitudes exceeding 17500ft. MD thesis, University of Cambridge, pp. 66–9.

Ward, M.P. (1973) Periodic respiration. *Ann. R. Coll. Surg. Engl.* **52**, 330–4.

Ward, M.P. (1974) Frostbite. *BMJ* **1**, 67–70.

Ward, M.P. (1975) *Mountain Medicine, a Clinical Study of Cold and High Altitude,* Crosby Lockwood Staples, London.

Ward, M.P. (1983) The Kongur Massif in Southern Xinjiang. *Geogr. J.* **149**, 137–52.

Ward, M.P. (1987) Cold, hypoxia and dehydration, in *Hypoxia and Cold* (eds. J.R. Sutton, C.S. Houston and G. Coates), Prager, New York, pp. 475–86.

Ward, M.P. (1990) Tibet: human and medical geography. *J. Wilderness Med.* **1**, 36–46.

Ward, M.P. (1991) Medicine in Tibet. *J. Wilderness Med.* **2**, 198–205.

Ward, M.P. (1993a) The first ascent of Mount Everest. *BMJ* **306**, 1455–8.

Ward, M.P. (1993b) The first ascent of Mount Everest, 1953: the solution of the problem of the 'last thousand feet'. *J. Wilderness Med.* **4**, 312–18.

Ward, M.P. (1995) The height of Mount Everest. *Alpine J.* **100**, 30–3.

Ward, M.P. (1997) Everest 1951: the footprints attributed to the Yeti – myth and reality. *Wilderness Environ. Med.* **8**, 29–32.

Ward, M.P. (1998) The survey of India and the pundits: the secret exploration of the Himalaya and Central Asia. *Alpine J.* **103**, 59–79.

Ward, M.P. and Jackson, F.S. (1965) Medicine in Bhutan. *Lancet* **1**, 811–13.

Warren, C.B.M. (1939) Alveolar air on Mount Everest. *J. Physiol. (Lond.)* **96**, 34–5.

Washburn, B. (1962) Frostbite. What it is – and how to prevent it – emergency treatment. *N. Engl. J. Med.* **266**, 974–89.

Webb, P. (1986) After drop of body temperature during re-warming – an alternative explanation. *J. Appl. Physiol.* **60**, 385–90.

Wedin, B., Vanggaard, L. and Hirvonen, J. (1979) 'Paradoxical undressing' in fatal hypothermia. *J. Forensic Sci.* **24**, 543–53.

Wedzicha, J.A., Cotes, P.M., Empey, D.W. *et al.* (1985) Serum immunoreactive erythropoietin in hypoxic lung disease with and without polycythaemia. *Clin. Sci.* **69**, 413–22.

Weeke, J. and Gundersen, H.J.G. (1983) The effect of heating and cold cooling on serum T.S.H., G.H., and norepinephrine in resting normal man. *Acta Physiol. Scand.* **47**, 33–9.

Weibel, E.R. (1970) Morphometric estimation of pulmonary diffusion capacity. *Respir. Physiol.* **11**, 54–75.

Weil, J.V. (1986) Ventilatory control at high altitude, in *Handbook of Physiology,* Sec. 3, vol. II (eds. N.S. Cherniack and J.G. Widdicome), American Physiological Society, Bethesda, MD, pp. 703–27.

Weil, J.V., Byrne-Quinn, E., Sodal, I.E. *et al.* (1970) Hypoxic ventilatory drive in normal man. *J. Clin. Invest.* **49**, 1061–72.

Weil, J.V., Byrne-Quinn, E., Ingvar, E. *et al.* (1971) Acquired attenuation of chemoreceptor function in chronically hypoxic man at high altitude. *J. Clin. Invest.* **50**, 186–95.

Weil, J.V., Kryger, M.H. and Scoggin, C.H. (1978) Sleep and breathing at high altitude, in *Sleep Apnea Syndromes* (eds. C. Guilleminault and W. Dement), Liss, New York, pp. 119–36.

Weiss, E.A. (1991) Environmental heat illness, in *Proceedings of the First World Congress on Wilderness Medicine,* Wilderness Medical Society, Point Reyes Station, CA, pp. 347–57.

Weisse, A.B., Moschos, C.B., Frank, M.L. *et al.* (1975) Haemodynamic effects of staged haematocrit reduction in patients with stable cor pulmonale and severely elevated haematocrit. *Am. J. Med.* **58**, 92–8.

Weller, A.S., Millard, C.E., Stroud, M.A. *et al.* (1997) Physiological responses to a cold, wet and windy environment during prolonged intermittent walking. *Am. J. Physiol.* **272** (*Regulatory Integrative Comp. Physiol.* **41**) R226–33.

Welsh, C.H., Wagner, P.D., Reeves, J.T. *et al.* (1993) Operation Everest II: spirometric and radiographic changes in acclimatized humans at simulated high altitudes. *Am. Rev. Respir. Dis.* **147**, 1239–44.

Wessels, C. (1924) *Early Jesuit Travellers in Central Asia, 1603–1721,* Nijhoff, The Hague, p. 54.

West, J.B. (1962a) Diffusing capacity of the lung for carbon monoxide at high altitude. *J. Appl. Physiol.* **17**, 421–6.

West, J.B. (1962b) Regional differences in gas exchange in the lung of erect man. *J. Appl. Physiol.* **17**, 893–8.

West, J.B. (1981) *High Altitude Physiology: Benchmark Papers in Physiology,* vol. 15, Hutchinson Ross, Stroudsburg, PA, p. 328.

West, J.B. (1982a) American Medical Research Expedition to Everest, 1981. *Physiologist* **25**, 36–8.

West, J.B. (1982b) Diffusion at high altitude. *Fed. Proc.* **41**, 2128–30.

West, J.B. (1983) Climbing Mt. Everest without oxygen: an analysis of maximal exercise during extreme hypoxia. *Respir. Physiol.* **52**, 265–79.

West, J.B. (1985a) *Everest – the Testing Place,* McGraw-Hill, New York.

West, J.B. (ed.) (1985b) *Best and Taylor's Physiological Basis of Medical Practice,* 11th edn, Williams and Wilkins, Baltimore, MD.

West, J.B. (1986a) Highest inhabitants in the world. *Nature* **324**, 517.

West, J.B. (1990) *Ventilation/Blood flow and Gas Exchange,* 5th edn, Blackwell Scientific, Oxford.

West, J.B. (1986c) Lactate during exercise at extreme altitude. *Fed. Proc.* **45**, 2953–7.

West, J.B. (1987) Alexander M. Kellas and the physiological challenge of Mount Everest. *J. Appl. Physiol.* **63**, 3–11.

West, J.B. (1988a) Rate of ventilatory acclimatization to extreme altitude. *Respir. Physiol.* **74**, 323–33.

West, J.B. (1988b) Tolerable limits to hypoxia on high mountains, in *Hypoxia: the Tolerable Limits* (eds. J.R. Sutton, C.S. Houston and G. Coates), Benchmark Press, Indianapolis, pp. 353–62.

West, J.B. (1993a) Acclimatization and tolerance to extreme altitude. *J. Wilderness Med.* **4**, 17–26.

West, J.B. (1993b) The Silver Hut expedition, high-altitude field expeditions, and low-pressure chamber simulations, in *Hypoxia and Molecular Medicine* (eds. J.R. Sutton, C.S. Houston and G. Coates), Queen City Printers, Burlington, VT, pp. 190–202.

West, J.B. (1995) Oxygen enrichment of room air to relieve the hypoxia of high altitude. *Respir. Physiol.* **99**, 225–32.

West, J.B. (1996a) Prediction of barometric pressures at high altitudes with the use of model atmospheres. *J. Appl. Physiol.* **81**, 1850–4.

West, J.B. (1996b) T.H. Ravenhill and his contributions to mountain sickness. *J. Appl. Physiol.* **80**, 715–24.

West, J.B. (1997) Fire hazard in oxygen-enriched atmospheres at low barometric pressures. *Aviat. Space Envir. Med.* **68**, 159–62.

West, J.B. (1998) *High Life: a History of High-Altitude Physiology and Medicine*, Oxford University Press, New York.

West, J.B. (1999a) Barometric pressures on Mt. Everest: new data and physiological significance. *J. Appl. Physiol.* **86**, 1062–6.

West, J.B. (1999b) Review of Pugh paper – a commentary. *Wilderness Environ. Med.* **10**, 250–1.

West, J.B. (2000) *Respiratory Physiology – The Essentials,* 6th edn, Williams & Wilkins, Baltimore, MD.

West, J.B., Boyer, S.J., Graber, D.J. *et al.* (1983c) Maximal exercise at extreme altitudes on Mount Everest. *J. Appl. Physiol.* **55**, 688–98.

West, J.B., Colice, G.L., Lee, Y.-J. *et al.* (1995) Pathogenesis of high-altitude pulmonary edema: direct evidence of stress failure of pulmonary capillaries. *Eur. Respir. J.* **8**, 523–9.

West, J.B., Hackett, P.H., Maret, K.H. *et al.* (1983b) Pulmonary gas exchange on the summit of Mount Everest. *J. Appl. Physiol.* **55**, 678–87.

West, J.B., Lahiri, S., Gill, M.B. *et al.* (1962) Arterial oxygen saturation during exercise at high altitude. *J. Appl. Physiol.* **17**, 617–21.

West, J.B., Lahiri, S., Maret, K.H., Peters, R.M. Jr and Pizzo, C.J. (1983a) Barometric pressures at extreme altitudes on Mt. Everest: physiological significance. *J. Appl. Physiol.* **54**, 1188–94.

West, J.B. and Mathieu-Costello, O. (1992a) High altitude pulmonary edema is caused by stress failure of pulmonary capillaries. *Intl. J. Sports Med.* **13** (Suppl. 1), S54–8.

West, J.B. and Mathieu-Costello, O. (1992b) Strength of the pulmonary blood–gas barrier. *Respir. Physiol.* **88**, 141–8.

West, J.B. and Mathieu-Costello, O. (1992c) Stress failure of pulmonary capillaries: role in lung and heart disease. *Lancet,* **340**, 762–7.

West, J.B., Mathieu-Costello, O., Jones, J.H. *et al.* (1993) Stress failure of pulmonary capillaries in racehorses with exercise-induced pulmonary hemorrhage. *J. Appl. Physiol.* **75**, 1097–109.

West, J.B., Peters, R.M., Aksnes, G., Maret, K.H., Milledge, J.S. and Schoene, R.B. (1986) Nocturnal periodic breathing at altitudes of 6300 and 8050 m. *J. Appl. Physiol.* **61**, 280–7.

West, J.B., Tsukimoto, K., Mathieu-Costello, O. and Prediletto, R. (1991) Stress failure in pulmonary capillaries. *J. Appl. Physiol.* **70**, 1731–42.

West, J.B. and Wagner, P.D. (1977) Pulmonary gas exchange, in *Bioengineering Aspects of the Lung* (ed. J.B. West), Dekker, New York, pp. 361–457.

West, J.B. and Wagner, P.D. (1980) Predicted gas exchange on the summit of Mt Everest. *Respir. Physiol.* **42**, 1–16.

Westendorp, R.G.J., Frölich, M. and Meinders, A.E. (1993) What to tell steroid substituted patients about the effects of high altitude? *Lancet* **342**, 310–11.

Westerterp, K.R., Kayser, B., Brouns, F. *et al.* (1992) Energy expenditure climbing Mt. Everest. *J. Appl. Physiol.* **73**, 1815–19.

Westerterp, K.R., Kayser, B., Wouters, L., Le Trong, J.-L. and J.-P. Richalet (1994) Energy balance at high altitude of 6,542 m. *J. Appl. Physiol.* **77**, 862–6.

Westerterp, K.R., Robach, P., Wouters, L. and Richalet, J.-P. (1996) Water balance and acute mountain sickness before and after arrival at high-altitude of 4,350 m. *J. Appl. Physiol.* **80**, 1968–72.

Westerterp-Plantegna, M.S., Westerterp, K.R., Rubbens, M., Verwegen, C.R., Richalet, J.-P. and Gordette, B. (1999) Appetite at high altitude [(Operation Everest III Comex-97)]: a simulated ascent of Mount Everest. *J. Appl. Physiol.* **87**, 391–9.

Weston, A.R., Karamizrak, O., Smith, A. *et. al* (1999) African runners who lived at sea level exhibited greater fatigue resistance, lower lactate accumulation and higher oxidative activity. *J. Appl. Physiol.* **86**, 915–23.

Whayne, T.F. and Severinghaus, J.W. (1968) Experimental hypoxic pulmonary edema in the rat. *J. Appl. Physiol.* **25**, 729–32.

Whittaker, S.R.F. and Winton, F.R. (1933) The apparent viscosity of blood flowing in the isolated hind limb of the dog and its variation with corpuscular concentration. *J. Physiol.* **78**, 339–69.

Whittembury, J., Lozano, R. and Monge, C.C. (1968) Influence of cell concentration in the electrometric determination of blood pH. *Acta Physiol. Lat. Am.* **18**, 263–5.

WHO (1996) *World Health Statistics Annual 1995*, World Health Organization, Geneva.

Whymper, E. (1891–1892) *Travels Among the Great Andes of the Equator,* John Murray, London.

Wickwire, J. (1982) Pulmonary embolus and/or pneumonia on K2, in *Hypoxia, Man at Altitude* (eds. J.R. Sutton, N.L. Jones and C.S. Houston), Thieme Stratton, New York, pp. 173–6.

Wiedman, M. and Tabin, G.C. (1999) High-altitude retinopathy and altitude illness. *Ophthalmology* **106**, 1924–6.

Wielicki, K. (1985) Broad peak climbed in one day. *Alpine J.* **90**, 61–3.

Wiles, P.G., Grant, P.J., Jones, R.G. *et al.* (1986) Lowered skin blood flow at exhaustion. *Lancet* **2**, 295.

Wilkerson, J.A., Bangs, C.C. and Hayward, J.S. (1986) *Hypothermia, Frostbite and Other Cold Injuries,* The Mountaineers, Seattle, p. 45.

Wilkins, D.C. (1973) Acclimation to heat in the Antarctic, in *Polar Human Biology* (eds. O.G. Edholm and E.K.E. Gunderson), Heinemann Medical, London, pp. 171–81.

Wilkinson, R., Milledge, J.S. and Landon, M.J. (1993) Microalbuminuria in chronic obstructive lung disease. *BMJ* **307**, 239–40.

Will, D.H., McMurty, I.F., Reeves, T.J. *et al.* (1978) Cold-induced pulmonary hypertension in cattle. *J. Appl. Physiol.* **45**, 469–73.

Williams, E.S. (1961) Salivary electrolyte composition at high altitude. *Clin. Sci.* **21**, 37–42.

Williams, E.S. (1975) Mountaineering and the endocrine system, in *Mountain Medicine and Physiology* (eds. C. Clarke, M. Ward and E. Williams), Proceedings of a Symposium for Mountaineers, Expedition Doctors and Physiologists, Alpine Club, London, pp. 38–44.

Williams, E.S., Ward, M.P., Milledge, J.S. *et al.* (1979) Effect of the exercise of seven consecutive days hill-walking on fluid homeostasis. *Clin. Sci.* **56**, 305–16.

Willison, J.R., Thomas, D.J., DuBoulay, G.H. *et al.* (1980) Effects of high haematocrit on alertness. *Lancet* **1**, 846–8.

Winearls, C.G., Oliver, D.O., Pippard, M.J. *et al.* (1986) Effect of human erythropoietin derived from recombinant DNA on the anaemia of patients maintained by chronic haemodialysis. *Lancet* **2**, 1175–7.

Winslow, R.M., Chapman, K.W., Gibson, C.C. *et al.* (1989) Different haematologic response to hypoxia in Sherpas and Quechua Indians. *J. Appl. Physiol.* **66**, 1561–9.

Winslow, R.M. and Monge C.C. (1987) *Hypoxia, Polycythemia, and Chronic Mountain Sickness*, Johns Hopkins University Press, Baltimore, MD.

Winslow, R.M., Monge, C.C., Brown, E.G. *et al.* (1985) Effects of hemodilution on O_2 transport in high-altitude polycythemia. *J. Appl. Physiol.* **59**, 1495–502.

Winslow, R.M., Monge, C.C., Statham, N.J. *et al.* (1981) Variability of oxygen affinity of blood: human subjects native to high altitude. *J. Appl. Physiol.* **51**, 1411–16.

Winslow, R.M., Samaja, M. and West, J.B. (1984) Red cell function at extreme altitude on Mount Everest. *J. Appl. Physiol.* **56**, 109–16.

Winter, R.J.D., Davidson, A.C., Treacher, D.F. *et al.* (1987b) Plasma atrial natriuretic factor in chronically hypoxaemic patients with pulmonary hypertension. *Clin. Sci.* **73**, 51P.

Winter, R.J.D., Melaegros, L., Pervez, S. *et al.* (1987a) Plasma atrial natriuretic factor and ultrastructure of atrial specific granules following chronic hypoxia in rats. *Clin. Sci.* **72**, 26P.

Winter, R.J.D., Meleagros, L., Pervez, S. *et al.* (1989) Atrial natriuretic peptide levels in plasma and in cardiac tissues after chronic hypoxia in rats. *Clin. Sci.* **76**, 95–101.

Winterborn, M., Bradwell, A.R., Chesner, I. and Jones, G. (1986) Mechanisms of proteinuria at high altitude. *Clin. Sci.* **70**, 58P.

Winterstein, H. (1911) Die Regulierung der Atmung durch das Blut. *Pflügers Arch. Ges. Physiol.* **138**, 167–84.

Winterstein, H. (1915) Neue Untersuchungen über die physikalisch-chemische Regulierung der Atmung. *Biochem. Z.* **70**, 45–73.

Wittenberg, J.B. (1959) Oxygen transport: a new function proposed for myoglobin. *Biol. Bull.* **117**, 402–3.

Wohns, R.N.W. (1987) Transient ischemic attacks at high altitude, in *Hypoxia and Cold* (eds. J.R. Sutton, C.S. Houston and G. Coates), Praeger, New York, p. 536.

Wolde-Gebriel, Z., Demeke, T., West, C.E. and Van der Haar, F. (1993) Goitre in Ethiopia. *Br. J. Nutr.* **69**, 257–68.

Wolfel, E.E., Groves, B.M., Brooks, G.A. *et al.* (1991) Oxygen transport during steady state submaximal exercise in chronic hypoxia. *J. Appl. Physiol.* **70**, 1129–36.

Wolff, C.B. (1980) Normal ventilation in chronic hypoxia. *J. Physiol.* **308**, 118–19P.

Wolff, C.B. (2000) Cerebral blood flow and oxygen delivery at high altitude. *High Alt. Med. Biol.* **1**, 33–8.

Wright, A.D., Imray, C.H., Morrissey, M.S., Marchbanks, R.J. and Bradwell, A.R. (1995) Intracranial pressure at high altitude and acute mountain sickness. *Clin. Sci.* **89**, 201–4.

Wu, T.Y. (1994a) Low prevalence of systemic hypertension in Tibetan native highlanders. *ISMM Newsletter* **4**(1), 5–7.

Wu, T. (1994b) Children on the Tibetan plateau. *ISMM Newsletter* **4**(3), 5–6.

Wu, T.Y. (2000) Take note of altitude gastrointestinal bleeding. *ISMM Newsletter* **10**(2), 9–10.

Wu, T-Y. and Liu, Y.R. (1995) High altitude heart disease. *Chin. J. Pediatr.* **6**, 348–50.

Wu, T-Y., Zhang, Q., Jin, B. *et al.* (1992) Chronic mountain sickness (Monge's disease): an observation in

Quinghai-Tibet plateau, in *High Altitude Medicine* (eds. G. Ueda, J.T. Reeves and M. Sekiguchi), Sinshu University Press, Matsumoto, pp. 314–24.

Wylie, A. (1881) Notes on the Western Regions. Translated from the *Tsëen Han Shoo Book 96, Part 1. J. R. Anthropol. Inst.* **10**, 20–73.

Xu, F. and Severinghaus, J.W. (1998) Rat brain VEGF expression in alveolar hypoxia: possible role in high-altitude cerebral edema. *J. Appl. Physiol.* **85**, 53–7.

Yamaguchi, S., Matsuzawa, S., Yoshikawa, S. *et al.* (1991) Effect of acclimatization and deacclimatization on hypoxic ventilatory response. *Jpn. J. Mount. Med.* **11**, 77–84.

Yamamoto, W.S. and Edwards, M.W. (1960) Homeostasis of carbon dioxide during intra-venous infusion of carbon dioxide. *J. Appl. Physiol.* **15**, 807–18.

Yanagidaira, Y., Sakai, A., Kashimura, O. *et al.* (1994) The effects of prolonged exposure to cold on hypoxic pulmonary hypertension in rats. *J. Wilderness Med.* **5**, 11–19.

Yaron, M., Waldman, N., Niermeyer, S. *et al.* (1998) The diagnosis of acute mountain sickness in preverbal children. *Arch. Pediatr. Adolesc. Med.* **152**, 683–7.

Yoneda, I. and Watanabe, Y. (1997) Comparison of altitude tolerance and hypoxia symptoms between non-smokers and habitual smokers. *Aviat. Space Environ. Med* **68**, 807–11.

Young, A.J., Castellani, J.W., O'Brian, C. *et al.* (1998) Exertional fatigue, sleeplessness and negative energy balance increases susceptibility to hypothermia. *J. Appl. Physiol.* **85**, 1210–17.

Young, A.J., Muza, S.R., Sawka, M.N. *et al.* (1986) Human thermo-regulatory responses to cold air are altered by repeated cold water immersion. *J. Appl. Physiol.* **60**, 1542–8.

Young, P.M., Rose, M.S., Sutton, J.R. *et al.* (1989) Operation Everest II: plasma lipid and hormonal responses during a simulated ascent of Mt Everest. *J. Appl. Physiol.* **66**, 1430–5.

Young, A.J., Sawka, M.N., Muza, S.R. *et al.* (1996) Effects of erythrocyte infusion on $\dot{V}_{O_2 max}$ at high altitude. *J. Appl. Physiol.* **81**, 252–9.

Zacarian, S.A. (1985) Cryogenics: the cryolesions and the pathogenesis of cryonecrosis, in *Cryosurgery for Skin and Cutaneous Diseases,* Mosby, St Louis, MO.

Zaccaria, M., Rocco, S., Noventa, D. *et al.* (1998) Sodium regulating hormones at high altitude: basal and post-exercise levels. *J. Clin. Endocrinol. Metab.* **83**(2), 570–4.

Zangger, T. (1899) On the danger of high altitudes for patients with arteriosclerosis. *Lancet* **1**, 1628–9.

Zangger, T. (1903) On the danger of railway trips to high altitudes especially for elderly patients. *Lancet* **1**, 1730–5.

Zhang, Y.B. (1985) *An Introduction to Medical Research in Qinghai*, High Altitude Medical Research Institute, Qinghai, China.

Zhongyuan, S., Deming, Z., Changming, L. and Miaoshen, Q. (1983) Changes of electroencephalogram under acute hypoxia and relationship between tolerant ability to hypoxia and adaptation ability to high altitudes. *Sci. Sin.* **26**, 58–69.

Zhongyuan, S., Xuehan, N., Shoucheng, Z. *et al.* (1980) Electrocardiogram made on ascending the mount Qomolangma from 50 m A.S.L. *Sci. Sin.* **23**, 1316–25.

Zhuang, J., Droma, T., Sun, S. *et al.* (1993) Hypoxic ventilatory responsiveness in Tibetan compared with Han residents of 3,658 m. *J. Appl. Physiol.* **74**, 303–11.

Zimmerman, G.A. and Crapo, R.O. (1980) Adult respiratory distress syndrome secondary to high altitude pulmonary edema. *West. J. Med.* **133**, 335–7.

Zuntz, N., Loewy, A., Müller, F. and Caspari, W. (1906) *Höhenklima und Bergwanderungen in ihrer Wirkung auf den Menschen,* Bong, Berlin. An English translation of the relevant passages can be found in *High Altitude Physiology* (ed. J.B. West), Hutchinson Ross, Stroudsburg, PA, 1981.

Index

NOTE: this index covers pages 1–364 (pages 1–21 cover the historical background). American English spelling is used, eg 'edema'. Page numbers in italics refer to figures or tables.

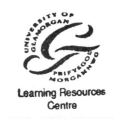